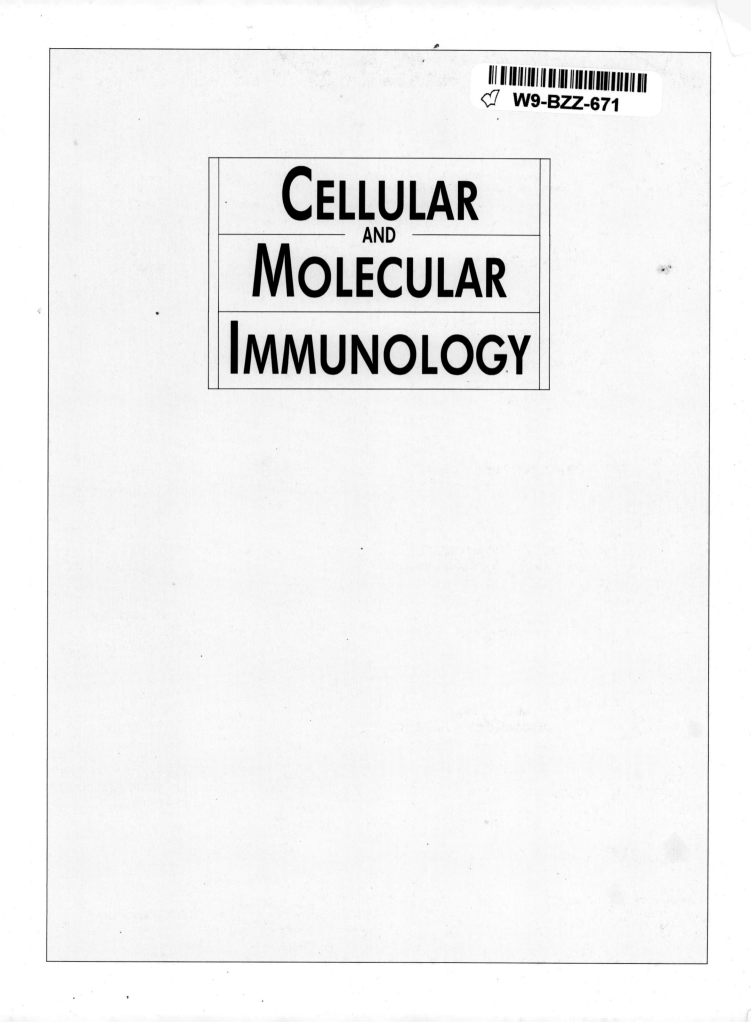

CELLULAR
AND
MOLECULAR
IMMUNOLOGY

SAUNDERS TEXT AND REVIEW SERIES

CELLULAR
AND
MOLECULAR
IMMUNOLOGY

SECOND EDITION

ABUL K. ABBAS, M.B.B.S.
Professor of Pathology
Harvard Medical School and Brigham and Women's Hospital
Boston, Massachusetts

ANDREW H. LICHTMAN, M.D., Ph.D.
Assistant Professor of Pathology
Harvard Medical School and Brigham and Women's Hospital
Boston, Massachusetts

JORDAN S. POBER, M.D., Ph.D.
Professor of Pathology, Immunobiology, and Biology
Yale University School of Medicine
New Haven, Connecticut

W.B. SAUNDERS COMPANY
A Division of Harcourt Brace & Company

Philadelphia   London   Toronto   Montreal   Sydney   Tokyo

W.B. SAUNDERS COMPANY
A Division of Harcourt Brace & Company

The Curtis Center
Independence Square West
Philadelphia, Pennsylvania 19106

Library of Congress Cataloging-in-Publication Data

Abbas, Abul K.
   Cellular and molecular immunology / Abul K. Abbas, Jordan S. Pober,
Andrew H. Lichtman. — 2nd ed.
      p.   cm.
   Includes bibliographical references and index.
   ISBN 0-7216-5505-X
   1. Cellular immunity. 2. Molecular immunology. I. Lichtman,
Andrew H.   II. Pober, Jordan S.   III. Title.   IV. Title: Cellular
and molecular immunology.
   [DNLM: 1. Immunity, Cellular. 2. Lymphocytes—immunology.   QW
568 A122c 1994]
   QR185.5.A23   1994
   616.07′9—dc20
DNLM/DLC   93-50216

Cellular and Molecular Immunology, 2nd edition

ISBN 0–7216–5505–X

I.E. ISBN 0–7216–5290–5

Printed in the United States of America.

Last digit is the print number: 9   8   7   6   5   4   3

To

Ann, Jonathan, Rehana

Sheila, Eben, Ariella, Amos, Ezra

Barbara, Jeremy, Jonathan

PREFACE

The principal goals of the second edition of *Cellular and Molecular Immunology* are essentially the same as those of the first—to convey the principles of immunology by providing students with an understanding of the experimental observations that have led to the formulation of these principles, and to describe the mechanisms and pathogenesis of immunologic disorders. We have continued to emphasize the interpretations of key experimental and clinical observations because this approach best enables students to appreciate the implications of new findings as they emerge. Understanding the evolution of immunologic concepts also should make the book useful for physicians and researchers who are interested in immunology as a scientific discipline. New information has been added to virtually every chapter in the second edition, reflecting the remarkable pace of progress in analyzing and understanding the immune system. A new chapter (Chapter 11) has been added to update the field of lymphocyte recirculation and discuss immune responses at different anatomic sites. Concepts of self-tolerance and autoimmunity have been combined into another new chapter (Chapter 19) to provide a more coherent discussion of these topics. We have condensed or deleted old material to minimize the expansion of the book and keep it at an appropriate size for a one-semester course.

As with the first edition, many individuals have been of invaluable help. Eric Martz, of the University of Massachusetts, read the entire book and gave us insightful suggestions for changes and improvements. Individual chapters were reviewed by the following immunologists, who are listed here in alphabetical order: Thierry Boon, Don Capra, Mark Davis, Doug Fearon, Eli Gilboa, Hugh McDevitt, Roberto Poljak, Peter Sayles, Hans Schreiber, Al Sheffer, and John Tew. Their candid critiques and suggestions have greatly helped our task. Many individuals on the staff of W.B. Saunders have played key roles. In particular, William Schmitt, our editor, has been a source of support and calm throughout the preparation of the book; Risa Clow has again done a marvelous job with the illustrations; and Arlene Friday has superbly copy-edited a manuscript that undoubtedly presented a challenge for any editor. In addition, we appreciate the important contributions of Nellie McGrew, developmental editor, Peter Faber, production manager, and Paul Fry, designer.

In closing, we would like to add that we have been gratified by the generous comments of reviewers and colleagues and by the acceptance of the first edition in many medical, graduate, and undergraduate courses. We hope this edition will continue to convey a coherent understanding of immunology as well as some of the excitement of immunology as an area of scientific research.

ABUL K. ABBAS
ANDREW H. LICHTMAN
JORDAN S. POBER

PREFACE
TO THE FIRST EDITION

Cellular and Molecular Immunology is intended as an introductory textbook primarily for students of medicine and related disciplines. This book evolved from a course we teach to first-year medical students at Harvard Medical School who are enrolled in the joint Harvard–MIT M.D. program in Health Sciences and Technology. The impetus for writing this book is the remarkable development of immunology as a science and the equally remarkable effect that this science has had upon clinical medicine. Over the past 20 years, the field of immunology has undergone radical changes. We can now identify the specific cells and molecules that are the essential components of the immune system, and we can predict the functions of these components based on a limited number of general principles. Students and practitioners of medicine need to be conversant with these advances in order to understand the immunologic diseases and to use the rapidly emerging methods of diagnosis and therapy that are based on immunologic approaches.

Accordingly, we believe that there is a need for a new textbook that should meet two major goals. The first and foremost is to convey an accurate and up-to-date understanding of the immune system. This book emphasizes the organizing principles of immunology and is not intended to be simply a compendium of facts. The principles of immunology are derived from the shared interpretations of key experiments. To enable the student to appreciate the basis of modern immunology, these key experiments and their interpretations are described, usually in summary or schematic form. The discussion of experimental studies also serves to illustrate the evolution of immunology as a science and, we hope, to convey some of the excitement that accompanies scientific discoveries. The most important methods used in experimental analyses are described in "boxes," which are separated from the main text. As an aid to students, each chapter concludes with a list of recent review articles that may serve as a bridge to the primary scientific reports. In addition, we have listed selected research papers that present experimental studies described in the text.

The second goal is to provide students of medicine with an appreciation of how immunologic principles are being applied to understand human diseases. The importance of the immune system in clinical medicine is greatest in two broad areas—defense against infections, and diseases due to abnormal immune responses. These and other connections between immunology and medicine are highlighted throughout the book. More detailed descriptions of selected clinical disorders that illustrate important points have also been included in the boxes.

The book is organized into four sections, each focusing on different aspects of immunology. Section I presents an introduction to the cells and tissues of the immune system. Section II examines the molecular mechanisms used by the immune system to recognize antigens and the process of activation of the immune system that results from antigen recognition. Section III describes the means by which the stimulated immune system eliminates foreign molecules, cells, and organisms. Section IV is specifically devoted to clinical problems that are primarily immunologic or in which modern immunology has made a major contribution.

This book would not have been possible without the help and support of many individuals. Foremost among these were colleagues who provided invaluable constructive criticisms. Dr. Geoffrey Sunshine, of Tufts University School of Medicine, and Hal Burstein, an M.D.–Ph.D. candidate at Harvard Medical School, read the entire book and guided us through many problems of clarity and consistency. Individual chapters or topics were reviewed by the following immunologists, who are listed here in alphabetical order: Drs. Hugh Auchincloss, J. Latham Claflin, Robert Colvin, George Eisenbarth, Vic Engelhard, Frank Fitch, Steven Galli, Richard Hodes, Keith James, Stephanie James, Anne Marshak-Rothstein, Rick Mitchell, Harry Orr, David Parker, Jose Quintans, Ray Redline, Alan Sher, Richard Titus, and Janis Weis. We consider ourselves fortunate that we have been able to draw upon such a wealth of expertise. Valuable input also came from the first-year medical students on whom we first tried out the approach that is the cornerstone of this book.

We owe a great debt to many members of the staff of W.B. Saunders Company. In particular, Marty Wonsiewicz and Rosanne Hallowell, editors, and Risa Clow, illustrator, have shown extraordinary dedication and have been very much a part of the planning and writing of this book. Important contributions have also been made by Carol Robins, copy editor; Pat Morrison, Assistant Manager of Illustration and Design; Paul Fry, designer; and Pete Faber, production manager.

Many thanks are also due to Mary Jane Tawa, David Lence, and Jim Throp, who typed most of the manuscript, and to Pam Battaglino for hand-drawn illustrations.

Finally, we are grateful to the people who faithfully supported us even when we were not available for them—the members of our laboratories, who kept our research projects alive and well; Dr. Ramzi Cotran, our department chairman, whose indulgence was more than we could have asked for; and, above all, our families, who were tolerant of our many demands and awaited the completion of the book with an eagerness that matched our own.

ABUL K. ABBAS
ANDREW H. LICHTMAN
JORDAN S. POBER

CONTENTS

SECTION I

INTRODUCTION TO IMMUNOLOGY

The first two chapters introduce the nomenclature of immunology and the components of the immune system. Chapter 1 describes different categories of immune responses and their general properties, and introduces the fundamental principles that govern all immune responses. Chapter 2 is devoted to a description of the cells and tissues of the immune system, with an emphasis on their anatomic organization and structure-function relationships. This will set the stage for a more thorough discussion of the individual cells that participate in immune responses and how the immune system recognizes and responds to antigens.

CHAPTER ONE

GENERAL

PROPERTIES OF

IMMUNE

RESPONSES

The term immunity is derived from the Latin word *immunitas,* which referred to the exemption from various civic duties and legal prosecution offered to Roman senators during their tenures in office. Historically, immunity meant protection from disease, and, more specifically, infectious disease. The cells and molecules responsible for immunity constitute the **immune system,** and their collective and coordinated response to the introduction of foreign substances is the **immune response.** We now know that many of the mechanisms of resistance to infections are also involved in the individual's response to non-infectious foreign substances. Furthermore, mechanisms that normally protect individuals from infections and eliminate foreign substances are themselves capable of causing tissue injury and disease in some situations. Therefore, a more inclusive and modern definition of immunity is a reaction to foreign substances, including microbes, as well as macromolecules such as proteins and polysaccharides, without implying a physiologic or pathologic consequence of such a reaction. Immunology is the study of immunity in this broader sense and of the cellular and molecular events that occur after an organism encounters microbes and other foreign macromolecules.

Historians often credit Thucydides, in Athens during the fifth century B.C., as having first mentioned immunity to an infection that he called "plague" (but that was probably not the bubonic plague we recognize today). The concept of immunity may have existed long before, as suggested by the ancient Chinese custom of making children inhale powders made from the crusts of skin lesions of patients recovering from smallpox. Immunology, in its modern form, is an experimental science, in which explanations of immunologic phenomena are based on experimental observations and the conclusions drawn from them. The evolution of immunology as an experimental discipline has depended on our ability to manipulate the function of the immune system under controlled conditions. Historically, the first clear example of this, and one that remains among the most dramatic ever recorded, was Edward Jenner's successful vaccination against smallpox. Jenner, an English physician, noticed that milkmaids who had recovered from cowpox never contracted the more serious smallpox. Based on this observation, he injected the material from a cowpox pustule into the arm of an 8-year-old boy. When this boy was later intentionally inoculated with smallpox, the disease did not develop. Jenner's landmark treatise on **vaccination** (Latin *vaccinus,* of or from cows) was published in 1798. It led to the widespread acceptance of this method for inducing immunity to infectious diseases. An eloquent testament to the importance and progress of immunology was the announcement by the World Health Organization in 1980 that smallpox was the first infectious disease that had been eradicated worldwide by a program of vaccination.

In the last 25 years, there has been a remarkable transformation in our understanding of the immune system and its functions. Advances in cell culture techniques, recombinant DNA methodology, and protein biochemistry have changed immunology from a largely descriptive science into one in which diverse immune phenomena can be tied together coherently and explained in quite precise structural and biochemical terms. This chapter outlines the general features of immune responses and introduces the concepts that form the cornerstones of modern immunology and that recur throughout the remainder of this book.

NATURAL AND ACQUIRED IMMUNITY

Healthy individuals protect themselves against microbes by means of many different mechanisms. These include physical barriers, phagocytic cells and eosinophils in the blood and tissues, a class of lymphocytes called natural killer (NK) cells, and various blood-borne molecules, all of which participate in defending individuals from a potentially hostile environment. All of these defense mechanisms are present prior to exposure to infectious microbes or other foreign macromolecules, are not enhanced by such exposures, and do not discriminate among most foreign substances. These are the components of **natural** (also called **native** or **innate**) **immunity.** Other defense mechanisms are induced or stimulated by exposure to foreign substances, are exquisitely specific for distinct macromolecules, and increase in magnitude and defensive capabilities with each successive exposure to a particular macromolecule. These mechanisms constitute **acquired,** or **specific, immunity** (Table 1–1). Foreign substances that induce specific immunity are called **antigens.** By convention, immunology is the study of specific immunity, and "immune responses" refer to responses that are specific for different inducing antigens.

The specific immune response is one component of an integrated system of host defense in which numerous cells and molecules function cooperatively. The specific immune system has retained many of the mechanisms of natural immunity that are necessary for eliminating foreign invaders and has added to them two important additional properties:

First, *the specific immune system "remembers" each encounter with a microbe or foreign antigen, so*

TABLE 1–1. Features of Natural and Specific (Acquired) Immunity

	Natural	Specific (Acquired)
Physicochemical barriers	Skin, mucous membranes	Cutaneous and mucosal immune systems; antibody in mucosal secretions
Circulating molecules	Complement	Antibodies
Cells	Phagocytes (macrophages, neutrophils), natural killer cells	Lymphocytes
Soluble mediators active on other cells	Macrophage-derived cytokines, e.g., α and β interferons, tumor necrosis factor	Lymphocyte-derived cytokines, e.g., interferon-γ

that subsequent encounters stimulate increasingly effective defense mechanisms. This is called immunologic memory, and is the basis of protective vaccination against infectious diseases.

Second, *the specific immune response amplifies the protective mechanisms of natural immunity, directs or focuses these mechanisms to the sites of antigen entry, and thus makes them better able to eliminate foreign antigens.*

The concept that specific immune responses serve to enhance natural immunity is also reflected in the phylogeny of defense mechanisms (Box 1–1). Prior to the evolution of vertebrates, host defense against foreign invaders was mediated largely by the mechanisms of natural immunity, including phagocytic cells and circulating molecules that resemble components of the mammalian complement system (see Chapter 15). Specific immunity consisting of **lymphocytes** and their secreted products, such as **antibodies,** appeared in vertebrates and is clearly present in fish. Whereas phagocytes and complement cannot distinguish between distinct antigens and are not specifically enhanced by repeated exposures to the same antigen, lymphocytes and antibodies are highly specific and their production or expansion is stimulated by foreign antigens. Nevertheless, in order to carry out their function of defending the host by eliminating foreign antigens, both lymphocytes and antibodies require the participation of phagocytes and complement. The skin and mucosal surfaces are major components of the natural immune system because they serve as physical barriers to the external environment. Specific immune responses at these surfaces enhance their natural immune function. These and other examples of the cooperation between the specific immune system and the mechanisms of natural immunity are described in much more detail in subsequent chapters.

TYPES OF SPECIFIC IMMUNITY

Specific immune responses are normally stimulated when an individual is exposed to a foreign antigen. The form of immunity that is induced by this process of immunization is called **active immunity** because the immunized individual plays an active role in responding to the antigen. Specific immunity can also be conferred upon an individual by transferring cells or serum from a specifically immunized individual. The recipient of such an **adoptive transfer** becomes resistant, or immune, to the particular antigen without ever having been exposed to or having ever responded to that antigen. Therefore, this form of immunity is called **passive immunity.** Passive immunization is a useful method for conferring resistance rapidly, without having to wait for an active immune response to develop. For instance, passive immunization against snake venoms by the administration of antibodies from immunized individuals is a life-saving treatment for potentially lethal snake bites. The technique of adoptive transfer of specific immunity has also made it possible

to define the various cells and molecules that are responsible for mediating immune responses.

Specific immune responses are classified into two types, based on the components of the immune system that mediate the response (Fig. 1–1):

1. **Humoral immunity** is mediated by molecules in the blood that are responsible for specific recognition and elimination of antigens; these are called **antibodies.** It can be transferred to unimmunized (also called "naive") individuals by cell-free portions of the blood, i.e., plasma or serum.

2. **Cell-mediated immunity,** also called **cellular immunity,** is mediated by cells called **T lymphocytes.** It can be transferred to naive individuals with cells from an immunized individual but not with plasma or serum.

Clinically, immunity cannot be measured by transferring cells or antibodies, or by testing an individual's resistance to an infection. Therefore, immunity is actually assayed by determining whether individuals who have been previously exposed to a foreign substance manifest a detectable reaction when re-exposed to, or challenged with, that substance. Such a reaction is an indication of "sensitivity" to challenge, and individuals who have been exposed to a foreign substance are said to be "sensitized." Diseases caused by abnormal or excessive immune reactions are called "hypersensitivity diseases."

The first definitive experimental demonstration of humoral immunity was provided by Emil von Behring and Shibasaburo Kitasato in 1890. They showed that if serum from animals who had recovered from diptheria infection was transferred to naive animals, the recipients became specifically resistant to diphtheria infection. The active components of the serum were called **antitoxins** because they neutralized the pathologic effects of the bacterial toxin. In the early 1900s, Karl Landsteiner and other investigators showed that not only toxins but also other, non-microbial substances could induce humoral immunity. From such studies arose the more general term **antibodies** for the serum proteins that mediate humoral immunity. Substances that bound antibodies and generated the production of antibodies were then called **antigens.** (The properties of antibodies and antigens are described in Chapter 3.) In 1900, Paul Ehrlich provided a theoretical framework of the specificity of antigen-antibody reactions, the experimental proof for which came over the next 50 years from the work of Landsteiner and others using simple chemicals as antigens. Ehrlich's theories of the physicochemical complementarity of antigens and antibodies are remarkable for their prescience. This early emphasis on antibodies led to the general acceptance of the **humoral theory of immunity,** according to which immunity is mediated by substances present in body fluids (humors).

The **cellular theory of immunity,** which stated that host cells were the principal mediators of immunity, was championed initially by Elie Metchnikoff. His demonstration of phagocytes surrounding a thorn stuck into a translucent starfish larva, published in 1893, was perhaps the first experimental evidence that

BOX 1–1. EVOLUTION OF THE IMMUNE SYSTEM

Mechanisms for defending the host against foreign invaders and for healing injured self tissues are present in some form in all members of the enormously diverse and large numbers of phyla of invertebrates. These mechanisms constitute natural immunity. The more discriminating and specialized defense mechanisms that constitute specific or acquired immunity are generally found in vertebrates only. Various cells in invertebrates respond to microbes by enclosing these infectious agents within aggregates and destroying them. These responding cells resemble phagocytes and have been called phagocytic amebocytes in acelomates, hemocytes in molluscs and arthropods, coelomocytes in annelids, and blood leukocytes in tunicates. Invertebrates do not contain antigen-specific lymphocytes and do not produce immunoglobulin molecules or complement proteins. However, they contain a number of soluble molecules that bind to and lyse microbes. These molecules include lectin-like proteins, which bind to carbohydrates on microbial cell walls and agglutinate the microbes, and numerous lytic and antimicrobial factors such as lysozyme, which is also produced by neutrophils in higher organisms. Phagocytes in some invertebrates may be capable of secreting cytokines that resemble macrophage-derived cytokines in the vertebrates. Thus, *host defense in invertebrates is mediated by the cells and molecules that resemble the effector mechanisms of natural immunity in higher organisms.*

Many studies have shown that invertebrates are capable of rejecting foreign tissue transplants, or allografts. If sponges (Porifera) from two different colonies are parabiosed by being mechanically held together, they become necrotic in 1 to 2 weeks, whereas sponges from the same colony become fused and continue to grow. Earthworms (annelids) and starfish (echinoderms) also reject tissue grafts from other species of the phyla. These rejection reactions are mediated mainly by phagocyte-like cells. They differ from graft rejection in vertebrates in that specific memory for the grafted tissue is either not generated or is difficult to demonstrate. Nevertheless, such results indicate that even invertebrates must express cell surface molecules that distinguish self from non-self, and such molecules may be the precursors of histocompatibility molecules in vertebrates.

The various components of the mammalian immune system appear to have arisen virtually together in phylogeny and have become increasingly specialized with evolution (see Table). Thus, of the cardinal features of specific immune responses, *specificity, memory, self/non-self discrimination, and a capacity for self-limitation are present in the lowest vertebrates, and diversity of antigen recognition increases progressively in the higher species.* All vertebrates contain antibody molecules. Fishes have only one type of antibody, called IgM; this number increases to two types in anuran amphibians like *Xenopus*, and to seven or eight in mammals. The diversity of antibodies is much lower in *Xenopus* than in mammals, even though the genes coding for antibodies are structurally similar. Lymphocytes that have some characteristics of both B and T cells are probably present in the earliest vertebrates, such as lampreys, and become specialized into functionally and phenotypically distinct subsets in amphibia and most clearly in birds and mammals. The major histocompatibility complex, which is a genetic locus that controls graft rejection and T lymphocyte antigen recognition, is present in some of the more advanced species of amphibians and fishes and in all birds and mammals. Its absence from some amphibians and fishes and all reptiles suggests that these histocompatibility genes have evolved independently on several occasions during vertebrate phylogeny. The earliest organized lymphoid tissues detected during evolution are the gut-associated lymphoid tissues; spleen, thymus, and lymph nodes (see Chapter 2) are found in higher vertebrates.

	Natural Immunity		Acquired (Specific) Immunity		
	Phagocytosis	*NK Cells*	*Antibodies*	*T and B Lymphocytes*	*Lymph Nodes*
INVERTEBRATES					
Protozoa	+	—	—	—	—
Sponges	+	—	—	—	—
Annelids	+	+	—	—	—
Arthropods	+	—	—	—	—
VERTEBRATES					
Elasmobranchs (sharks, skates, rays)	+	+	+(IgM only)	+	—
Teleosts (common fish)	+	+	+(IgM, ? other)	+	—
Amphibians	+	+	+(2 or 3 classes)	+	—
Reptiles	+	+	+(3 classes)	+	—
Birds	+	+	+(3 classes)	+	—
Mammals	+	+	+(7 or 8 classes)	+	+(some species)

Abbreviation: NK, natural killer.
Key: +, present; —, absent.

cells responded to foreign invaders. Sir Almroth Wright's observation in the early 1900s that factors in immune serum enhanced the phagocytosis of bacteria, a process known as **opsonization,** lent support to the belief that antibodies merely prepared microbes for ingestion by phagocytes. These early "cellularists" were unable to prove that specific protective immunity could be mediated by cells. In 1942, Landsteiner and Merrill Chase reported that skin reactions to different chemicals (a type of "sensitization") could be transferred to naive animals with cells but not with serum from specifically immunized animals. The cellular theory of immunity became firmly established in the 1950s, when George Mackaness showed that resistance to an intracellular bacterium, *Listeria monocytogenes*, could also be adoptively transferred with cells but not with serum. We now know that the specificity of cell-mediated immunity is due to lymphocytes, which often function in concert with other cells such as **phagocytes** to control or eliminate microbes.

Adoptive transfer of specific immunity is one of the principal techniques for analyzing immune responses. It is now complemented by *in vitro* experiments, in which the cells of the immune system can be stimulated by defined antigens and the development of specific immune responses can be examined. As we shall discuss in subsequent chapters, such studies have shown that *humoral immunity and cell-mediated im-munity are mediated by responses of distinct types of lymphocytes.* Some, called **B lymphocytes,** respond to foreign antigens by developing into antibody-producing cells, whereas others, called **T lymphocytes,** are the mediators of cellular immunity. Humoral immunity is the principal defense mechanism against extracellular microbes and their secreted toxins because antibodies can bind to these and assist in their destruction. In contrast, obligate intracellular microbes such as viruses and some bacteria proliferate inside host cells, where they are inaccessible to circulating antibodies. Defense against such infections is due to cell-mediated immunity, which functions by inducing and promoting the intracellular destruction of microbes or the lysis of infected cells (Fig. 1–1).

CARDINAL FEATURES OF IMMUNE RESPONSES

Humoral and cell-mediated immune responses to all antigens have a number of fundamental properties. The experimental analysis of the immune response is, in fact, an attempt to provide molecular and mechanistic explanations for these cardinal features of specific immunity.

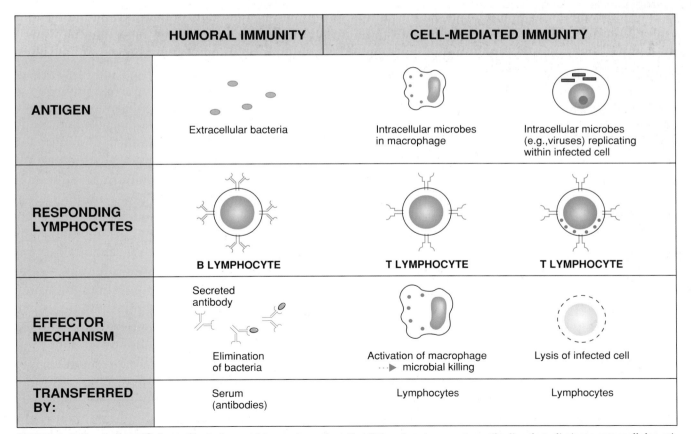

	HUMORAL IMMUNITY	CELL-MEDIATED IMMUNITY	
ANTIGEN	Extracellular bacteria	Intracellular microbes in macrophage	Intracellular microbes (e.g.,viruses) replicating within infected cell
RESPONDING LYMPHOCYTES	B LYMPHOCYTE	T LYMPHOCYTE	T LYMPHOCYTE
EFFECTOR MECHANISM	Secreted antibody — Elimination of bacteria	Activation of macrophage ···▶ microbial killing	Lysis of infected cell
TRANSFERRED BY:	Serum (antibodies)	Lymphocytes	Lymphocytes

FIGURE 1–1. Forms of specific immunity. *In humoral immunity, cells called B lymphocytes secrete antibodies that eliminate extracellular microbes. In cell-mediated immunity, T lymphocytes activate macrophage to kill intracellular microbes or destroy infected cells (e.g., virus-infected cells).*

1. *Specificity*. Immune responses are specific for distinct antigens (Fig. 1–2). In fact, immune responses are specific for different structural components of complex protein, polysaccharide and other antigens. The portions of such antigens that are specifically recognized by individual lymphocytes are called **determinants,** or **epitopes.** This fine specificity exists because individual B and T lymphocytes that respond to foreign antigens express membrane receptors that distinguish subtle differences between distinct antigens. Antigen-specific lymphocytes develop without antigenic stimulation, so that clones of cells with different antigen receptors and specificities are available in unimmunized individuals to recognize and respond to exposure to foreign antigens. This concept is the basic tenet of the **clonal selection hypothesis,** which is discussed in more detail later in this chapter.

2. *Diversity*. The total number of antigenic specificities of the lymphocytes in an individual, called the **lymphocyte repertoire,** is extremely large. It is estimated that the mammalian immune system can discriminate at least 10^9 distinct antigenic determinants. This extraordinary diversity of the repertoire is a result of variability in the structures of the antigen-binding sites of lymphocyte receptors for antigens. In other words, different clones of lymphocytes differ in the structures of their antigen receptors and, therefore, in their specificity for antigens, creating a total repertoire that is extremely diverse. One of the most important advances in immunology has been the elucidation of the molecular mechanisms that produce such structural diversity. These mechanisms are discussed in Chapters 4 and 8.

3. *Memory*. Exposure of the immune system to a foreign antigen enhances its ability to respond again to that antigen. Thus, responses to second and subsequent exposures to the same antigen, called **secondary immune responses,** are usually more rapid, larger, and often qualitatively different from the first, or primary, immune responses to that antigen (Fig. 1–2). This property of specific immunity is called **immunologic memory.** Several features of lymphocytes are responsible for memory:

a. Lymphocytes proliferate when stimulated by antigens, and the progeny of a particular antigen-responsive lymphocyte has the same antigen receptors and, hence, specificity as the original cell. Therefore, each exposure to antigen expands the clone(s) of lymphocytes specific for that antigen.

b. Memory cells, which are lymphocytes that have previously responded to antigenic stimulation, survive for prolonged periods even in the absence of the antigen. Thus, memory cells are prepared to respond rapidly to antigenic challenge.

c. As we shall see in Chapters 4 and 9, memory B cells respond to lower concentrations of antigens and produce antibodies that bind antigen with higher affinity than do previously unstimulated B cells. This is only one of several qualitative differences between primary and secondary antibody responses.

4. *Self-limitation*. All normal immune responses wane with time after antigen stimulation (Fig. 1–2). There are several reasons why immune responses are self-limited.

a. The first, and probably most important, is that immune responses that are induced by antigens function to eliminate the antigen. This results in the elimination of the stimulus for lymphocyte activation.

b. Lymphocytes perform their functions for brief periods after antigenic stimulation, after which

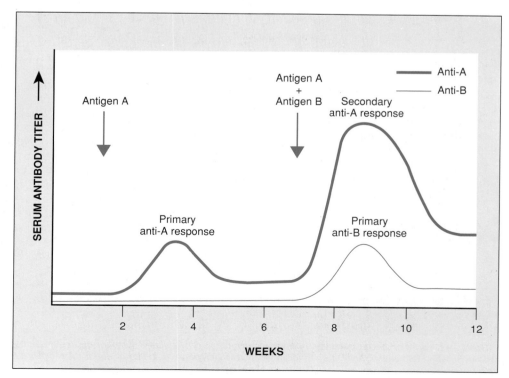

FIGURE 1–2. Specificity, memory, and self-limitation of immune responses. *Antigens A and B induce the production of different antibodies (specificity). The secondary response to antigen A is more rapid and larger than the primary response (memory). Antibody levels, or titers, decline with time after each immunization (self-limitation).*

these cells become quiescent, develop into memory cells, or differentiate into end-cells with short half-lives.

c. Antigens and the immune responses to these antigens stimulate a number of mechanisms whose principal function is feedback regulation of the response itself. These regulatory mechanisms are discussed in Chapter 10.

5. *Discrimination of self from non-self.* One of the most remarkable properties of the immune system is its ability to distinguish between foreign antigens and self antigens. Thus, the lymphocytes in each individual are able to recognize and respond to many foreign antigens but are normally unresponsive to the potentially antigenic substances present in that individual. Immunologic unresponsiveness is also called **tolerance.** Self-tolerance is an acquired process that has to be learned by the lymphocytes of each individual. It occurs in part because lymphocytes pass through a stage in their development when encounter with antigen leads to their death or inactivation. Thus, potentially self-recognizing lymphocytes come into contact with self antigens at this stage of functional immaturity and are prevented from developing to a stage at which they would be able to respond to self antigens. A great deal is now known about the selection processes that are responsible for self-tolerance, and these will be discussed in Chapters 8 and 19. Abnormalities in the induction or maintenance of self-tolerance lead to immune responses against self (autologous) antigens, and debilitating diseases that are called **autoimmune diseases.** The generation and pathologic consequences of autoimmunity are described in Chapter 19.

These five cardinal features of specific immunity are necessary if the immune system is to perform its normal function of host defense. Specificity and memory enable the immune system to mount heightened responses to persistent or recurring stimulation with the same antigen and thus to combat infections that are prolonged or occur repeatedly. Diversity is essential if the immune system is to defend individuals against the many potential pathogens in the environment. Self-limitation allows the system to return to a state of rest after it eliminates each foreign antigen, thus enabling it to respond optimally to other antigens that the individual encounters. Self-tolerance and the ability to distinguish between self and non-self are vital for preventing reactions against one's own cells and tissues while maintaining a diverse repertoire of lymphocytes specific for foreign antigens.

PHASES OF IMMUNE RESPONSES

All immune responses are initiated by the recognition of foreign antigens. This leads to activation of the lymphocytes that specifically recognize the antigen, and culminates in the development of mechanisms that mediate the physiologic effect of the response, namely elimination of the antigen. Thus, specific immune responses may be divided into (1) the **cognitive phase,** (2) the **activation phase,** and (3) the **effector phase**

(Fig. 1–3). Throughout this book, we will discuss the mechanisms of specific immunity in the context of these three phases.

Cognitive Phase

The cognitive phase of immune responses consists of the binding of foreign antigens to specific receptors on mature lymphocytes that exist prior to antigenic stimulation. B lymphocytes, the cells of humoral immunity, express antibody molecules on their surfaces that can bind foreign proteins, polysaccharides, or lipids in soluble form. T lymphocytes, which are responsible for cell-mediated immunity, express receptors that recognize only short peptide sequences in protein antigens. Moreover, T lymphocytes have the unique property of recognizing and responding only to peptide antigens that are present on the surfaces of other cells. The structural basis of antigen recognition by T cells and its physiologic implications are discussed in Chapter 6.

Activation Phase

The activation phase of immune responses is the sequence of events induced in lymphocytes as a consequence of specific antigen recognition. All lymphocytes undergo two major changes in response to antigens. First, they proliferate, leading to expansion of the clones of antigen-specific lymphocytes and amplification of the protective response. Second, lymphocytes differentiate from cells whose primary function is cognitive to cells that function to eliminate foreign antigens. Thus, antigen-recognizing B lymphocytes differentiate into antibody-secreting cells, and the secreted antibody binds the soluble (extracellular) antigen and triggers the mechanisms that eliminate the antigen. Some T lymphocytes differentiate into cells that activate phagocytes to kill intracellular microbes, and other T lymphocytes directly lyse cells that are producing foreign antigens such as viral proteins. The ability of T cells to recognize cell-bound antigens focuses T cell responses in such a way that cell-mediated immunity is effective against intracellular microbes. A general feature of lymphocyte activation is that it usually requires two types of signals: the first is provided by the antigen, and the second by other cells, which may be **"helper cells"** or **"accessory cells."** The nature of these stimuli and the sequence of T and B cell activation are discussed in Chapters 7 and 9.

Two aspects of lymphocyte activation are important in order to allow the small number of cells that respond to any one antigen to perform the many functions that lead to elimination of the antigen. First, immunization and antigen recognition trigger numerous amplification mechanisms that rapidly expand the specifically responding cells and, to a lesser extent, bystander cells as well. Second, lymphocytes preferentially migrate to sites of antigen administration and immune responses. The cellular and biochemical mechanisms of amplification and lymphocyte migration are discussed in later chapters.

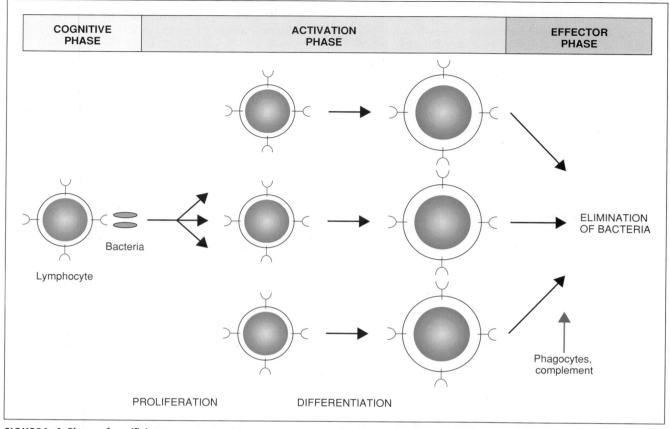

COGNITIVE PHASE	ACTIVATION PHASE	EFFECTOR PHASE

Bacteria

Lymphocyte

ELIMINATION OF BACTERIA

Phagocytes, complement

PROLIFERATION   DIFFERENTIATION

FIGURE 1–3. Phases of specific immune responses. *Immune responses consist of three phases:* cognitive *(antigen recognition),* activation *(proliferation and differentiation of lymphocytes), and* effector *(elimination of antigen). This example illustrates an immune response to bacteria, but the same phases are seen in all specific immune responses. Since this applies to both B and T lymphocytes, the lymphocytes shown can be of either class.*

Effector Phase

The effector phase of immune responses is the stage at which lymphocytes that have been specifically activated by antigens perform the functions that lead to elimination of the antigen. Lymphocytes that function in the effector phase of immune responses are called **effector cells.** Many effector functions require the participation of other, non-lymphoid cells (which are also often referred to as "effector cells") and defense mechanisms that are also operative in natural immunity. For instance, antibodies bind to foreign antigens and enhance their phagocytosis by blood neutrophils and mononuclear phagocytes. Antibodies also activate a system of plasma proteins termed **complement,** which participates in the lysis and phagocytosis of microbes (see Chapter 15). Other antibodies stimulate the degranulation of mast cells and the release of mediators, which combat infections and are responsible for the vascular components of acute inflammation (see Chapter 14). Activated T lymphocytes secrete protein hormones, called **cytokines,** which enhance the functions of phagocytes and stimulate inflammatory responses (see Chapters 12 and 13). Phagocytes, complement, mast cells, cytokines, and the leukocytes that mediate

inflammation are all components of natural immunity, because they do not specifically recognize or distinguish between different foreign antigens, and they are all involved in defense against microbes, even without specific immune responses. Thus, the effector phase of specific immunity illustrates a fundamental concept that was emphasized earlier in this chapter—that specific immune responses serve to amplify and focus onto foreign antigens a variety of effector mechanisms that are also functional in the absence of lymphocyte activation (Fig. 1–4).

THE CLONAL SELECTION HYPOTHESIS

From the initial demonstration that the immune system could respond specifically to a vast number of foreign antigens, the problem of explaining how such a diverse repertoire could be generated and maintained was appreciated by immunologists. Two mutually exclusive hypotheses were proposed to explain the specificity and diversity of immune responses, even before there was a clear understanding of the importance of

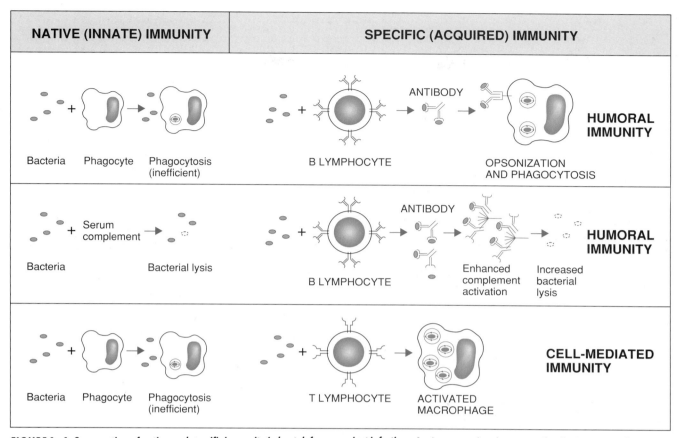

NATIVE (INNATE) IMMUNITY	SPECIFIC (ACQUIRED) IMMUNITY

Bacteria   Phagocyte   Phagocytosis (inefficient)

B LYMPHOCYTE   ANTIBODY   OPSONIZATION AND PHAGOCYTOSIS   **HUMORAL IMMUNITY**

Bacteria   Serum complement   Bacterial lysis

B LYMPHOCYTE   ANTIBODY   Enhanced complement activation   Increased bacterial lysis   **HUMORAL IMMUNITY**

Bacteria   Phagocyte   Phagocytosis (inefficient)

T LYMPHOCYTE   ACTIVATED MACROPHAGE   **CELL-MEDIATED IMMUNITY**

FIGURE 1–4. Cooperation of native and specific immunity in host defense against infections. *In the examples shown, antibodies promote phagocytosis or activate serum complement to kill microbes, and T lymphocytes enhance the phagocytic and microbicidal functions of macrophages.*

lymphocytes in antigen recognition. According to the instructional theory, immunocompetent cells and antibodies acquired their specificity after the introduction of antigen by changing the conformation of antigen-binding receptors, so that these became capable of recognizing the antigen. The alternative view, which we now know is correct, was first suggested by Niels Jerne in 1955, modified by David Talmadge and Macfarlane Burnet, and most clearly enunciated by Burnet in 1957. The key postulates of this theory, called the **clonal section hypothesis,** have been convincingly proved by a variety of experiments, and form the cornerstone of the current concept of lymphocyte specificity and antigen recognition. In essence, the clonal selection hypothesis states the following (Fig. 1–5):

1. *Every individual contains numerous clonally derived lymphocytes, each clone having arisen from a single precursor and being capable of recognizing and responding to a distinct antigenic determinant.* Thus, the development of antigen-specific clones of lymphocytes occurs prior to and independent of exposure to antigen. The cells constituting each clone have identical antigen receptors, which are different from the receptors on the cells of all other clones. Although it is difficult to place an upper limit on the number of antigenic determinants that can be recognized by the mam-

malian immune system, a frequently used estimate is in the order of 10^9. This is a reasonable approximation of the potential number of antigen receptor proteins that can be produced, and may, therefore, reflect the number of distinct clones of lymphocytes present in each individual.

2. *Antigen selects a specific pre-existing clone and activates it,* leading to its proliferation and its differentiation into effector and memory cells. The observation that a secondary immune response is more rapid and larger than the primary response is explained by the clonal expansion of antigen-specific lymphocytes as a result of priming (first immunization) with antigen. Because the clones that respond to any one antigen are a small fraction of the total lymphocytes in an individual, blood lymphocyte counts do not change significantly during most immune responses.

Many lines of evidence prove that both B and T lymphocytes with diverse receptors and specificities exist prior to the introduction of antigen, and clones with distinct specificities are selectively activated by different antigens.

1. If lymphocytes isolated from an immunized animal are cultured at limiting dilution with antigen such that each culture well initially contains only one antibody-producing B cell, antibody of only one specificity

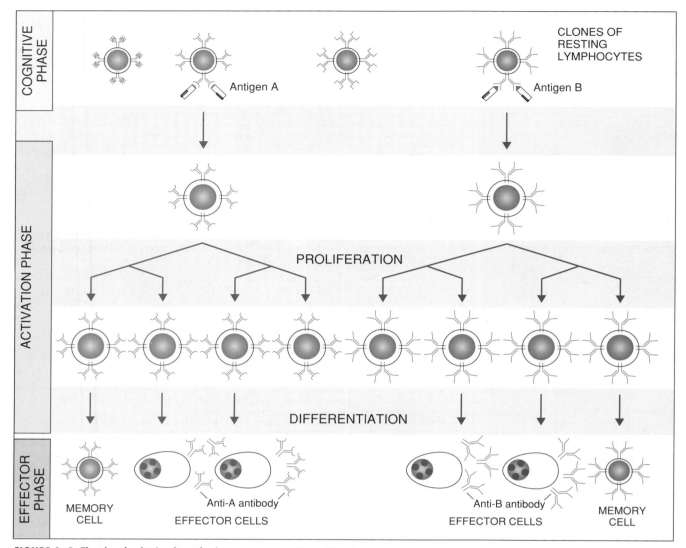

FIGURE 1-5. *The clonal selection hypothesis.* Each antigen (A or B) selects a pre-existing clone of specific lymphocytes and stimulates its proliferation and differentiation. The diagram shows only B lymphocytes giving rise to antibody-secreting cells and memory cells, but the same principle applies to T lymphocytes as well.

can be detected in each well even if the lymphocytes were exposed to multiple antigens.

2. Different antigens bind to different lymphocytes, and no two structurally distinct foreign antigens bind to the same cell.

3. If an animal is injected with an antigen to which a highly radioactive tag is attached, that antigen binds to specific lymphocytes. The lymphocytes, being radiosensitive, are killed. Injection of such an antigen makes the animal incapable of responding to that antigen (until new lymphocytes develop), but the animal responds normally to all other structurally different antigens.

4. In lymphocytes with distinct specificities, the antigen receptors have structurally different combining sites. This has been established by nucleotide and amino acid sequencing of receptors isolated from lymphocyte clones.

5. Each monoclonal lymphoid tumor or cell line contains a set of antigen receptor genes and expresses antigen receptor proteins that are unique and different from all other monoclonal populations.

The specific immune system is remarkable for its complexity and diversity. Immune responses require the coordinated and precisely regulated interplay of many different cells and secreted molecules. Perhaps the greatest achievement of modern immunology is the application of a reductionist approach to analyzing the complexity of the immune system. As we shall see throughout this book, it is now possible to separate the interacting components of the immune system and to dissect their properties and functions individually. Such analyses have led to a clear understanding of the molecular basis of specific antigen recognition, so that the essential features of the cognitive phase of humoral and cell-mediated immune responses are known. In particular, the structure of B and T lymphocyte receptors for antigens is now understood, and the molecular genetic basis of the expression of diverse antigen receptors is known. The antigenic epitopes of numerous model protein antigens that are recognized by lymphocytes have been completely defined. The selection of the lymphocyte repertoire and the mechanisms responsible for discrimination between self and non-self are being elucidated, so that approaches for analyzing autoimmune diseases are becoming feasible. We have also learned a great deal about lymphocyte surface proteins and biochemical signals involved in the proliferative and differentiative responses of these cells to foreign antigens. Among the most impressive advances is the identification of the cytokines that mediate many of the effector functions of lymphocytes and are responsible for the communications among cells of the immune system that serve to amplify and regulate immune responses. The potential use of cytokines as biological response modifiers for treating human diseases is one of the exciting applications of this basic research. Thus, immunology has progressed from a science of phenomena to one of defined genes, molecules, and cells. The challenge in the years to come is to apply our knowledge of these molecules and cells to understand how physiologic immune responses are initiated and regulated in normal individuals and how responses become deficient or aberrant, leading to pathologic tissue injury and clinical diseases.

SUMMARY

The specific immune response is initiated by the recognition of foreign antigens by specific lymphocytes, which respond by proliferating and differentiating into effector cells whose function is to eliminate the antigen. The effector phase of specific immunity requires the participation of various defense mechanisms, including the complement system, phagocytes, inflammatory cells, and cytokines, that are also operative in natural immunity. The specific immune response amplifies the mechanisms of natural immunity and enhances their function, particularly upon repeated exposures to the same foreign antigen. The immune system possesses several properties that are of fundamental importance for its normal functions. These include specificity for distinct antigens, diversity of antigen recognition, memory for antigen exposure, self-limitation, and the ability to discriminate between self and foreign antigens.

In the remainder of this book we describe the biology of lymphocytes, in particular, the structural basis of antigen recognition by lymphocytes, their stimulation leading to the development of effector cells, their regulation, the nature of effector mechanisms, and the abnormalities that lead to diseases of deficient or excessive immunity.

SELECTED READINGS

Burnet, F. M. A modification of Jerne's theory of antibody production using the concept of clonal selection. Australian Journal of Science 20:67–69, 1957.

Jerne, N. K. The natural-selection theory of antibody formation. Proceedings of the National Academy of Sciences USA 41:849–857, 1955.

Reinisch, C. L., and G. W. Litman. Evolutionary immunobiology. Immunology Today 10:278–281, 1989.

Silverstein, A. M. A History of Immunology. Academic Press, San Diego, 1989.

CELLS AND TISSUES

OF THE IMMUNE

SYSTEM

The cells of the immune system are normally present as circulating cells in the blood and lymph, as anatomically defined collections in lymphoid organs, and as scattered cells in virtually all tissues except the central nervous system. The anatomic organization of these cells and their ability to circulate and exchange among the blood, lymph, and tissues are of critical importance for the generation of immune responses. The immune system has to be able to respond to a very large number of foreign antigens introduced at any site in the body, and only a small number of lymphocytes specifically recognize and respond to any one antigen. These lymphocytes not only must locate foreign antigens but also have to activate the many effector mechanisms that are required to eliminate these antigens. The ability of the immune system to optimally perform its protective functions is dependent on several properties of its constituent cells and tissues. These include the following:

1. The cells of the immune system are concentrated in organs that are optimal sites for antigen-induced lymphocyte growth and differentiation.

2. Lymphocytes migrate and exchange between the circulation and tissues, home to sites of antigen exposure, and are retained at these sites.

3. Bidirectional interactions between antigen-specific lymphocytes and other cells that are involved in the cognitive and effector phases of immune responses serve to optimize these responses.

4. Multiple amplification loops magnify the effects of stimulating the few lymphocytes that are specific for any one antigen.

This chapter describes the morphology of the cells and tissues of the immune system, with an emphasis on the ways in which their structural characteristics reflect or contribute to their functions. The circulation of lymphocytes and the functional anatomy of immune responses are discussed in Chapter 11, after the description of the cellular and biochemical bases of antigen recognition and lymphocyte activation.

Lymphocytes are the cells that specifically recognize and respond to foreign antigens. However, both the cognitive and activation phases of immune responses depend on non-lymphoid cells, called **accessory cells,** which are not specific for different antigens and whose functions will be described in greater detail in later chapters. Mononuclear phagocytes, dendritic cells, and several other cell populations function as accessory cells in the induction of immune responses. The activation of lymphocytes leads to the generation of numerous effector mechanisms. Many of these effector mechanisms require the participation of **effector cells,** such as mononuclear phagocytes and other leukocytes (white blood cells). In some situations, antigen-stimulated lymphocytes themselves function as effector cells. Lymphocytes and effector cells are present in the blood, from where they can migrate to peripheral sites of antigen exposure and function to eliminate the antigen. Lymphocytes and accessory cells are also organized in anatomically discrete lymphoid organs, where they interact with one another to initiate and amplify immune responses. The cellular constituents of the blood are listed in Table 2–1. We will describe first the properties of the individual cell types and then the functional anatomy of lymphoid organs.

LYMPHOCYTES

The *specificity of immune responses is due to lymphocytes,* which are the only cells in the body capable of specifically recognizing and distinguishing different antigenic determinants. This has been established by several lines of evidence:

1. Adoptive transfer of specific humoral and cell-mediated immunity from immunized to naive individuals can be achieved only by lymphocytes or their secreted products.

2. Some congenital and acquired immunodeficiencies are associated with reduction of lymphocytes in the peripheral circulation and in lymphoid tissues. Furthermore, selective depletion of lymphocytes with drugs, irradiation, or cell type–specific antibodies leads to impaired immune responses.

3. Lymphocytes are often found in increased numbers at sites of immunization and/or in lymphoid tissues that drain these sites.

TABLE 2–1.   Normal Blood Cell Counts

	Number per mm^3 (Mean ± S.D.)	Per Cent of Leukocytes	
		Mean	*95 Per Cent Range*
White blood cells (×10^3) (leukocytes)	7.25 ± 1.7		
Neutrophils		55	34.6–71.4
Eosinophils		3	0 – 7.8
Basophils		0.5	0 – 1.8
Lymphocytes		35	19.6–52.7
Monocytes		6.5	2.4–11.8
Red blood cells (×10^6) (erythrocytes)	5.0 ± 0.35		
Platelets (×10^3)	248 ± 50		

Abbreviation: S.D., standard deviation.

4. Stimulation of lymphocytes by antigens in culture leads to responses *in vitro* that show many of the characteristics of immune responses induced under more physiologic conditions *in vivo*.

5. Most importantly, specific high-affinity receptors for antigens are produced by lymphocytes and no other cells.

Lymphocyte Development and Heterogeneity

The **small lymphocyte** is 8 to 10 micrometers (μm) in diameter and has a large nucleus with dense heterochromatin. There is a thin rim of cytoplasm that contains a few mitochondria, ribosomes, and lysosomes but no specialized organelles (Fig. 2–1). This bland morphologic pattern provides no clues to the remarkable functional capabilities of lymphocytes. Like all blood cells, lymphocytes originate in the bone marrow. This was first demonstrated by experiments with radiation-induced bone marrow chimeras. Lymphocytes and bone marrow stem cells are radiosensitive and are killed by high doses of γ-irradiation. If an irradiated mouse of one inbred strain is injected with bone marrow cells of another strain that can be distinguished from the host, all the lymphocytes that develop subsequently are derived from the bone marrow cells of the donor (Fig. 2–2). Such approaches have proved useful for defining the maturation of lymphocytes and other blood cells. In the initial stages of their development, lymphocytes do not produce surface receptors for antigens and are, therefore, unresponsive to antigens. As they mature, they begin to express antigen receptors, become responsive to antigenic stimulation, and develop into different functional classes.

Lymphocytes consist of distinct subsets that are quite different in their functions and protein products, even though they all appear morphologically similar (Table 2–2 and Fig. 2–3). One class of lymphocytes consists of **B lymphocytes**, so called because in birds they were first shown to mature in an organ called the bursa of Fabricius. In mammals, there is no anatomic equivalent of the bursa, and the early stages of B cell maturation occur in the bone marrow. Thus, "B" lymphocyte refers to bursa- or bone marrow–derived. *B lymphocytes are the only cells capable of producing antibodies.* The antigen receptors of B lymphocytes are membrane-bound forms of antibodies. Interaction of antigens with these membrane antibody molecules initiates the sequence of B cell activation, which culminates in the development of effector cells that actively secrete antibody molecules (see Chapter 9).

The second major class of lymphocytes consists of **T lymphocytes,** whose precursors arise in the bone marrow and then migrate to and mature in the thymus (the name "T" lymphocyte referring to thymus-derived). T lymphocytes are further subdivided into functionally distinct populations, the best defined of which are **helper T cells** and **cytolytic (or cytotoxic) T cells** (Fig. 2–3). T cells do not produce antibody molecules. Their antigen receptors are membrane molecules distinct from but structurally related to antibodies (see Chapter 7). Helper and cytolytic T lymphocytes have an unusual specificity for antigens—they recognize only peptide antigens attached to proteins that are encoded in the major histocompatibility complex (MHC) and expressed on the surfaces of other cells. As a result, these T cells recognize and respond to cell surface–associated but not soluble antigens (see Chapter 6). In response to antigenic stimulation, helper T cells secrete protein hormones called **cytokines,** whose function is to promote the proliferation and differentiation of the T

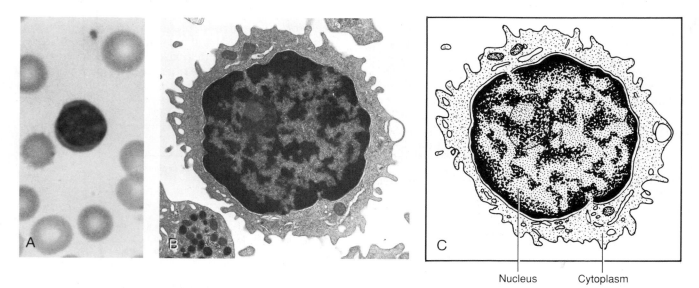

Nucleus   Cytoplasm

FIGURE 2–1. Morphology of a small lymphocyte.
A. *Light micrograph of a lymphocyte in a peripheral blood smear.*
B. *Electron micrograph of a small lymphocyte. (Courtesy of Dr. Noel Weidner, Department of Pathology, Brigham and Women's Hospital, Boston.)*
C. *Schematic diagram of the lymphocyte depicted in B, illustrating the large nucleus and scant cytoplasm with few organelles.*

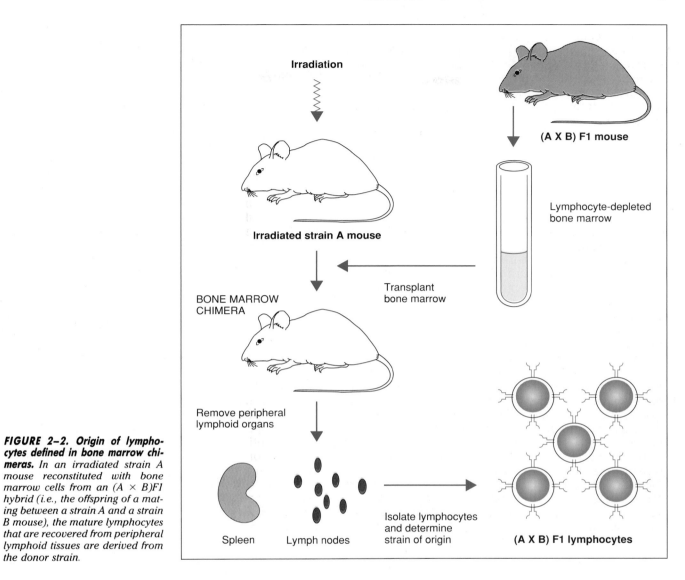

FIGURE 2-2. Origin of lymphocytes defined in bone marrow chimeras. *In an irradiated strain A mouse reconstituted with bone marrow cells from an (A × B)F1 hybrid (i.e., the offspring of a mating between a strain A and a strain B mouse), the mature lymphocytes that are recovered from peripheral lymphoid tissues are derived from the donor strain.*

TABLE 2-2.   Lymphocyte Classes

Class	Functions	Antigen Receptor	Selected Phenotypic Markers	Per Cent of Total Lymphocytes		
				Blood	*Lymph Node*	*Spleen*
B LYMPHOCYTES	Antibody production (humoral immunity)	Surface antibody (immunoglobulin)	Fc receptors; class II MHC	10–15	20–25	40–45
T LYMPHOCYTES Helper	Stimuli for B cell growth and differentiation (humoral immunity) Macrophage activation by secreted cytokines (cell-mediated immunity)	$\alpha\beta$ heterodimers	CD3$^+$ CD4$^+$, CD8$^-$	50–60*	50–60	50–60
Cytolytic	Lysis of virus-infected cells, tumor cells, allografts Macrophage activation by secreted cytokines (cell-mediated immunity)	$\alpha\beta$ heterodimers	CD3$^+$ CD4$^-$CD8$^+$	20–25	15–20	10–15
NATURAL KILLER CELLS	Lysis of virus-infected cells, tumor cells; antibody dependent cellular cytotoxicity	?	Fc receptor for IgG (CD16)	~10	Rare	~10

* In most tissues, ratio of CD4$^+$CD8$^-$ to CD8$^+$CD4$^-$ cells is about 2:1.

Some T lymphocytes function to inhibit immune responses; these are called "supressor cells," but it is unclear if they are a distinct subpopulation of T lymphocytes.

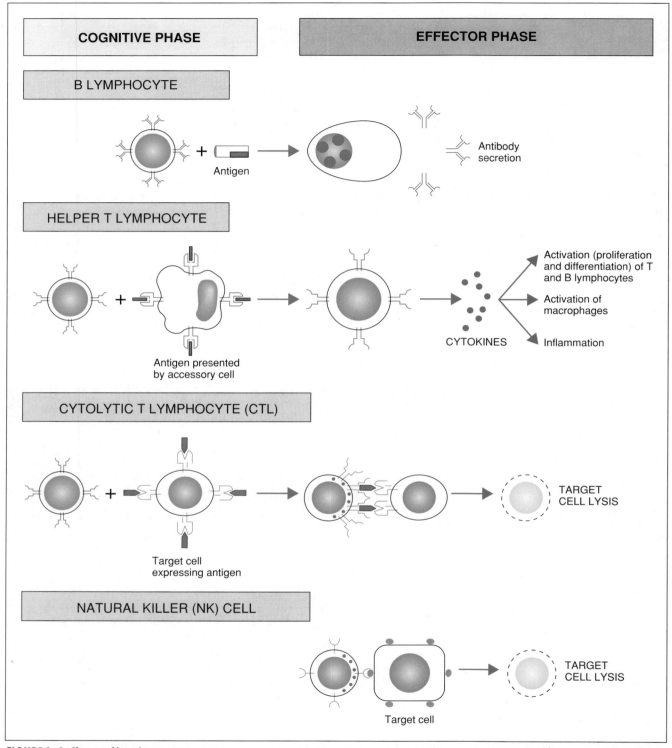

FIGURE 2–3. Classes of lymphocytes. *B lymphocytes recognize soluble antigens and develop into antibody-secreting cells. Helper T lymphocytes recognize antigens on the surfaces of accessory cells and secrete cytokines, which stimulate different components of immunity and inflammation. Cytolytic T lymphocytes recognize antigens on target cells and lyse these targets. Natural killer cells use receptors that are not yet identified to recognize and lyse targets.*

cells as well as other cells, including B cells and macrophages. Cytokines also recruit and activate inflammatory leukocytes, including macrophages and granulocytes, providing important links between specific T cell immunity and natural immunity. Cytolytic T lymphocytes (CTLs) lyse cells that produce foreign antigens,

such as cells infected by viruses and other intracellular microbes. The mechanisms of action and physiologic functions of these T cell populations are described in detail in later chapters. In addition to providing helper and cytolytic functions, T cells may also inhibit immune responses. There is, at present, considerable controversy about the nature and physiologic roles of these so-called "suppressor T cells." In fact, it is not clear whether suppression of immune responses is mediated by a distinct T cell subset or by cells that, under various situations, can function as helper or cytolytic cells (see Chapter 10).

The most important advance in the identification and analysis of these T cell subsets has been the discovery that *functionally distinct populations express different membrane proteins.* These proteins serve as phenotypic markers of different lymphocyte populations. For instance, most helper T cells express a surface protein called CD4, and most CTLs express a different marker called CD8. Antibodies against such markers can, therefore, be used to identify and isolate various lymphocyte populations. Many of the surface proteins that were initially recognized as phenotypic markers for various lymphocyte subpopulations turned out, upon further analysis, to play important roles in the biologic functions of these cells. In this book, we use the unified CD nomenclature for lymphocyte markers. CD stands for "cluster of differentiation" and refers to a molecule recognized by a "cluster" of monoclonal anti-bodies that can be used to identify the lineage or stage of differentiation of lymphocytes and thus to distinguish one class of lymphocyte from another (Box 2–1). CD proteins were first used for subclassifying T cells, but different CD molecules recognized by specific antibodies now serve as useful markers of B cells and other leukocytes that participate in immune and inflammatory responses. Examples of some CD proteins are mentioned in Table 2–2 and the biochemistry and functions of the most important ones are described in later chapters. A current list of known CD markers for leukocytes is provided in the Appendix, p. 431.

The third major class of lymphocytes does not express markers for either T or B cells and was, therefore, initially called the **null cell** population. It is now apparent that most null cells are large lymphocytes with numerous cytoplasmic granules that are capable of lysing a variety of tumor- and virus-infected cells without overt antigenic stimulation. As a result, these lymphocytes are called **large granular lymphocytes** or **natural killer (NK) cells,** designations that define a morphologic or functional group whose ontogeny and specificity are incompletely understood. The properties

---

BOX 2–1. LYMPHOCYTE MARKERS: THE CD NOMENCLATURE

From the time that functionally and developmentally distinct classes of lymphocytes were recognized, immunologists have attempted to develop methods for distinguishing them. The basic approach was to produce antibodies that would selectively recognize different subpopulations. This was initially done by raising "alloantibodies," i.e., antibodies that might recognize allelic forms of cell surface proteins, by immunizing inbred strains of mice with lymphocytes from other strains. Such techniques were remarkably successful and led to the development of antibodies that reacted with murine T cells (anti–Thy-1 antibodies) and even against functionally different subsets of T lymphocytes (anti–Lyt-1 and –Lyt-2 antibodies). The limitations of this approach, however, are obvious, since it is only useful for cell surface proteins that exist in allelic forms. Other approaches that met with some success but also have major limitations included searching for lymphocyte-specific autoantibodies in patients with autoimmune diseases. The advent of hybridoma technology gave such analyses a tremendous boost, and the most dramatic development was the production of monoclonal antibodies that reacted specifically and selectively with defined populations of lymphocytes, first human and subsequently in many other species. (Alloantibodies and monoclonal antibodies are described in Chapter 3.)

The cell surface molecules recognized by monoclonal antibodies are called "antigens," since antibodies can be raised against them, or "markers," since they identify and discriminate between ("mark") different cell populations. These markers can be grouped into several categories—some are specific for cells of a particular lineage or maturational pathway, and the expression of others varies according to the state of activation or differentiation of the same cells. Biochemical analyses of cell surface proteins recognized by different monoclonal antibodies in the same species or even in different species demonstrated that in many instances these antibodies were specific for the same evolutionar-ily conserved cellular proteins. Considerable confusion was created because these surface markers were initially named according to the antibodies that reacted with them. In order to resolve this, a uniform nomenclature system was adopted, initially for human leukocytes. According to this system, a surface marker that identifies a particular lineage or differentiation stage, that has a defined structure, and that is recognized by a group ("cluster") of monoclonal antibodies is called a member of a **cluster of differentiation.** Thus, all leukocyte surface antigens whose structures are defined are given a "CD" designation, i.e., CD1, CD2, etc. Although this nomenclature was originally used for human leukocyte antigens, it is now common practice to refer to homologous markers in other species and on cells other than leukocytes by the same CD designation. Newly developed monoclonal antibodies are periodically exchanged among laboratories, and the antigens recognized are assigned to existing CD structures or introduced as new "workshop" candidates ("CDw").

The value of CD antigens in classifying lymphocytes is enormous. For instance, most helper T lymphocytes are CD3$^+$CD4$^+$CD8$^-$, and most CTLs are CD3$^+$CD4$^-$CD8$^+$. This has allowed immunologists to identify the cells participating in various immune responses, isolate them, and individually analyze their specificities, response patterns, and effector functions. Such antibodies have also been used to define specific alterations in particular subsets of lymphocytes that might be occurring in various diseases. Further investigations of the effects of monoclonal antibodies on lymphocyte function have shown that these surface proteins are not merely phenotypic markers but are themselves involved in a variety of lymphocyte responses. The two most frequent functions attributed to various CD antigens are (1) to promote cell-cell interactions and adhesion, and (2) to transduce signals that lead to lymphocyte activation. Examples of both types of functions are described in Chapter 7.

and functions of NK cells are discussed in more detail in Chapter 13.

Morphologic Changes Associated with Lymphocyte Activation

Lymphocytes undergo a well-defined pattern of changes upon activation. It is technically difficult to study the responses of lymphocytes to antigens because only a very small fraction of the total population is specific for any one antigen. Immunologists have overcome this problem by using **polyclonal activators,** e.g., antibodies against antigen receptors, that stimulate many B or T lymphocytes irrespective of antigenic specificity. It is generally assumed that polyclonal activators mimic antigens; i.e., the changes induced by the former in many lymphocytes are similar to the changes induced by antigens in antigen-specific clones.

Prior to antigenic or polyclonal stimulation, small lymphocytes are in a state of rest, or in the G_0 stage of the cell cycle. If resting lymphocytes do not encounter antigen, they probably die within a few days or weeks, and the population is maintained at a steady-state level by the development of new cells from precursors in the bone marrow. In response to antigenic (or polyclonal) stimulation, resting small lymphocytes enter the G_1 stage of the cell cycle. They become larger and are called large lymphocytes, or **lymphoblasts.** These cells are 10 to 12 μm in diameter and have a wider rim of cytoplasm, more organelles, and increased amounts of cytoplasmic ribonucleic acid (RNA) compared with unstimulated small lymphocytes. Progression to the S phase of the cell cycle continues, and the activated large lymphocytes divide. This sequence of events is called **blast transformation.** Mitotic division is responsible for proliferation of the antigen-responsive clones of lymphocytes. Subsequent to or in concert with proliferation, the stimulated lymphocytes differentiate from a cognitive stage at which they recognize antigen to an effector stage at which they function to eliminate the antigen. Differentiated helper T cells have essentially the same morphologic appearance as small or large lymphocytes. Differentiated CTLs may contain increased numbers of cytolytic granules whose contents include proteins that lyse target cells. Antibody-producing B cells often differentiate into specialized forms called **plasma cells.** Plasma cells are found only in lymphoid organs and at sites of immune responses and normally do not circulate in the blood or lymph. They have a characteristic morphology with eccentric nuclei, abundant cytoplasm, and distinct perinuclear haloes (Fig. 2–4). Under the electron microscope, the cytoplasm can be seen to contain dense rough endoplasmic reticulum, which is the site where antibodies (and other secreted and membrane proteins) are synthesized. There is also a large Golgi complex, which stains poorly with routinely used histologic stains and is responsible for the perinuclear halo; antibody molecules are converted to their final forms and packaged for secretion in this organelle. Plasma cells are believed to be terminally differentiated cells with little or no capacity for mitotic division, and are, in essence, factories for the synthesis and secretion of antibody molecules. It is estimated that half or more of the messenger

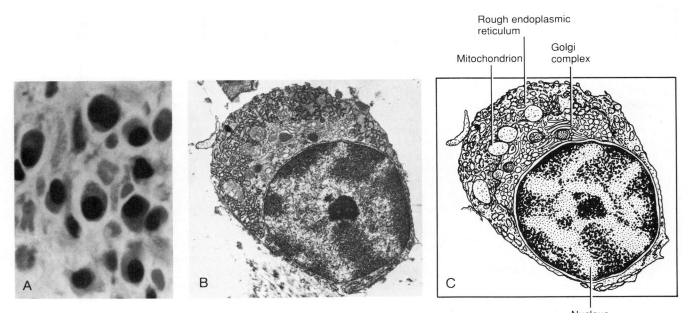

Rough endoplasmic reticulum

Golgi complex

Mitochondrion

Nucleus

FIGURE 2–4. Morphology of plasma cells.
A. *Light micrograph of plasma cells in tissues.*
B. *Electron micrograph of a plasma cell. (Courtesy of Dr. Noel Weidner, Department of Pathology, Brigham and Women's Hospital, Boston.)*
C. *Schematic diagram of the plasma cell depicted in B, illustrating the eccentric nucleus with a "cartwheel" pattern of chromatin, the abundant cisternae of the rough endoplasmic reticulum, and the prominent Golgi complex.*

RNA (mRNA) in plasma cells codes for antibody proteins.

Some of the progeny of antigen-stimulated B and T lymphocytes do not differentiate into effector cells. Instead, they become **memory lymphocytes,** which are capable of surviving for long periods, perhaps 20 years or more, apparently in the absence of antigenic stimulation. Memory cells are functionally quiescent, i.e., they do not produce effector molecules unless they are stimulated by antigens. The stimuli that determine whether a progeny of an activated T or B lymphocyte will become an effector cell or a memory cell are not known. The development of memory cells is crucial to the success of vaccination as a method of providing long-lived immunity against infections. It is believed that memory cells are morphologically similar to small lymphocytes. However, the characteristics of memory cells are not fully known, because these cells are defined by their survival and until recently there were virtually no phenotypic markers to clearly distinguish them from resting or recently activated lymphocytes. It is now appreciated that most naive and memory T cells express different surface proteins. Naive T cells that have not been exposed to their specific antigens express a 200 kD isoform of a surface molecule called CD45 that contains a segment encoded by an exon designated "A". This CD45 isoform can be recognized by antibodies specific for the A encoded segment, and is therefore called CD45RA (for "restricted A"). CD45RA⁺ naive T cells also express high levels of the peripheral lymph node homing receptor but low levels of other surface proteins involved in cell-cell adhesion. In contrast, most activated and memory T cells express a 180 kD isoform of CD45 in which the A exon has been spliced out; this isoform is called CD45RO. Memory T cells also express low levels of the peripheral lymph node homing receptor, but higher levels of other adhesion molecules. The significance of these differences will be discussed in Chapter 11, when we describe lymphocyte recirculation and homing to various tissues. It is not established whether the phenotypes of memory cells are fixed or whether some CD45RO⁺ cells may revert to expressing the CD45RA isoform.

MONONUCLEAR PHAGOCYTES

The **mononuclear phagocyte system** constitutes the second major cell population of the immune system and consists of cells that have a common lineage whose primary function is phagocytosis. In the early 20th century, morphologists observed that certain cells took up dyes injected intravenously (called "vital dyes," since they stained live cells). Aschoff identified these cells as macrophages in connective tissues, microglia in the central nervous system, endothelial cells lining vascular sinusoids, and reticular cells of lymphoid organs, and suggested that these varied cell types functioned in host defense by phagocytosis of foreign invaders such as microbes. He grouped them collectively into the **reticuloendothelial system** (RES). It is now clear that the pinocytosis of which the endothelial and reticular cells are capable is fundamentally different from the active phagocytosis of macrophages. It is, therefore, more appropriate to classify monocytes and macrophages as members of the mononuclear phagocyte system.

Development

All the cells of the mononuclear phagocyte system originate in bone marrow and, after maturation and subsequent activation, can achieve varied morphologic forms (Fig. 2–5). The first cell type that enters the peripheral blood after leaving the marrow is incompletely

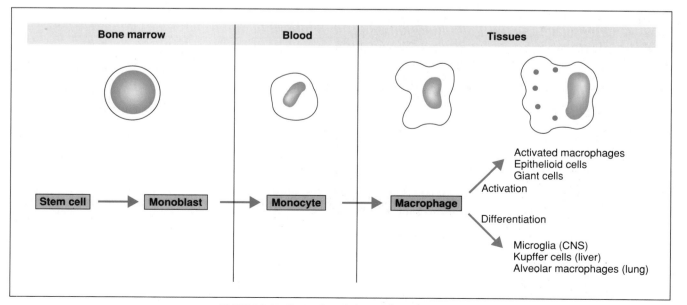

FIGURE 2–5. Maturation of mononuclear phagocytes.

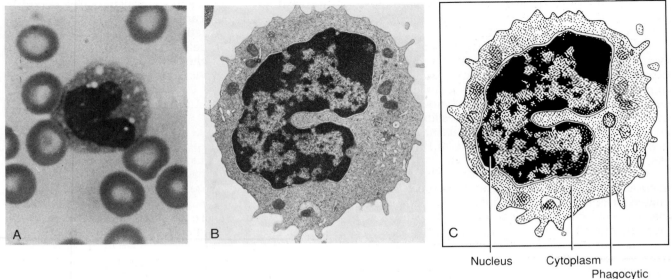

Nucleus   Cytoplasm
                    Phagocytic
                    vacuole

FIGURE 2–6. Morphology of mononuclear phagocytes.
A. *Light micrograph of a monocyte in a peripheral blood smear.*
B. *Electron micrograph of a peripheral blood monocyte. (Courtesy of Dr. Noel Weidner, Department of Pathology, Brigham and Women's Hospital, Boston.)*
C. *Schematic diagram of the monocyte depicted in B, illustrating the characteristic nucleus, scant cytoplasmic organelles, and phagocytic vacuoles.*

differentiated and is called the **monocyte.** Monocytes are 10 to 15 μm in diameter, and they have bean-shaped nuclei and finely granular cytoplasm containing lysosomes, phagocytic vacuoles, and cytoskeletal filaments (Fig. 2–6). Once they settle in tissues, these cells mature and become **macrophages,** which are also called "histiocytes." Macrophages can be activated by a variety of stimuli and may assume different forms. Some develop abundant cytoplasm and are called **epithelioid cells** because of their resemblance to epithelial cells of the skin. Macrophages can fuse to form polykarons, also termed **multinucleate giant cells.** Macrophages are found in all organs and connective tissues, and have been given special names to designate specific locations. For instance, in the central nervous system they are the "microglia"; when lining the vascular sinusoids of the liver, they are called "Kupffer cells"; in pulmonary airways, they are the "alveolar macrophages"; and multinucleate phagocytes in bone are called "osteoclasts."

Activation and Function

Mononuclear phagocytes represent the clearest example of a cell population that is critical for natural immunity but has also become adapted to play a central role in specific acquired immunity. Macrophages perform many of their functions in host defense prior to the development of specific immunity; these same functions become more efficient at sites of immune responses. This illustrates a concept that was introduced in Chapter 1, namely that the immune response imparts specificity to and enhances defense mechanisms that

are operative even in the absence of specific antigen recognition by lymphocytes.

The principal *functions of mononuclear phagocytes in natural immunity* include the following:

1. Macrophages phagocytose foreign particles, such as microbes, macromolecules, including antigens, and even self tissues that are injured or dead, such as senescent erythrocytes. Macrophage recognition of foreign substances and injured tissues may involve receptors for phospholipids and sugars, but the precise mechanisms are not well understood. Phagocytosed substances are degraded within macrophages by lysosomal enzymes. Macrophages function as the principal "scavenger cells" of the body. In addition, the cells secrete enzymes, reactive oxygen species, nitric oxide (in mice), and lipid-derived mediators such as prostaglandins, all of which serve to kill microbes and control the spread of infections, and can injure even normal tissues in the immediate vicinity.

2. Macrophages produce cytokines that recruit other inflammatory cells, especially neutrophils, and are responsible for many of the systemic effects of inflammation, such as fever. Macrophages also produce growth factors for fibroblasts and vascular endothelium that promote the repair of injured tissues.

Mononuclear phagocytes function as both accessory and effector cells in immune responses. They play the following important roles in the cognitive, activation, and effector phases of specific immunity.

1. Macrophages display foreign antigens on their surface in a form that can be recognized by antigen-specific T lymphocytes. This function of macrophages as **antigen-presenting cells** (APCs) is described in

Chapter 6. Macrophages also express proteins that promote T cell activation. Thus, *macrophages function as accessory cells in lymphocyte activation.*

2. In the effector phase of certain cell-mediated immune responses, antigen-stimulated T cells secrete cytokines that activate macrophages. Such activated macrophages are more efficient at performing phagocytic, degradative, and cytocidal functions than are unstimulated cells, and are thus better able to destroy phagocytosed antigens. Thus, *macrophages are among the principal effector cells of cell-mediated immunity* (see Chapter 13).

3. In the effector phase of humoral immune responses, foreign antigens, such as microbes, become coated, or opsonized, by antibody molecules and complement proteins. Because macrophages express surface receptors for antibodies and for certain complement proteins, they bind and phagocytose opsonized particles much more avidly than uncoated particles (see Chapter 3). *Thus, macrophages participate in the elimination of foreign antigens by humoral immune responses.*

The ability of macrophages and lymphocytes to stimulate each other's functions provides an important amplification mechanism for specific immunity. The mechanisms and physiologic consequences of the bidirectional interactions between immunocompetent lymphocytes and non-lymphoid accessory and effector cells will be referred to in many sections of this book.

DENDRITIC CELLS

Dendritic cells are accessory cells that play important roles in the induction of immune responses. These cells are identified morphologically as cells with membranous or spine-like projections. There are two types of dendritic cells that have different properties and functions. **Interdigitating dendritic cells,** which are usually called simply "dendritic cells," are present in the interstitium of most organs, are abundant in T cell–rich areas of lymph nodes and spleen, and are scattered throughout the epidermis of the skin, where they are called **Langerhans cells.** Langerhans cells contain an unusual cytoplasmic organelle called the Birbeck granule, whose function is unknown. These interdigitating dendritic cells are thought to arise from marrow precursors and are related in lineage to mononuclear phagocytes. They are extremely efficient at presenting protein antigens to CD4$^+$ helper T cells (see Chapter 6). Langerhans cells are capable of picking up antigens that enter via the skin and transporting these antigens to draining lymph nodes, where immune responses are initiated. In fact, many of the dendritic cells in lymphoid organs and interstitial tissues may have arisen from Langerhans cells, which migrate from the skin into tissues after picking up antigens. The second type of dendritic cells are called **follicular dendritic cells** because they are present in the germinal centers of lymphoid follicles in the lymph nodes, spleen, and mu-

cosa-associated lymphoid tissues. Follicular dendritic cells are not derived from precursors in the bone marrow and are unrelated to interdigitating dendritic cells. Follicular dendritic cells trap antigens complexed to antibodies or complement products and display these antigens on their surfaces for recognition by B lymphocytes. The functions of interdigitating and follicular dendritic cells in immune responses are discussed in more detail in Chapters 6 and 9.

GRANULOCYTES

In addition to lymphocytes and mononuclear phagocytes, other blood leukocytes, which are called **granulocytes** because they contain abundant cytoplasmic granules, participate in the effector phase of specific immune responses. The details of the morphology, biochemistry, and functions of granulocytes are beyond the scope of this book. These leukocytes are often referred to as **inflammatory cells,** because they play important roles in inflammation and natural immunity, and function to eliminate microbes and dead tissues. However, like macrophages, granulocytes are stimulated by T cell–derived cytokines and phagocytose opsonized particles, so that these cells serve important effector functions in specific immune responses as well.

Peripheral blood contains three types of granulocytes, which are classified according to the staining characteristics of their predominant granules.

Neutrophils, also called **polymorphonuclear leukocytes** because of their multilobed, morphologically diverse nuclei, are the most numerous. They respond rapidly to chemotactic stimuli, phagocytose and destroy foreign particles, such as microbes, can be activated by cytokines produced primarily by macrophages and endothelial cells, and are the major cell population in the acute inflammatory response. Neutrophils also possess receptors for a type of antibody called IgG and for complement proteins, and they migrate to and accumulate at sites of complement activation. Therefore, they avidly phagocytose opsonized particles and function as effector cells of humoral immunity.

Eosinophils are thought to function mainly in defense against certain types of infectious agents. Eosinophils express receptors for a class of antibody called IgE and are able to bind avidly to IgE-coated particles. They are particularly effective at destroying infectious agents that stimulate the production of IgE, such as helminthic parasites. In fact, helminths may be relatively resistant to the lysosomal enzymes of neutrophils and macrophages, but are often killed by the specialized granule proteins of eosinophils. Eosinophils are also abundant at sites of immediate hypersensitivity (allergic) reactions; in this setting, eosinophils contribute to tissue injury and inflammation (see Chapter 14). The growth and differentiation of eosinophils are stimulated by a helper T cell–derived cytokine called interleukin-5, and T cell activation may contribute to eosinophil accumulation at sites of parasitic infestation and allergic reactions.

Basophils are the circulating counterparts of tissue mast cells. Both basophils and mast cells express high-affinity receptors for IgE and, therefore, avidly bind free IgE antibodies. Subsequent interaction of antigens with these bound IgE molecules stimulates basophils and mast cells to secrete their granule contents, which are the chemical mediators of immediate hypersensitivity (see Chapter 14). Thus, these granulocytes are effector cells of IgE-mediated immediate hypersensitivity.

FUNCTIONAL ANATOMY OF LYMPHOID TISSUES

In order to optimize cellular interactions necessary for the cognitive and activation phases of specific immune responses, the majority of lymphocytes, mononuclear phagocytes, and other accessory cells are localized and concentrated in anatomically defined tissues or organs, which are also the sites where foreign antigens are transported and concentrated. Such anatomic compartmentalization is not fixed because, as discussed in Chapter 11, many lymphocytes recirculate and constantly exchange between the circulation and tissues. Lymphoid tissues can be classified into two groups: (1) the **generative organs** are the ones in which lymphocytes arise and mature and where lymphocytes capable of recognizing self antigens are deleted or inactivated, and (2) the **peripheral organs** are the sites where mature lymphocytes respond to foreign antigens (Fig. 2–7). Included in the generative lymphoid organs of mammals are the bone marrow, where all the lymphocytes arise, and the thymus, where T cells mature and reach a stage of functional competence. In birds, another generative organ is the bursa of Fabricius, the site of B cell maturation; the bursal equivalent in mammals is the bone marrow itself. The peripheral lymphoid tissues include the lymph nodes, spleen, mucosa-associated lymphoid tissues, and the cutaneous immune system. In addition, poorly defined aggregates of lymphocytes are found in connective tissues and in virtually all organs except the central nervous system.

Bone Marrow

During fetal life, the generation of all blood cells, called **hematopoiesis,** occurs initially in blood islands and then in liver and spleen. This function is gradually taken over by the bone marrow and increasingly by the marrow of the flat bones, so that by puberty hematopoiesis occurs mostly in the sternum, vertebrae, iliac bones, and ribs. The red marrow that is found in these bones consists of a sponge-like reticular framework located between long trabeculae. The spaces in this framework are filled with fat cells and the precursors of blood cells, which mature and exit via the dense network of vascular sinuses to become part of the circulatory system.

All the blood cells originate from a common **stem cell** that becomes committed to differentiate along particular lineages, i.e., erythroid, megakaryocytic, granulocytic, monocytic, and lymphocytic (Fig. 2–8). The proliferation and maturation of precursor cells in the bone marrow are stimulated by cytokines. Many of these cytokines are also called "colony-stimulating factors" (CSFs) because they are assayed by their ability to stimulate the growth and development of various leukocyte colonies from marrow cells. Hematopoietic cy-

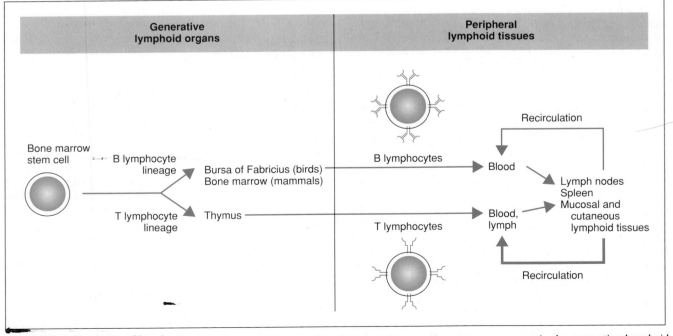

FIGURE 2–7. Maturation of lymphocytes. *Development of mature lymphocytes prior to antigen exposure occurs in the generative lymphoid organs, and immune responses to foreign antigens occur in the peripheral lymphoid tissues.*

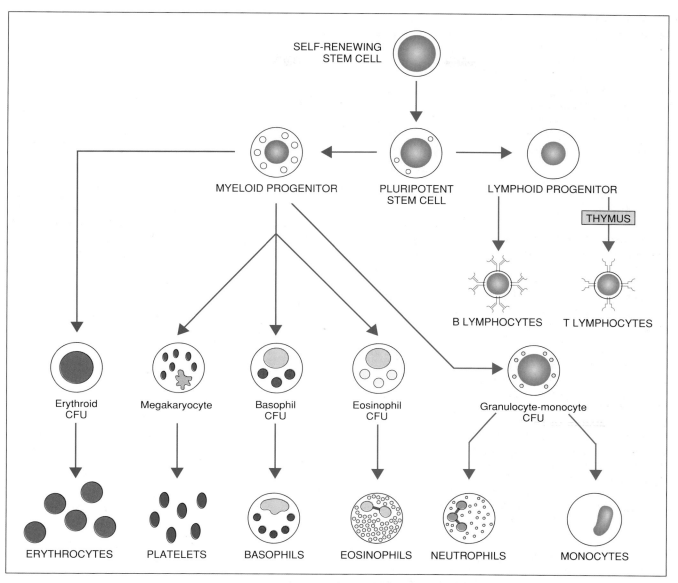

FIGURE 2–8. Maturation of blood cells: the hematopoietic "tree."

tokines are produced by stromal cells and macrophages in the bone marrow, thus providing the local environment for hematopoiesis, and by antigen-stimulated T lymphocytes, providing a mechanism for replenishing leukocytes that may be consumed during immune and inflammatory reactions. Different cytokines promote the proliferation and maturation of different lineages of bone marrow precursor cells (see Chapter 12). Little is known about the nature of the uncommitted stem cell or the mechanisms that regulate its commitment to specific lineages. In 1988, techniques for reconstituting the immune system of congenitally immunodeficient mice with human lymphohematopoietic stem cells were described. These immunodeficient mice lack T and B lymphocytes, and after the implantation of human hematopoietic tissues, mature human lymphocytes develop in the animals and populate the circulation and peripheral lymphoid tissues. Such approaches hold great promise for more

precise identification and characterization of stem cells and their developmental pathways.

The marrow contains mature B lymphocytes, which have developed from progenitor cells (see Chapter 4). There are also numerous antibody-secreting plasma cells, which develop in peripheral lymphoid tissues as a consequence of antigenic stimulation of B cells and then migrate to the marrow. The maturation of T lymphocytes occurs not in the bone marrow but in the thymus.

Thymus

The thymus is a bilobed organ situated in the anterior mediastinum. Each lobe is divided into multiple lobules by fibrous septa, and each lobule consists of an outer cortex and an inner medulla (Fig. 2–9). The cortex contains a dense collection of T lymphocytes, and

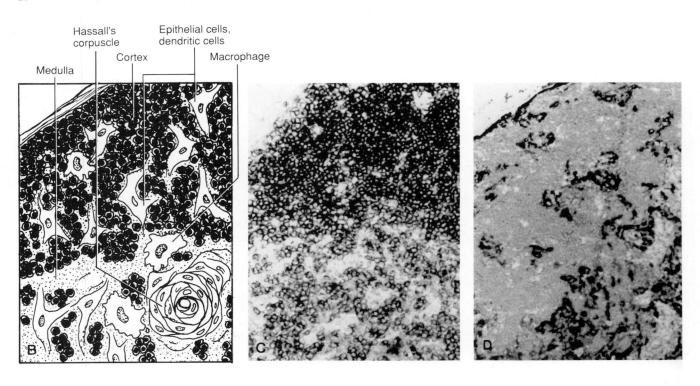

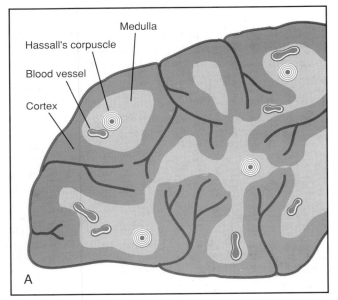

FIGURE 2–9. Morphology of the thymus.

A. *Schematic diagram of the thymus, illustrating a portion of a lobe divided into multiple lobules by fibrous trabecula.*

B. *Diagram of the edge of a lobule showing the cells of the cortex and medulla.*

C. *T lymphocytes in the cortex of the thymus, detected by an immunoperoxidase stain with an antibody specific for T cells. (Immunoperoxidase staining is described in Chapter 3; positive cells appear dark.) (Courtesy of Dr. G. S. Pinkus, Department of Pathology, Brigham and Women's Hospital, Boston.)*

D. *Epithelial cells scattered throughout the cortex and medulla, detected by an immunoperoxidase stain specific for keratin, an intracellular intermediate filament protein. (Courtesy of Dr. G. S. Pinkus, Department of Pathology, Brigham and Women's Hospital, Boston.)*

the lighter-staining medulla is more sparsely populated with lymphocytes. Scattered throughout the thymus are non-lymphoid epithelial cells, which have abundant cytoplasm, as well as bone marrow–derived dendritic cells and macrophages. In the medulla are structures called Hassall's corpuscles, which are composed of tightly packed whorls of epithelial cells that may be remnants of degenerating cells. The thymus has a rich

vascular supply and efferent lymphatic vessels that drain into mediastinal lymph nodes.

The lymphocytes in the thymus, also called **thymocytes,** are T lymphocytes at various stages of maturation. Precursors that are committed to the T cell lineage enter the thymic cortex via blood vessels. It is not known whether B cell precursors enter the thymus and fail to survive or whether there are mechanisms that ensure that only cells committed to developing into T lymphocytes can enter the thymus. The most immature thymocytes do not express receptors for antigens or surface markers, including CD4 and CD8, that are characteristic of the mature phenotype. These immature cells migrate from the cortex toward the medulla and come into contact with epithelial cells, macrophages, and dendritic cells. Efficient contact may occur in lymphoepithelial complexes in which lymphocytes are found closely apposed to the invaginated plasma membranes of large epithelial cells called "nurse cells." En route to the medulla, thymocytes begin to express receptors for antigens and surface markers that are present on mature, peripheral T lymphocytes. Thus, the medulla contains mostly mature T cells, and only mature CD4$^+$ or CD8$^+$ T cells exit the thymus and enter the blood, lymph, and peripheral lymphoid tissues.

From the large number of primitive T cells that enters the thymus, many cells that might recognize self antigens do not survive, whereas cells whose receptors are specific for foreign antigens are stimulated to mature. These selection processes, which are critical for the ability of the immune system to discriminate between self and non-self, are described in considerable detail in Chapter 8.

Lymph Nodes

Lymph nodes are small nodular aggregates of lymphoid tissue situated along lymphatic channels throughout the body. Epithelia, such as the skin and the mucosa of the gastrointestinal and respiratory tracts, as well as connective tissues and most organs have a lymphatic drainage. Antigens that enter through any of these portals end up in lymphatic vessels and are transported to lymph nodes (see Chapter 11). Thus, the lymphatic system provides a mechanism for antigen collection, and the cells in the lymph nodes "sample" the lymph for the presence of foreign antigenic material.

Each lymph node is surrounded by a fibrous capsule that is pierced by numerous afferent lymphatics, which empty the lymph into a subcapsular sinus (Fig. 2–10). The node consists of an outer cortex in which there are aggregates of cells constituting the **follicles,** some of which contain central areas called **germinal centers,** which stain lightly with commonly used histologic stains, and outer regions called **mantle zones.** Follicles without germinal centers are called primary follicles, and those with germinal centers are secondary follicles. The inner medulla contains less dense lymphocytes and mononuclear phagocytes scattered among lymphatic and vascular sinusoids. Lymphocytes and accessory cells are often found in close proximity but do not form intercellular junctions, which is important for maintaining the ability of the lymphocytes to migrate and recirculate between the lymph, blood, and tissues. The lymph that enters the subcapsular sinus percolates through the cortex and medulla and exits via a single efferent lymphatic located in the hilum of the node. In addition, each node has a vascular supply with afferent and efferent vessels at the hilum.

Different classes of lymphocytes and non-lymphoid accessory cells are sequestered in particular areas of the node. Follicles are the B cell–rich areas of lymph nodes (Fig. 2–10). Primary follicles contain predominantly mature, resting B lymphocytes that have apparently not been stimulated recently by antigens. The germinal centers, which develop in response to stimulation by helper T cell–dependent protein antigens, contain numerous large lymphocytes. *Germinal centers are the sites where antigen-stimulated B cells proliferate and give rise to progeny that produce antibodies with high affinities for the antigen.* Follicular dendritic cells, which reside in germinal centers, display antigens on their surfaces and function to selectively activate B cells that bind the antigen with high affinities. Fully differentiated plasma cells develop outside the germinal centers and may migrate out of lymph nodes to other tissues. The processes of B lymphocyte stimulation and antibody production are described in more detail in Chapter 9.

The T lymphocytes are located predominantly between the follicles and in the deep cortex, called the parafollicular areas (Fig. 2–10). Most of these T cells are CD4$^+$ helper T cells, intermingled with relatively sparse CD8$^+$ cells. Naive T lymphocytes, which have not been stimulated by their specific foreign antigens, enter each lymph node either via the lymph or through specialized venules lined by cuboidal endothelium, called **high endothelial venules,** that are abundant in T cell–rich zones. Here the T cells encounter foreign antigens that have been transported to the node in the lymph. Interdigitating dendritic cells, which are also abundant in the T cell areas, as well as other accessory cells present the antigens to naive helper T cells. Thus, the *lymph nodes are the sites where T cell responses to lymph-borne protein antigens are initiated.*

The medulla contains scattered lymphocytes, large numbers of macrophages and dendritic cells, and, in nodes draining sites of immunization, numerous plasma cells, all of which are interspersed with lymphatic channels.

The mechanisms responsible for the anatomic sequestration of different classes of lymphocytes in distinct areas of the node are unclear. One possibility is that compartmentalization is maintained by specific adhesions of different lymphocytes to stromal cells or extracellular matrix proteins. The anatomic organization of lymph nodes provides multiple sites for interactions between accessory cells and lymphocytes and between different classes of lymphocytes. Dendritic cells located in T cell–rich areas present antigens to CD4$^+$ helper T cells. Follicular dendritic cells in germinal centers present antigens to activated and memory B cells. B lymphocytes that enter the node from the blood must traverse helper T cell–rich zones en route to follicles, thus maximizing the chances for cooperative T cell–B cell interactions (see Chapter 9). It is, therefore, not surprising that the organization of various cell populations in lymph nodes is critical for the generation of immune responses (see Chapter 11). The structure of lymph nodes is not fixed, but changes with antigen exposure. For instance, germinal centers develop within 1 week after immunization, and gradually regress after the antigenic stimulus is eliminated.

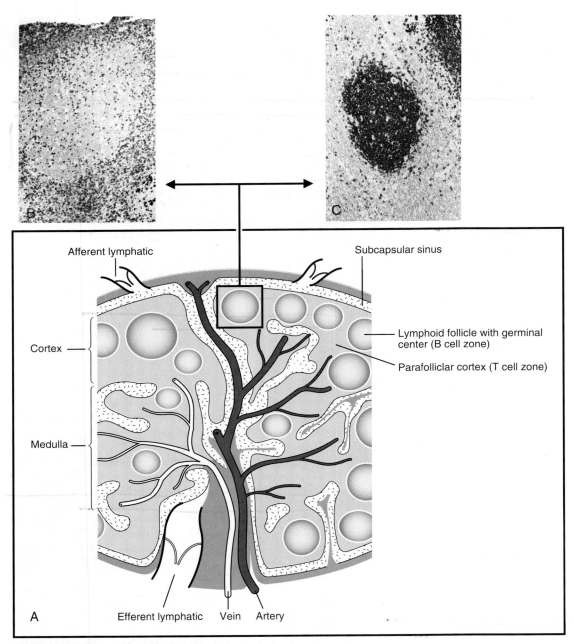

FIGURE 2–10. Morphology of a lymph node.

A. *Schematic diagram of a lymph node showing the distinct cortex with lymphoid follicles and dense lymphocytes and the medulla with lymphatic cords and vessels.*

B. *T lymphocytes in the parafollicular region of the cortex, detected by an immunoperoxidase stain with an antibody specific for T cells. (Courtesy of Dr. G. S. Pinkus, Department of Pathology, Brigham and Women's Hospital, Boston.)*

C. *B lymphocytes in a follicle in the cortex, detected by an immunoperoxidase stain with an antibody specific for B cells. (Courtesy of Dr. G. S. Pinkus, Department of Pathology, Brigham and Women's Hospital, Boston.)*

Spleen

The spleen is an organ weighing about 150 gm in adults, located in the left upper quadrant of the abdomen. It is supplied by a single splenic artery, which pierces the capsule at the hilum and divides into progressively smaller branches that remain surrounded by protective and supporting fibrous trabeculae (Fig.

2–11). Small arterioles are surrounded by cuffs of lymphocytes, called **periarteriolar lymphoid sheaths,** to which are attached the lymphoid follicles, some of which contain germinal centers. The periarteriolar lymphoid sheaths and follicles are surrounded by a rim of lymphocytes and macrophages, called the **marginal zone.** These dense lymphoid tissues constitute the **white pulp** of the spleen. The arterioles ultimately end in vascular sinusoids, scattered among which are large numbers of erythrocytes, macrophages, dendritic cells, sparse lymphocytes, and plasma cells; these constitute the **red pulp.** The sinusoids end in venules that drain into the splenic vein, which carries blood out of the spleen and into the portal circulation.

Lymphocytes and accessory cells are anatomically segregated in the spleen as they are in lymph nodes (Fig. 2–11). The periarteriolar sheaths contain mainly T lymphocytes, about two thirds of which are of the CD4+ helper class and one third are CD8+. The follicles and germinal centers are the predominantly B cell zones,

FIGURE 2–11. Morphology of the spleen.

A. *Schematic diagram of the spleen. Note that the white pulp, made up of dense lymphoid tissues in periarteriolar sheaths and follicles, is intermingled with the red pulp, composed of vascular sinusoids and scattered cells.*

B. *T lymphocytes in the periarteriolar lymphoid sheath, detected by an immunoperoxidase stain with an antibody specific for T cells. (Courtesy of Dr. G. S. Pinkus, Department of Pathology, Brigham and Women's Hospital, Boston.)*

C. *B lymphocytes in a lymphoid follicle, detected by an immunoperoxidase stain with an antibody specific for B cells. (Courtesy of Dr. G. S. Pinkus, Department of Pathology, Brigham and Women's Hospital, Boston.)*

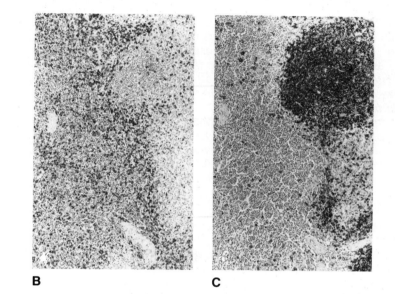

B

C

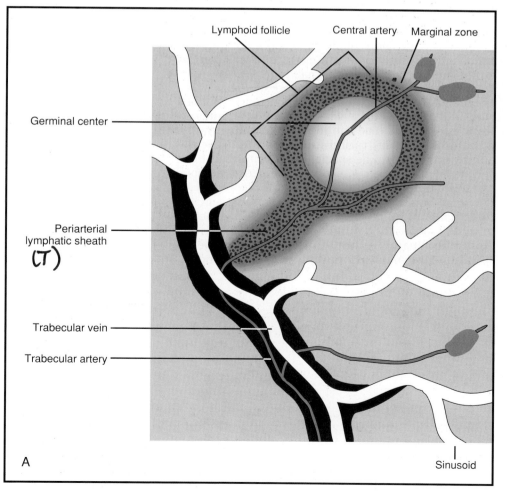

Lymphoid follicle   Central artery   Marginal zone

Germinal center

Periarterial lymphatic sheath (T)

Trabecular vein

Trabecular artery

A

Sinusoid

having the same anatomic features and functions as in lymph nodes. The marginal zones contain both B lymphocytes and CD4$^+$ helper T cells. Antigens and lymphocytes enter the spleen through the vascular sinusoids; the spleen lacks high endothelial venules. Activation of B cells is initiated in the marginal zones, which are adjacent to helper T cells in lymphoid sheaths. Activated B cells subsequently migrate into germinal centers or into the red pulp (see Chapter 9).

In principle, the function of the spleen and its responses to antigens are much like those of lymph nodes, the essential difference being that *the spleen is the major site of immune responses to blood-borne antigens, whereas lymph nodes are involved in responses to antigens in the lymph.* The spleen is also an important "filter" for the blood; its red pulp macrophages are responsible for clearing the blood of unwanted foreign substances and senescent erythrocytes even in the absence of specific immunity.

Other Peripheral Lymphoid Tissues

In addition to the lymph nodes and spleen, lymphocytes are found either scattered or in aggregates in many tissues. Some of these collections are anatomically well organized and have unique properties. Located beneath the mucosa of the gastrointestinal and respiratory tracts are aggregates of lymphocytes and accessory cells that resemble lymph nodes in structure and function. These aggregates include Peyer's patches in the lamina propria of the small intestine, tonsils in the pharynx, and submucosal lymphoid follicles in the appendix and throughout the upper airways. The lymphoid tissues in these sites constitute the **mucosal immune system.** The **cutaneous immune system** consists of lymphocytes and accessory cells in the epidermis and dermis. The specialized structural features and functions of the cutaneous and mucosal immune systems are described in Chapter 11.

In addition to these normal lymphoid organs, **ectopic lymphoid tissues** can develop at sites of strong immune responses. A striking example of this is the disease rheumatoid arthritis, in which an immune response in the synovium ultimately leads to destruction of the cartilage and bone in joints. In severe cases, synovial tissues contain well-developed lymphoid follicles with prominent germinal centers.

Summary

The principal cellular constituents of the immune system are lymphocytes, mononuclear phagocytes, and related accessory cells. Lymphocytes are the only immunocompetent cells capable of specific recognition of antigens. They are morphologically homogeneous but consist of distinct subsets that perform different functions and can be distinguished phenotypically. Mononuclear phagocytes are critical for host defense in the absence of specific immunity and have also evolved into key participants in the cognitive, activation, and effector phases of specific immune responses. Lymphocytes originate in the bone marrow, mature in different generative organs, and are located in anatomically defined peripheral lymphoid tissues. The structural organization of lymphoid tissues optimizes intimate contact and short-range interactions between the cell populations that cooperate in the generation of immune responses.

Selected Readings

Bhan, A. K., and I. Bhan. In situ characterization of human lymphoid cells using monoclonal antibodies. *In* M. Miyasaka and Z. Trnka (eds.). Differentiation Antigens in Lymphohemopoietic Tissues. M. Dekker, New York and Basel, 1988, pp. 13–46.

Brekelmans, P., and W. van Ewijk. Phenotypic characterization of murine thymic microenvironments. Seminars in Immunology 2:13–24, 1990.

Heinen, E., N. Corwann, and C. Kinet-Denoel. The lymph follicle: a hard nut to crack. Immunology Today 9:240–243, 1988.

Ikuta, K., N. Uchida, J. Friedman, and I. L. Weissman. Lymphocyte development from stem cells. Annual Review of Immunology 10:759–783, 1992.

Mackay, C. R. Immunological memory. Advances in Immunology 53:217–265, 1993.

McCune, J. M., H. Kaneshima, M. Lieberman, I. L. Weissman, and R. Namikawa. The scid-hu mouse: current status and potential applications. Current Topics in Microbiology and Immunology. 152:183–194, 1989.

Osmond, D. G. The turnover of B-cell populations. Immunology Today 14:34–37, 1993.

LYMPHOCYTE

SPECIFICITY AND

ACTIVATION

The initial phases of specific immune responses are the specific recognition of antigen by lymphocytes and the responses of lymphocytes to antigenic stimulation. This section is devoted to a discussion of the cellular and molecular basis of antigen recognition and lymphocyte activation.

We will begin with antibodies, which are the antigen receptors and effector molecules of B lymphocytes, because the structure and production of antibodies are understood in great detail. Chapter 3 describes the molecular structure of antibodies and how these proteins recognize antigens and perform their effector functions. Chapter 4 deals with the structure and expression of antibody genes, the generation of antibody diversity, and the development of the B cell repertoire.

Before continuing with a discussion of antibody production, the next four chapters will consider antigen recognition by T cells, which play a central role in all immune responses to protein antigens, including antibody responses. In Chapter 5 we will describe the genetics and biochemistry of the major histocompatibility complex (MHC), whose products are integral components of the ligands that T cells specifically recognize. Chapter 6 discusses the association of foreign antigens with MHC molecules and the biochemistry and physiologic significance of antigen presentation. Chapter 7 deals with the structure of the T cell antigen receptor, the role of other T cell surface proteins in responses to antigens, and the mechanisms of T lymphocyte activation. The expression of T cell receptor genes and the development of mature T lymphocytes in the thymus are described in Chapter 8.

We will return to humoral immunity in Chapter 9 and discuss the responses of B lymphocytes to antigens and to stimuli provided by helper T cells. Chapter 10 describes how these immune responses are regulated and the phenomenon of immunologic tolerance to foreign antigens. Finally, in Chapter 11 we will describe the development of immune responses at the organismal level and the special features of immune responses at different anatomic sites.

ANTIBODIES AND

ANTIGENS

One of the earliest experimental demonstrations of acquired immunity was the induction of humoral immunity to microbial toxins. The protective effects of humoral immunity are now known to be mediated by a family of structurally related glycoproteins called **antibodies** (commonly written as Ab). *Antibodies always initiate their biologic effects by binding to antigens.* Antibodies are not enzymes and, except in unusual circumstances, do not modify the covalent structure of antigens. Antibody binding to antigen, although entirely non-covalent, is nevertheless exquisitely specific for one antigen versus another and often very strong. Antibodies, major histocompatibility complex (MHC) molecules (see Chapter 5), and T cell antigen receptors (see Chapter 7) constitute the three classes of molecules used by the immune system to specifically recognize antigens. Of these three, antibodies are distinguished by the widest range of antigenic structures they can recognize, by the greatest ability to distinguish between different antigens, and by the greatest strength of binding to antigen. Antibodies are also the best studied of these antigen-binding molecules. Therefore, we will begin our discussion of how the immune system specifically recognizes antigens by describing in molecular terms how antibodies perform this function.

Antibodies are produced in a membrane-bound form by B lymphocytes, and these membrane molecules function as B cell receptors for antigens. *The interaction of antigen with membrane antibodies on B cells constitutes the cognitive phase of humoral immunity.* Antibodies are also produced in a secreted form by the progeny of B cells that differentiate in response to antigenic stimulation. *These secreted antibodies bind to antigens and trigger several of the effector functions of the immune system.* The specificity of the effector phase is due to the antigen-antibody interaction, but the effector functions themselves are usually not specific for the eliciting antigen. In fact, these functions are often mediated by portions of the antibody molecule that are spatially distinct from the site of antigen binding. In this chapter, we will also describe the structural features of antibody molecules that underlie their effector functions. Finally, we will describe how antibodies can be used as laboratory reagents to analyze biologic systems, including the immune system itself.

MOLECULAR STRUCTURE OF ANTIBODIES

Structural analyses of antibody molecules involving the efforts of many laboratories have been in progress for more than 50 years. Early studies were performed with naturally occurring mixtures of antibodies present in the blood of immunized individuals. Blood contains many different antibodies, each derived from a particular clone of B cells and each having a distinct structure and specificity for antigen. Nevertheless, antibodies are sufficiently similar to each other that Michael Heidelberger and colleagues were able to purify mixtures of antibodies from blood, laying the groundwork for subsequent structural studies. Working with

these mixtures, immunologists were able to deduce the overall structure of antibody molecules. However, the molecular heterogeneity of these polyclonal antibodies interfered with more detailed analysis of antibody structure, such as amino acid sequence determination. The key methodological breakthrough in this endeavor was the discovery that patients or animals with multiple myeloma, a monoclonal tumor of antibody-secreting plasma cells, often have high levels of biochemically identical antibodies or portions of antibodies in their blood or urine, providing a source of individual antibody molecules of a single (albeit usually unknown) specificity. In 1975, Georges Kohler and Cesar Milstein described a method for immortalizing individual antibody-secreting cells from an immunized animal, permitting the selection of individual **monoclonal antibodies** of predetermined specificity (Box 3–1). The availability of homogeneous populations of antibodies and antibody-producing cells permitted complete amino acid sequence determination of several individual antibody molecules and, eventually, molecular cloning and genetic analysis of antibodies. These studies have culminated in the x-ray crystallographic determinations of the three-dimensional structure of several antibody molecules and, in a few cases, of antibody with bound antigen. As a result, we now know more about the structure of antibody molecules than about any other element of the immune system. This portion of the chapter describes the purification of antibody molecules and their general structural features.

Natural Distribution and Purification of Antibody Molecules

Although antibodies were first isolated from the fluid portion of the blood, they are found in several distinct anatomic locations:

1. Antibodies are present within cytoplasmic membrane-bound compartments (endoplasmic reticulum and Golgi apparatus) and on the surface of B lymphocytes, which are the only cells that synthesize antibody molecules.

2. Antibodies are present in the plasma (fluid portion) of the blood and, to a lesser extent, in the interstitial fluid of the tissues where secreted antibody from B cells accumulates.

3. Antibodies are present on the surface of certain immune effector cells, such as mononuclear phagocytes, natural killer (NK) cells, and mast cells, which do not synthesize antibody but have specific receptors for binding antibody molecules.

4. Antibodies are present in secretory fluids such as mucus and milk, into which certain types of antibody molecules are specifically transported.

When blood or plasma forms a clot, antibodies remain in the residual fluid, called **serum.** A sample of serum that contains a large number of antibody molecules that bind to a particular antigen is commonly called an **antiserum.** (The study of antibodies and

BOX 3–1. HYBRIDOMAS AND MONOCLONAL ANTIBODIES

The technique of producing virtually unlimited quantities of a single antibody specific for a particular antigenic determinant has revolutionized immunology and has had a far-reaching impact on research in diverse fields as well as in clinical medicine. This technique is based on the fact that each B lymphocyte produces antibody of a single specificity. Therefore, each monoclonal tumor derived from a B lymphocyte, called a **myeloma**, produces only one antibody. Such tumors occur spontaneously in humans and can be induced experimentally by various treatments in mice. Myeloma-derived homogeneous antibodies have proved invaluable for elucidating the structure of Ig proteins, and Ig genes were first isolated from myelomas. However, most myelomas secrete antibodies of unknown antigenic specificities, because the transformation process that gives rise to these tumors affects B lymphocytes randomly and it is not possible to predict the specificity of any randomly transformed clone of B cells. Many attempts have been made to produce homogeneous or monoclonal antibodies of known specificity. Since normal B lymphocytes cannot grow indefinitely, such attempts have focused on immortalizing B cells that produce a specific antibody. The first and now generally used technique for doing this was described by Georges Kohler and Cesar Milstein in 1975. The method involves cell fusion or **somatic cell hybridization** between a normal antibody-producing B cell and a myeloma line, and selection of fused cells that secrete antibody of the desired specificity derived from the normal B cell. Such fusion-derived immortalized antibody-producing cell lines are called **hybridomas**, and the antibodies they produce are **monoclonal antibodies.**

The success of this technique depended on the development of cultured myeloma lines that would grow in normal culture medium but would not grow in a defined "selection" medium because they lacked a functional gene(s) required for DNA synthesis in this selection medium. Fusing normal cells to these defective myeloma fusion partners would provide the necessary gene(s) from the normal cells, so that only the somatic cell hybrids would continue to grow in the selection medium. Moreover, genes from the myeloma cell make such hybrids immortal. Cell lines that can be used as fusion partners are created by inducing defects in nucleotide synthesis pathways (Fig. A). Normal animal cells synthesize purine nucleotides and thymidylate *de novo* from phosphoribosyl pyrophosphate and uridylate, respectively, in several steps, one of which involves the transfer of a methyl or formyl group from activated tetrahydrofolate. Anti-folate drugs, such as aminopterin, block the reactivation of tetrahydrofolate, thereby inhibiting the synthesis of purine and thymidylate. Since these are necessary components of DNA, aminopterin blocks DNA synthesis via the *de novo* pathway. Aminopterin-treated cells can use a salvage pathway in which purine is synthesized from exogenously supplied hypoxanthine using the enzyme hypoxanthine-guanine phosphoribosyltransferase (HGPRT) and thymidylate is synthesized from thymidine using the enzyme thymidine kinase (TK). Therefore, cells grow normally in the presence of aminopterin if the culture medium is also supplemented with hypoxanthine and thymidine (called HAT medium). Cell lines, however, can be made defective in HGPRT if they are mutagenized and selected in thioguanine or azaguanine, which are analogs of normal metabolites that function as substrates for HGPRT but give rise to nonfunctional purines. Similarly, cells can be made defective in TK by mutagenesis and selection in bromodeoxyuridine, which is metabolized by TK to form a light-sensitive, lethal product. Such HGPRT- or TK-negative cells cannot use the salvage pathway and will, therefore, die in HAT medium. If normal cells are fused to HGPRT-negative or TK-negative cells, the normal cells provide the necessary enzyme(s), so that the hybrids synthesize DNA and grow in HAT medium.

This principle was applied to the generation of antibody-producing hybridomas by first developing HGPRT-negative and/or TK-negative myeloma lines. Myeloma lines are the best fusion partners for B cells, since like cells tend to fuse and give rise to stable hybrids more efficiently than unlike cells. Kohler and Milstein fused an HGPRT-defective mouse myeloma line to normal B cells from mice immunized with a known antigen, using Sendai virus, which expresses an envelope protein ("fusion protein") that fuses cells together. Hybrids were selected for growth in HAT medium; under these conditions, unfused myeloma cells die because they cannot use the salvage pathway and the B cells cannot survive for more than 1 to 2 weeks because they are not immortalized, so that only hybrids will grow (Fig. B). More recent advances in this basic technique include the use of myeloma lines that do not produce their own Ig and the use of polyethyelene

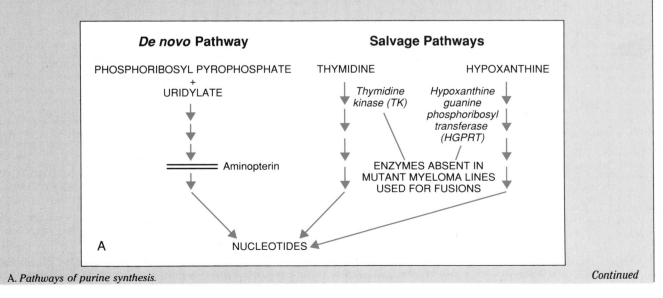

De novo Pathway

PHOSPHORIBOSYL PYROPHOSPHATE
+
URIDYLATE

━━ Aminopterin

Salvage Pathways

THYMIDINE

Thymidine kinase (TK)

HYPOXANTHINE

Hypoxanthine guanine phosphoribosyl transferase (HGPRT)

ENZYMES ABSENT IN MUTANT MYELOMA LINES USED FOR FUSIONS

A   NUCLEOTIDES

A. Pathways of purine synthesis.

Continued

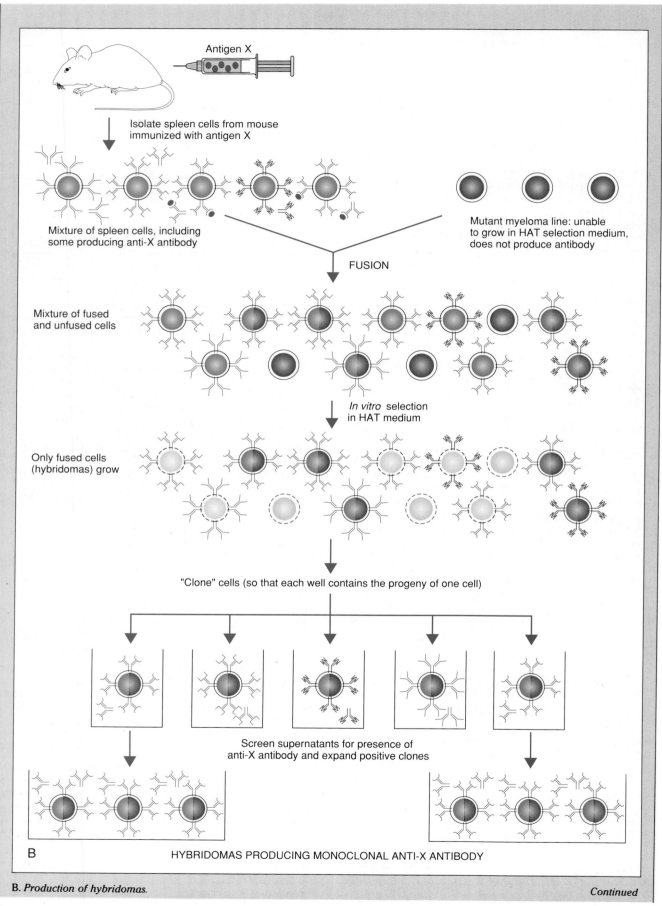

Antigen X

Isolate spleen cells from mouse immunized with antigen X

Mixture of spleen cells, including some producing anti-X antibody

Mutant myeloma line: unable to grow in HAT selection medium, does not produce antibody

FUSION

Mixture of fused and unfused cells

In vitro selection in HAT medium

Only fused cells (hybridomas) grow

"Clone" cells (so that each well contains the progeny of one cell)

Screen supernatants for presence of anti-X antibody and expand positive clones

B

HYBRIDOMAS PRODUCING MONOCLONAL ANTI-X ANTIBODY

B. *Production of hybridomas.*

Continued

glycol instead of Sendai virus as the fusing agent because of technical ease. The fused cells are cultured at a concentration at which each culture well is expected to contain only one hybridoma cell. The culture supernatant from each well in which growing cells are detected is then tested for the presence of antibody reactive with the antigen used for immunization. The screening method depends on the antigen being used. For soluble antigens, the usual technique is RIA or ELISA; and for cell surface antigens, a variety of assays for antibody binding to viable cells can be used (see Laboratory Uses of Antibodies later in this chapter). Once positive wells are identified, i.e., wells containing hybridomas producing the desired antibody, the cells are cloned in semisolid agar or by limiting dilution, and clones producing the antibody are isolated by another round of screening. These cloned hybridomas produce monoclonal antibodies of a desired specificity. Hybridomas can be grown in large volumes or as ascitic tumors in syngeneic mice in order to produce large quantities of monoclonal antibodies.

Two features of this somatic cell hybridization make it extremely valuable. First, it is the best method for producing a monoclonal antibody against a known antigenic determinant. Second, it can be used to identify unknown antigens present in a mixture because each hybridoma is specific for only one antigenic determinant. For instance, if several hybridomas are produced that secrete antibodies that bind to the surface of a particular cell, each hybridoma clone will secrete an antibody specific for only one surface antigenic determinant. These monoclonal antibodies can then be used to purify different cell surface molecules, some of which may be known molecules and others that may not have been identified previously. Some of the commonest applications of hybridomas and monoclonal antibodies include the following:

1. *Identification of phenotypic markers unique to particular cell types.* The basis for the modern classification of lymphocytes and mononuclear phagocytes is the binding of population-specific monoclonal antibodies. These have been used to define "clusters of differentiation" for various cell types (see Chapter 2).

2. *Immunodiagnosis.* The diagnosis of many infectious and systemic diseases relies upon the detection of specific antigens and/or antibodies in the circulation or in tissues, using monoclonal antibodies in immunoassays.

3. *Tumor diagnosis and therapy.* Tumor-specific monoclonal antibodies are used for detection of tumors by imaging techniques and for immunotherapy of tumors *in vivo*.

4. *Functional analysis of cell surface and secreted molecules.* In immunologic research, monoclonal antibodies that bind to cell surface molecules and either stimulate or inhibit particular cellular functions are invaluable tools for defining the functions of surface molecules, including receptors for antigens. Antibodies that neutralize cytokines are routinely used for detecting the presence and functional roles of these protein hormones *in vitro* and *in vivo*.

At present, hybridomas are most often produced by fusing HAT-sensitive mouse myelomas with B cells from immunized mice, rats, or hamsters. The same principle is used to generate mouse T cell hybridomas, by fusing T cells with a HAT-sensitive, T cell–derived tumor line; uses of such monoclonal T cell populations are described in Chapter 7. Attempts are being made to generate human monoclonal antibodies, primarily for administration to patients, by developing human myeloma lines as fusion partners. (It is a general rule that the stability of hybrids is low if cells from species that are far apart in evolution are fused, and this is presumably why human B cells do not form hybridomas with mouse myeloma lines at high efficiency.) As we shall discuss later in the chapter, only small portions of the antibody molecule are responsible for binding to antigen; the remainder of the antibody molecule can be thought of as a "framework." This structural organization allows the DNA segments encoding the antigen-binding sites from a murine monoclonal antibody to be "stitched" into a cDNA encoding a human myeloma protein, creating a hybrid gene. When expressed, the resultant hybrid protein, which retains antigen specificity, is referred to as a "humanized antibody." Humanized antibodies offer an alternative strategy for generating monoclonal antibodies that may be safely administered to patients.

---

their reactions with antigens is therefore classically called **serology.**) The number of antibody molecules in a serum specific for a particular antigen is often measured by serially diluting the serum until binding can no longer be observed; sera with a large number of antibody molecules specific for a particular antigen are said to be "strong" or have a "high titer."

Plasma or serum glycoproteins are traditionally separated by solubility characteristics into albumins and globulins and may be further separated by migration in an electric field, a process called **electrophoresis** (Fig. 3–1). Elvin Kabat and colleagues demonstrated that most antibodies are found in the third fastest migrating group of globulins, named **gamma globulins** for the third letter of the Greek alphabet. Another common name for antibody is **immunoglobulin** (Ig), referring to the immunity-conferring portion of the gamma globulin fraction. The terms immunoglobulin and antibody are used interchangeably throughout this book.

Currently, antibody molecules are generally purified from plasma or other natural fluids by a two-step procedure. The first step is to precipitate antibodies from the biologic fluid by adding a concentration of ammonium sulfate that ranges from 40 to 50 per cent of saturation. Under these conditions, albumin and most small molecules remain in solution, so that partially purified antibody can be collected in a pellet by centrifugation. The antibody-containing pellet is redissolved in buffer and then purified by **chromatography.** Homogeneous antibodies can be isolated from other proteins in the pellet by size *(gel filtration chromatography)*, charge *(ion exchange chromatography)*, or specific binding to an antibody-binding molecule such as staphylococcal protein A. When the antibody of interest in the biologic fluid is specific for a known antigen, the antigen can be immobilized on a column matrix and used to bind the antibody, a method called *affinity chromatography*. In all cases, antibody can be removed from the column matrix by a suitable change in buffer conditions. In the case of affinity chromatography, release often involves temporary and reversible denaturation with a salt solution such as magnesium chloride or with a change in pH. Many such chromatographic procedures, especially gel filtration and ion exchange chromatography, are now routinely run under high pressure using special column matrices to achieve

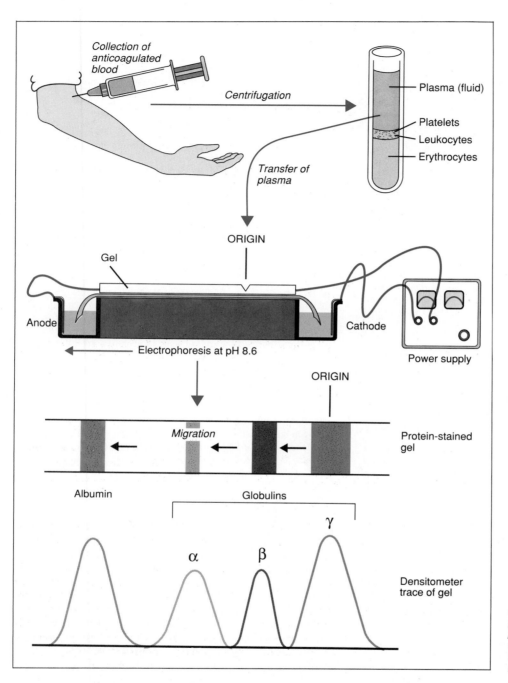

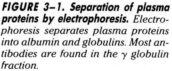

FIGURE 3–1. Separation of plasma proteins by electrophoresis. *Electrophoresis separates plasma proteins into albumin and globulins. Most antibodies are found in the γ globulin fraction.*

rapid and highly resolved separations. This technique is called *high-pressure liquid chromatography* (HPLC).

Overview of Antibody Structure

A number of the structural and functional features of antibodies were determined from the early studies of these molecules:

1. *All antibody molecules are similar in overall structure, accounting for certain common physicochemical features, such as charge and solubility.* These common properties may be exploited as a basis for the purification of antibody molecules from fluids such as

blood. *All antibodies have a common core structure of two identical light chains (each about 24 kilodaltons [kD]) and two identical heavy chains (about 55 or 70 kD)* (Fig. 3–2). One light chain is attached to each heavy chain, and the two heavy chains are attached to each other. Both the light chains and the heavy chains contain a series of repeating, homologous units, each about 110 amino acid residues in length, which fold independently in a common globular motif, called an **immunoglobulin domain.** All Ig domains contain two layers of β-pleated sheet with three or four strands of antiparallel polypeptide chain. Certain Ig domains, such as those comprising variable regions (see later), have

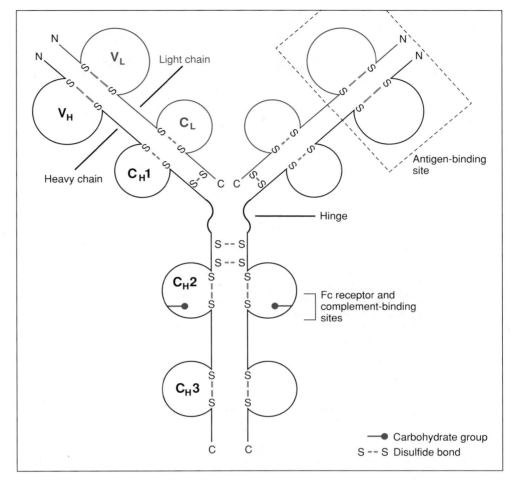

FIGURE 3-2. Schematic diagram of an immunoglobulin molecule. *In this drawing of an IgG molecule, the antigen-binding sites are formed by the juxtaposition of V_L and V_H domains. The locations of complement and Fc receptor–binding sites within the heavy chain constant regions are approximations. S--S refers to intrachain and interchain disulfide bonds; N and C refer to amino and carboxy termini of the polypeptide chains, respectively.*

an extra strand in each of the two layers. As will be discussed in Chapter 7, many other proteins of importance in the immune system contain regions that use the same folding motif and show structural relatedness to Ig amino acid sequences. All molecules that contain this motif are said to belong to the **Ig superfamily,** and all of the gene segments encoding the Ig-like domains are believed to have evolved from the same common ancestral gene (see Chapter 7, Box 7–2).

2. Despite their overall similarity, *antibody molecules can be readily divided into a small number of distinct classes and subclasses, based on minor differences in physicochemical characteristics such as size, charge, and solubility and on their behavior as antigens* (Box 3–2). In humans, the classes of antibody molecules are called IgA, IgD, IgE, IgG, and IgM, and members of each class are said to have the same isotype (Table 3–1). IgA and IgG isotypes can be further subdivided into closely related subclasses, or subtypes, called IgA1 and IgA2, and IgG1, IgG2, IgG3, and IgG4, respectively. In certain instances, it will be convenient to refer to studies of mouse antibody. Mice have the same general isotypes as humans, but the IgG isotype is divided into the IgG1, IgG2a, IgG2b, and IgG3 subclasses in mice. The heavy chains of all antibody molecules of an isotype or subtype share extensive regions of amino acid sequence identity but differ from antibodies be-

longing to other isotypes or subtypes. Heavy chains are designated by the letter of the Greek alphabet corresponding to the overall isotype of the antibody: IgA1 contains $\alpha1$ heavy chains; IgA2, $\alpha2$; IgD, δ; IgE, ϵ; IgG1, $\gamma1$; IgG2, $\gamma2$; IgG3, $\gamma3$, IgG4, $\gamma4$; and IgM, μ. The shared regions of heavy chain amino acid sequences are responsible for both the common physicochemical properties and the common antigenic properties of antibodies of the same isotype. In addition, the shared regions of the heavy chains provide members of each isotype with common abilities to bind to certain cell surface receptors or to other macromolecules like complement and thereby activate particular immune effector functions. Thus, the separation of antibody molecules into isotypes and subtypes on the basis of common structural features also separates antibodies according to which set of effector functions they commonly activate. In other words, *different effector functions of antibodies are mediated by distinct isotypes and subtypes.* As we shall see later, there are two isotypes of antibody light chains, called κ and λ. The light chains, however, do not mediate or influence the effector functions of antibodies.

3. *There are more than 1×10^7, and perhaps as many as 10^9, structurally different antibody molecules in every individual, each with unique amino acid sequences in their antigen-combining sites.* This extraor-

BOX 3–2.   ANTI-IMMUNOGLOBULIN ANTIBODIES

Antibody molecules are proteins and therefore can be antigenic. Immunologists have exploited this fact to produce antibodies specific for Ig molecules that can be used as reagents to analyze the structure and function of Ig molecules. In order to obtain an anti-antibody response, it is necessary that the Ig molecules used to immunize an animal be recognized in whole or in part as foreign. The simplest approach is to immunize one species, e.g., rabbit, with Ig molecules of a second species, e.g., mouse. Populations of antibodies generated by such cross-species immunizations are largely specific for epitopes present in the constant regions of light or heavy chains. Such sera can be used to define the **isotype** of an antibody.

When an animal is immunized with Ig molecules derived from another animal of the same species, the immune response is confined to epitopes of the immunizing Ig that are absent or uncommon on the Ig molecules of the responder animal. Two types of determinants have been defined by this approach. First, determinants may be formed by minor structural differences (polymorphisms) in amino acid sequences located in the conserved portions of Ig molecules. Ig genes that encode such polymorphic structures are inherited as mendelian alleles. (The concepts of **polymorphism** and **allelic genes** are discussed more fully in Chapter 5.) Determinants on Ig molecules that differ among animals that have inherited different alleles are called **allotopes.** All antibody molecules that share a particular allotope are said to belong to the same **allotype.** Most allotopes are located in the constant regions of light or heavy chains, but some are found in the framework portions of variable regions. Allotypic differences have no functional significance, but they have been important in the study of Ig genetics. For example, allotypes detected by anti-Ig antibodies were initially used to locate the position of Ig genes by linkage analysis. In addition, the remarkable observation that, in homozygous animals, all of the heavy chains of a particular isotype (e.g., IgM) share the same allotype even though the V regions of these antibodies have different amino acid sequences provided the first evidence that the constant portions of all Ig molecules of a particular isotype are encoded by a single gene that is separate from the genes encoding V regions. As will be discussed in Chapter 4, we now know that this surprising conclusion is correct.

The second type of determinant on antibody molecules that can be recognized as foreign by other animals of the same species is that formed largely or entirely by the hypervariable regions of an Ig variable domain. When a homogeneous population of antibody molecules, e.g., a myeloma protein or a monoclonal antibody, is used as an immunogen, antibodies are produced that react with the hypervariable loops. These determinants are recognized as "foreign" because they are usually present in very small quantities in any given animal, i.e., at too low a level to induce self-tolerance (see Chapter 19). Such determinants on individual antibody molecules are **idiotopes**, and all antibody molecules that share an idiotope are said to belong to the same **idiotype.** The term idiotype is also used to describe the shared idiotope. As will be discussed in Chapter 4, hypervariable sequences that form idiotopes arise both from inherited germline diversity and from somatic events. Individual idiotopes that arise from somatic events are rare and may define the products of one or a few clones of antibody-producing B cells. Idiotopes that arise from the germline are less rare and, in some cases, may be present on the majority of antibody molecules that recognize a particular antigen (**dominant idiotopes**). Unlike allotopes, idiotopes may be functionally significant because they may be involved in regulation of B cell functions. The theory of lymphocyte regulation through antibody-binding idiotopes expressed on membrane Ig molecules, called the **network hypothesis,** is discussed further in Chapter 10.

In addition to experimentally elicited anti-Ig antibodies, immunologists have also been interested in naturally occurring antibodies reactive with self Ig molecules. Small quantities of anti-idiotypic antibodies may be found in normal individuals. Anti-Ig antibodies are particularly prevalent in an autoimmune disease called rheumatoid arthritis (see Chapter 20), in which setting they are known as **rheumatoid factor.** Rheumatoid factor is usually an IgM antibody that reacts with the constant regions of self IgG. The significance of rheumatoid factor in the pathogenesis of rheumatoid arthritis is unknown.

---

dinary diversity of structure (whose generation is explained in Chapter 4) accounts for the extraordinary specificity of antibodies for antigens, because each amino acid difference may produce a difference in antigen binding. In theory, such extensive sequence diversity poses a structural problem because the three-dimensional structure of any protein is completely determined by its amino acid sequence and certain sequences are incapable of folding into soluble, stable proteins. In an antibody molecule, this problem is

TABLE 3–1.   Human Antibody Isotypes*

Antibody	Subtypes	H Chain (Designation)	H Chain Domains (Number)	Hinge	Tail Piece	Serum Concentration (mg/ml)	Secretory Form	Molecular Weight of Secretory Form (kD)
IgA	IgA1	$\alpha 1$	4	Yes	Yes	3	Monomer, dimer, trimer	150, 300, or 400
	IgA2	$\alpha 2$	4	Yes	Yes	0.5	Monomer, dimer, trimer	150, 300, or 400
IgD	None	δ	4	Yes	Yes	Trace	—	180
IgE	None	ϵ	5	No	No	Trace	Monomer	190
IgG	IgG1	$\gamma 1$	4	Yes	No	9	Monomer	150
	IgG2	$\gamma 2$	4	Yes	No	3	Monomer	150
	IgG3	$\gamma 3$	4	Yes	No	1	Monomer	150
	IgG4	$\gamma 4$	4	Yes	No	0.5	Monomer	150
IgM	None	μ	5	No	Yes	1.5	Pentamer	950

* Multimeric forms of IgA and IgM are associated with J chain via the tail piece region of the heavy chain. IgA in mucus is also associated with secretory piece.

solved by confining the sequence diversity to three short stretches within the amino terminal domains of the heavy and light chains. The amino acid sequences of the amino terminal domains are called **variable (V) regions,** to distinguish them from the more conserved **constant (C) regions** of the remainder of each chain. The highly divergent stretches within the V regions are called **hypervariable regions,** and they are held in place by more conserved **framework regions.** In an intact immunoglobulin, the three hypervariable regions of a light chain and the three hypervariable regions of a heavy chain can be brought together in three-dimensional space to form an antigen-binding surface. Because these sequences form a surface complementary to the three-dimensional surface of a bound antigen, the hypervariable regions are called **complementarity-determining regions** (CDRs).

With this overview of antibody structure and function in mind, we will now consider antibody structure in greater detail.

Detailed View of Antibody Structure

LIGHT CHAIN STRUCTURE

All antibody light chains fall into one of two classes or isotypes, κ and λ. Each member of a light-chain isotype shares complete amino acid sequence identity of the carboxy terminal C region with all other members of that isotype. In humans, antibodies with κ and λ light chains are present in about equal number. In mice, κ-containing antibodies are about ten times more frequent than λ-containing antibodies. There are no known differences in function between κ-containing and λ-containing antibodies.

Each light chain, whether κ or λ, is folded into separate V and C domains corresponding to the amino terminal and carboxy terminal halves of the polypeptide, respectively (Fig. 3–3). Each domain is about 110 amino acids long. As noted above, most of the amino acid sequence variation among different light chains is confined to three separate locations in the V region. These three hypervariable segments, or CDRs, are each about ten amino acids long (Fig. 3–4). Proceeding from the amino terminus, these regions are the CDR1, CDR2, and CDR3, respectively. CDR3 is the most variable of the CDRs, and, as will be discussed in Chapter 4, there are more genetic mechanisms for generating sequence diversity in this region than in CDR1 and CDR2. V region folding into an Ig domain is mostly determined by the sequence of the framework regions adjacent to the CDRs. Within the framework regions, certain amino residues and certain structural features are very highly conserved. For example, all V region sequences contain an internal disulfide loop of about 90 amino acid residues. Other portions of the framework regions differ between κ and λ chains. When V_κ or V_λ regions fold into an Ig domain, the CDRs are present on the surface as projecting loops (Fig. 3–3). Recent studies suggest that each CDR (except CDR3 of the heavy chain) folds similarly, regardless of the precise amino acid sequence, suggesting that there are conserved ("canonical") structural features within the hypervariable segments of antibodies. Sequence differences among the CDRs of different antibody molecules result in unique chemical structures being projected at the surfaces of the projecting loops. As we shall discuss shortly, these *variations in surface structure account for specificity for antigens.*

The carboxy terminus of the C region of the light chain also folds into an Ig domain. Although C_κ and C_λ differ in exact amino acid sequence, they are structurally related, or homologous, to each other and, to a lesser extent, to V_κ and V_λ.

FIGURE 3–3. Polypeptide folding into Ig domains in a human antibody light chain. *The V and C regions each independently fold into Ig domains. The white arrows represent polypeptide arranged in β-pleated sheets, the dark blue bars are intrachain disulfide bonds, and the numbers indicate the positions of amino acid residues counting from the amino (N) terminus. The CDR1, CDR2, and CDR3 loops of the V region, colored in light blue, are brought together to form the antigen-binding surface of the light chain. (Adapted with permission from Edmundson, A. B., K. R. Ely, E. E. Abola, M. Schiffer, and N. Panagiotopoulos. Rotational allostery and divergent evolution of domains in immunoglobulin light chains. Biochemistry 14:3953–3961, 1975. Copyright 1975, American Chemical Society.)*

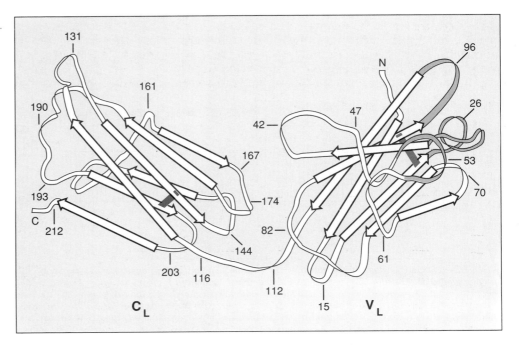

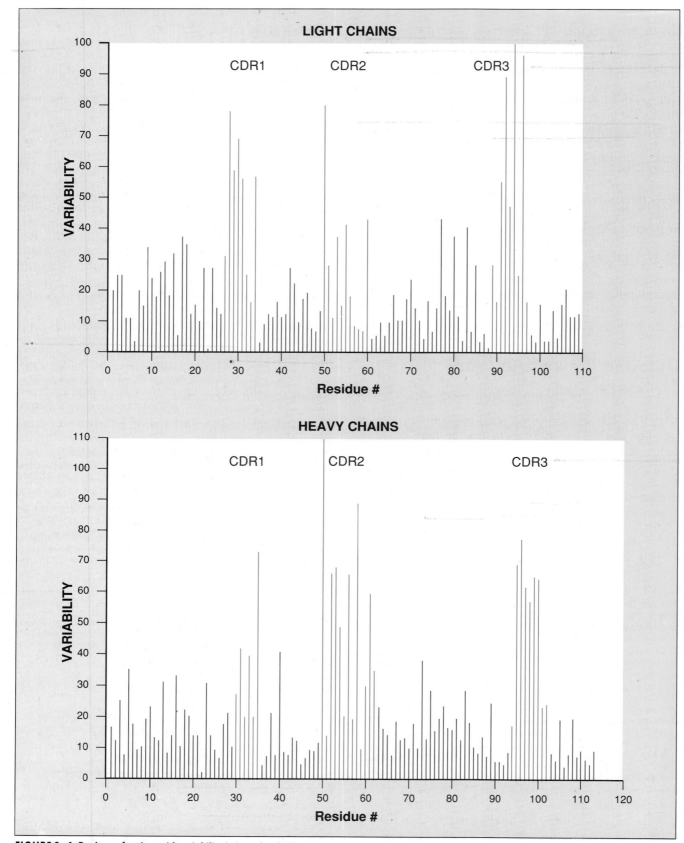

FIGURE 3–4. Regions of amino acid variability in Ig molecules. *The histograms depict the extent of variability, defined as the number of differences in each amino acid residue among various independently sequenced Ig heavy and light chains, plotted against amino acid residue number, measured from the amino terminus. This method of analysis, developed by Elvin Kabat and Tai Te Wu, indicates that the most variable residues are clustered in three "hypervariable" regions, colored in blue, corresponding to the three CDRs shown in Figure 3–3. (Courtesy of Dr. E. A. Kabat, Department of Microbiology, Columbia University College of Physicians and Surgeons, New York.)*

HEAVY CHAIN STRUCTURE

All heavy chain polypeptides, regardless of antibody isotype, contain a tandem series of segments, each approximately 110 amino acid residues in length. These segments are homologous to each other, and all undergo characteristic folding into 12 kD Ig domains. As in light chains, the amino terminal variable, or V_H, domain displays the greatest sequence variation among heavy chains, and the most variable residues are concentrated into three short (up to ten amino acid residue) stretches called CDR1, CDR2, and CDR3 (Fig. 3–4). Also similar to light chains, the heavy chain CDR3 shows greater variability in sequence and folding pattern than CDR1 or CDR2.

The remainder of the heavy chain, which forms the constant (C) region, differs among isotypes; however, it is invariant among the member antibodies within a particular isotype. In IgM and IgE antibodies, the constant region folds to form four tandem Ig domains. In IgG, IgA, and IgD antibodies, the shorter constant regions form three Ig domains. (In the mouse, the δ chain gene has undergone a deletion such that the constant region forms only two Ig domains.)

In γ, α, and δ heavy chains, there is a nonglobular segment, containing from about ten (in $\alpha 1$, $\alpha 2$, $\gamma 1$, $\gamma 2$, and $\gamma 4$) to over 60 (in $\gamma 3$ and δ) amino acid residues, located between the first and second constant region domains (called $C_H 1$ and $C_H 2$, respectively). Although portions of this sequence form rodlike helical structures, other portions assume a random and flexible conformation, permitting molecular motion between $C_H 1$ and $C_H 2$. For this reason, this segment of the heavy chain is called the **hinge.** Some of the greatest differences between the constant regions of the IgG subclasses are concentrated in the hinge. For steric reasons, antibody subtypes with flexible hinges may be better able to use more than one antigen-binding site to attach to a particular antigen; as discussed later in this chapter, binding involving more than one attachment point will increase the strength of attachment.

All heavy chains may be expressed in one of two molecular forms that differ in amino acid sequence on the carboxy terminal side of the last C_H domain. The secretory form, found in blood plasma, terminates with a sequence containing charged and hydrophilic amino acid residues. The membrane form, found only on the plasma membrane of the B lymphocyte that synthesized the antibody, has distinct carboxy terminal sequences that include approximately 26 uncharged, hydrophobic side chains followed by variable numbers of charged (usually basic) amino acid residues that form the cytoplasmic segments (Fig. 3–5). This structural motif is characteristic of transmembrane proteins. The hydrophobic residues are believed to form an α-helix, which extends across the hydrophobic portion of the membrane lipid bilayer; the basic side chains of the cytoplasmic amino acids interact with the phospholipid head groups on the cytoplasmic surface of the membrane. In membrane IgM or IgD, the extreme carboxy terminus or cytoplasmic portion of the heavy chain is very short, only three amino acid residues; in membrane IgG or IgE, it is somewhat longer, up to about 30 amino acid residues in length.

The secretory forms of μ, α, and δ heavy chains, but not γ or ϵ, have additional extended nonglobular sequences on the carboxyterminal side of the last C_H domain. These extensions are called **tail pieces.** In secreted IgM and IgA molecules, the tail pieces contribute toward intermolecular interactions that result in the formation of multimeric Ig molecules. Specifically, IgM forms a pentamer, containing ten heavy chains and ten light chains, and IgA can form dimers containing four heavy chains and four light chains, or trimers, containing six heavy chains and six light chains (Fig. 3–6). Little is known about the usual form of circulating IgD because it is normally present in only trace amounts in the blood. Multimeric IgM and IgA also contain an additional 15 kD polypeptide, called the **joining (J) chain,** which is disulfide-bonded to the tail pieces, stabilizing the multimer. All membrane Ig molecules, regardless of isotype, are believed to be monomeric, containing two heavy and two light chains.

All heavy chains are characteristically N-glycosylated; that is, the polypeptide contains N-linked oligosaccharide groups attached to asparagine side chains. The location of oligosaccharides may vary in different Ig isotypes. The precise composition of the oligosaccharides is not fully determined by the polypeptide sequence and may also vary with the physiologic state of the host at the time of antibody synthesis.

ASSOCIATION OF LIGHT AND HEAVY CHAINS

The basic pattern of chain association in all antibody molecules is that each light chain is attached to a heavy chain and each heavy chain pairs with another heavy chain. The association between light and heavy chains involves both covalent and non-covalent interactions (see Fig. 3–2). Covalent interactions are in the form of disulfide bonds between the carboxy terminus of the light chain and the $C_H 1$ domain of the heavy chain. The exact position of the heavy chain cysteine that participates in disulfide bond formation varies with the isotype. Non-covalent interactions arise primarily from hydrophobic interactions between V_L and V_H domains and between the C_L domain and the $C_H 1$ domain. This association of V_L and V_H domains produces a spatial apposition such that the juxtaposed V domains can each contribute to the binding of antigen (see Plate I, opposite page 50).

The pairing of heavy chains is best understood from studies of IgG molecules. As in the case of light and heavy chain association, both covalent and non-covalent interactions are involved. Heavy chains form interchain disulfide bonds in the region near the carboxy terminus of the hinge. Extensive non-covalent interactions occur between the $C_H 3$ domains. In contrast, there is little favorable interaction between the polypeptides of the $C_H 2$ domains. Some of the N-linked oligosaccharides are located in a physical gap formed between these portions of the chain and may positively interact with each other, contributing to interchain associations. The length and flexibility of the hinge re-

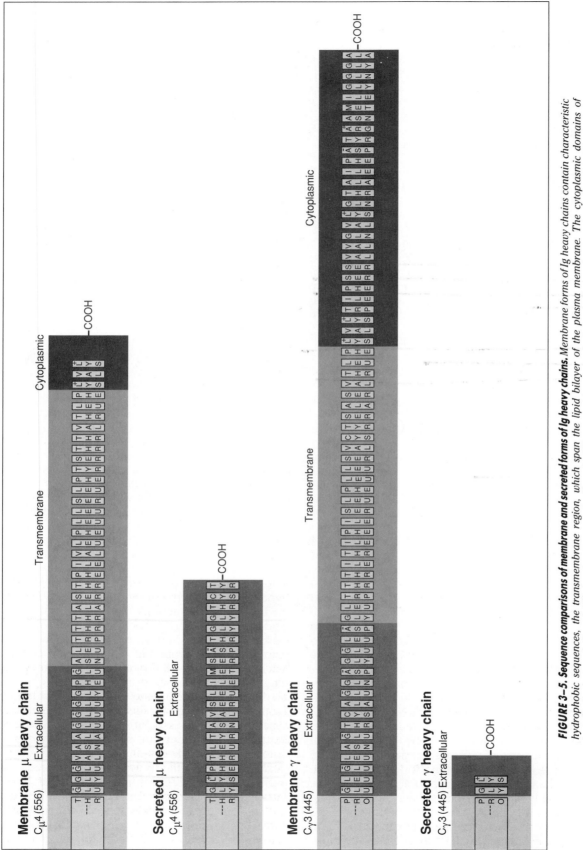

FIGURE 3–5. Sequence comparisons of membrane and secreted forms of Ig heavy chains. *Membrane forms of Ig heavy chains contain characteristic hydrophobic sequences, the transmembrane region, which span the lipid bilayer of the plasma membrane. The cytoplasmic domains of membrane heavy chains of different isotypes are significantly different: μ contains only three residues, whereas γ3 contains 28. The carboxy termini of secreted forms also differ among isotypes: μ has a long tail piece involved in pentamer formation, whereas γ3 does not. Amino acids are shown in the three-letter code, and charged residues are marked + or −; the numbers in parentheses mark the amino acid residue number of the carboxy terminus of the last Ig domain (i.e., $C_\mu 4$ or $C_\gamma 3$).*

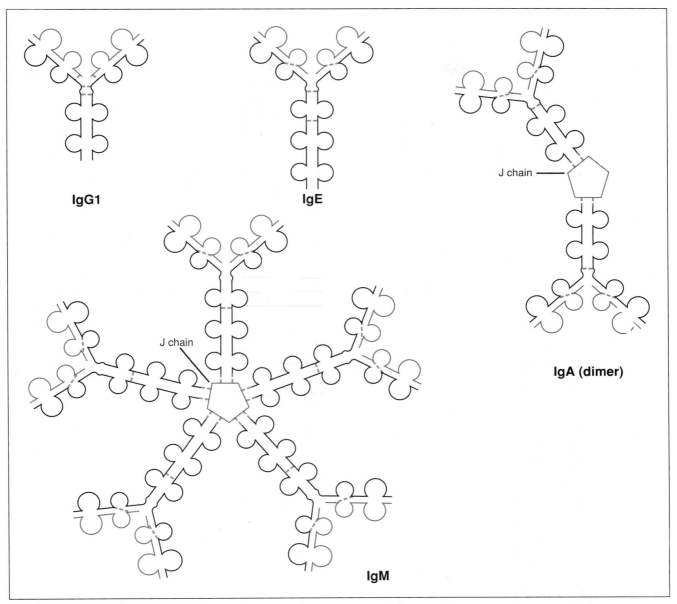

FIGURE 3–6. Schematic diagrams of various Ig isotypes. *IgG and IgE circulate as monomers, whereas secreted forms of IgA and IgM are dimers and pentamers, respectively, stabilized by the J chain. (Some IgA molecules are trimers, not shown.)*

gions differ significantly among IgG subclasses because, as noted above, most of the amino acid sequence differences among the four subclasses are located in the hinge region. These sequence differences lead to very different overall shapes among the IgG subtypes, as depicted in Figure 3–7.

These structural features of chain association explain the results of the classical limited proteolysis studies of rabbit IgG conducted by Rodney Porter and colleagues. The theory of limited proteolysis is that globular or rodlike domains of folded proteins are more resistant to the peptide-bond cleaving actions of proteolytic enzymes than are extended, flexible regions of polypeptide. In IgG molecules, the most susceptible region is therefore the hinge located between $C_\gamma 1$ and $C_\gamma 2$ of the heavy chain. The proteolytic enzyme papain pref-

erentially cleaves rabbit IgG molecules into three separate pieces (Fig. 3–8). Two of the pieces are identical to each other and consist of an intact light chain associated with a V_H–$C_\gamma 1$ fragment of the heavy chain. These fragments each retain the ability to bind antigen, a function of the V_L and V_H domains, and are therefore called **Fab** (fragment, antigen-binding). The third piece contains identical fragments of the γ heavy chain composed of the $C_\gamma 2$ and $C_\gamma 3$ domains. This piece of IgG has a propensity to self-associate and to crystallize into a lattice. It is therefore called **Fc** (fragment, crystalline). Lattice formation depends upon a uniformity of structure. The propensity of Fc regions to form a lattice reflects the presence of common amino acid sequences of the $C_\gamma 2$ and $C_\gamma 3$ domains shared by all antibodies of the same subtype. As we shall discuss later in this chap-

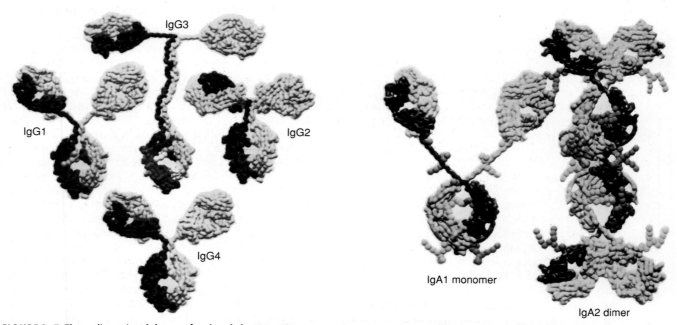

FIGURE 3–7. Three-dimensional shapes of various Ig isotypes. *These computer-generated space-filling models of different Ig isotypes illustrate that the shapes of antibody molecules are quite distinct, largely owing to differences in the lengths of the hinge regions. (Courtesy of Dr. R. S. H. Pumphrey, Regional Immunology Service, St. Mary's Hospital, Manchester.)*

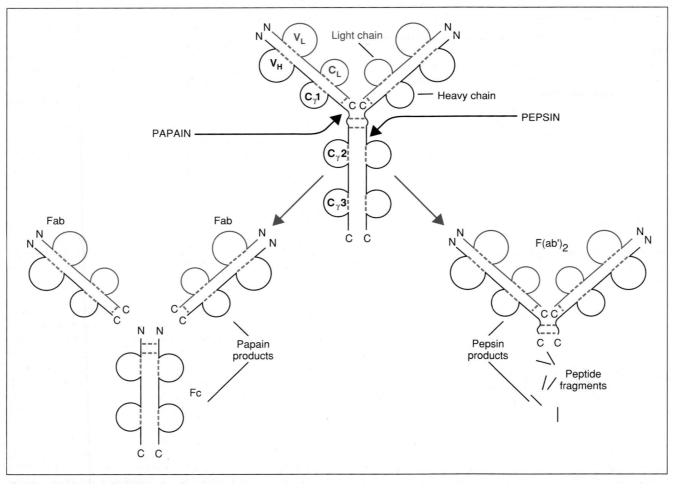

FIGURE 3–8. Proteolytic fragments of an IgG molecule. *Sites of papain and pepsin cleavage are indicated by arrows. Papain digestion allows separation of two antigen-binding regions (the Fab fragments) from the portion of the IgG molecule that activates complement and binds to Fc receptors (the Fc fragment). Pepsin generates a single bivalent antigen-binding fragment [F(ab')₂] with higher avidity for antigen than the two monovalent Fab fragments produced by papain cleavage.*

ter, many of the effector functions of immunoglobulins are mediated by the Fc portions of the molecule.

Different results are obtained when the proteolytic enzyme pepsin is used instead of papain to cleave rabbit IgG molecules (Fig. 3–8). In this case, under limiting conditions of enzyme concentrations and time, proteolysis is restricted to the carboxy terminus of the hinge region near the $C_\gamma 2$ domain such that the antigen-binding fragment of IgG retains the hinge and the interchain disulfide bonds. Fab fragments containing the heavy chain hinge are called Fab′; when the interchain disulfide bonds are intact, the two Fab′ fragments remain associated in a form called **F(ab′)₂.** The Fc fragment is often extensively degraded and does not survive proteolysis by pepsin. Fab and F(ab′)₂ are often useful as experimental tools because they can bind to antigens without activating Fc-dependent effector mechanisms.

These proteolysis experiments are not readily extended to other antibody isotypes such as IgM. In fact, they are not even applicable to all IgG molecules in many species other than rabbit. However, the basic organization of the Ig molecule that Porter deduced from his studies of rabbit IgG is common to all Ig molecules of all isotypes and of all species. These features may be summarized as follows:

1. Each $V_L V_H$ pairing forms an independent antigen-binding site. Thus, all monomeric IgG molecules have two separate antigen-binding sites, and secreted pentameric IgM molecules have ten separate antigen-binding sites (see Figs. 3–2 and 3–6).

2. The structure of the hinge region (or lack of one in certain isotypes) sterically determines how many binding sites of a single antibody molecule can simultaneously interact with antigen molecules, e.g., on a cell surface.

3. The Fc portion of an antibody molecule is spatially distinct from and functions independently of the antigen-binding site formed by the Fab regions. Since Fc regions activate immune effector functions, the kinds of effector functions activated by a particular Ig molecule are largely independent of the specificity for antigen and instead depend primarily on the isotype of the antibody.

ANTIBODY BINDING OF ANTIGENS

In the preceding sections, we have developed a general description of the structure of antibody molecules. Now we will turn to a more detailed discussion of the structural basis and physicochemical characteristics of antigen binding.

Structural Aspects of Biologic Antigens

An **antigen** can be defined as any substance that may be specifically bound by an antibody molecule. This differs from the original (historical) definition of antigen as a molecule that generates an antibody. We now know that almost every kind of biologic molecule, including simple intermediary metabolites, sugars, lipids, autacoids, and hormones as well as macromolecules such as complex carbohydrates, phospholipids, nucleic acids, and proteins, can serve as antigens. However, only macromolecules can initiate lymphocyte activation necessary for an antibody response. Molecules that generate immune responses are called **immunogens.** (Although technically less precise, the more inclusive term "antigens" is still commonly used to refer to "immunogens.") In order to generate antibodies specific for small molecules, immunologists commonly attach such small molecules to macromolecules before immunization. In this system, the small molecule is called a **hapten** and the macromolecule, usually a foreign protein, is called a **carrier.** The hapten-carrier complex, unlike free hapten, can act as an immunogen.

In general, macromolecules are much bigger than the antigen-binding region of an antibody molecule. Therefore, an antibody binds to only a specific portion of the macromolecule, called a **determinant,** or **epitope.** These two words are synonymous and are used interchangeably throughout the book. A hapten may be thought of as an exogenous determinant that is attached to a macromolecule.

Macromolecules typically contain multiple determinants, each of which, by definition, can be bound by an antibody. In some cases, the determinants are spatially well separated, and two individual antibody molecules can be bound to the same antigen molecule without influencing each other; such determinants are said to be non-overlapping. In other cases, the first antibody bound to an antigen may sterically interfere with the binding of the second, and the determinants of the antigen are said to be overlapping. In rarer cases, binding of the first antibody may cause a conformational change in the structure of the antigen, influencing the binding of the second antibody by means other than steric hindrance. Such interactions are called allosteric effects.

In the case of phospholipids or of complex carbohydrates, the antigenic determinants are entirely a function of the covalent structure of the macromolecule. However, in the case of nucleic acids, and even more so in the case of proteins, the non-covalent folding of the macromolecule may also contribute to the formation of determinants. In proteins, epitopes formed by adjacent amino acid residues in the covalent sequence are called **linear determinants** (Fig. 3–9). It is estimated that, in a protein antigen, the size of the linear determinant that forms contacts with specific antibody is about six amino acids long. Linear determinants may be accessible to antibodies in the native folded protein if they appear on the surface or in a region of extended conformation. More often, linear determinants may be inaccessible in the native conformation and appear only when the protein is denatured. In contrast, **conformational determinants** are formed by amino acid residues from separated portions of the linear amino acid sequence that are spatially juxtaposed only upon folding (Fig. 3–9). In theory, denatured proteins could transiently give rise to conformational

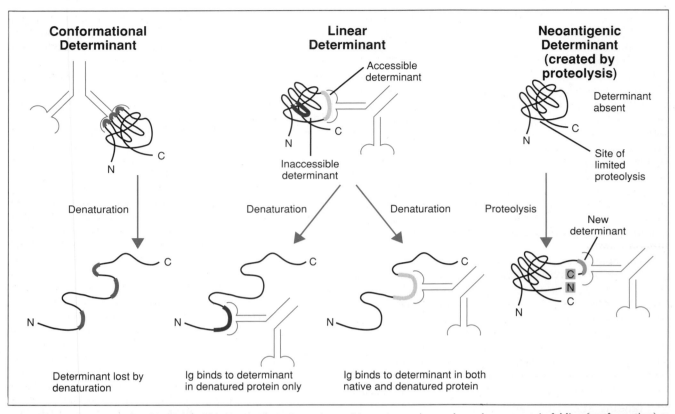

FIGURE 3–9. The nature of antigenic determinants. *Antigenic determinants (shown in gray) may depend upon protein folding (conformation) as well as upon covalent structure. Some linear determinants are accessible in native proteins, whereas others are exposed only upon protein unfolding. Neodeterminants arise from covalent modifications such as peptide bond cleavage.*

determinants; however, such determinants are too short-lived unless they are maintained by energetically favorable interactions such as those found in native proteins. Thus, antibodies specific for certain linear determinants and antibodies specific for conformational determinants can be used to ascertain whether a protein is denatured or in its native conformation, respectively. When there is more than one stable conformation, antibodies may be specific for one or the other. The energy of antibody binding may actually alter the relative stability of the two conformations, shifting the dynamic equilibrium.

Proteins may be subjected to covalent modifications such as phosphorylation or specific proteolysis. These modifications, by altering the covalent structure, can produce new antigenic epitopes. Such epitopes, called **neoantigenic determinants,** may be recognized by specific antibodies (Fig. 3–9).

At the beginning of this chapter, we made the general assertion that antibodies are not enzymes. However, certain antigen-binding sites may coincidentally resemble the active sites of enzymes and function to catalyze reactions. It should be emphasized that this is an area of intense research activity as a means of designing enzymes but is unlikely to play much of a role in normal immunity.

A final consideration about macromolecules as antigens is that proteins, nucleic acids, and complex carbohydrates may have internally repetitive structures, forming more than one identical determinant per molecule. For proteins, such structures commonly arise from polymerization of monomeric units. Molecules with repetitive structures are said to be **multivalent** and can interact with more than one binding site on an individual antibody or with more than one antibody.

Structural Basis of Antigen Binding

The limited proteolysis of antibody molecules described above indicated that the antigen-binding region of antibody is contained within the Fab fragment. Several lines of evidence provide a more precise localization of this function to the hypervariable regions of V_L and V_H.

1. V_L and V_H vary among antibodies of different antigenic specificity, and most of this variation is confined to the hypervariable regions.

2. Changes in the hypervariable regions, either by spontaneous mutation or by specifically directed mutagenesis, can alter antigen-binding specificity.

3. Crystallographic analysis of many antibody structures reveals that the hypervariable regions form extended loops that are exposed on the surface of the antibody and are thus able to interact with antigen.

4. Crystallographic analysis of a limited number of

antigen-antibody complexes shows that the amino acid residues of the hypervariable regions form extensive contact with bound antigen. The most extensive contact is with the third hypervariable region, the most variable of the three. (See Plate I.)

The assignment of antigen-binding specificity to the hypervariable regions led to the alternative name for these sequences as complementarity-determining regions described earlier in the chapter. *The amino acid sequences of the CDRs are primarily responsible for the specificity of antigen binding.* However, it should be noted that antigen-binding is not completely a function of the CDRs. Some framework region residues also may contact the antigen. Moreover, in binding of some antigens, one or more of the CDRs may be outside the region of contact with antigen, thus not participating in antigen binding.

The original models for antigen binding, based on analogy to enzymes, proposed that antibodies contained clefts for binding antigens. Indeed, some of the earliest characterized antibody-antigen complexes involved small carbohydrate antigens, and the antibodies that were studied did have clefts lined by amino acid residues of the hypervariable regions. However, more recently analyzed antibody-antigen complexes have revealed that native protein antigens may interact with a more planar antibody-combining site. This is critical for recognition of native proteins, as globular protein antigens are unlikely to fit into clefts. As will be discussed in Chapters 5 and 6, this is a key difference between the antigen-binding sites of antibody molecules and those of certain other antigen-binding molecules of the immune system, namely MHC molecules, which cannot bind to native globular proteins.

Affinity and Avidity of Antigen Binding

To describe the physicochemical characteristics of antigen binding to antibody, we will first consider a simplified system consisting of an antigen that has only one determinant per molecule and a population of identical antibody molecules specific for this determinant. When this antigen and antibody are mixed in solution, antigen-antibody complexes constantly form and spontaneously dissociate. After a period of time, the rate of complex formation will exactly equal the rate of complex dissociation and a state of **dynamic equilibrium** will have been reached. If antibody is present at much lower concentration than antigen, the proportion of antibody molecules that have bound antigen at equilibrium is determined by two factors: the concentration of antigen molecules and the strength of the binding interaction. (The strength of the binding interaction is also influenced by other factors such as temperature and solvent conditions, but to simplify the analysis, we will hold these constant.) Under such conditions, the concentration of antigen that allows one half of the antibodies to be in complex with antigen and leaves one half free is a measure of the strength, or **affinity,** of

the binding interaction. This concentration of antigen, measured in molarity, is called the **dissociation constant** (K_d) of the interaction. *A smaller K_d means a greater affinity;* i.e., a lower concentration of antigen is needed to reach half maximal occupancy. Affinity may also be represented by the reciprocal of the dissociation constant (i.e., $1/K_d$), which is called the **association constant** (K_a); since K_a is the reciprocal of K_d, a larger K_a signifies greater affinity. It is important to note that affinity depends on both the antibody and the antigen. A given antibody molecule can have different affinities for different related antigens.

The K_d of antigen binding can be measured directly for small antigens (e.g., haptens) by means of equilibrium dialysis (Fig. 3–10). In this method, a solution of antibody is confined within a "semipermeable" membrane of porous cellulose and is immersed in a solution containing the antigen. (Semipermeable in this context means that small molecules, like antigen, can pass freely through the membrane pores, but that macromolecules, like antibody, cannot.) If no antibody were present within the membrane, the antigen in the bathing solution would enter the membrane-bound compartment until the concentration of antigen within the membrane-bound compartment became exactly the same as that outside. Another way to view the system is that, at dynamic equilibrium, antigen enters and leaves the membrane-bound compartment at exactly the same rate. However, when antibody is present inside the membrane, the net amount of antigen inside the membrane at equilibrium increases by the quantity that is bound to antibody. This occurs because only unbound antigen can diffuse across the membrane, and, at equilibrium, it is the unbound concentration of antigen that must be identical inside and outside the membrane. The extent of the increase in antigen inside the membrane depends on the antigen concentration, on the antibody concentration, and on the K_d of the binding interaction. By measuring the antigen and antibody concentrations, by spectroscopy or by other means, the K_d can be calculated.

An alternative way to determine the K_d is by measuring the rates of antigen-antibody complex formation and dissociation. These rates depend on the concentrations of antibody and antigen, on the affinity of the interaction, and on certain geometric parameters that equally influence the rate in both directions. All parameters except the concentrations can be summarized as rate constants, and both the **on rate constant** (k_{on}) and the **off rate constant** (k_{off}) can be calculated experimentally by determining the concentrations and the actual rates of association or dissociation, respectively. The ratio of k_{off}/k_{on} allows one to cancel out all of the parameters not related to affinity and is exactly equal to the dissociation constant K_d. Thus, one can measure K_d at equilibrium by equilibrium dialysis or calculate K_d from rate constants measured under non-equilibrium conditions.

So far we have considered only the situation in which the antigen contains a single determinant and thus can interact with a single antibody-combining site. For antibodies specific for natural antigens, the K_d usu-

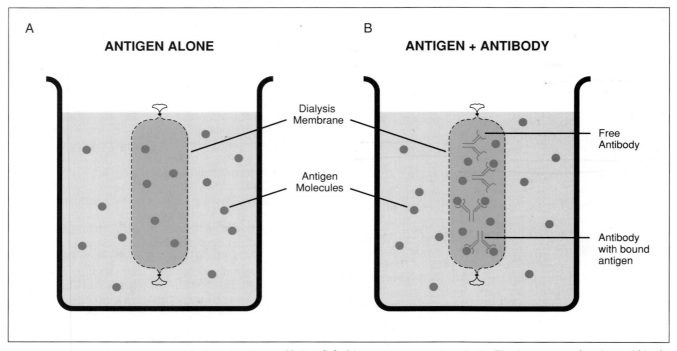

FIGURE 3–10. Analysis of antigen-antibody binding by equilibrium dialysis. *In the presence of antibody (B), the amount of antigen within the dialysis membrane is increased compared with the absence of antibody (A). As described in the text, this difference, caused by antibody binding of antigen, can be used to measure the affinity of the antibody for the antigen. This experiment can only be performed when the antigen is a small molecule (e.g., a hapten) capable of freely crossing the dialysis membrane.*

ally varies from about 10^{-7} M to 10^{-11} M. In a natural serum, there will be a mixture of such antibodies with different affinities for the specific antigen, depending primarily upon the precise amino acid sequences of the CDRs. (The average affinity of the antibody molecules in a population will increase with repeated immunization, a phenomenon called **affinity maturation;** this is discussed in Chapter 4.) Natural antigens, as opposed to small haptens, usually contain more than one determinant and therefore bind more than one antibody molecule. Moreover, multivalent antigens will have more than one copy of a particular determinant. (Multivalency may arise because a macromolecule may be multimeric or may have an internal repeating structure.) A cell surface will also be multivalent by virtue of having multiple copies of a particular surface antigen. Unless inhibited by steric constraints, a single antibody may be able to attach to a single multivalent antigen by more than one binding site. For IgG or IgE, this attachment can involve, at most, two binding sites because there are only two combining regions per antibody molecule, one on each Fab. For IgM, however, a single antibody may bind at up to ten different sites! Although the affinity of any one site will be unchanged, the overall strength of attachment must take into account binding at all of the sites. This overall strength of attachment is called the **avidity** and will be much stronger than the affinity of any given site. Mathematically, the strength of the avidity increases almost geometrically (rather than additively) for each occupied site. Thus, a low-affinity IgM molecule can still bind very tightly to a multivalent antigen because many low-affinity interactions can produce a single high-avidity interaction.

Multivalent interactions between antigen and antibody are of biologic significance. If a multivalent antigen is mixed with a specific antibody in a test tube, the two will associate to form **immune complexes** (Fig. 3–11). At the correct concentrations, called a "zone of equivalence," antibody and antigen form an extensively cross-linked network of non-covalently attached molecules such that most or all of the antigen and antibody molecules are complexed into large masses. Similar complexes form when macromolecular "monovalent" antigens are incubated with antisera containing several different antibodies, each specific for different determinants on the antigen. Although the primary non-covalent interactions involve the Fab portions of the antibody and antigen, Fc-Fc associations between antibody molecules may also contribute. Thus, intact IgG molecules may form larger complexes than F(ab')$_2$, despite similar specific antigen-binding properties.

Immune complexes can be dissociated into smaller aggregates either by increasing the concentration of antigen so that free antigen molecules will displace cross-linked antigen from antibody-combining sites ("zone of antigen excess") or by increasing antibody so that free antibody molecules will displace cross-linked antibody from antigen determinants ("zone of antibody excess"). If a "zone of equivalence" is reached *in vivo,* large immune complexes can form in the circulation. If such complexes are trapped in tissue (or form in tissue), they can initiate an inflamma-

PLATE I

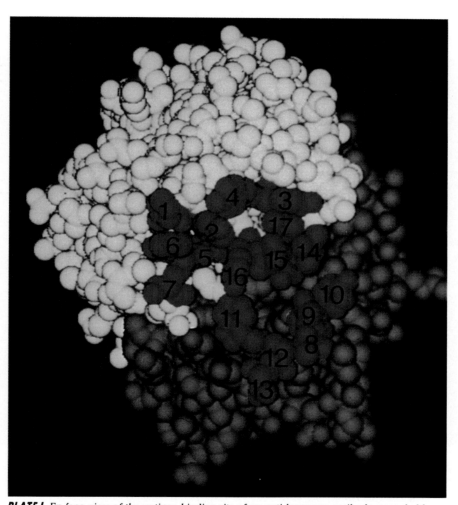

PLATE I. En face *view of the antigen-binding site of an anti-lysozyme antibody, revealed by x-ray crystallography of an antigen-antibody complex. In this space-filling model, the variable regions of the heavy and light chains are shown in blue and yellow, respectively. The numbered side chains in red indicate amino acid residues in the complementarity-determining regions (CDRs) of the light chain (1–7) and heavy chain (8–17) that contact the protein antigen on this planar surface. (Courtesy of Dr. R. J. Poljak, Pasteur Institute, Paris, France, and reproduced with permission from A. G. Amit, R. A. Mariuzza, S. E. V. Phillips, and R. J. Poljak. Three-dimensional structure of an antigen-antibody complex at 2.8 Å resolution. Science 233:747–753, 1986. Copyright 1986 by the AAAS.)*

PLATE II

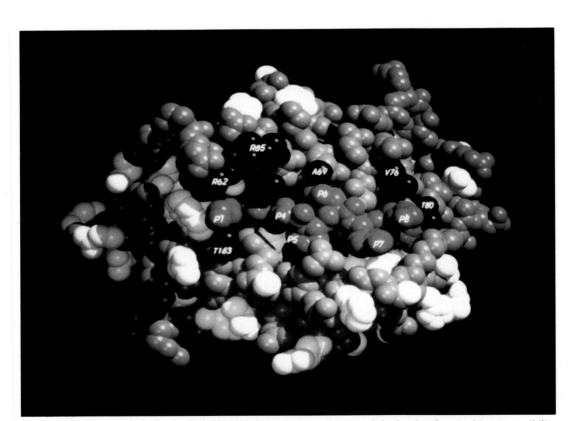

PLATE II. En face *view of a foreign peptide occupying the antigen-binding cleft of a class I major histocompatibility complex (MHC) molecule (HLA-Aw68) as revealed by x-ray crystallography. In this space-filling model, the peptide (residues 91–99 of the influenza virus nucleoprotein) is colored orange. The α-helix formed by the α1 domain of the class I molecule is shown on the top, and the α-helix formed by the α2 domain is shown on the bottom of the picture. Polymorphic residues of the MHC molecule that extend upward (and contribute to T cell recognition) are colored maroon, whereas nonpolymorphic and invariant residues are colored light and dark blue, respectively. The amino acid residues of the peptide that extend out of the cleft, and contribute to determinants recognized by T cells, are labeled P1, P4, P5, P6, P7, and P8, corresponding to the position of the residue with respect to the amino terminus of the peptide. The labels on the polymorphic MHC amino acid residues indicate both the identity of the amino acid side chain (in the single letter code) and the position of the residue with respect to the amino terminus of the class I heavy chain. (Courtesy of Dr. D. C. Wiley, Harvard University, Cambridge, MA, and reproduced with permission from M. L. Silver, H-C. Guo, J. L. Strominger, and D. C. Wiley. Atomic structure of a human MHC molecule presenting an influenza peptide. Nature 360:367–369, 1992. Copyright 1992 by Macmillan Magazines Ltd.)*

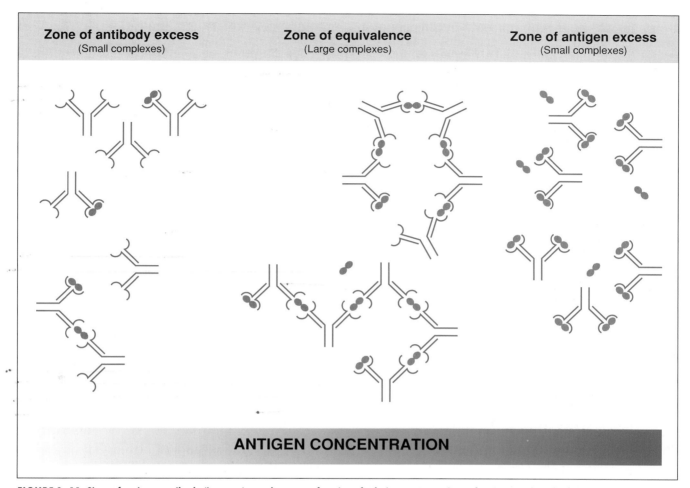

Zone of antibody excess	Zone of equivalence	Zone of antigen excess
(Small complexes)	(Large complexes)	(Small complexes)

ANTIGEN CONCENTRATION

FIGURE 3–11. Sizes of antigen-antibody (immune) complexes as a function of relative concentrations of antigen and antibody. *Large complexes are formed at concentrations of multivalent antigens and antibodies that are termed the "zone of equivalence"; the complexes are smaller in relative antigen or antibody excess.*

tory reaction resulting in "immune complex diseases" (see Chapter 20).

EFFECTOR FUNCTIONS OF ANTIBODIES

The effector function of an antibody is triggered by binding of antigen. Once antigen is bound, different consequences may ensue, depending on the structure, anatomic location, and isotype of the antibody. The following sections consider the various biologic effects of antibody binding to antigen.

Membrane Antibody As the B Cell Antigen Receptor

Resting B cells are activated to proliferate and secrete antibody by encounter with specific antigen. The specificity and recognition are provided by the membrane forms of antibody expressed on the B cell surface. At different points in the history of a B cell, differ-

ent heavy chain isotypes may be expressed. For example, immature B cells may express IgM, previously unstimulated mature B cells may express IgM and IgD, and previously stimulated memory B cells may express any isotype or subtype. As noted earlier, membrane Ig differs structurally from secreted Ig of the same isotype, in that membrane Ig contains an extra hydrophobic sequence of about 26 amino acids near the carboxy terminus (see Fig. 3–5). This sequence spans the hydrophobic region of the plasma membrane lipid bilayer so that the extreme carboxy terminal amino acids are located in the cytoplasm. Much evidence suggests that cross-linking of cell surface antibody by multivalent antigen may be an important signal that contributes to B cell activation. As will be discussed in Chapter 9, membrane Ig molecules associate with two other proteins (called $Ig\alpha$ and $Ig\beta$) that are involved in signal generation.

We have mentioned previously that the Ig molecules produced by any one B cell contain hypervariable regions that are different from those in Ig molecules produced by most or all other B cells (see Box 3–2). The unique determinants of Ig hypervariable regions are the **idiotopes,** and the collection of idiotopes on a particular antibody molecule constitutes its **idiotype.** Operationally, idiotypes may be defined as determinants (idiotopes) shared by multiple antibody molecules in a population. It has been postulated that during immune responses to antigens, anti-idiotypic antibodies specific for the responding lymphocytes are also produced. These anti-idiotypes bind to the surface Ig of the responding B cells and may regulate the magnitude of the immune response (see Chapter 10).

Neutralization of Antigen by Secreted Antibody

The initial discovery of antibodies arose by analyzing the humoral factors that protect immunized hosts against microbial toxins. Many injurious agents, such as toxins, drugs, viruses, bacteria, and other parasites, initiate cell injury by binding to specific cell surface receptors. Secreted antibodies can sterically hinder this interaction by binding to antigenic determinants on the agent (or, less commonly, on the cell receptor), thereby **neutralizing** the toxic or infectious process. This action may be mediated by antibodies of any isotype and experimentally can also be mediated by Fab or F(ab')$_2$ fragments.

Isotype-Specific Functions of Antibodies

Many functions of antibody molecules are mediated by their Fc portions and are, therefore, specific for particular isotypes or subtypes. As will be seen in Chapter 4, B cells may undergo **heavy chain isotype switching,** allowing the same antigen-binding specificity to be expressed at different times as part of Ig molecules of different isotypes. As a consequence, the same antibody specificity for antigen can be utilized to activate different effector functions. Although the V regions of antibodies are responsible for the specificity and diversity of humoral immunity, the availability of multiple C regions in different isotypes provides an additional measure of adaptability. The production of various heavy chain isotypes serves to direct the humoral immune response along different functional and anatomic pathways, involving diverse interactions with the body's mechanisms of natural immunity and inflammation.

ACTIVATION OF COMPLEMENT BY IGG AND IGM

The **complement system** consists of a family of serum proteins that can be activated by a proteolytic cascade to generate effector molecules. The name complement refers to a heat-labile serum component that was needed to "complement" the function of heat-stable antibody in order to produce lysis of certain target cells. The complement system mediates many of the cytolytic and inflammatory effects of humoral immunity

(Chapter 15). Here we will focus upon the ability of antibody to activate the complement system.

One sequence of complement activation, called the **classical complement pathway,** is triggered when a complement protein binds to the Fc region of antigen-complexed IgG or IgM. Neither free IgG nor IgM binds the first protein involved in complement activation, called C1q, so that complement is not activated by circulating free antibody. In the case of IgG, it is believed that the affinity of C1q is insufficient to bind to a single Fcγ region. However, C1q can bind to aggregated Fcγ present in immune complexes or to the clusters of Fcγ regions formed when multiple IgG molecules bind to antigens on a cell surface. The interaction of C1q occurs through the $C_\gamma 2$ domain of the IgG molecule. Different IgG subtypes are variously able to initiate this reaction. For example, IgG3 efficiently activates complement, IgG1 somewhat less so, IgG2 poorly, and IgG4 not at all. (In mice, IgG2a, IgG2b, and IgG3 all activate complement, but IgG1 does not.)

Activation of complement by IgM differs from activation by IgG. Secreted IgM is already pentameric in its native form in the circulation. However, C1q is sterically hindered from binding by the three-dimensional structure of circulating IgM. The binding of IgM to a planar (e.g., cell) surface is postulated to change the conformation of the antibody, allowing access of C1q to the Fc regions. C1q binding may then occur to the $C_\mu 3$ domain (the one that most resembles $C_\gamma 2$).

OPSONIZATION BY IGG FOR ENHANCED PHAGOCYTOSIS

Both mononuclear phagocytes and granulocytes have the ability to ingest particulate matter as a prelude to intracellular killing and degradation. The ingestion process of particulate matter, called **phagocytosis,** involves attachment of surface membrane to the foreign material and then "zipping up" of membrane around it. The efficiency of the process is markedly improved if the membrane of the phagocytic cell can attach itself with specificity to the object undergoing phagocytosis (Fig. 3–12).

Both mononuclear phagocytes and neutrophils express receptors for the Fc portions of IgG molecules. In fact, at least three distinct types of Fcγ receptors are expressed, each with different affinities and selectivities for different IgG subtypes (Box 3–3). Recent studies have revealed that each of the three types of IgG Fc receptor molecules is actually a subfamily of several structurally related proteins encoded by different genes. It is interesting that all three classes of IgG Fc receptors on leukocytes (written FcγR) contain Ig-like domains and are thus members of the Ig superfamily. When IgG molecules bind to and coat antigenic particles, a process called **opsonization,** the bound IgG is recognized by the FcγR molecules on the leukocyte, serving to enhance the efficiency of phagocytosis. Both high- and low-affinity FcγRs contribute to phagocytosis, and the IgG subtypes that bind best to these receptors (IgG1 and IgG3) are most efficient for promoting phagocytosis.

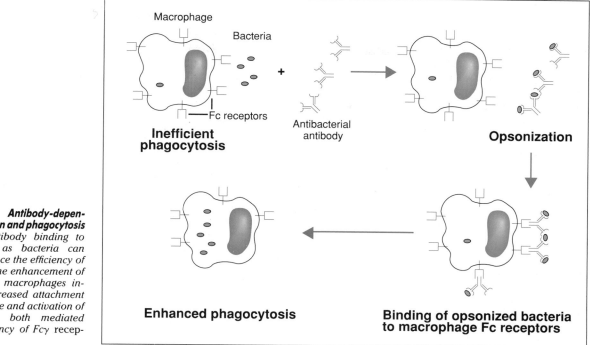

Macrophage

Bacteria

Fc receptors

Inefficient phagocytosis

Antibacterial antibody

Opsonization

Enhanced phagocytosis

Binding of opsonized bacteria to macrophage Fc receptors

FIGURE 3–12. Antibody-dependent opsonization and phagocytosis of bacteria. Antibody binding to particles such as bacteria can markedly enhance the efficiency of phagocytosis. The enhancement of phagocytosis in macrophages involves both increased attachment to the cell surface and activation of the phagocyte, both mediated through occupancy of Fcγ receptors.

It should be noted that a fragment derived from the third component of complement (C3b) can also opsonize particles for phagocytosis through binding to a leukocyte receptor for C3b. Since C3b can be generated and attached to cells as a consequence of the classical pathway of complement activation, IgM binding can indirectly lead to opsonization and enhanced phagocytosis.

Opsonization may lead to more than merely increasing the binding of the particulate matter to phagocytes. Both high- and low-affinity FcγRs also appear to be involved in metabolic activation of phagocytes, increasing the efficiency of the subsequent intracellular degradation of ingested particles.

ANTIBODY-DEPENDENT CELL-MEDIATED CYTOTOXICITY TARGETED BY IgG, IgE, AND IgA

Several different leukocyte populations other than cytolytic T lymphocytes (CTLs), including neutrophils, eosinophils, mononuclear phagocytes, and especially natural killer (NK) cells, are capable of lysing various target cell types. In many cases, killing of target cells requires that the target cell be precoated with specific IgG, and the lytic process is called **antibody-dependent cell-mediated cytotoxicity** (ADCC) (Fig. 3–13A). Recognition of bound antibody occurs through a low-affinity receptor for Fcγ on the leukocyte, called FcγRIII or CD16. In the case of NK cells, the predominant cellular mediators of ADCC, it is now appreciated that IgG serves two distinct functions. First, it provides cognitive function; i.e., those target cells that have bound IgG will be preferentially killed compared with those not

displaying IgG. Second, the occupancy (and perhaps aggregation) of FcγRIII serves to activate the NK cell to synthesize and secrete cytokines such as tumor necrosis factor and interferon-γ as well as to discharge their granules. These released cytokines and granule proteins probably mediate the cytolytic functions of this cell type (see Chapters 12 and 13).

Since CD16 is a low-affinity receptor and more efficiently binds aggregated IgG than monomeric IgG, monomeric IgG in plasma neither activates NK cells nor competes effectively with cell-bound IgG for recognition. *Thus, ADCC occurs only when the target cell is precoated with antibody.*

Eosinophils mediate a special type of ADCC directed against parasites such as helminths. Helminths are relatively resistant to lysis by neutrophils and mononuclear phagocytes, but they can be killed by a basic protein present in the granules of eosinophils. In this case, IgE rather than IgG serves as the principal isotype that provides recognition and effector cell activation because eosinophils express Fc receptors for IgE antibodies. Eosinophils may also use IgA to direct ADCC.

IMMEDIATE HYPERSENSITIVITY TRIGGERED BY IgE

Mast cells and basophils express high-affinity receptors for the Fc portion of IgE molecules. The structure and function of this IgE receptor, called FcεRI, are described in Chapter 14. Because of their high affinity, FcεRI receptors are occupied by IgE monomer in the absence of antigen, a key difference from FcγRIII involved in ADCC (Fig. 3–13B). The introduction of specific antigen causes aggregation of the IgE molecule and

BOX 3-3. CELLULAR RECEPTORS FOR IgG (FcγR)

The cell surface receptors for the Fc portion of IgG molecules are now known to consist of three subfamilies of related molecules, designated FcγRI, II, and III. FcγRI (CD64) is derived from a single gene in both humans and mice. The functional receptor consists of a single transmembrane polypeptide of about 40 kD. The large extracellular amino terminal region of FcγRI folds into three tandem Ig domains that extend into a 21 amino acid residue transmembrane segment and an ~60 amino acid residue carboxy terminal intracellular region. This intracellular region may exist in two different forms, arising from alternatively spliced transcripts. FcγRI is the only high-affinity receptor for the Fc portions of IgG molecules, and it binds human IgG1 or IgG3 antibodies with a K_d of 10^{-8} to 10^{-9}M. The affinity for IgG4 or IgG2 antibodies is much lower.

Members of the FcγRII subfamily (CDw32) are encoded by at least three separate genes in humans, but probably by only one gene in mice. The functional receptor consists of a single chain transmembrane polypeptide of about 30 kD. The large extracellular amino terminal region forms two tandem Ig domains. The extracellular domain extends into a 23 amino acid residue transmembrane segment and a carboxy terminal intracellular region of 50 to 80 amino acid residues. Sequence variations in the intracellular portions of the molecule, accounting for the variability in length, arise both from use of different genes and from alternative splicing of RNA. The affinity of FcγRII for human IgG1 or IgG3 antibodies is relatively weak, i.e., K_d greater than 10^{-7}M, and is essentially nonexistent for IgG2 or IgG4 antibodies.

Members of the FcγRIII subfamily (CD16) are encoded by two genes in humans and by only one gene in mice. One of the human genes encodes a 33 kD transmembrane polypeptide, whereas the other encodes a 29 kD phosphatidylinositol-linked protein. Both forms have extracellular amino terminal regions that fold into two tandem Ig domains. In the transmembrane form, the extracellular region folds into a 23 amino acid residue transmembrane domain and a 25 amino acid residue intracellular region. The affinity of FcγRIII for IgG molecules is similar to that of FcγRII. A unique feature of the transmembrane form of FcγRIII is that it associates with other transmembrane polypeptides known to be involved in signaling. Specifically, it may associate with homodimers of the γ chain of the high affinity receptor for IgE (FcεRI, see Chapter 15), with homodimers of the ζ chain of the T cell receptor complex (see Chapter 7), or with heterodimers formed between the γ and ζ chains.

Both FcγRI and FcγRII are thought to participate in phagocytosis and in signaling in mononuclear phagocytes and neutrophils. FcγRI expression may be up-regulated by inflammatory cytokines, and its increased expression may enhance the efficiency of these processes at sites of antigenic stimulation and inflammation, i.e., where cytokines are made. One particular isoform of FcγRII (called FcγRIIB) is expressed largely on B lymphocytes, where it may mediate antibody feedback (Chapter 10). Perhaps the best correlation of isoform with function is the unique expression of the transmembrane form of FcγRIII (FcγRIIIA) in NK cells, where it mediates ADCC. In contrast, expression of the phosphatidylinositol-linked form of FcγRIII (FcγRIIIB) is restricted to neutrophils, where it may contribute to phagocytosis but not ADCC.

Human Cellular Receptors for IgG

Family	CD	Affinity for IgG	Cell Distribution	Function
FcγRI	64	High ($K_d = 10^9$M)	Activated phagocytes	Phagocytosis
FcγRIIA	CDw32	Low ($K_d > 10^{-7}$M)	Phagocytes	Phagocytosis
FcγRIIB	CDw32	Low ($K_d > 10^{-7}$M)	B cells	Antibody feedback
FcγRIIIA	CD16	Low ($K_d > 10^{-7}$M)	NK cells	ADCC
FcγRIIIB	CD16	Low ($K_d > 10^{-7}$M)	Neutrophils	Phagocytosis

its receptor. This clustering, in turn, causes the mast cell or basophil to release inflammatory and vasoactive mediators (e.g., histamine) from preformed storage granules, and to synthesize and secrete lipid-derived mediators (e.g., leukotrienes, prostaglandins, and platelet activating factor) and cytokines *de novo*. The consequence of the release of these mediators is a vascular and inflammatory response called **immediate hypersensitivity,** which is discussed in Chapter 14.

MUCOSAL IMMUNITY MEDIATED BY IGA

Although IgA is a relatively unimportant component of systemic humoral immunity, it plays a key role in mucosal immunity. This is because IgA alone of the various isotypes can be selectively transported across mucosal barriers into the lumens of mucosa-lined organs. More IgA is synthesized by a normal individual than any other isotype, but because synthesis occurs mainly in mucosal lymphoid tissues and transport into the mucosal lumen is so efficient, IgA constitutes less than one quarter of the antibody in plasma. Epithelial cells of organs such as the intestine express specific Fc receptors for dimeric IgA molecules. This FcαR receptor is commonly called the **poly-Ig receptor** or **secretory component.** Initially, secretory component binds IgA on the basal surface of the epithelial cell that is facing the blood. Bound IgA is passaged through the cell to the mucosal surface by vesicular transport. Surprisingly, IgA is not simply released from its receptor. Rather, secretory component itself is specifically cleaved, leaving a bound secretory component peptide (called **secretory piece**) attached to the dimeric IgA

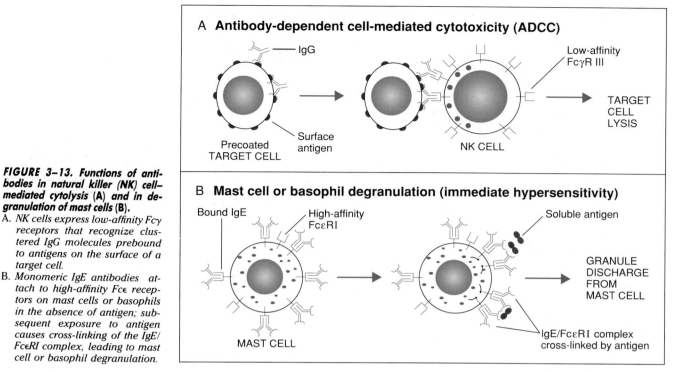

A **Antibody-dependent cell-mediated cytotoxicity (ADCC)**

IgG

Low-affinity
FcγR III

TARGET
CELL
LYSIS

Precoated
TARGET CELL

Surface
antigen

NK CELL

B **Mast cell or basophil degranulation (immediate hypersensitivity)**

Bound IgE

High-affinity
FcεRI

Soluble antigen

GRANULE
DISCHARGE
FROM
MAST CELL

MAST CELL

IgE/FcεRI complex
cross-linked by antigen

*FIGURE 3–13. Functions of antibodies in natural killer (NK) cell–mediated cytolysis (**A**) and in degranulation of mast cells (**B**).*
A. *NK cells express low-affinity Fcγ receptors that recognize clustered IgG molecules prebound to antigens on the surface of a target cell.*
B. *Monomeric IgE antibodies attach to high-affinity Fcε receptors on mast cells or basophils in the absence of antigen; subsequent exposure to antigen causes cross-linking of the IgE/FcεRI complex, leading to mast cell or basophil degranulation.*

molecule. Once in mucosal secretions, IgA functions to neutralize injurious agents (see Chapter 11).

NEONATAL IMMUNITY MEDIATED BY MATERNAL IGG

Neonatal mammals often lack the ability to mount an effective immune response against microbes. However, maternally produced antibodies can provide a protective action. Maternal IgG is transported across the placenta and enters the fetal circulation. In addition, maternal IgA is secreted into breast milk, where it can neutralize pathogenic organisms that attempt to colonize the infant's gut. Maternal IgG is also present in breast milk. IgG is specifically taken up from the gut lumen into the blood of the neonate, the opposite direction of IgA secretion. A distinct receptor for IgG has been identified that mediates this transport function. Interestingly, this receptor is unique among Fc receptors in that it structurally resembles a class I MHC molecule (see Chapter 5).

FEEDBACK INHIBITION OF IMMUNE RESPONSES MEDIATED BY IGG

Various lymphocyte populations express Fc receptors for different Ig isotypes. These receptors are believed to modulate lymphocyte function independent of antigenic specificity. The best example of this phenomenon is the binding of aggregated IgG or IgG-containing antibody-antigen complexes to FcγRII on B cells, which may inhibit activation of these B cells, a process called **antibody feedback** (see Chapter 10).

LABORATORY USES OF ANTIBODIES

This portion of the chapter describes how antibodies may be used as tools in research and in clinical diagnosis. Historically, many of the uses of antibody depended upon the ability of antibody and specific antigen to form large immune complexes. Immunochemists could detect antigen by observing the formation of such complexes in solution by light scattering. In addition, specific antigens could be purified from solutions containing mixtures of molecules by collecting the specific immune complexes by centrifugation or by precipitation of antibody with chemical agents. The presence of antigen could be detected by allowing antibody-antigen precipitates to form in gels. In the classic "double-diffusion" method of Ouchterlony, antigen and antibody were allowed to diffuse into gels from separate but nearby wells and a "precipitin line" of insoluble immune complexes would form at the point where the concentrations of diffusing antibody and antigen reached a zone of equivalence (Fig. 3–14). The position of the precipitin line provided information about antigen concentration, and comparisons of the precipitin lines formed by different antigen solutions allowed structural inferences about antigenic similarities or differences to be made. However, very little direct structural information could be learned about the antigens by these methods. In a later technique, the antigen solution could first be separated by electrophoresis under non-denaturing conditions and then allowed to diffuse into an antibody-containing gel. The extent of migration during electrophoresis provided additional information about the structure of the antigen. These meth-

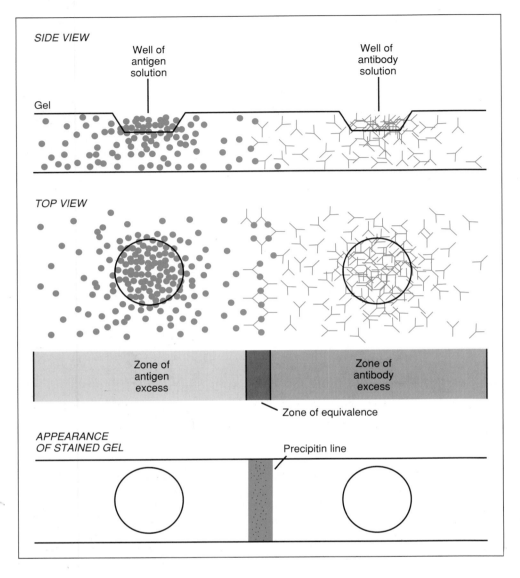

SIDE VIEW

Well of antigen solution

Well of antibody solution

Gel

TOP VIEW

Zone of antigen excess

Zone of antibody excess

Zone of equivalence

APPEARANCE OF STAINED GEL

Precipitin line

FIGURE 3–14. Analysis of the binding of antigen and antibody by agar gel diffusion (Ouchterlony technique). *Diffusion of antibody and antigen leads to a zone of equivalence, where large insoluble immune complexes form and can be detected as a precipitin line.*

ods were of great importance in early studies, but now have been almost entirely replaced by simpler methods based on immobilized antibodies or antigens. In the remainder of this chapter, we describe four common applications of antibodies in widespread current use.

Quantitation of Antigen

Immunologic methods of quantifying antigen concentration provide exquisite sensitivity and specificity and have become standard techniques for both research and clinical applications. All modern immunochemical methods of quantitation are based upon having a simple and accurate method for measuring the quantity of indicator molecules. When the indicator molecule is labeled with a radioisotope, as first introduced by Rosalyn Yalow and colleagues, it may be quantified by counting radioactive decay events in a scintillation counter; the assay is called a **radioimmunoassay** (RIA). When the indicator molecule is cova-

lently coupled to an enzyme, it may be quantified by determining with a spectrophotometer the initial rate at which the enzyme converts a clear substrate to a colored product; the assay is called an **enzyme-linked immunosorbent assay** (ELISA). Several variations of RIA and ELISA are in common use.

DIRECT RIA (Fig. 3–15)

A fixed quantity of antibody is attached to a solid support. The immobilized antibody will bind a finite portion of added radiolabeled indicator antigen. How much antigen binds depends on the antigen concentration and on the affinity of the antibody for the antigen. In the assay, the test solution of unknown antigen concentration is compared with a series of standard solutions containing known concentrations of unlabeled antigen for their ability to inhibit competitively the binding of the radiolabeled indicator antigen to the immobilized antibody. The greater the content of competing antigen in the test or standard solution, the less

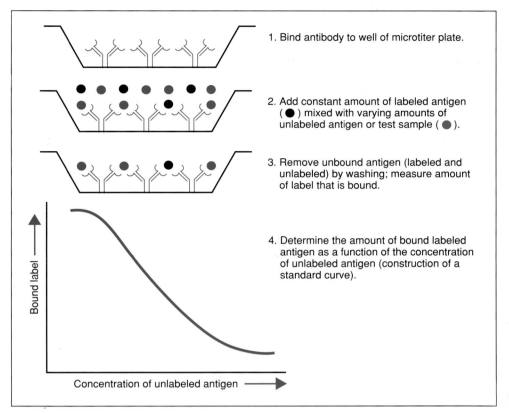

1. Bind antibody to well of microtiter plate.

2. Add constant amount of labeled antigen (●) mixed with varying amounts of unlabeled antigen or test sample (●).

3. Remove unbound antigen (labeled and unlabeled) by washing; measure amount of label that is bound.

4. Determine the amount of bound labeled antigen as a function of the concentration of unlabeled antigen (construction of a standard curve).

FIGURE 3–15. Direct radioimmunoassay (RIA). With a fixed amount of immobilized antibody, the amount of labeled antigen bound decreases as the concentration of competing unlabeled antigen is increased, allowing quantification of unlabeled antigen.

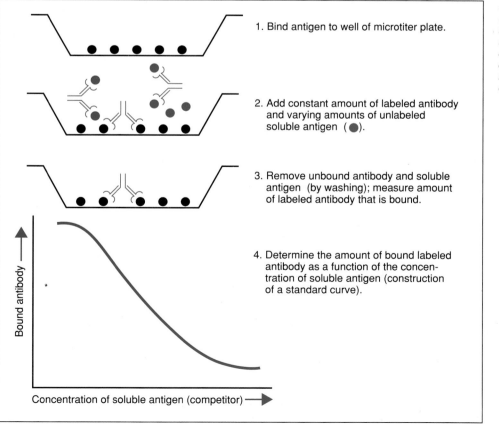

1. Bind antigen to well of microtiter plate.

2. Add constant amount of labeled antibody and varying amounts of unlabeled soluble antigen (●).

3. Remove unbound antibody and soluble antigen (by washing); measure amount of labeled antibody that is bound.

4. Determine the amount of bound labeled antibody as a function of the concentration of soluble antigen (construction of a standard curve).

FIGURE 3–16. Competitive ELISA or RIA. With a fixed amount of immobilized antigen, the amount of labeled antibody bound decreases as the concentration of unlabeled antigen (competitive inhibitor) is increased, allowing quantification of unlabeled antigen.

radiolabeled indicator antigen is bound. The results for the standard solutions of known antigen concentration are used to derive an inhibition curve as a function of antigen concentration, from which the concentration in the test sample can be inferred.

COMPETITIVE ELISA OR RIA (Fig. 3–16)

A fixed quantity of antigen is attached to a solid support, and a fixed quantity of indicator antibody in solution is then allowed to bind to the antigen. The amount of bound indicator antibody is measured using a covalently linked enzyme or radioisotope; the label may be attached directly to the indicator antibody, or it may be attached to a secondary antibody (e.g., rabbit anti-mouse Ig when the primary indicator antibody is mouse anti-antigen). The test solution of unknown antigen concentrations is compared with a series of stan-

dard solutions of known concentrations of antigen to inhibit competitively the binding of the indicator antibody. The greater the content of antigen in the test or standard solution, the less antibody is bound. The results from the standard solutions of known antigen concentration are used to derive an inhibition curve as a function of antigen concentration, from which the concentration in the test sample can be inferred.

SANDWICH ELISA OR RIA (Fig. 3–17)

A fixed quantity of one antibody is attached to a solid support. A test solution of unknown antigen concentration or a series of standard solutions of known concentrations of antigen is allowed to bind. Unbound antigen is removed, and a second population of enzyme-linked or radiolabeled indicator antibodies is al-

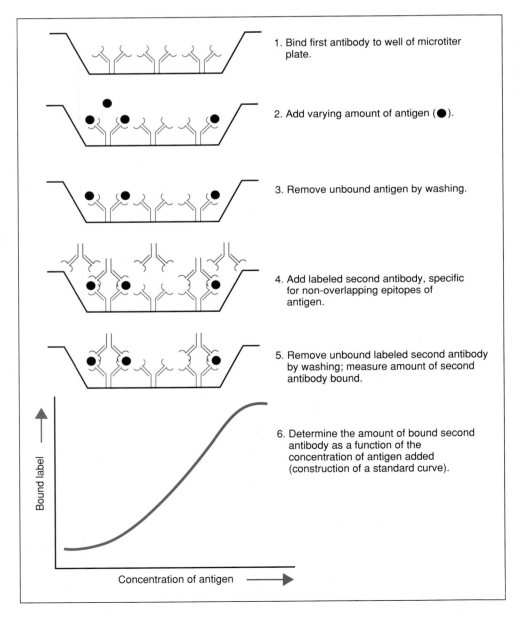

1. Bind first antibody to well of microtiter plate.

2. Add varying amount of antigen (●).

3. Remove unbound antigen by washing.

4. Add labeled second antibody, specific for non-overlapping epitopes of antigen.

5. Remove unbound labeled second antibody by washing; measure amount of second antibody bound.

6. Determine the amount of bound second antibody as a function of the concentration of antigen added (construction of a standard curve).

Bound label

Concentration of antigen

FIGURE 3–17. Sandwich ELISA or RIA. *With a fixed amount of one immobilized antibody, the binding of a second, labeled antibody increases as the concentration of antigen increases, allowing quantification of antigen.*

lowed to bind. The more antigen in the test or standard solutions, the more enzyme-linked or radiolabeled second antibody will bind. The results from the standard solutions are used to construct a binding curve for second antibody as a function of antigen concentration, from which the quantity of antigen in the test solution may be inferred. When this test is performed with two antibodies, it is essential that these antibodies see non-overlapping determinants on the antigen; otherwise, the second antibody cannot bind.

Identification and Characterization of Protein Antigens

The two major approaches used by immunochemists to identify and characterize protein antigens are immunoprecipitation and Western blotting.

IMMUNOPRECIPITATION (Fig. 3–18)

An antibody directed against one protein antigen in a mixture of proteins is used to isolate the specific antigen from the mixture. In most modern procedures, the antibody is attached to a solid phase particle (e.g., an agarose bead), either by direct chemical coupling or indirectly. Indirect coupling may be achieved by means of an attached "second antibody" such as rabbit anti-mouse Ig antibody or by means of some other protein with specific affinity for the Fc portion of Ig molecules, such as protein A or protein G from staphylococcal bacteria. After the antibody-coated beads are incubated with the solution of antigen, unbound molecules are separated from the bead-antibody-antigen complex by washing. Specific antigen is then released (eluted) from the antibody by changing pH or by other solvent conditions that reduce the affinity of binding. Large quantities of antigen can be purified by this procedure of affinity chromatography. (Recall that affinity chromatography is also used as a method for purifying antibody molecules; see p. 37.) The purified antigen can then be analyzed by conventional protein chemical techniques. Alternatively, a small amount of radiolabeled protein can be purified, and the characteristics of the macromolecule can be inferred from the behavior of the radioactive label in analytical separation techniques such as polyacrylamide gel electrophoresis or isoelectric focusing (Box 3–4).

WESTERN BLOTTING (Fig. 3–19)

If the protein antigen to be characterized is in a mixture with other antigens, it may be first subjected to analytical separation, typically by sodium dodecyl sulfate (SDS)–polyacrylamide gel electrophoresis, so that the positions of different proteins in the gel are a function of their molecular sizes. The array of separated proteins is then transferred from the separating gel to a support membrane by capillary action (blotting) or by electrophoresis, such that the membrane acquires a replica of the array of separated macromolecules present in the gel. SDS is displaced from the protein during the transfer process, and native antigenic determinants are often regained as the protein refolds. The position of the antigen on the membrane can then be detected by binding of labeled antibody, thus providing information about antigen size. Both enzyme-linked and radiolabeled antibodies are commonly used.

The technique of transferring proteins from a gel to a membrane is called Western blotting as a biochemist's joke. Southern is the last name of the scientist who first blotted deoxyribonucleic acid (DNA) from a separating gel to a membrane, a technique since called Southern blotting. By analogy, "Northern blotting" was applied to the technique of transferring ribonucleic acid (RNA) from a gel to a membrane, and "Western blotting" was applied to protein transfer. A more detailed description of both Southern and Northern blotting will be presented in Box 4–2, Chapter 4.

Cell Surface Labeling and Separation

Antibodies are commonly used to characterize, identify, and separate cell populations. In these methods, the antibody can be radiolabeled, enzyme linked, or, most commonly, fluorescently labeled. In the case of fluorescent labels, the amount of bound antibody on every individual cell in a population is measured by passing suspended cells one at a time through a fluorimeter. This ability to analyze identical cells more than compensates for the fact that fluorescence intensity is always an arbitrary quantity and, unlike radioactivity or absorbance, cannot be related to an absolute number of molecules except by comparison with known standards. The flowing cells can also be differentially deflected by electromagnetic fields whose strength and direction are varied according to the measured intensity of the fluorescence signal, thereby allowing one to separate cell populations according to surface antibody binding (Fig. 3–20). The instrument that performs this task is called a **fluorescence-activated cell sorter** (FACS). Modern FACS instruments routinely allow simultaneous detection of three or more different fluorescent signals, each attached to a different antibody, permitting analysis or separation of cells according to any specified combination of surface antibody-binding patterns. A more rapid but less rigorous separation can be accomplished by allowing cells to attach to antibodies bound to plates ("panning") or to magnetic beads.

Localization of Antigen Within Tissues or Cells

Antibodies can be used to identify the anatomic distribution of an antigen within a tissue or within compartments of a cell. The common principle behind these techniques is that a label is attached to the specific antibody and that the position of the label in the

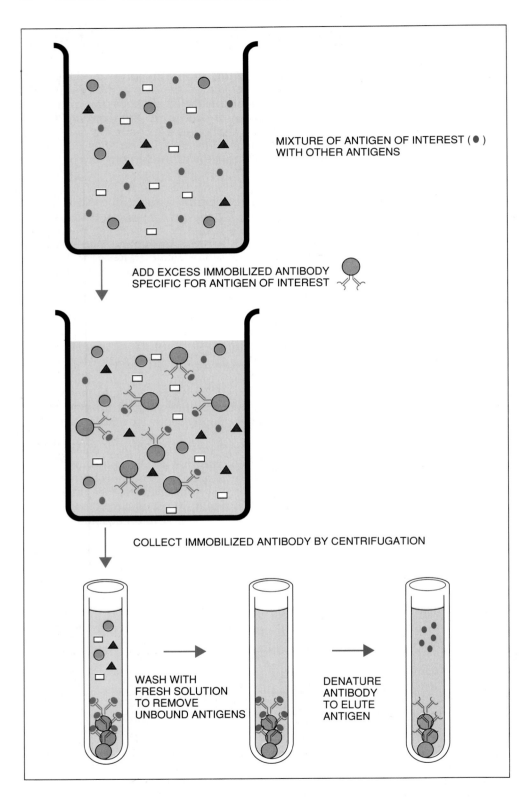

MIXTURE OF ANTIGEN OF INTEREST (●)
WITH OTHER ANTIGENS

ADD EXCESS IMMOBILIZED ANTIBODY
SPECIFIC FOR ANTIGEN OF INTEREST

COLLECT IMMOBILIZED ANTIBODY BY CENTRIFUGATION

WASH WITH
FRESH SOLUTION
TO REMOVE
UNBOUND ANTIGENS

DENATURE
ANTIBODY
TO ELUTE
ANTIGEN

FIGURE 3–18. Isolation of an antigen by immunoprecipitation. *Immunoprecipitation can be used as a means of purification, as a means of quantification, or as a means of identification of an antigen. Antigens purified by immunoprecipitation are often analyzed by polyacrylamide gel electrophoresis (see Box 3–4).*

tissue or cell, determined with a suitable microscope, is used to infer the position of the antigen. In the earliest version of this method, called **immunofluorescence,** the antibody was labeled with a fluorescent moiety and allowed to bind to a monolayer of cells or to a frozen section of a tissue. The stained cells or tissues were

examined with a fluorescence microscope to locate the antibody. Although extremely sensitive, the fluorescence microscope is not an ideal tool for identifying the normal unstained structures of the cell or tissue. Thus, it is often difficult to interpret precisely where the label has been localized. This problem may be overcome by

BOX 3-4.   POLYACRYLAMIDE GEL ELECTROPHORESIS OF PROTEINS

Analytical separation of proteins by size is routinely accomplished by electrophoresis through cross-linked polyacrylamide gels in the presence of SDS, an ionic detergent. Dodecyl sulfate binds to proteins in proportion to their molecular size, and the net negative charge of the bound detergent overwhelms the intrinsic charge of the protein. The bound dodecyl sulfate also causes refolding of the protein, after disruption of any intrachain disulfide bonds, into semirigid rods of length proportional to molecular size. As a result, both hydrodynamic resistance and net charge become entirely functions of molecular size, and consequently, migration to the anode in an applied electric field is also a function only of size. *Stated simply, smaller proteins migrate faster.* The size of an unknown protein can be determined by comparing the distance migrated in an SDS-polyacrylamide gel with the migration of known size standards electrophoresed in parallel lanes of the same gel. In general, the gel porosity is made sufficiently large to prevent sieving effects, but size resolution can be further enhanced by using gradients of cross-linked polyacrylamide concentration to introduce a small sieving effect. By this technique, one can accurately determine the size of any protein from about 5000 to 250,000 or more daltons. Some inaccuracies in molecular size determination can be introduced by extensive post-translational modifications (e.g., glycosylation or sulfation) or by the presence of hydophobic regions that disproportionately bind dodecyl sulfate.

An alternative analytical separation strategy is based upon isoelectric point. When proteins are electrophoresed through a pre-formed or self-generating pH gradient, they will migrate until they reach their isoelectric point, i.e., the condition of zero net charge. This separation technique is called **isoelectric focusing** and is also conveniently performed in polyacrylamide gels.

An optimal analytical separation scheme has been developed that combines these techniques. One first separates proteins by isoelectric focusing in one dimension and then subjects the initially separated array of proteins to SDS-polyacrylamide gel electrophoresis in the second, orthogonal direction. Such two-dimensional (2-D) gels can resolve more than one thousand separate proteins from a typical cell!

Once separated, the positions of the proteins in the gel are localized by staining. A common technique is to fix the proteins in place by denaturing solvents and then to stain them with a dye such as Coomassie blue or to use the fixed protein as a nidus for *in situ* reduction of silver ("silver staining"). Alternatively, radiolabeled proteins can be detected by dehydrating fixed gels and using the dried gel to expose photographic x-ray film (autoradiography). Finally, as discussed in the text, proteins separated by electrophoresis may be transferred by capillary action (blotting) or electrophoresis from the gel to a membrane where they can be stained by immunochemical procedures (Western blotting).

---

use of a confocal fluorescence microscope. Alternatively, antibodies may be coupled to enzymes that convert colorless substrates to colored insoluble substances that precipitate at the position of the enzyme. A conventional light microscope may then be used to localize the antibody in a stained cell or tissue. The most common variant of this method utilizes the enzyme horseradish peroxidase, and the method is commonly referred to as the **immunoperoxidase technique.** Examples of this method have been shown in Chapter 2. Another commonly used enzyme is alkaline phosphatase. Different antibodies, coupled to different enzymes, may be used in conjunction to produce simultaneous "two color" localizations of different antigens. In other variations, antibody can be coupled to an electron-dense probe, such as colloidal gold, and the location of antibody can be determined subcellularly by means of an electron microscope, a technique called **immunoelectron microscopy.** Different sized gold particles have been used for simultaneous localization of different antigens at the ultrastructural level.

In all immunomicroscopic methods, signals may be enhanced by using "sandwich" techniques. For example, instead of attaching horseradish peroxidase to a specific mouse antibody directed against the antigen of interest, it can be attached to a second antibody (e.g., rabbit anti-mouse Ig antibody) that is used to bind to the first, unlabeled antibody. When the label is attached directly to the specific, primary antibody, the method is referred to as **direct;** when the label is attached to a secondary or even tertiary antibody, the method is **indirect.** In some cases, molecules other than antibody can be used in indirect methods. For example, staphy-

lococcal protein A, which binds to IgG, or avidin, which binds to primary antibodies labeled with biotin, can be coupled to enzymes.

SUMMARY

Antibodies, or immunoglobulins, are a family of structurally related glycoproteins produced by B lymphocytes that function as the mediators of specific humoral immunity. All antibodies have a common core structure of two identical light chains and two identical heavy chains. Each chain consists of multiple independently folded domains of about 110 amino acids containing conserved intrachain disulfide bonds. The N-terminal domains of heavy and light chains form the variable regions of antibody molecules, which differ among antibodies of different specificities. The variable (V) regions of heavy and light chains each contain three separate hypervariable regions of about ten amino acids that are spatially assembled to form the antigen-combining site of the antibody molecule. Light chains contain one constant (C) region domain, and heavy chains contain three or four, which are similar in antibodies of the same class (isotype) and subclass but differ among antibodies of different classes and subclasses. Most of the effector functions of antibodies are mediated by the C regions of the heavy chains, but these functions are triggered by binding of antigens to the spatially distant combining site in the variable region.

Macromolecular antigens contain multiple epitopes, or determinants, each of which may be recog-

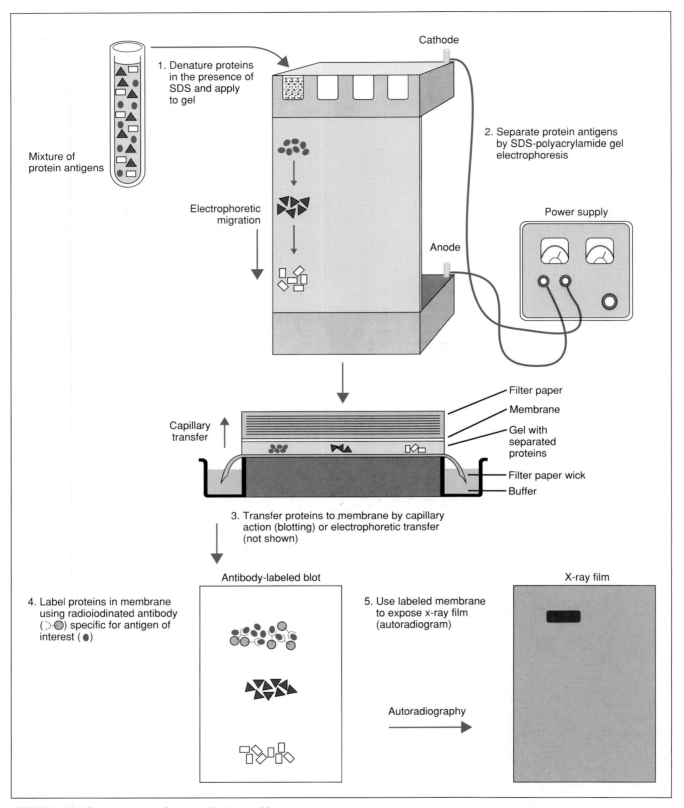

FIGURE 3–19. Characterization of antigens by Western blotting. *Protein antigens, separated by polyacrylamide gel electrophoresis and transferred to a membrane, can be labeled with radioactive or (not shown) enzyme-coupled antibodies. Analysis of an antigen by Western blotting provides information similar to that obtained from immunoprecipitation followed by polyacrylamide gel electrophoresis. Some antibodies work only in one or the other technique.*

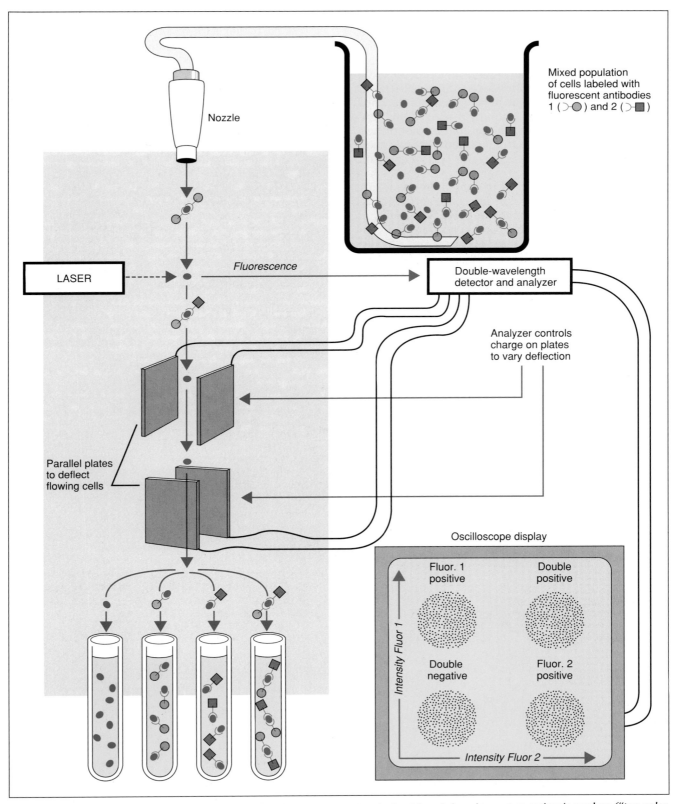

FIGURE 3–20. The principle of fluorescence-activated cell sorting. *The separation depicted here is based upon two antigenic markers ("two-color sorting"). Modern instruments can routinely separate cell populations based upon three or more markers.*

nized by an antibody. The affinity of the interaction between the combining site of a single antibody molecule and a single epitope is measured as a dissociation constant (K_d). Multivalent antigens contain multiple identical epitopes to which identical antibody molecules can bind. When multivalent antigens react with antibodies, a zone of equivalence may be reached, where the relative concentrations of antigen and antibody favor the formation of large immune complexes. In zones of antigen excess or antibody excess, these extensively cross-linked aggregates dissociate into smaller complexes.

Antibodies are produced in membrane-associated and secreted forms. Membrane Ig, on the surface of a B cell, is the B cell receptor for antigen. Secreted antibody molecules neutralize antigens, activate the complement system, and opsonize antigens and enhance their phagocytosis by various cells. In addition, different antibody isotypes bind to Fc receptors on eosinophils, mast cells, and natural killer cells and stimulate the functions of these cells as a consequence of antigen binding. Other Fc receptors on epithelial and placental cells mediate transepithelial transport of IgA and IgG antibodies, respectively.

Antibodies are also invaluable tools in the laboratory. Radioimmunoassay and enzyme-linked immunosorbent assay are used to quantify antigens in solution. Immunoprecipitation and Western blotting are used for the purification and structural analysis of protein antigens. Fluorescence-activated cell sorting is used to identify, characterize, and purify cell populations that express particular surface antigens. Immunomicroscopic techniques such as immunofluorescence and immunoperoxidase are used to identify and localize antigens in cells and tissues.

SELECTED READINGS

Alzari, P. M., M. Lascombe, and R. J. Poljak. Three-dimensional structure of antibodies. Annual Review of Immunology 6:555–580, 1988.

Amit, A. G., R. A. Mariuzza, S. E. V. Phillips, and R. J. Poljak. Three-dimensional structure of an antigen-antibody complex at 2.8 A resolution. Science 233:747–753, 1986.

Burton, D. R. Structure and function of antibodies. *In* F. Calabi and M. S. Neuberger (eds.). Molecular Genetics of Immunoglobulins. Elsevier Science Publishers, Amsterdam, 1987.

Burton, D. R., and J. M. Woof. Human antibody effector function. Advances in Immunology 51:1–84, 1992.

Davies, D. R., and E. A. Padlan. Antibody-antigen complexes. Annual Review of Biochemistry 59:439–473, 1990.

Johnstone, A., and R. Thorpe. Immunochemistry in Practice, 2nd ed. Blackwell Scientific Publishers, Oxford, 1987.

Kohler, G., and C. Milstein. Continuous cultures of fused cells secreting antibody of predefined specificity. Nature 256:495–497, 1975.

Porter, R. R. The hydrolysis of rabbit γ-globulin and antibodies by crystalline papain. Biochemical Journal 73:119, 1959.

Ravetch, J. V., and J.-P. Kinet. Fc receptors. Annual Review of Immunology 9:457–492, 1991.

Wu, T. T., and E. A. Kabat. An analysis of the sequences of the variable regions of Bence Jones proteins and myeloma light chains and their implications for antibody complementarity. Journal of Experimental Medicine 132:211–250, 1970.

CHAPTER FOUR

MATURATION OF B LYMPHOCYTES AND EXPRESSION OF IMMUNOGLOBULIN GENES

Antibodies, or immunoglobulins (Igs), are synthesized exclusively by B lymphocytes. Therefore, the humoral immune response to a foreign antigen reflects the types of Ig produced by the B cells that are stimulated by that antigen. At different stages of their maturation, B cells provide both cognitive and effector functions in the humoral immune response. Membrane Ig-expressing B cells are the cognitive cells, since they specifically recognize and respond to antigens. Following antigenic stimulation, they differentiate into effector cells that secrete Ig. Elucidation of the mechanisms of antibody synthesis has been one of the major advances in immunology during the last 15 years. This chapter describes the molecular genetic basis of humoral immune responses, with particular reference to the organization and expression of Ig genes, the differentiation of B lymphocytes, and the mechanisms by which antibody diversity is generated. The cellular interactions and extrinsic stimuli that lead to B cell proliferation and differentiation, including the functions of helper T cells in specific antibody responses, will be discussed in Chapter 9.

GENERAL FEATURES OF ANTIBODY PRODUCTION

The first analyses of specific antibody responses to foreign antigens were initiated in the early 1900s and focused on the types of antibodies produced in a person or experimental animal exposed to bacteria or microbial toxins. The total population of antibody specificities that an individual can produce is called the **antibody repertoire** and is a reflection of all the B cell clones capable of Ig synthesis and secretion in response to antigenic stimulation. During its life, each B lymphocyte and its clonal progeny go through a series of well-defined maturational or differentiative stages, each of which has a characteristic pattern of Ig production. Attempts to understand the development of B lymphocytes ultimately led to the isolation of Ig genes and to analyses of their expression and regulation. Much of our current understanding of B cell ontogeny, especially the regulation of Ig gene expression, is based on analyses of B cells during fetal life and of tumors that correspond to distinct maturational stages of B lymphocytes. Such tumors appear spontaneously in man and in experimental animals and can also be induced by oncogenic viruses *in vivo* and *in vitro*. Recently, methods have been developed for culturing mouse bone marrow stem cells on monolayers of marrow stromal cells and matrices. Such techniques are useful for defining the ontogeny of normal untransformed B cells.

Diversity of the Antibody Repertoire

The **primary antibody repertoire** consists of all the antibodies that an individual can produce in response to the first (primary) immunization with different antigens. It is determined by the number of B cell clones (estimated to be $>10^9$ in each individual) that exist prior to immunization and express membrane Ig molecules with distinct specificities for antigens. As the clonal selection hypothesis predicted, lymphocytes specific for different antigens develop before the introduction of these antigens. It follows, therefore, that *the information needed to generate the enormously diverse repertoire of antibodies is present in the DNA of each individual*. If, however, each Ig heavy and light chain were produced by an individual gene, more than one third of the genome that can code for functional proteins would be required to generate 10^9 antibody specificities. This is clearly not the case, and as we shall see later in this chapter, each Ig heavy chain and light chain polypeptide is not encoded by a discrete DNA sequence in the germline. Instead, B lymphocytes have developed remarkably effective genetic mechanisms for generating a large and highly diverse repertoire from a pool of Ig genes that is of more limited size.

Maturation of B Lymphocytes

All B lymphocytes arise in the bone marrow from a stem cell that does not produce Ig but is committed to the B cell lineage (Fig. 4–1). The earliest cell type that synthesizes a detectable Ig gene product contains cytoplasmic μ heavy chains composed of variable (V) and constant (C) regions. This cell is called the **pre–B lymphocyte** and is found only in hematopoietic tissues, such as the bone marrow and fetal liver. It does not express functional, fully assembled membrane IgM, since surface expression requires synthesis of both heavy and light chains. Therefore, pre–B cells cannot recognize or respond to antigen. Some of the μ heavy chains in pre–B cells associate with proteins called "surrogate light chains," which are structurally homologous to κ and λ light chains but are invariant, i.e., they do not have V regions and are identical in all B cells. Complexes of μ and surrogate light chains may be expressed on the cell surface at low levels, and are postulated to play a role in stimulating the subsequent production of κ or λ light chains and the continued maturation of B cells. Although this process is not well understood, the importance of surrogate light chains is underscored by studies of mice deficient in these proteins. For instance, "knockout" of the gene encoding one of the surrogate light chains, called $\lambda 5$, by homologous recombination (Box 4–1) results in markedly reduced development of mature B cells.

At the next identifiable stage in B cell maturation, κ or λ light chains are also produced. These associate with μ heavy chains, and then the assembled IgM molecules are expressed on the cell surface, where they function as specific receptors for antigens. The expression of surface Ig requires its association with several other proteins, which are discussed later in the chapter. IgM-bearing B cells that are recently derived from marrow precursors are called **immature B lymphocytes** because they do not proliferate and differentiate in response to antigens. In fact, their encounter with anti-

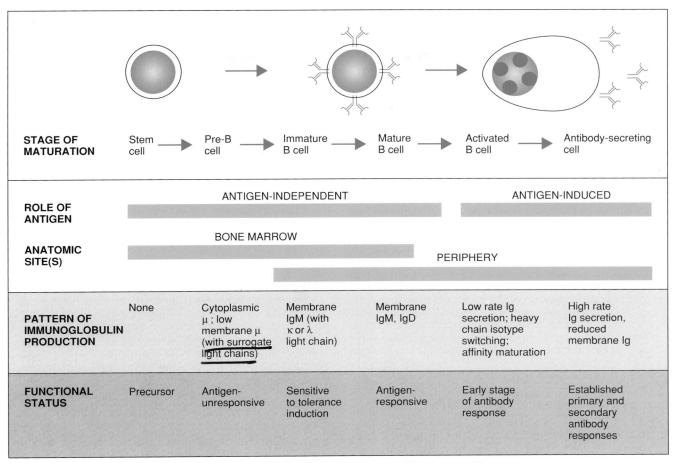

STAGE OF MATURATION	Stem cell →	Pre-B cell →	Immature B cell →	Mature B cell →	Activated B cell →	Antibody-secreting cell
ROLE OF ANTIGEN	ANTIGEN-INDEPENDENT				ANTIGEN-INDUCED	
ANATOMIC SITE(S)	BONE MARROW			PERIPHERY		
PATTERN OF IMMUNOGLOBULIN PRODUCTION	None	Cytoplasmic μ ; low membrane μ (with surrogate light chains)	Membrane IgM (with κ or λ light chain)	Membrane IgM, IgD	Low rate Ig secretion; heavy chain isotype switching; affinity maturation	High rate Ig secretion, reduced membrane Ig
FUNCTIONAL STATUS	Precursor	Antigen-unresponsive	Sensitive to tolerance induction	Antigen-responsive	Early stage of antibody response	Established primary and secondary antibody responses

FIGURE 4–1. Sequence of B lymphocyte maturation and antigen-induced differentiation.

gens such as self antigens may lead to cell death or functional unresponsiveness (tolerance) rather than activation. This property is important for maintaining tolerance to self antigens that the B cells encounter during their maturation in the bone marrow (see Chapter 19). Once a B cell expresses a complete heavy or light chain, it cannot produce another heavy or light chain containing a different V region. The stimuli that drive maturation of pre–B cells to immature and then mature B cells are incompletely defined. Interleukin-7 (IL-7), a cytokine produced by bone marrow stromal cells, is a growth factor for pre–B cells. Adhesive interactions between developing B cells and marrow stromal cells are also important in the maturation process. In addition, an immunodeficiency disease called X-linked agammaglobulinemia, in which cells fail to develop beyond the pre-B stage (see Chapter 21), is due to a mutation in a tyrosine kinase of the *src* family, suggesting that this enzyme plays a key role in B cell maturation.

Having acquired a complete Ig and, therefore, a specificity, B cells migrate out of the bone marrow and can be found in the peripheral circulation and lymphoid tissues. They continue to mature, even in the absence of antigenic stimulation. **Mature B cells** coexpress μ and δ heavy chains in association with the original κ or λ light chain and, therefore, produce both membrane IgM and IgD. Both classes of membrane Ig

have the same V region and hence the same antigen specificity. Such cells are responsive to antigens. It is possible that some B cells may acquire functional responsiveness to antigenic stimulation without expressing IgD. Although maturation to this stage does not require overt exposure to antigen, it is believed that unless these B lymphocytes encounter antigen, they die in a few days or weeks. It is estimated that an adult mouse (having a body weight of ~20 gm) produces 5×10^7 B cells daily from progenitors in the bone marrow. Of these, only 1 to 2×10^6 survive and enter the circulation and peripheral lymphoid tissues, serving to maintain the peripheral pool of ~5×10^8 mature B cells.

Once the mature B cells are stimulated by antigens (and other signals that will be described in Chapter 9), they are called **activated B lymphocytes.** Activated B cells proliferate and differentiate, producing an increasing proportion of their Ig in a secreted form and progressively less in a membrane-bound form. Some of the progeny of activated B cells undergo **heavy chain class (isotype) switching** and begin to express Ig heavy chain classes other than μ and δ, e.g., γ, α, or ε. Other activated B lymphocytes may not secrete antibody but instead persist as membrane Ig–expressing **memory cells.** Memory cells survive for weeks or months without further antigenic stimulation and actively recirculate between the blood, lymph, and lymphoid organs. The stimulation of memory B cells by

BOX 4–1. TRANSGENIC MICE AND TARGETED GENE KNOCKOUTS

Two important methods for studying the functional effects of specific gene products *in vivo* are the creation of transgenic mice, which over-express a particular gene in a defined tissue(s), and gene knockout mice, in which a targeted mutation is used to ablate the function of a particular gene. Both techniques have been widely employed to analyze many biologic phenomena. As we shall see throughout this book, transgenic and knockout mice are providing valuable information about the development of the immune system and the functions of a variety of proteins in immune responses.

To create **transgenic mice**, foreign DNA sequences, called **transgenes**, are introduced into the pronuclei of fertilized mouse eggs, and the eggs are implanted into the oviducts of pseudopregnant females. Usually, if a few hundred copies of a gene are injected into pronuclei, about 25 per cent of the mice that are born are transgenic. One to 50 copies of the transgene insert in tandem into a random site of breakage in a chromosome, and are subsequently inherited as a simple mendelian trait. Because integration usually occurs before DNA replication, most (about 75%) of the transgenic pups carry the transgene in all their cells, including germ cells. In most cases, integration of the foreign DNA does not disrupt normal function. Also, each founder mouse carrying the transgene is a heterozygote, from which homozygous lines can be bred.

The great value of transgenic technology is that it can be used to express genes in particular tissues by attaching coding sequences of the gene to regulatory sequences that normally drive the expression of genes selectively in that tissue. For instance, lymphoid promoters and enhancers can be used to over-express genes in lymphocytes, and the insulin promoter to express genes in the β cells of pancreatic islets. Examples of the utility of these methods for studying the immune system will be mentioned in many chapters of this book. Transgenes can also be expressed under the control of inducible promoters, such as the metallothionine promoter, which responds to heavy metals. In these cases, transcription of the transgene can be controlled at will by administering the inducing agent.

The most definitive way of establishing the obligatory function of a gene *in vivo* is the creation of **knockout mice** by targeted mutation or disruption of the gene. This technique relies on the phenomenon of **homologous recombination**. If an exogenous gene is inserted into a cell, e.g., by electroporation, it can integrate randomly into the cell's genome. However, if the gene contains sequences that are homologous to an endogenous gene, it will preferentially recombine with and replace endogenous sequences. To select for cells that have undergone homologous recombination, a drug-based selection strategy is employed. The fragment of homologous DNA to be inserted into a cell is placed in a vector typically containing a neomycin resistance gene and a viral thymidine kinase (TK) gene (see figure). This "targeting vector" is constructed in such a way that the neomycin resistance gene is always inserted but the TK gene is lost only if homologous recom-

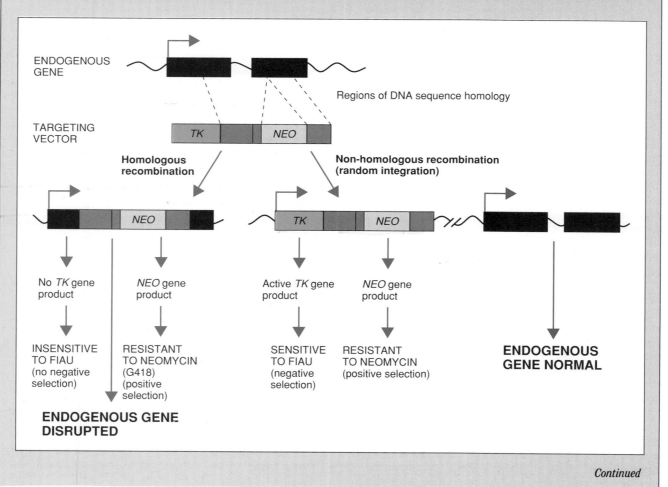

Continued

bination occurs. The vector is introduced into cells, and the cells are grown in neomycin and in FIAU, a drug that is metabolized by TK to generate a lethal product. Cells in which the gene is integrated randomly will be resistant to neomycin but will be killed by FIAU, whereas cells in which homologous recombination has occurred will be resistant to both drugs. This "positive-negative selection" ensures that the inserted gene in surviving cells has undergone homologous recombination with endogenous sequences. The presence of the inserted DNA in the middle of an endogenous gene usually disrupts the coding sequences and ablates expression and/or function of that gene. In addition, targeting vectors can be designed such that homologous recombination will lead to deletion of one or more exons of the endogenous gene.

To generate a mouse carrying a targeted gene disruption or mutation, a targeting vector is used to first disrupt the gene in a murine embryonic stem (ES) cell line. ES cells are pluripotent cells, derived from mouse embryos, that can be propagated and induced to differentiate in culture, or can be incorporated into a mouse blastocyst, which may be implanted in a pseudopregnant mother and carried to term. Importantly, the progeny of the ES cells develop normally into mature tissues, which will express exogenous genes that have been transfected into the ES cells. Thus, the targeting vector designed to disrupt a particular gene is inserted into ES cells, and colonies in which homologous recombination has occurred (on one chromosome) are selected with drugs, as described above. The presence of the desired recombi-

nation is verified by analysis of DNA, using techniques such as Southern blot hybridization or the polymerase chain reaction (PCR). The selected ES cells are injected into blastocysts, which are implanted into pseudopregnant females. Mice that develop will be chimeric for a heterozygous disruption or mutation, i.e., some of the tissues will be derived from the ES cells and others from the remainder of the normal blastocyst. Usually, the germ cells are also chimeric, but since these are haploid, only some will contain the chromosome copy with the disrupted (mutated) gene. If chimeric mice are mated with normal (wild-type) animals, and either sperm or eggs containing the chromosome with the mutation fuse with the wild-type partner, all cells in the offspring derived from such a zygote will be heterozygous for the mutation (so-called "germline transmission"). Such heterozygous mice can be mated to yield animals that will be homozygous for the mutation with a frequency that is predictable based on simple mendelian segregation. Such "knockout mice" are deficient in the expression of the targeted gene.

Knockout mice have opened new approaches for analyzing the functions of a wide variety of molecules. They have also led to an appreciation that many important gene products are "redundant", in that lack of expression of one gene may be compensated by other gene products.

(This box is partly the courtesy of Dr. Arlene H. Sharpe, Department of Pathology, Harvard Medical School and Brigham and Women's Hospital, Boston.)

---

antigen leads to the secondary antibody response. Memory B cells generally express Ig molecules whose affinities for antigens are higher than those of their unstimulated clonal precursors. Antigen-induced differentiation of mature or memory B lymphocytes culminates in the development of **antibody-secreting cells,** some of which can be morphologically identified as plasma cells. In the blood or lymphoid tissues of normal individuals, the majority of B cells are IgM$^+$ or IgM$^+$IgD$^+$.

Throughout their lives, the members of each B cell clone express the same V region and maintain essentially the same antigen specificity. However, subtle changes in antibody V regions do occur during responses to antigens. In particular, the average affinity of the secreted antibody and of membrane Ig on antigen-specific B cells increases after antigenic stimulation and is substantially higher in secondary than in primary antibody responses. This is called **affinity maturation** and is a property of humoral immune responses to protein antigens. Affinity maturation is measured at the population level, i.e., at the level of the entire antibody response. It arises from small mutations in the DNA coding for Ig V regions in individual, antigen-stimulated B lymphocytes, leading to an increase in the affinity of Ig produced by these cells. The mechanisms and consequences of somatic mutations in Ig genes are discussed later in this chapter.

Two other features of Ig production by B cells are noteworthy. First, each B cell clone and its progeny are specific for only one antigenic determinant. It is, therefore, necessary for each B cell to express only one set of Ig heavy and light chain V genes throughout its life,

even though all heterozygous individuals inherit two sets of Ig genes, one from each parent. A single specificity is maintained because only one of the two parental alleles of Ig is expressed by each B cell clone from its earliest maturational stage. This phenomenon is called **allelic exclusion** and is characteristic of both B and T lymphocyte receptors for antigens. Second, each B cell clone produces either a κ or a λ light chain but not both, and although heavy chain class switching occurs following activation, switches from one light chain class to the other do not occur throughout the life of each clone. This is called **light chain isotype exclusion.**

In summary, analyses of the antibody repertoire and B lymphocyte maturation and differentiation have led to the following general conclusions.

1. Each clone of B cells produces one set of Ig heavy chain and light chain V regions, and different clones produce Igs with different V regions.

2. During the life history of each clone, the same heavy chain V region is expressed in association with membrane or secreted forms of C regions and with C regions of different isotypes. In contrast, the light chain C region remains the same.

3. The specificities of V regions in each B cell and its progeny remain essentially unaltered but are "fine-tuned" after antigenic stimulation, leading to affinity maturation.

Molecular biologic analyses have proved invaluable for elucidating the mechanisms of antibody production, including the generation of diversity, allelic exclusion, Ig secretion, heavy chain isotype switching, and affinity maturation. It is now clear that these processes are regulated by changes in the organization of Ig genes and by the transcription and translation of these genes. In the remainder of this chapter, we will focus on the expression of Ig genes, beginning with the earliest events in committed B lymphocytes and proceeding through the various stages of B cell maturation and differentiation.

REARRANGEMENT OF IMMUNOGLOBULIN GENES
Discovery of Ig Gene Rearrangement

The first hypothesis about the organization of the genes that coded for different portions of Ig molecules was proposed even before B lymphocytes were recognized as antibody-producing cells. It was known in the 1950s that each chain of antibody molecules consisted of highly diverse V regions, which accounted for the specificities of antibodies, and relatively invariant C regions. Moreover, each C region had to be the product of a single allelic gene locus because in any individual the C regions present in all the antibodies of a particular isotype, irrespective of their antigenic specificities, contained sequences that were inherited in mendelian fashion. (These sequences constitute the allotypes of antibodies and have been described in Box 3–2, Chapter 3.) This apparent diversity of V regions and constancy of C regions of antibody molecules created a paradox, since the V and C regions made up one poly-

peptide chain and it was believed at that time that one protein was always encoded by one gene. Therefore, one would have to propose that only the variable portion of this putative gene was subject to extensive alterations or mutations. Realizing this paradox, Dreyer and Bennett postulated in 1965 that each antibody chain was actually encoded by at least two genes, one variable and the other constant, and the two became joined at the level of the DNA or messenger RNA (mRNA) to give rise to functional Ig proteins.

Formal proof of this hypothesis came over a decade later. In a landmark study, Susumu Tonegawa and his colleagues demonstrated that the structure of Ig genes in the cells of an antibody-producing tumor, called a myeloma or plasmacytoma, is different from that in embryonic tissues or in non-lymphoid tissues not committed to Ig production. This observation is best demonstrated by a technique called Southern blot hybridization, which is used to examine the sizes of DNA fragments produced by enzymatic digestion of genomic DNA (Box 4–2). By this method, it has been shown that *the sizes of DNA fragments containing Ig genes are different in cells that do and do not make antibody* (Fig. 4–2). The explanation for these different sizes is that V and C regions for any Ig light (L) or heavy (H) chain are encoded by different gene segments that are located far apart in embryonic cells and are brought close together in cells committed to antibody synthesis, i.e., B lymphocytes. *Thus, Ig genes undergo a process of somatic DNA recombination or rearrangement during B cell ontogeny.* These findings provided the first clear molecular explanation for the production of antibodies. The current concepts are best understood by describing the unrearranged, or germline, configuration of Ig genes, and then the pattern and mechanisms of their rearrangement during B cell development.

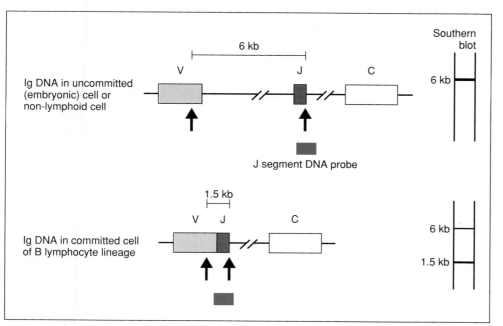

FIGURE 4–2. Detection of Ig gene rearrangement by Southern blot hybridization. *In this hypothetical example, genomic DNA from an embryonic or non-lymphoid cell is cut by a restriction enzyme at sites shown by bold arrows, producing a 6 kb fragment that is detected by Southern blot hybridization using a J segment–specific DNA probe. In a clone of B cells, the same enzyme generates a 1.5 kb fragment, because VJ rearrangement has led to the deletion of the DNA between the rearranged gene segments. (Note that a 6 kb band persists in the B cells; this band is derived from the unrearranged allelic locus.)*

BOX 4-2.   SOUTHERN BLOT HYBRIDIZATION

This technique, introduced by E. M. Southern, is used to characterize the organization of DNA surrounding a specific nucleic acid sequence, e.g., a particular gene. In a typical experiment, genomic DNA is chemically extracted from the nuclei of isolated cells or from whole tissues. At this point, the DNA will be present in extremely long segments and must be broken down into small fragments for analysis. This is accomplished by enzymatic cleavage with **restriction endonucleases**. (These bacterial enzymes are so named because they function to restrict the sur-

vival of foreign bacterial DNA in a host strain and because they cleave DNA at specific internal sites as opposed to digesting DNA from the ends as an exonuclease would.) Restriction endonucleases cleave double-stranded DNA only at positions of particular symmetric nucleotide sequences, usually about 6 bp in length. Such sequences are called **restriction sites**, and each site is uniquely recognized by a particular restriction endonuclease. Within the genome of an individual, restriction sites are present at the same positions in every cell, barring somatic mutation or

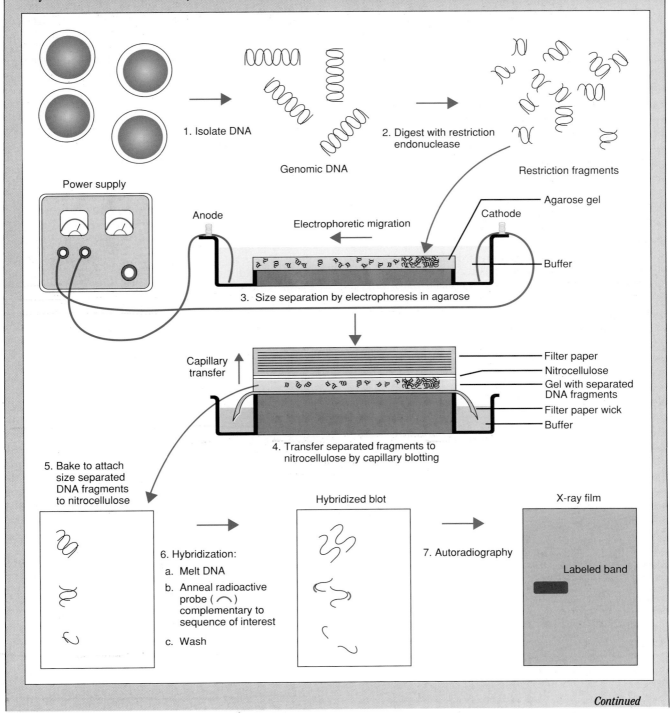

Continued

DNA rearrangement. Complete digestion with a particular enzyme leads to cleavage of the genomic DNA, giving rise to an array of DNA fragments ranging from about 0.5 to 10 kb in size. Different restriction endonucleases produce different arrays of **restriction fragments,** but each enzyme generally produces the same fragments from the DNA of every cell from an individual. This, of course, is not the case when one examines genes that rearrange in different ways in different clones of cells, such as Ig and T cell receptor genes.

To analyze the fragments, the digested DNA is separated according to size by electrophoresis in an agarose gel. The separated fragments are transferred by capillary action (blotting) from the gel to a membrane of nitrocellulose or nylon. Each fragment is then attached in place to the membrane by heating or ultraviolet irradiation. The net result is that the array of fragments is arranged by size on the membrane. Any particular nucleic acid sequence, such as a gene of interest, will be present on one or a few unique-sized fragments, depending only on the choice of restriction endonuclease and the distances between the relevant restriction sites that flank the gene or are located within the gene.

The analysis is completed by ascertaining the size of the restriction fragment(s) that contains the gene of interest. This is accomplished by nucleic acid **hybridization.** Double-stranded DNA can be "melted" into single-stranded DNA by changing temperature and solvent conditions. When the temperature is lowered, single-stranded DNA will reanneal to form double-stranded DNA. The rate at which reannealing of a sequence occurs is determined by the concentration of DNA containing complementary nucleic acid sequences present in the system. In the Southern blot hybridization technique, the DNA on the membrane is melted and then allowed to reanneal in the presence of a solution containing a large excess of single-stranded DNA (probe) with a sequence complementary to the gene of interest. The probe is typically labeled with radioactive phosphorus. It preferentially anneals to the melted DNA on the membrane only at the position of the restriction fragment that contains the complementary sequence. After excess probe is removed by washing, the location of the bound probe is determined by autoradiography and compared with the positions of DNA fragments of known size. By varying the conditions of the hybridization and of the subsequent washing steps, one can control the quantity of probe that remains bound as a function of sequence complementarity. Practically, this means that at "high stringency" the probe may need to be an exact complement of the gene of interest, whereas at "low stringency" one can identify related but non-identical sequences.

Restriction sites are generally located at the same positions in the genomes of all individuals of a species. Occasionally, this is not true and a particular restriction site is present only in or near some allelic forms of a gene. This variability in the presence of a particular restriction site leads to variability in the length of the restriction fragment that is detected by Southern blot hybridization using a probe that hybridizes near the variable restriction site. The length of the fragment is inherited as a mendelian allele, and its variation among individuals is described as a **restriction fragment length polymorphism (RFLP).** Southern blotting for RFLPs is now commonly used to study the inheritance of nearby ("linked") genes.

Nucleic acid electrophoresis, blotting, and hybridization with DNA probes have also been used to analyze mRNA molecules. In this case, mRNA is isolated from the cell of interest and subjected to electrophoresis without digestion; mRNA is already single-stranded, and the gel electrophoresis is run under denaturing conditions to prevent internal hybridization. The position of probe binding can indicate the size of the mRNA (rather than of a restriction fragment of DNA), and the extent of probe binding correlates with the abundance of mRNA present in the cell. This technique for RNA analysis is now universally referred to as **Northern blotting,** a biochemist's joke alluding to the DNA blotting technique introduced by Southern that now bears his name.

Genomic Organization of Immunoglobulin Genes

The organization of Ig genes* in the germline is fundamentally similar in all species studied. Genes encoding the two light chains, κ and λ, and the single locus containing the various heavy chain genes are located on different chromosomes. Each set has a similar basic organization, which is illustrated for mouse and human Ig genes in Figures 4–3 and 4–4, respectively.

The Ig heavy and light chain loci are composed of multiple genes that give rise to the V and C regions of the proteins, separated by stretches of non-coding DNA. At the 5′ end of each Ig locus are the **V region exons,** each about 300 base-pairs (bp) long, separated from one another by non-coding DNA of varying lengths. About 90 bp 5′ of each V region exon is a small (60 to 90 bp long) exon that encodes the translation initiation signal and 20 to 30 amino terminal residues of the translated protein. These residues are moderately hydrophobic and make up the **signal** (or **leader) peptides.** Signal sequences are found in secreted and transmembrane proteins, and are involved in guiding the emerging polypeptides during their synthesis on ribosomes into the lumen of the endoplasmic reticulum. Here, the signal sequences are rapidly cleaved and lost from the mature proteins, probably before translation is complete. The numbers of V genes (used here synonymously with V region exons) in the mouse vary from two for λ chains to about 1000 for heavy chains and can be found over large stretches of genomic DNA, at least 1000 to 2000 kilobases (kb) long (Figs. 4–3 and 4–4). In humans, each H or L chain locus contains ~100 to 200 V genes. In all species examined to date, V genes

---

*In Ig (and T cell receptor) loci, the term "gene" usually refers to the DNA encoding the complete H or L chain polypeptide. As we shall discuss presently, each H or L chain gene consists of multiple "gene segments" that code for V, C, and other regions, and are separated from one another in the genome by large stretches of DNA that are never transcribed. Each V and C gene segment is further composed of coding sequences that are present in the mature mRNA; these are called **exons.** For instance, each C_H gene segment that gives rise to a heavy chain C region is composed of five to six exons. Exons are separated by pieces of DNA, called **introns,** that are transcribed and present in the primary (nuclear) RNA but are absent from the mRNA. The removal of introns from the primary transcript is the process of RNA **splicing.** Sometimes, the terms "gene," "gene segment," and "exon" are used interchangeably. For instance, "V gene" might refer to the gene segment coding for the complete V region of an Ig heavy or light chain, which actually consists of a V region exon and additional segments (J and D, as we shall see later), or "V gene" might refer to a V region exon only (as in "V gene families," discussed in this chapter).

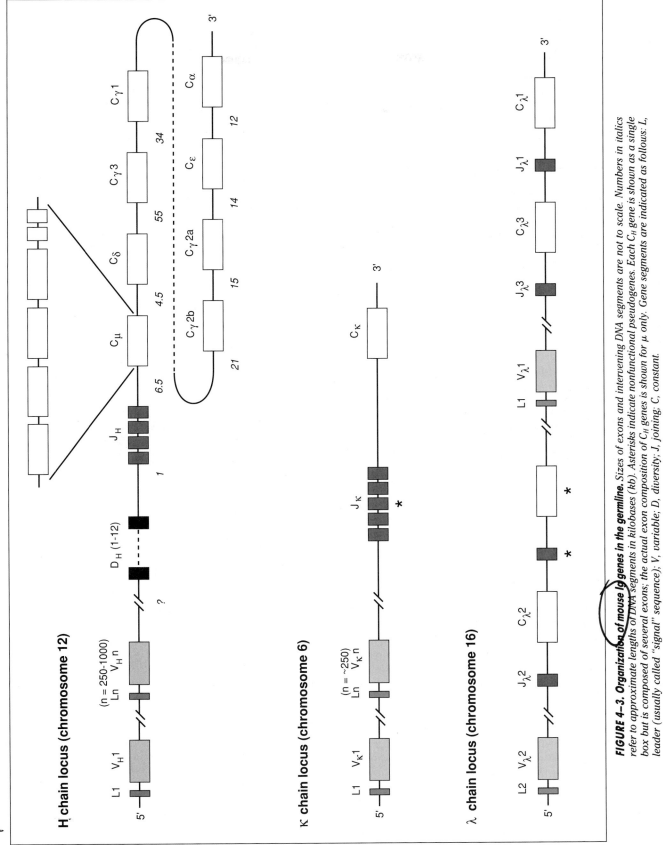

FIGURE 4–3. Organization of mouse Ig genes in the germline. *Sizes of exons and intervening DNA segments are not to scale. Numbers in italics refer to approximate lengths of DNA segments in kilobases (kb). Asterisks indicate nonfunctional pseudogenes. Each C$_H$ gene is shown as a single box but is composed of several exons; the actual exon composition of C$_H$ genes is shown for μ only. Gene segments are indicated as follows: L, leader (usually called "signal" sequence); V, variable; D, diversity; J, joining; C, constant.*

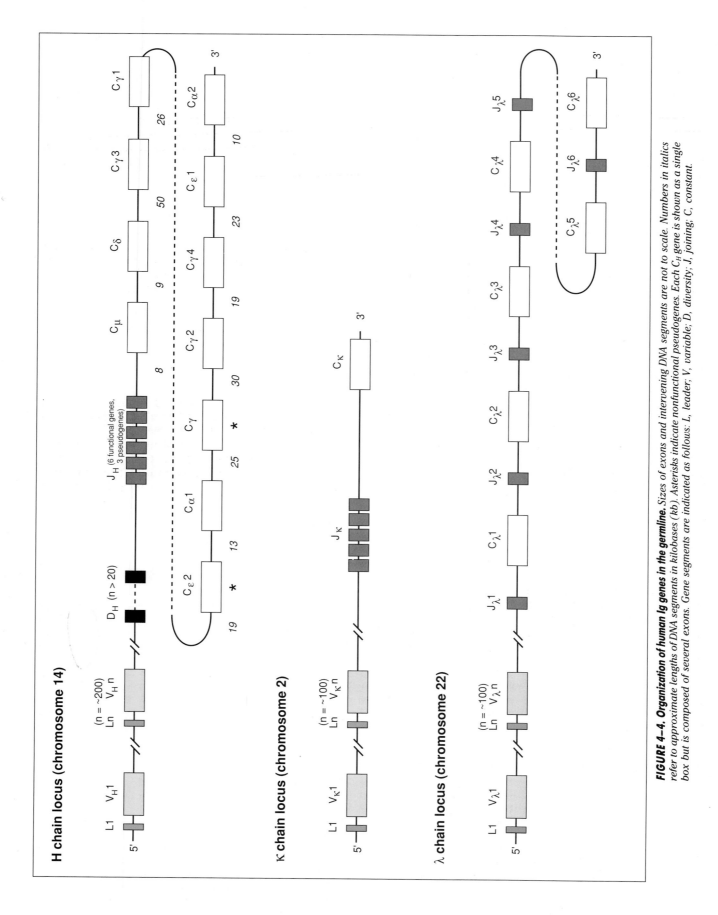

FIGURE 4–4. Organization of human Ig genes in the germline. Sizes of exons and intervening DNA segments are not to scale. Numbers in italics refer to approximate lengths of DNA segments in kilobases (kb). Asterisks indicate nonfunctional pseudogenes. Each C_H gene is shown as a single box but is composed of several exons. Gene segments are indicated as follows: L, leader; V, variable; D, diversity; J, joining; C, constant.

are organized into multiple **families.** The members of each family are identical at 70 to 80 per cent of their nucleotide sequences. Each family is thought to have originated by duplication of a single V gene exon. In the mouse H chain there are at least nine V gene (V_H) families, each consisting of two to 60 members. The sizes and complexities of V gene families in other Ig loci and other species are not fully known yet.

At varying distances 3′ of the V genes are the **C region genes.** In both mice and humans, the κ light chain locus has a single C gene, λ has three to six, and the genes for heavy chain C regions (C_H) of different isotypes are arranged in a tandem array whose order is characteristic for each species. Each heavy chain C region gene actually consists of three to four exons (each similar in size to a V region exon) that make up the complete C region, and smaller exons that code for the carboxy terminal ends, including the transmembrane and cytoplasmic domains of the heavy chains. Between the V and C genes, and separated by introns of varying lengths, are additional coding sequences, 30 to 50 bp long, which make up the **joining (J) segments** and, in the H chain locus only, the **diversity (D) segments.** The J and D gene segments code for the carboxy terminal ends of the V regions, including the third hypervariable (complementarity-determining) regions of antibody molecules. Thus, in an Ig light chain protein (κ or λ), the variable region is encoded by the V and J exons, and the constant region by a C exon (which does not have transmembrane or cytoplasmic segments). In the heavy chain protein, the variable region is encoded by the V, D, and J exons. The constant region of the protein is derived from the multiple C exons and, for membrane-associated heavy chains, the exons encoding the transmembrane and cytoplasmic domains (Fig. 4–5).

Based on the tandem organization of V and C genes in each Ig locus and on the structural homologies between them, it is likely that these genes evolved from repeated duplication of a primordial gene. Each V and C exon codes for an individual domain of an antibody molecule. Other proteins that contain Ig-like disulfide-bonded domains are considered to be members of the Ig gene superfamily (see Box 7–2, Chapter 7) and are encoded by genes that are homologous to Ig V and C genes.

Although the introns and the non-coding DNA sequences between exons are not expressed in mature mRNA, they play an important role in the production of antibodies. As we shall see later, recognition sequences that dictate rearrangement of various exons are present in the non-coding DNA, and nucleotide sequences that regulate transcription and RNA splicing are located in the introns.

Sequence of Immunoglobulin Gene Rearrangement

All cells except B lymphocytes contain Ig genes in the germline configuration, and only B lymphocytes express these genes in functionally rearranged forms, capable of giving rise to functional proteins. *DNA rearrangements in Ig gene loci occur in a precise order*; this explains the pattern of B cell maturation described earlier (see Fig. 4–1). The first rearrangement involves the

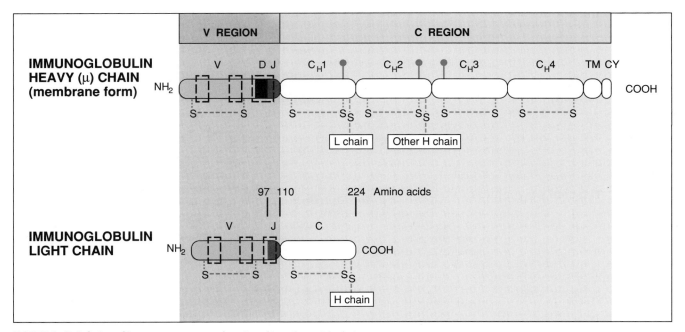

FIGURE 4–5. Relation of Ig gene segments to domains of Ig polypeptide chains. *The V and C regions of Ig polypeptides are encoded by different gene segments. The locations of intrachain and interchain disulfide bonds (S—S) and of carbohydrates (⌐) as shown are approximate. Areas in dashed boxes indicate hypervariable (complementarity determining) regions. In the μ chain, transmembrane (TM) and cytoplasmic (CY) domains are encoded by separate exons. In the light chain, numbers refer to positions of amino acids; see Figure 3–3 for the locations of these residues in the three-dimensional structure.*

heavy chain locus and leads to the joining of one D and one J segment with deletion of the intervening DNA (Fig. 4–6). The D segments 5' of the rearranged D and the J segments 3' of the rearranged J are not affected by this recombination (D1 and J2–4 in Fig. 4–6). DJ rearrangement may actually occur prior to commitment of a lymphoid precursor to the B cell lineage, because

about 20 per cent of T cell–derived tumors contain DJ rearrangements in Ig heavy chain loci. Following the DJ rearrangement, one of the many V genes is joined to the DJ complex, giving rise to a rearranged VDJ gene. At this stage, all D segments 5' of the rearranged D are also deleted. This VDJ recombination occurs only in cells committed to become B lymphocytes and is a

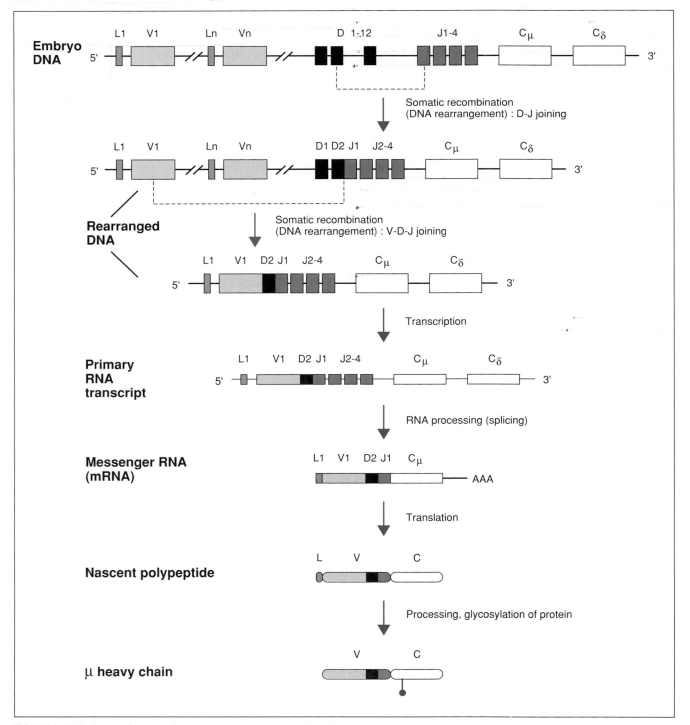

FIGURE 4–6. Sequence of gene rearrangement, transcription, and synthesis of the mouse Ig μ heavy chain. *In this example, the V region of the μ chain is encoded by the exons V1, D2, and J1. V genes are indicated as V1 to Vn; C_H genes 3' of Cδ are not shown; the location of carbohydrates (↑) is schematic; and gene segments and distances between them are not shown to scale.*

critical control point in Ig expression because only the rearranged V gene is subsequently transcribed. The C region genes remain separated from this VDJ complex by an intron (presumably containing the unrearranged J segments), and the primary (nuclear) RNA transcript has the same organization. It is not known whether all the C regions are expressed in the primary transcript. Subsequent processing of the RNA leads to splicing out of the intron between the VDJ complex and the most proximal C region gene, which is C_μ, giving rise to a functional mRNA for the μ heavy chain. Multiple adenine nucleotides, called poly-A tails, are added to one of several consensus polyadenylation sites located 3' of the C_μ RNA. Genes coding for other C_H classes also have 3' polyadenylation sites, which are utilized when these C regions are expressed (see below). It is thought that cleavage of the primary RNA transcript and splicing are tightly coupled to polyadenylation, since most func-

tional, complete mRNAs have poly-A tails. How these events are coordinately regulated is not known. Translation of the μ heavy chain mRNA leads to production of the μ protein, giving rise to the "cytoplasmic μ only" phenotype of the pre–B lymphocyte.

② The next somatic DNA recombination involves a light chain locus (κ and then λ; see below) and follows an essentially similar sequence (Fig. 4–7). One V segment is joined to one J segment, forming a VJ complex, which remains separated from the C region by an intron, and this gives rise to the primary RNA transcript. Splicing of the intron from the primary transcript joins the C gene to the VJ complex, forming an mRNA that is translated to produce the κ or λ protein. The light chain assembles with the previously synthesized μ in the endoplasmic reticulum to form the complete membrane IgM molecule, which is expressed on the cell surface, and the cell is now an immature B lymphocyte.

FIGURE 4–7. Sequence of gene rearrangement, transcription, and synthesis of mouse Igκ light chain. *In this example, the V region of the κ chain is encoded by the exons V1 and J1. V genes are indicated as V1 to Vn; the location of carbohydrates (†) is schematic; and gene segments and distances between them are not shown to scale.*

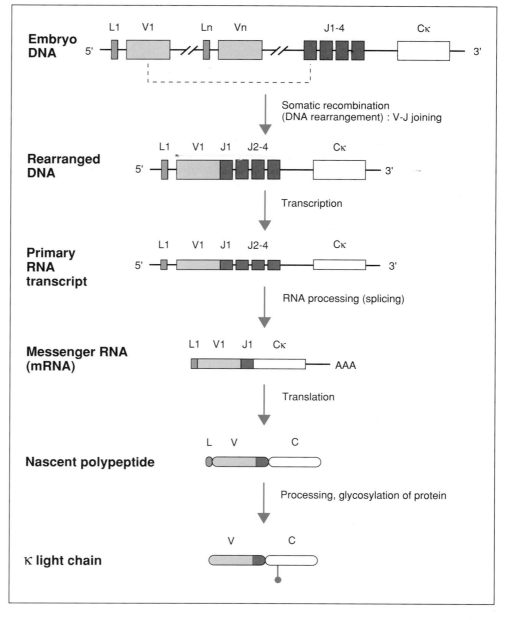

Rearrangements of Ig genes are the essential first steps in the production of antibodies. *In addition, the μ heavy chain protein that is synthesized in a developing B cell itself regulates the somatic recombination of Ig genes in two ways (Fig. 4–8):*

1. First, the μ protein produced by the rearranged gene on one chromosome irreversibly inhibits rearrangement on the other chromosome, accounting for allelic exclusion of Ig heavy chains. Heavy chain genes on the second allelic chromosome will rearrange only if the first rearrangement is nonproductive. Such nonproductive DNA rearrangements may be due to deletions, mutations, or frameshifts during recombination that generate stop codons. Thus, in any B cell, one heavy chain allele is productively rearranged and expressed, and the other is in the germline configuration or is aberrantly rearranged. If both alleles undergo nonproductive recombinations, the cell cannot produce Ig, will be unable to recognize and respond to antigens, and apparently dies. This occurs frequently, and is one of the reasons why only a small fraction of the cells tnat arise from B cell progenitors develop into mature B lymphocytes. Studies with transgenic mice (see Box 4–1) have shown that the membrane but not the secreted form of the μ protein suppresses heavy chain gene rearrangement and is responsible for allelic exclusion; however, the precise mechanism of this suppression is unknown.

2. A second effect of the production of a μ protein in a pre–B cell may be *stimulation of light chain gene rearrangement.* This has been suggested by analyses of pre-B tumor lines in which VJ$_\kappa$ rearrangements spontaneously occur in culture. Such light chain DNA recombinations are seen only in daughter cells of the original clone that synthesize μ protein. Again, the molecular signals by which the μ protein stimulates light chain gene rearrangement are not known. However, light chain gene rearrangement does occur in mice in which the μ gene is knocked out, indicating that the μ protein is not an obligatory stimulus for the rearrangement of light chain genes.

Rearrangement of light chain genes occurs first in the κ locus (Fig. 4–9). If the κ rearrangement is productive, giving rise to a κ protein, subsequent rearrangement of the λ light chain is blocked. Rearrangement of the λ locus occurs only if the rearranged κ genes on both parental chromosomes are unable to code for a functional protein. This explains why an individual B cell clone can produce only one of the two types of light chains during its life (light chain isotype exclusion). It also accounts for the observation that in κ-producing B cells, the λ genes are in a germline or unrearranged configuration, whereas in λ-producing B cells, the κ genes on both chromosomes are either deleted or aberrantly recombined. As in the heavy chain locus, functional rearrangement involving either light chain locus on one of the two parental chromosomes actively prevents rearrangement at the other allele, accounting for allelic exclusion of light chains in individual B cells. Also, as for heavy chains, if one allele undergoes nonfunctional rearrangement, DNA recombination can occur on the other allele; however, if both alleles of both κ and λ chains are nonfunctional, that cell apparently dies.

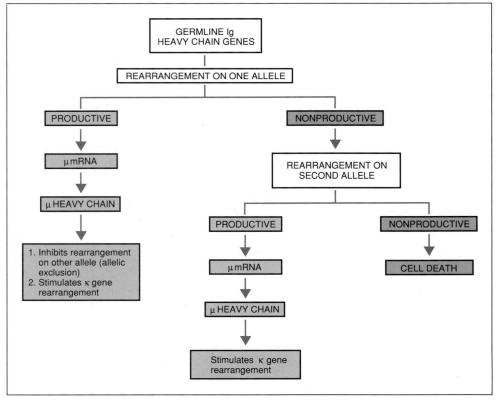

FIGURE 4–8. Order of rearrangement and expression of Ig heavy chain (μ) genes. *The consequences of productive (functional) and nonproductive (aberrant) rearrangements of Ig heavy chain genes on the two allelic chromosomes are shown. The μ chain is the first Ig protein produced in a developing B lymphocyte.*

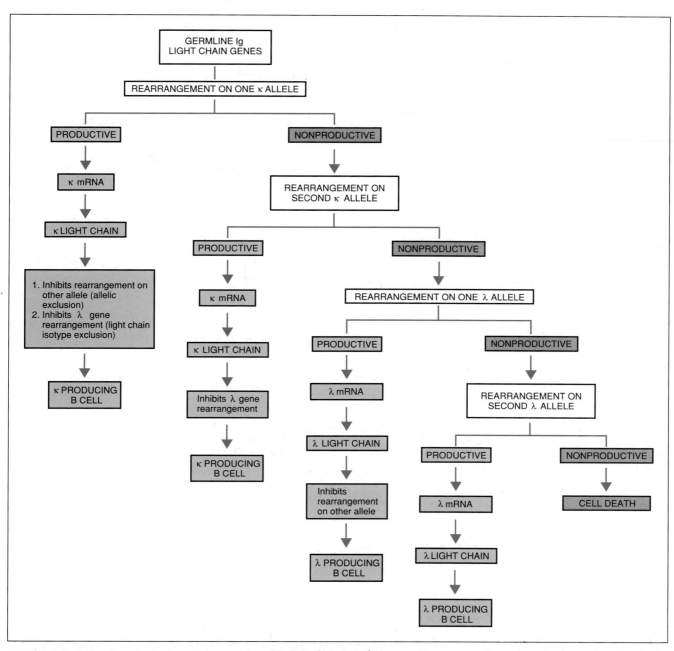

FIGURE 4–9. Order of rearrangement and expression of Ig light chain (κ and λ) genes. *The consequences of productive and nonproductive rearrangements of Ig κ and λ chain genes on the two allelic chromosomes are shown.*

Mechanisms of Immunoglobulin Gene Rearrangement

Rearrangement of Ig (and, as we shall discuss in Chapter 8, T cell receptor) genes occurs principally by a mechanism of excision (looping out) of the DNA between various gene segments followed by ligation of these segments. In the κ locus, some V exons are in a 3′ to 5′ orientation in the germline. These exons can recombine with downstream J gene segments by a process of inversion, in which the V gene segment is in-verted and joined to the J segment without deletion of the intervening DNA.

Ig gene rearrangement is a special kind of recombi-nation involving non-homologous gene segments that is mediated by a system of enzymes. The enzymes that mediate V-D-J or V-J joining actually comprise both lymphocyte-specific activities, which are called **recom-binases,** and more generalized activities, such as ex-onucleases and DNA ligases, that are present in all cells. The lymphocyte-specific recombinases recognize specific DNA **recognition sequences** located in the intervening DNA 3′ of each V exon and 5′ of each J segment and flanking both sides of each D segment (Fig. 4–10). The recognition sequences are highly conserved stretches of seven or nine nucleotides separated by non-conserved 12 or 23 nucleotide spacers. The location of these recognition sequences in a light chain gene allows recombinases to bring the V and J exons into apposition, forming a loop of intervening DNA. The intervening DNA is then excised, and the ends of the V and J exons are annealed to complete the rearrangement process. This same basic mechanism is responsible for DJ and VDJ recombinations in the H chain locus.

Some features of recombinases have been deduced by transfecting fragments of germline Ig genes into various tumors or cell lines and following the spontaneous rearrangement of these genes:

1. Recombinases are cell type–specific. They are active in lymphocytes but not in non-lymphoid cells such as fibroblasts. This may explain why Ig gene rearrangement is observed only in B lymphocytes. It is, however, unlikely to be the complete answer, because the same or similar recombinases appear to act on Ig

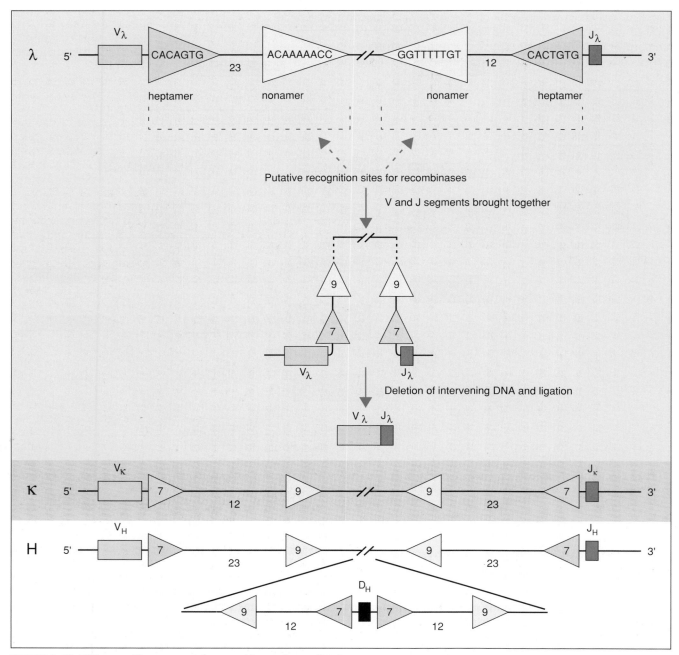

FIGURE 4–10. DNA recognition sequences for recombinases that mediate Ig gene rearrangement. *Conserved heptamer (7 bp) and nonamer (9 bp) sequences, separated by 12 or 23 base pair spacers, are located adjacent to V and J exons (for κ and λ loci), or V, D, and J exons (in the H chain locus). Recombinases presumably recognize these regions and bring the exons together, forming loops of non-coding intervening DNA that are excised and the exons are joined. Alternatively, the exons can be joined by a process of inversion, followed by excision and ligation. (Adapted with permission from Tonegawa, S. Somatic generation of antibody diversity. Nature 302:575–581, 1983. Copyright © 1983, Macmillan Magazines Ltd.)*

and T cell receptor genes *in vitro*, and yet *in vivo* complete, functional rearrangements of Ig genes occur only in B cells, and of T cell receptor genes only in T lymphocytes.

2. Recombinases function only at the early developmental stages of B cells. They are active in immature B cells such as pre-B lines and tumors, but not in antibody-secreting cells like myelomas. Therefore, cells already producing functional antibodies cannot rearrange additional Ig genes and cannot alter their specificity.

Recently, two genes that stimulate Ig gene recombination, called recombination activating genes 1 and 2 (RAG-1 and RAG-2), have been identified in pre–B and immature T cells. It is not known whether these two genes code for the recombinases themselves or for proteins that regulate recombinase function. Knockout of RAG-1 or RAG-2 from mice genes leads to a failure to produce both Ig and T cell receptor proteins, and a complete lack of mature B and T lymphocytes.

Rearrangement of Ig genes during B cell development is also controlled by accessibility of the DNA to recombinases. In eukaryotic cells, most regions of DNA are covered by proteins, condensed into a structure called chromatin, which prevent the uncontrolled expression of genes. Early in B cell maturation, the chromatin structure of Ig genes opens, so that the genes become accessible to recombinases. This allows the functional rearrangement and subsequent transcription of complete Ig genes.

Generation of the Antibody Repertoire

Several different genetic mechanisms contribute to the diversity of membrane-bound and secreted antibodies in each individual. The estimated contribution of each of these mechanisms to the total repertoire of antibodies is summarized in Table 4–1.

TABLE 4–1. Mechanisms Contributing to the Generation of Primary Antibody Diversity in the Mouse*

	H	κ	λ
Germline genes*			
V gene segments	250–1000	250	2
J segments	4	4	3
D segments	12	0	0
Combinatorial joining			
V × J (×D)	10,000–40,000	1000	6
H-L chain associations			
H × κ	$1–4 \times 10^7$		
H × λ	$5–10 \times 10^4$		
Total potential repertoire with junctional diversity	$10^9–10^{11}$		

* Numbers of gene segments and the contribution of junctional diversity are estimates. The mouse is unusual among all species examined because of the low number of V_λ genes and the limited diversity in antibodies with λ light chains. Apart from this, other mammals (including humans) are similar. Somatic mutations may further increase diversity in secondary responses.

1. *Multiple germline genes.* Both heavy chains and light chains may be encoded by multiple germline V genes, which have different sequences and produce Ig molecules with different specificities. Because D genes and J genes also encode portions of the antigen-binding regions of Ig molecules, the utilization of different germline D and J genes also contributes to diversity. The amount of diversity generated at a particular Ig locus correlates with the number of gene segments at that locus. For instance, in mice, 90 to 95 per cent of antibodies that are produced contain κ light chains, and the λ-containing antibodies recognize a quite restricted set of antigens. In mice, the λ locus contains only two functional V genes. In humans, on the other hand, the κ and λ loci contain roughly equal numbers of V genes, are equally represented in antibodies produced, and are similar in their diversity.

2. *Combinatorial diversity.* The somatic recombination of Ig DNA participates in the generation of antibody diversity in several ways. The combinatorial associations of different V, D, and J gene segments lead to a large potential for generating different antibody specificities. The maximum possible number of combinations is the product of the number of V, D (if present), and J exons at each locus. Every clone of B cells and its progeny express a unique combination of V, D, and J genes. One corollary of this observation is that every monoclonal tumor derived from a B cell is also different from all other tumors. Therefore, the pattern of Ig gene rearrangement is a useful marker for assessing the clonality of B cell–derived lymphomas and leukemias (Box 4–3). Because of combinatorial diversity, *antibody molecules show the greatest diversity at the junctions of V and C regions* in both heavy and light chains. These junctions form the third hypervariable region, or CDR3, which is the most important portion of the Ig molecule for binding antigen and for determining the specificities of antibodies (see Chapter 3). The CDR3 of heavy and light chains is actually encoded in a large part by J and/or D gene segments.

3. *Junctional diversity.* Even the same set of germline V, D, and J gene segments can generate different amino acid sequences at the junctions. This additional junctional diversity arises from two mechanisms:

a. The first is inaccurate or **imprecise DNA rearrangement,** which occurs because nucleotide sequences at the 3′ end of a V gene and the 5′ end of a J segment in a light chain, or at the ends of V, J, and D gene segments in a heavy chain, can each recombine at any of several nucleotides in the germline sequence. As long as the recombination does not generate nonfunctional DNA sequences, such as nonsense or stop codons, different nucleotide and, subsequently, amino acid sequences can arise (Fig. 4–11). Imprecise joining can also lead to recombinations that are out of frame so that the DNA cannot be transcribed, and this may be a price that is paid for generating diversity. B cells can occasionally compensate for out-of-frame joining events by deleting one or two nucleotides upstream of the joint.

b. The second mechanism for junctional diversity is **N region diversification.** Nucleotides, called N

BOX 4–3. IMMUNOGLOBULIN GENES IN B LYMPHOCYTE–DERIVED TUMORS

Since the presence of functionally rearranged Ig heavy and light chain genes is the *sine qua non* of a B lymphocyte, examination of tumors for the presence of such rearrangements has proved to be a useful diagnostic and analytical method. Perhaps the earliest significant result of such studies was that tumors that did not express phenotypic markers characteristic of a particular cell lineage could be classified unambiguously. For instance, the cell of origin of hairy cell leukemias was an issue of great debate until the demonstration that virutally all these tumors contained rearranged Ig genes, establishing their derivation from B lymphocytes. The expression of Ig proteins can also be used as a marker for the clonality of B cell tumors. This was initially done by analyzing the frequency of cells producing κ or λ light chains within a proliferative lesion of B lymphocytes. In humans, approximately half of all antibody molecules contain κ and half contain λ light chains. Therefore, if all the B cells in a lesion express either κ or λ, it is likely that this lesion is a monoclonal tumor. Conversely, if equal numbers of cells express κ and λ, the lesion is a polyclonal or non-neoplastic proliferation. This approach has been refined and tremendously improved by our ability to analyze Ig gene rearrangements by Southern blot hybridization, because every clone of B lymphocytes contains unique rearranged VJ and VDJ complexes in light chain and heavy chain loci, respectively. Thus, if genomic DNA from B cell tumors is isolated and digested with a panel of restriction enzymes, and then Southern blots are probed with cDNA probes for J or C regions, the pattern of restriction fragments containing these genes is unique for each clonally derived tumor. This pattern is reflected in the bands detected by Southern blot hybridization. Provided that a sufficiently large panel of restriction enzymes is used, no two tumors will exhibit identical bands. If the lesion being studied is not a tumor but a polyclonal hyperplasia of B lymphocytes, no one rearrangement is present in enough cells to give a discernible band, and a smear of DNA fragments will be visible in Southern blots. Such a distinction between hyperplastic and neoplastic lesions has important therapeutic implications. Moreover, the identification of a unique restriction fragment pattern of a B cell tumor is useful for determining if recurrences in patients are due to new tumors or to growth of tumor cells that resisted treatment. Similarly, if circulating tumor cells develop in the blood of patients with lymphoma initially confined to lymphoid organs, Southern blot analysis can establish whether or not this reflects conversion of the original lymphoma to a leukemic growth phase. A more recent and much more sensitive variation of this approach employs the polymerase chain reaction (PCR; see Box 5–2, Chapter 5). If the N region of a particular B cell tumor is known, PCR analysis using primers spanning these N sequences can be done to identify very small numbers of residual or recurrent tumor cells, because the N region of each B cell clone has a unique sequence.

---

sequences, which are not present in the Ig loci, can be added to the junctions of rearranged VJ or VDJ genes. This addition of new nucleotides is a random process mediated by an enzyme called terminal deoxyribonucleotidyl transferase (TdT).

Because of junctional diversity, the number of different amino acid sequences that are present in the third hypervariable regions of antibody molecules is actually greater than the number of germline J and D segments present in the genome. As we shall see in Chapter 8, both junctional inaccuracies and N region addition are even more important for generating diversity in T cell antigen receptor genes than in Ig genes. In fact, T cell receptor loci contain fewer V genes than Ig loci, and yet the potential for diversity is greater in T cell antigen receptors than in antibody molecules.

4. *Combinations of H and L chain proteins.* In addition to these mechanisms operative at the level of Ig genes, the combination of different H and L chain proteins in different B cells also contributes to diversity of the repertoire, because the V region of each chain participates in antigen recognition.

5. *Somatic mutations.* Changes in antigen-binding specificity as a result of somatic mutations in V genes can lead to a vast potential for generating additional diversity. This process is described later in the chapter.

The expression of different germline V, D, and J genes, combinatorial VJ and VDJ associations, junctional diversity, and H–L chain associations all occur prior to antigenic stimulation. These are the mechanisms responsible for the diversity of the primary, or naive, B cell repertoire. Therefore, in primary antibody responses to multideterminant antigens, multiple antigen-reactive B cell clones expressing different V genes and VJ_L and VDJ_H combinations may be stimulated. This may give rise to specific antibodies with a wide range of affinities for the antigen. In contrast, the secondary antibody response to the same antigen is dominated by only a few of the clones that were stimulated by the first immunization. These clones contain numerous somatic mutations in their Ig V genes (described below), and the cells producing Ig with the highest affinities for antigen are preferentially activated. As a result, the secondary response often consists of a more restricted population of antibodies with a higher average affinity for the antigen.

A practical application of the elucidation of the molecular basis of antibody diversity is the construction of antibodies by *in vitro* techniques. In theory, the mechanisms that generated a diverse antibody repertoire can be replicated in a genetically engineered microorganism that expresses recombinases. This will allow an antibody repertoire to be generated from germline genes in the laboratory, without immunization of individuals. Such an approach could replace hybridoma technology as a means of producing monoclonal antibodies, and is not limited to a particular species of animal. Although this is not yet feasible, some molecular approaches for generating antibodies have been initiated. In one example, the cDNAs encoding the heavy and light chains of a human anti-tetanus toxoid IgG were isolated from a hybridoma. The heavy chain cDNA was terminated after the $C_\lambda 1$ domain, leaving the cod-

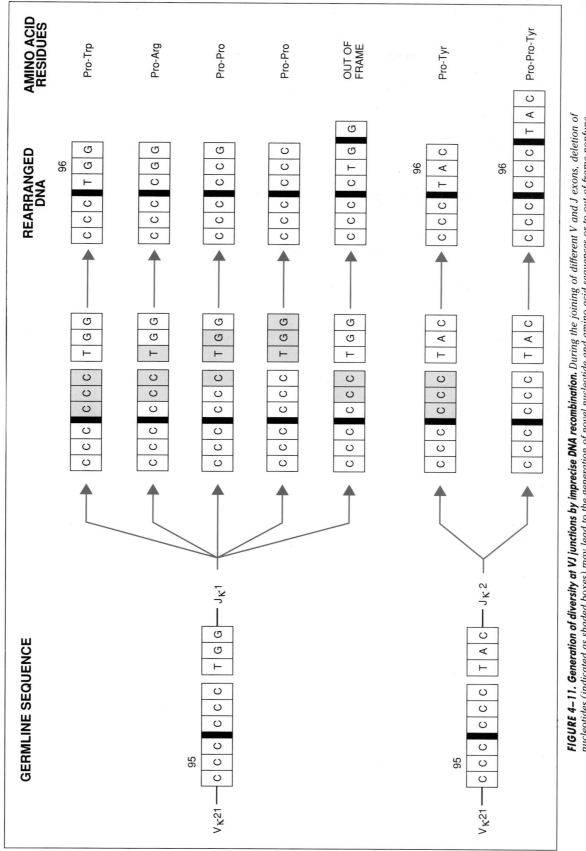

FIGURE 4–11. Generation of diversity at VJ junctions by imprecise DNA recombination. *During the joining of different V and J exons, deletion of nucleotides (indicated as shaded boxes) may lead to the generation of novel nucleotide and amino acid sequences or to out-of-frame nonfunctional recombinations. All the indicated amino acid sequences have been detected in different $V_\kappa 21$ containing mouse antibodies. Two examples are shown, one in which $J_\kappa 1$ was used and another in which $J_\kappa 2$ was used. (Adapted with permission from Weigert, M., R. Perry, D. Kelley, T. Hunkapiller, J. Schilling, and L. Hood. The joining of V and J gene segments creates antibody diversity. Nature 283:497–499, 1980. Copyright © 1980, Macmillan Magazines Ltd.)*

ing information for the Fab fragment. As we discussed in Chapter 3, the heavy chain CDR3 is the most diverse of the six hypervariable regions in Ig and is the only CDR that does not require conserved structural features for folding. It is also, as we discussed above, a major contributor to the diversity of the antibody repertoire. Using molecular techniques, the CDR3 of the V_H cDNA was replaced with random DNA sequences, generating a library of 5×10^7 different members. Each mutated V_H segment and the wild type light chain cDNA were both ligated into a bacteriophage to generate fusion products between the Ig segments and phage coat proteins. Collectively, these modified phages constitute a library of mutant heavy chain molecules, and each phage clone in the library will express on its coat a unique Fab molecule not expressed on other phage clones. Phages producing the recombinant Fab molecules were selected for binding to a hapten (fluorescein) that was not recognized by the original Fab. This experiment demonstrates that antibodies with new specificities can be generated *in vitro* and identified by antigen binding. This "combinatorial library" approach has the potential to replace immunization as a means of producing specific antibodies for laboratory or therapeutic uses.

EXPRESSION OF DIFFERENT CLASSES AND TYPES OF IMMUNOGLOBULINS

The molecular genetic events in the early life of a B cell, which we have described in the previous portion of the chapter, lead to the appearance of cells that express a membrane-associated IgM molecule. This IgM consists of μ heavy chains derived from one of the two parental chromosomes, complexed with κ or λ light chains also derived from one allele. The subsequent changes in Ig gene expression, other than mutations,

occur only in the constant regions of heavy chains and result in the production of membrane or secreted forms of heavy chains of various isotypes. Many of these changes lead to alterations in the functions of the antibody produced by the B cell, but the antigenic specificity of each Ig-producing B cell clone is retained. For instance, the switch in Ig production from a membrane to a secreted form converts the B cell from a cognitive to an effector cell. Because different Ig heavy chain isotypes perform distinct effector functions, heavy chain class switching is important for the elimination of microbes that are susceptible to different effector mechanisms (see Chapter 3). We now know in considerable detail how the clonal progeny of a membrane IgM-producing B cell can express different types of Ig molecules with the same antigen-binding regions as the original, or parent, cell, and how subtle changes in Ig genes after antigenic stimulation lead to increased affinity of antibodies.

Co-expression of IgM and IgD

The mature B lymphocyte is the functionally responsive stage in B cell maturation at which membrane-associated μ and δ heavy chains are co-expressed on the surface of each cell in association with κ or λ light chains. Both classes of Ig heavy chains on each cell have the same V region and, therefore, the same antigen specificity. Simultaneous expression of a single V_H with both C_μ and C_δ to form the two heavy chains occurs by alternative RNA splicing. A long primary RNA transcript is produced containing the rearranged VDJ complex as well as sequences encoded by both C_μ and C_δ genes (Fig. 4–12). If the introns are spliced out such that the VDJ complex is attached to the C_μ RNA, it gives rise to a μ mRNA. If however, the C_μ RNA is spliced out as well so that the VDJ complex becomes contiguous with C_δ, a δ mRNA is produced. Subsequent translation results in the synthesis of a

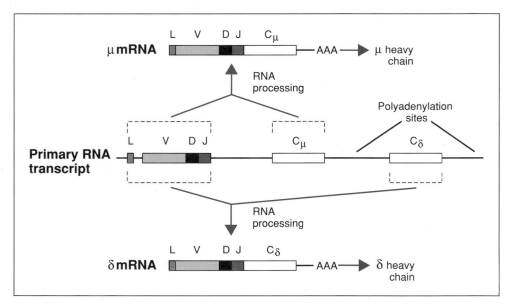

FIGURE 4–12. Co-expression of IgM and IgD in a B lymphocyte. *Alternative processing of a primary RNA transcript results in the formation of a μ or δ mRNA. Dashed lines indicate the H chain segments that are joined by RNA splicing.*

complete μ or δ heavy chain protein. *Thus, alternative splicing allows a B cell to simultaneously produce mature mRNAs of two different heavy chain isotypes.* The precise mechanisms that regulate the choice of polyadenylation and/or splice acceptor sites by which the rearranged VDJ is joined to C_μ or C_δ are not known, nor are the signals that determine when and why a B cell expresses both IgM and IgD rather than IgM alone.

Secretion of Immunoglobulin

Activation of a membrane Ig-expressing mature B lymphocyte by antigen leads to its proliferation and the induction of Ig secretion. Membrane and secreted Ig molecules differ at their carboxy termini (see Fig. 3–5, Chapter 3). For instance, in secreted μ, the $C_\mu 4$ domain is followed by a tail piece containing charged amino acids. In membrane μ, on the other hand, $C_\mu 4$ is followed by a short spacer, 26 hydrophobic transmembrane residues, and a cytoplasmic tail of three amino acids (lysine, valine, and lysine). *The transition from membrane to secreted heavy chain occurs at the level of mRNA processing.* This was first suggested by the observation that in tumors with membrane IgM, the size of the μ mRNA is about 2.7 kb, and in tumors with secreted IgM, it is about 2.4 kb. It is now believed that the primary RNA transcript in all IgM-producing B cells contains the rearranged VDJ, the four C_μ exons coding for the C region domains, a small exon immediately 3' of the fourth C_μ exon encoding the tail piece, and the two exons encoding the transmembrane and cytoplasmic domains. Alternative processing of this transcript, which is regulated by RNA cleavage and the choice of polyadenylation sites, determines whether or not the transmembrane and cytoplasmic exons are included in the mature mRNA (Fig. 4–13). If they are, the μ chain produced contains the amino acids that make up the transmembrane and cytoplasmic segments and is, therefore, anchored in the lipid bilayer of the plasma membrane. If, on the other hand, the transmembrane segment is excluded from the μ chain, the carboxy ter-

minus consists of about 20 amino acids constituting the tail piece. Since this protein does not have a stretch of hydrophobic amino acids or a positively charged cytoplasmic domain, it cannot remain anchored in the cell membrane and is secreted. Thus, each B cell can synthesize both membrane and secreted Ig. As differentiation proceeds, more and more of the Ig is secreted. All other C_H genes contain similar membrane exons, and all heavy chains can apparently be expressed in membrane-bound and secreted forms. The secretory form of the δ heavy chain is rarely made, however, so that IgD is usually present as a membrane-bound protein.

Heavy Chain Class (Isotype) Switching

After antigenic stimulation, mature IgM- and IgD-expressing B cells also undergo the process of heavy chain class (isotype) switching, allowing their progeny to produce antibodies with heavy chains of different classes, such as γ, α, and ϵ. The principal mechanism of isotype switching is a process called **switch recombination,** in which the rearranged VDJ gene segment recombines with a downstream C region gene and the intervening DNA is deleted. This phenomenon was first observed in myelomas, where it was found that cells producing one Ig isotype have deleted all rearranged C_H genes 5' of this isotype. Thus, if the C_μ and C_δ genes are deleted, the rearranged VDJ will be attached to the next C_H complex, giving rise to $\gamma 3$ heavy chains (in the mouse); subsequent deletion of all γ subclass-encoding genes will result in the production of ϵ heavy chains; and so on (Fig. 4–14A). These DNA recombination events are believed to occur at or near nucleotide sequences called **switch regions,** which are located in the introns at the 5' end of each C_H locus. Switch regions occupy distances of 1 to 10 kb and contain numerous tandem repeats of highly conserved DNA sequences, each of which is up to 52 bp long. The precise way they function is not known.

FIGURE 4–13. *Expression of membrane and secreted μ chains by B lymphocytes. Alternative processing of a primary RNA transcript results in the formation of a membrane or secreted μ mRNA. Dashed lines indicate the μ chain segments that are joined by RNA splicing. TM and CY refer to transmembrane and cytoplasmic segments, respectively. $C_\mu 1$, $C_\mu 2$, $C_\mu 3$, and $C_\mu 4$ are four exons of the C_μ gene.*

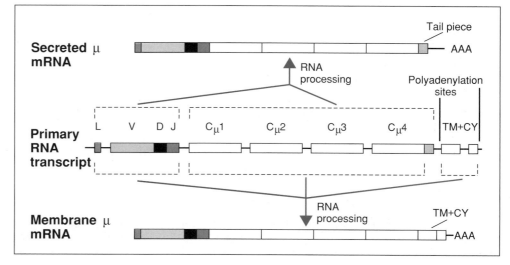

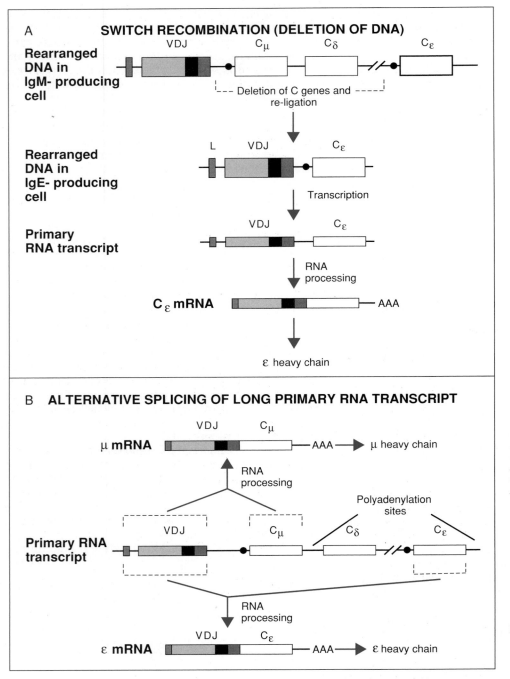

FIGURE 4-14. Mechanisms of heavy chain class (isotype) switching. *Heavy chain class (isotype) switching may be due to two mechanisms:*

A. *Switch recombination: Deletion of C_H genes, of which only C_μ and C_δ are shown, leads to recombination of the VDJ complex with the next, i.e., 3' C_H gene and expression of this gene, which is C_ϵ in the example shown. Switch regions are indicated by dark circles. (Note that the C_γ genes are located between C_δ and C_ϵ but are not shown.)*

B. *Alternative processing of a primary RNA transcript may lead to co-expression of multiple C_H genes, e.g., C_μ and C_ϵ.*

Occasionally, one observes co-expression of multiple heavy chain isotypes by single B cells in immunized animals or in antigen-stimulated cultures. This is inconsistent with switch recombination and deletion of intervening C region genes. An alternative mechanism for isotype switching is the production of a long primary transcript containing many or all C_H genes, followed by **alternative RNA splicing** and production of different mRNAs, much like the process that leads to co-expression of μ and δ or membrane and secreted Ig (Fig. 4–14B). It is possible that early during isotype switching in each B cell clone, alternative RNA splicing leads to co-expression of multiple heavy chain classes in individual cells. As differentiation proceeds, switch

recombination at the level of DNA results in the appearance of cells that produce only the more 3' heavy chain C regions. Throughout these differentiative events, the expressed VDJ complex and, therefore, the specificity of the Ig heavy chain remain unaltered (except, of course, for somatic mutations). Also, each B cell clone continues to produce only one light chain isotype, either κ or λ.

Heavy chain class switching is not a random process but is regulated by helper T cells and their secreted cytokines (see Chapter 9). For instance, the production of IgE is stimulated by a T cell–derived cytokine called interleukin-4 (IL-4), which is a necessary and sufficient "IgE switch factor." Similarly, the cytokine interferon-gamma (IFN-γ) selectively induces switching to IgG2a in mice. Cytokines induce switching to particular heavy chain isotypes by stimulating transcription through switch regions located 5' to C region genes, and this is followed by switch recombination of the rearranged VDJ complex to that C region (see Fig. 9–7, Chapter 9). The importance of switch regions in this process has been established by experiments showing that disruption of the switch region 5' of any C gene segment by homologous recombination prevents switching to and production of that isotype. Furthermore, the C_δ gene lacks a switch region, and switching to the IgD isotype does not occur after antigenic stimulation.

Somatic Mutations in Immunoglobulin Genes

After antigenic stimulation, the Ig heavy and light chain genes undergo another type of structural alteration, namely somatic mutations. *Somatic mutations in Ig genes involve primarily V gene segments and are principally responsible for the affinity maturation of antibodies.* In addition, mutations that alter antigen-binding specificities of Ig molecules can contribute to the generation of even more diversity of the B cell repertoire.

Comparison of V region amino acid and nucleotide sequences of IgM and IgG antibodies specific for the same antigen first revealed the existence of large numbers of point mutations in the IgG antibodies. Several features of the somatic mutations that occur in Ig genes have been established:

1. In the clonal progeny of B cells responding to a protein antigen or a hapten-protein conjugate, the numbers of mutations in heavy and light chain V genes are higher in IgG than in IgM antibodies, increase with time after the first immunization, and are even more frequent after secondary and tertiary immunizations (Fig. 4–15). These conclusions are based largely on comparisons of IgM- and IgG-producing antigen-specific hybridomas derived from B cells at different times after immunizations with the antigen.

2. Point mutations tend to be clustered in V region exons and adjacent flanking sequences of both H and L chains and are most numerous in the hypervariable regions (Fig. 4–15). One possible explanation for this localization of somatic mutations is that particular areas of the gene are mutation-sensitive. Alternatively, mutations may occur in rapidly proliferating B cells randomly throughout rearranged V genes, but only the ones involving antigen-combining sites lead to increased affinities of antibodies. B cells that produce antibodies of higher affinities are positively selected by antigen. This is because as the immune response develops, more antibody is produced and the concentration of available antigen decreases. Under these conditions, B cells that bind the antigen with higher affinity are preferentially stimulated. The germinal centers of lymphoid follicles in peripheral lymphoid tissues are the principal sites of somatic mutation in Ig V genes and subsequent selection of high-affinity antigen-specific B cells (see Chapter 9). Since mutations occur after antigenic stimulation, they tend to be more numerous in isotype-switched antibodies and in memory B cells. Therefore, memory B cells have higher average affinities for antigen than do naive cells.

3. Mutations may lead to loss of antigen-binding activity, so that B cells in which this happens become antigen-unresponsive and may die. Alternatively, as a result of somatic mutations, the Ig produced by a particular B cell may no longer be specific for the immunizing antigen but may acquire a new specificity for a different antigen. This is a potential mechanism for increasing the diversity of antibodies.

4. The somatic mutation rate is estimated to be 10^{-3} per V gene base pair per cell division, which is 10^3 to 10^4 times higher than the spontaneous rate of mutation in other mammalian genes. (For this reason, mutation in Ig V genes is also called "hypermutation.") Because the V genes of expressed heavy and light chains in each B cell contain a total of about 700 nucleotides, this implies that mutations will accumulate in expressed V regions at an average rate of almost one per cell division. It is estimated that as a result of somatic mutations, the nucleotide sequences of IgG antibodies derived from one clone of B cells can diverge 1 to 5 per cent from the original germline sequence. This usually translates to less than ten amino acid substitutions because some mutations may not change the V region amino acid sequence.

5. Affinity maturation is observed only in antibody responses to helper T cell–dependent protein antigens. Therefore, it is likely that T cells or their products are involved in stimulating mutational mechanisms or in selecting and stimulating B cells whose expressed V genes contain mutations that lead to increased antibody affinities (see Chapter 9).

The precise mechanisms of somatic mutations in Ig genes are poorly understood. Immunologists are actively searching for cell lines in which mutations can be induced *in vitro* by antigens and helper T cells or by T cell–derived cytokines. Such models should prove valuable for analyzing the extrinsic signals, enzymes, and regulatory mechanisms responsible for the extraordinarily high mutation rate in Ig V genes.

TRANSCRIPTIONAL AND TRANSLATIONAL CONTROL OF ANTIBODY PRODUCTION

The elucidation of the structure and expression of Ig genes during B cell maturation has been a remarkable milestone in the progress of immunology. More recently, attention has been devoted to a better understanding of the regulation of Ig gene expression. There are several reasons why this is an important area of scientific investigation. First, the production of Ig is an excellent example of the expression of cell type–

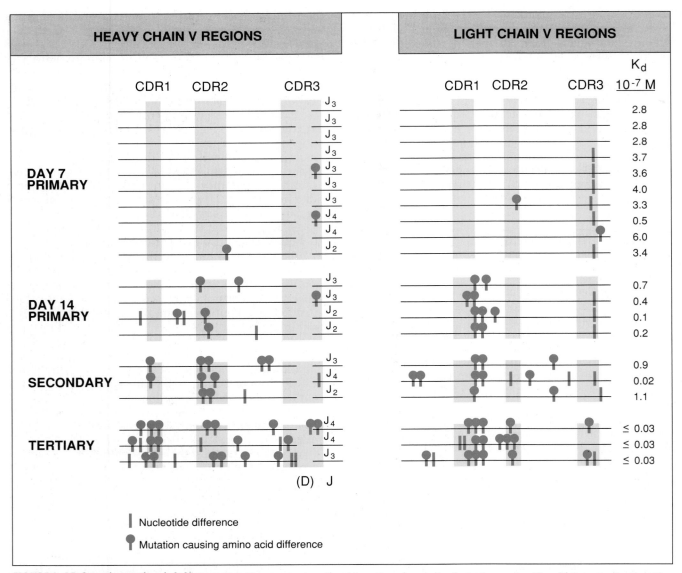

FIGURE 4–15. Somatic mutations in Ig V genes. *Hybridomas were produced from the spleen cells of mice immunized 7 or 14 days previously with a hapten, oxazolone, coupled to a protein, or from spleen cells obtained after secondary and tertiary immunizations with the same antigen. Hybridomas producing oxazolone-specific monoclonal antibodies were isolated, and the nucleotide sequences of the V genes encoding the Ig H and L chains were determined. Mutations in V genes increase with time after immunization and with repeated immunizations, and are clustered in the complementarity-determining regions (CDRs). The location of CDR3 in the heavy chains is approximate. The affinities of the antibodies also tend to increase with more mutations, as indicated by the lower dissociation constants (K_d) for hapten binding. Note that the use of different J segments also contributes to variability of antibodies. (Adapted with permission from Berek, C., and C. Milstein. Mutation drift and repertoire shift in the maturation of the immune response. Immunological Reviews 96:23–41, 1987. Munksgaard International Publishers Ltd, Copenhagen, Denmark.)*

specific, developmentally regulated genes. Second, changes in the pattern of Ig biosynthesis and secretion can be induced by well-defined external stimuli such as antigens, polyclonal activators, and helper T cells or T cell–derived cytokines (see Chapter 9). Finally, abnormalities in antibody production contribute to the pathogenesis of many diseases associated with deficient or excessive immune responses.

The general principles of transcriptional regulation of Ig genes are probably similar to those for other genes. Transcription is controlled primarily by *cis*-acting nucleotide sequences and by proteins that bind to these sequences. The production of antibodies is also

influenced by the rate of turnover of mRNAs, their translation, and the post-translational modification and assembly of heavy and light chains.

Cell Type–Specific Regulation of Immunoglobulin Gene Transcription

The transcription of most eukaryotic genes, including Ig genes, is regulated by two types of DNA sequences, called **promoters** and **enhancers**. The functions of these regulatory sequences have been defined by attaching the sequences to "reporter" genes, transfecting the constructs into cell lines, and monitoring the expression of the "reporter" mRNA and proteins. By mutating or deleting nucleotides within the regulatory sequences, it is possible to identify segments that function to varying degrees to control gene transcription.

Promoters are located immediately 5′ of the site where transcription is initiated, and their principal function is to ensure accurate and efficient transcrip-

---

BOX 4 – 4. NUCLEAR FACTORS AND THE REGULATION OF Ig GENE TRANSCRIPTION

The transcriptional activity of Ig genes, like that of other genes, is regulated by two *cis*-acting elements, promoters and enhancers. Deletion and mutational analyses have revealed the existence of several critical nucleotide sequences in Ig promoters and enhancers that are necessary for their function. Some of these sequences are active preferentially in B cells, whereas others stimulate transcription of a wide variety of genes in addition to Ig in diverse cell types. In general, the Ig heavy chain enhancer functions maximally in concert with the heavy chain promoter in B cells and serves to facilitate the formation of stable transcription-initiation complexes.

The functions of promoters and enhancers are controlled by **trans-acting nuclear factors**, also called **transcription factors**. These factors are DNA-binding proteins that bind to specific nucleotide sequences in promoters and enhancers and are capable of inhibiting or stimulating the transcription of nearby genes. In many cell types, particular DNA-binding proteins are induced or activated by stimuli that elicit biologic responses. Therefore, DNA-binding proteins may provide an important link between external stimulation of a cell and the subsequent response, which leads to specific changes in gene expression.

Several *assays* for DNA-binding proteins have been described; the three most widely used are

1. *DNA footprinting.* If a segment of DNA has a protein bound to it, that segment will be resistant to digestion by deoxyribonuclease (DNase). If a radioactively labeled DNA fragment (probe) is incubated with a putative DNA-binding protein, partially digested, and electrophoresed to separate fragments of different sizes, a DNA sequence that contains bound protein will resist enzymatic degradation and will produce a gap in the array of sized DNA fragments. Thus, each DNA sequence with associated protein will exhibit a characteristic "footprint."

2. *Methylation interference.* The same principle is used in an assay in which specific nucleotides are methylated, and attached methyl groups are detected by cleavage at methylated G residues and electrophoresis. Bound proteins interfere with methylation and, therefore, create detectable "gaps" in the pattern of methylation. If methylation is performed on intact cultured cells instead of isolated DNA, this assay is called "*in vivo* footprinting." It is used to identify genes with bound proteins in the cells.

3. *Electrophoretic mobility shift assay.* If a putative DNA-binding protein contained in a cell extract is incubated with a radioactively labeled target nucleotide sequence *in vitro* and then electrophoresed, the complex that is formed will migrate slowly in comparison to the nucleotide sequence alone. Thus, retardation of the target nucleotide indicates an increase in size as a consequence of the binding of a protein.

Using such assays, nuclear factors have been described that bind to several sites in the promoters and enhancers of Ig genes. Ig heavy chain promoters contain a conserved octanucleotide (ATGCAAAT) that is also present in the κ chain promoter, in reverse orientation in the Ig heavy chain enhancer, and in many non-Ig promoters as well. Transcription of Ig genes in B cells is critically dependent on the presence of an intact octamer motif in promoters. At least three proteins that specifically bind to the octamer have been isolated from nuclear extracts of mammalian cells. One, called Oct1 (or OTF1, for octamer transcription factor 1), is a ubiquitous mammalian transcription activator. Two others, Oct2 (OTF2A) and OTF2B, are lymphoid-specific and activate transcription of Ig genes. Oct2 has been molecularly cloned and has been shown to contain a domain homologous to a homeobox motif, which was originally identified as a component of *Drosophila* genes involved in morphogenesis. Expression of Oct2 cDNA in non-lymphoid cell lines strongly activates co-transfected "reporter" genes if these genes are linked to octamer-containing Ig promoter sequences. Such experiments provide formal proof of the specificity and transcriptional activity of DNA-binding proteins like Oct2. The mouse κ chain enhancer contains a 10 bp sequence that is the target of a DNA-binding protein called NF-κB (NF = nuclear factor). The NF-κB site is present in many other genes, such as the gene encoding the cytokine interleukin-2 and the α chain of the interleukin-2 receptor (Chapter 7).

NF-κB has some interesting properties, and is widely used as a model for studying transcription factors. In pre–B cells, NF-κB is a dimer of a 50 kD protein (p50) and a 65 kD protein (p65). In other cells, it may be a homodimer of p50 or p65, or may contain one of these associated with another member of this family of proteins (such as the cellular oncogene, *c-rel*). Several proteins have been shown to interact with NF-κB and to inhibit its activity. These inhibitors are called I-κB's. In unstimulated cells in which NF-κB is inactive, it resides in the cytoplasm bound to an I-κB. Certain stimuli activate the cellular enzyme protein kinase C, which phosphorylates I-κB and releases it from the NF-κB, allowing NF-κB to migrate to the cell nucleus and stimulate transcription of responsive genes. NF-κB is inactive in pre–B cells, which do not transcribe Ig κ genes constitutively. Treatment of the cells with lipopolysaccharide (LPS) activates protein kinase C, induces functional NF-κB, and stimulates κ gene transcription. NF-κB is also inactive or absent in myeloma cells that do actively synthesize κ chains, suggesting that this nuclear factor and, by implication, the κ enhancer may be required early in B cell differentiation to initiate κ gene transcription but are not needed to maintain transcription later in development.

Our understanding of transcription factors and the regulation of cell type–specific gene expression is still incomplete. Nevertheless, it is possible to come to some basic, albeit tentative, conclusions about the *general properties* of transcription factors.

1. Many transcription factors are widely distributed among different cell types and are not specific for particular genes.

2. Their activity may be inducible by external stimuli and may be related to the maturational stage of the cell.

3. They have positive and negative effects whose interplay determines the net level of gene transcription.

4. Although transcription factors are widely distributed, some of them do have effects that are cell type–specific and/or developmentally regulated. This may be because the binding sites on promoters and enhancers are unique and regulated, or because of endogenous inhibitors whose activity is specifically altered by cellular maturation or stimulation.

tion. The basic organization of Ig promoters is similar to promoters for other genes. Ig promoters contain AT-rich sequences, called TATA boxes, located immediately 5' of each V gene segment, which function to determine where transcription is initiated by RNA polymerase II. Most Ig promoters also contain numerous DNA sequences, including a conserved octanucleotide (which is also found in other genes), that stimulate transcription of adjacent genes preferentially in lymphoid cells and are believed to be the targets of nuclear DNA-binding proteins. Such proteins are derived from other distant genes and are, therefore, said to be *trans*-acting. They are postulated to play a prominent role in regulating transcription (Box 4–4).

Enhancer elements are DNA sequences whose major function is to increase the rate of transcription of linked genes. Enhancers function in an orientation-independent manner and, unlike promoters, are capable of enhancing transcription when situated at substantial distances upstream or downstream from the gene being transcribed. Many enhancers are tissue-specific; i.e., they function best in particular cell types and are maximally active in concert with the appropriate promoters. Enhancer elements have been identified in mouse and human heavy and light (κ) chain loci. One mouse heavy chain enhancer is located 3' of the J_H segments, and it is believed that a consequence of VDJ recombination is to bring the promoter located 5' of a V gene closer to this enhancer, permitting more efficient initiation of transcription (Fig. 4–16). Nuclear factors that are activated by external stimuli and bind to Ig heavy and κ chain enhancers have also been identified. The interactions of these protein factors with one another and with regulatory DNA sequences may be critical for stimulating cell type–specific Ig gene transcription in response to external signals and spontaneously during B cell maturation (Box 4–4). Recent experiments using gene knockout suggest that enhancers located 3' of Ig genes may also play a role in heavy chain isotype switching and in

somatic hypermutation. The mechanisms of these effects are not known.

Since Ig genes are transcriptionally active in B cells and are sites for multiple DNA recombinational events, foreign genes can be abnormally translocated to Ig loci and, as a result, may become transcriptionally active. For instance, in certain tumors of B cells, oncogenes are translocated to switch sites located 5' of heavy or light chain C region genes. Such chromosomal translocations are frequently accompanied by enhanced transcription of the oncogenes and are believed to be one of the factors causing the development of tumors of B lymphocytes (Box 4–5).

Regulation of Messenger RNA Turnover and Translation

The turnover rate of Ig mRNA changes during B cell differentiation and correlates with the quantity of Ig synthesized. For instance, the half-life of Ig mRNA in myelomas, which actively secrete large amounts of antibodies, is as long as 20 to 40 hours; in B cell lymphomas, which produce much lower quantities of Ig only in the membrane-bound form, the half-life is less than 6 hours. This may be one of the reasons why plasma cells contain 100 to 500 times more cytoplasmic Ig mRNA than do nonsecreting B lymphocytes. Moreover, if B lymphoma cell lines are stimulated to secrete more Ig, the level of steady-state Ig mRNA increases five to ten times more than the transcription rate, as measured by nuclear run-off assays. This implies that Ig mRNA is stabilized after stimulation and its half-life is prolonged. The mechanisms that control turnover of mRNA are largely unknown.

The importance of translational control in regulating Ig production is suggested by several observations. Mature B cells, despite containing about ten times more

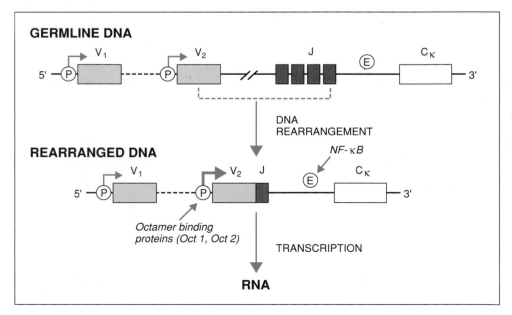

FIGURE 4–16. Transcriptional regulation of immunoglobulin genes. VDJ rearrangement brings promoter sequences (shown as ⓟ) close to the enhancer (E) located between the J and C loci, resulting in increased transcription of the rearranged V gene (V2, whose active promoter is indicated by a bold arrow). Also shown are the sites of binding of the nuclear factors Oct1, Oct2 and NF-κB.

BOX 4–5. CHROMOSOMAL TRANSLOCATIONS IN TUMORS OF B LYMPHOCYTES

Reciprocal chromosomal translocations in many tumors, including lymphomas and leukemias, were first noted by cytogeneticists in the 1960s, but their significance remained unknown until almost 20 years later. At this time, sequencing of switch regions 5' of C_H genes in B cell tumors revealed the presence of DNA segments that were not derived from Ig genes. This was first observed in two tumors derived from B lymphocytes, human Burkitt's lymphoma and murine myelomas. The "foreign" DNA was identified as a portion of the c-myc proto-oncogene, which is normally present on chromosome 8 in man. Proto-oncogenes are normal cellular genes that often code for proteins involved in cell growth and regulation, such as growth factors, receptors for growth factors, or transcription-activating factors. In normal cells, their expression is tightly regulated. When these genes are altered by mutations, inappropriately expressed, or incorporated into and reintroduced in cells by RNA retroviruses, they can become transcriptionally active and function as oncogenes. Such deregulation is postulated to be one of the mechanisms that lead to enhanced cellular growth and, ultimately, neoplastic transformation.

The most common translocation in Burkitt's lymphoma is t(8;14), involving the Ig heavy chain locus on chromosome 14; less commonly, t(2;8) or t(8;22) translocations are found, involving the κ or λ light chain loci, respectively. In all cases of Burkitt's lymphoma, c-myc is translocated from chromosome 8 to one of the Ig loci, which explains the reciprocal 8;14, 2;8, or 8;22 translocations detectable in these tumors. Because the Ig loci normally undergo several genetic rearrangements during B cell differentiation, they are likely sites for accidental translocations of distant genes. Detailed molecular analysis has revealed differences in the architecture of the translocations in different Burkitt's lymphomas, suggesting that rearrangements are sometimes catalyzed by isotype-switching enzymes and sometimes catalyzed by VDJ recombinase enzymes.

The product of the myc gene most likely acts as a nuclear regulatory factor controlling the transcription of genes required for cellular proliferation. Aberrant myc expression can lead to the development of malignant tumors, presumably by interfering with the normal control of cell growth. Other examples of the association of aberrant myc expression and tumors include the oncogenic potential of the avian myelocytomatosis virus, which carries a viral homolog of myc, the presence of multiple (amplified) copies of the myc gene in the genomes of many human tumors, and the development of B cell lymphomas in mice carrying a myc transgene linked to an Ig promoter.

An attractive hypothesis for the etiology of Burkitt's lymphomas is that translocations of myc into the Ig loci transcriptionally activate the cellular oncogene, leading to malignant transformation. In fact, these translocated myc genes are continually transcribed in Burkitt's lymphoma cell lines, but the unrearranged myc alleles in the same cells are not. Just how the myc gene becomes transcriptionally deregulated after translocation remains unknown. One possibility is that when myc is translocated to a site of active gene transcription, adjacent to Ig loci, the result is enhanced transcription of myc itself, and this leads to tumor development in the cells in which Ig genes are active, i.e., B lymphocytes. Although the regulatory components (promoters, enhancers) of the Ig genes can be very active, it is unknown whether they influence transcription of translocated myc genes. Several observations suggest that this is not the case. First, translocated myc genes may be in the opposite transcriptional orientation (i.e., 3' to 5') to the Ig genes. Second, the 5' IgH enhancer is often lost from the site of translocation. Third, the myc gene may end up quite distant from the Ig gene, out of the presumed range of influence of Ig regulatory sequences. Fourth, the myc gene is often translocated to the excluded allele, i.e., the functionally unrearranged, transcriptionally inactive Ig locus. It is also possible that translocation removes the myc gene from regulatory influences of genomic sequences that are left behind on chromosome 8. As a result, the myc gene becomes abnormally active. Although the precise mechanisms of myc deregulation are not yet known, these B cell tumors may illustrate a general concept that activation of cellular oncogenes, coupled with their location next to normal genes that are functional in particular cells, may be one of the mechanisms causing neoplastic transformation of these cells.

Other oncogenes and normal cellular genes are also involved in reciprocal chromosomal translocations in lymphomas and leukemias derived from cells other than B lymphocytes. Some examples are listed in the table. In T lymphocyte–derived tumors chromosomal translocations also often involve loci coding for antigen receptors. Some lymphocytic leukemias contain translocations that do not involve breakpoints at antigen receptor genes.

Type of Tumor	Chromosomal Translocations
B Cell–Derived	
Burkitt's lymphoma	t(8;14) (q24.1; q32.3) Less frequently, t(8;22) (q24.1; q11.2) or t(2;8) (p12; q24.1)
Intermediate lymphoma	t(11;14) (q13.3; q32.3)
Follicular lymphoma	t(14;18) (q32.3; q21.3)
T Cell–Derived	
Chronic lymphocytic leukemia	t(14;19) (q32.1; q13)
Acute lymphoblastic leukemia	t(8;14) (q24.1; q11.2) t(11;14)(p13;q11.2) t(7;9) (q34; q32) Numerous others reported

The above are illustrative examples of chromosomal translocations that have been characterized in human lymphomas and leukemias. Each translocation is indicated by the letter t. The first pair of numbers refers to the chromosomes involved, e.g., (8;14), and the second pair to the bands of each chromosome, e.g., (q24.1; q32.3). The normal chromosomal locations of antigen receptor genes (indicated in bold) are as follows: IgH 14q32.3; Igκ 2p12; Igλ 22q11.2; T cell receptor α 14q11.2; T cell receptor β 7q34; T cell receptor γ 7p15; and T cell receptor δ 14q11.

The normal location of the c-myc oncogene is 8q24.1. The bcl-2 gene at 18q21.3 produces a protein that prolongs the survival of cells. The bcl-1 gene at 11q13.3 encodes cyclin D1, a protein involved in cell cycle progression from the G1 to the S phase.

Courtesy of Dr. Jeffrey Sklar, Department of Pathology, Harvard Medical School and Brigham and Women's Hospital, Boston.

μ mRNA (for the membrane form) than δ mRNA, express more membrane IgD than IgM. Antibody-secreting cells often contain mRNAs for the membrane forms of heavy chains even when they do not express detectable membrane Ig. Such observations indicate that translation of Ig mRNA is a regulated process that varies according to the stage of B lymphocyte maturation and differentiation, but the control mechanisms are not yet identified.

Synthesis, Glycosylation, and Assembly of Immunoglobulin Molecules

Immunoglobulin heavy and light chains, like most secreted and membrane proteins, are synthesized on membrane-bound ribosomes in the rough endoplasmic reticulum. The 5′ signal peptides are cleaved co-translationally in the endoplasmic reticulum. The covalent association of heavy and light chains, created by the formation of disulfide bonds, probably occurs in the endoplasmic reticulum as well, where high-mannose oligosaccharides may be added to asparagine residues (N-linked glycosylation). Following synthesis, the polypeptide chains are directed into the cisternae of the Golgi complex, where the high-mannose carbohydrates are converted to their mature forms by the trimming of terminal mannose and the addition of other sugar side chains. Assembled antibody molecules are transported to the plasma membrane in vesicles, where they become anchored into the cell membrane or are secreted by a process of reverse pinocytosis. Moreover, other proteins that bind to Ig are coordinately regulated. For instance, the "J chains" attached to IgA and IgM (see Chapter 3) are believed to be important for the polymerization of the secreted forms of these antibodies (and are not related to J gene segments in Ig loci). In cells producing such antibodies, transcriptional activation of Ig heavy and light chains is accompanied by coordinate stimulation of J chain gene transcription and biosynthesis.

Intracellular Transport, Surface Expression, and Secretion of Immunoglobulins

The expression of membrane and secreted forms of Ig is also controlled by mechanisms that determine the intracellular fate of newly synthesized proteins. For instance, pre–B cells synthesize both the membrane and secreted forms of μ heavy chains but do not express significant quantities of either; i.e., most of the μ in pre–B cells is in the cytoplasm. It is thought that the secreted form of μ is retained intracellularly bound to proteins that reside within the lumen of the endoplasmic reticulum. One such protein has been given the rather uninformative designation "binding protein," or Bip. It is a member of the heat shock family of proteins

and acts as a chaperonin, the name given to molecules that conduct newly synthesized proteins among various intracellular compartments. Bip complexed to μ heavy chains may shuttle between the endoplasmic reticulum and a pre-Golgi compartment. This is one of the mechanisms that ensures that μ heavy chains of the secretory form are not secreted in pre–B cells, and probably also not in immature and mature B cells prior to activation by antigen. Another retention mechanism appears to involve the carboxy terminal tail piece that is found in the secretory forms of μ (and α) heavy chain proteins. These retention mechanisms are evidently turned off after antigen exposure, allowing Ig to be secreted. Although most of the studies of retention and secretion have focused on μ heavy chains, similar mechanisms are probably operative for other heavy chain isotypes.

Membrane-type μ heavy chains in pre–B cells bind to surrogate light chains and are rapidly degraded intracellularly. As the cells mature, the surrogate light chains are replaced by *bona fide* light chains (κ or λ), and this apparently protects the heavy chains from intracellular degradation. The result is expression of IgM on the surface of B cells. In mature B lymphocytes, IgM and IgD are present on the cell surface non-covalently associated with two other proteins, called Igα and Igβ. Thus, the antigen receptor of B cells is actually a complex of proteins, analogous to the T cell antigen receptor complex in T lymphocytes (see Chapter 7). Igα and Igβ serve the same two functions for Ig in B cells as the CD3 and ζ proteins do for T cell antigen receptors. These functions are assembly and expression of the complex in the plasma membrane, and the transduction of signals generated by binding of antigen to membrane Ig (see Chapter 9).

OTHER SURFACE MOLECULES OF B LYMPHOCYTES

In addition to the antigen receptor complex, B lymphocytes express a variety of cell surface proteins of immunologic significance. These have been identified by numerous techniques, the most useful of which is the production of monoclonal antibodies specific for B cells. Some of the important surface molecules of B cells are listed in Table 4–2; note that many of these are not unique to cells of the B lymphocyte lineage.

These surface proteins on B cells are important for several reasons:

1. They may be lineage- and maturation-specific phenotypic markers for B cells. Combinations of monoclonal antibodies reactive with B lymphocytes form clusters of differentiation that are expressed at different stages of B cell maturation (Fig. 4–17). To date, however, there are few available monoclonal antibodies that definitively distinguish between resting, activated, and memory B lymphocytes, all of which fall into the broad category of "mature B cells." Despite the production of numerous B cell–reactive monoclonal antibodies, the expression of endogenously synthesized mem-

TABLE 4–2. Selected Surface Molecules of B lymphocytes

Surface Molecule	Function/Significance
Immunoglobulin (Ig)	Antigen receptor
Class II MHC molecules	Role in helper T cell–B cell interactions
CD40	Role in helper T cell–B cell interactions
CD5 (Ly-1)	Marker for distinct subset of B cells
CD9	Marker for acute leukemias
CD10 (CALLA)	Marker for acute leukemias
CD19 (B4)	? Role in B cell activation
CD20 (B1)	? Role in B cell activation
CD22	? Role in B cell activation; binds to CD45R on T cells
B7 (also present on activated macrophages, dendritic cells)	Costimulator for T cell activation; binds to CD28 and CTLA-4 on T cells
CD45R (B220)	Form of leukocyte common antigen
CD72	? Role in T cell–B cell interactions; binds to CD5 on T cells
Complement receptors	
C3b receptor (CR1) (CD35)	? Regulation of B cell activation
C3d receptor (CR2) (CD21)	Receptor for Epstein-Barr virus (in primates); ? regulation of B cell activation
Fc receptors	
FcγRII (receptor for IgG)	Negative feedback control of B cell activation
Low-affinity FcεRII (CD23)	Unknown; induced by IL-4

brane Ig is the *sine qua non* of the B lymphocyte and remains the most reliable marker for cells of the B lymphocyte lineage. Recently, a great deal of attention has been given to a small subset of B cells that express CD5 (Ly-1), which was originally identified as a marker for a subset of T lymphocytes. Only 5 to 10 per cent of B cells in the blood and lymphoid organs are CD5[+], and these may express a quite limited repertoire of V genes. Surprisingly, virtually all B cell–derived chronic lymphocytic leukemias are CD5[+]. Moreover, CD5[+] B cells spontaneously secrete IgM antibodies that often react with self antigens, and these cells may be significantly expanded in autoimmune diseases. CD5[+] B cells do not develop in the bone marrow, and in mice large numbers of these cells are found as a self-renewing population in the peritoneum. It is, therefore, likely that this small subset of B lymphocytes has unique properties in terms of ontogeny, function, and role in disease.

2. Various surface molecules may function in B cell activation or regulation. We have already alluded to the function of membrane Ig as the B cell antigen receptor. In Chapter 9, we will describe the importance of contact between B lymphocytes and helper T cells in the induction of antibody responses against protein antigens. Class II MHC molecules and CD40 play key roles in mediating T-B cell contact, and several other molecules, including CD22 and CD72, have been postulated to be involved in this process as well. Antibodies specific for CD19, CD20, CD23, CD40, and type 1 and type 2 complement receptors (CR1 and CR2, respectively) have all been shown to stimulate or inhibit B lympho-

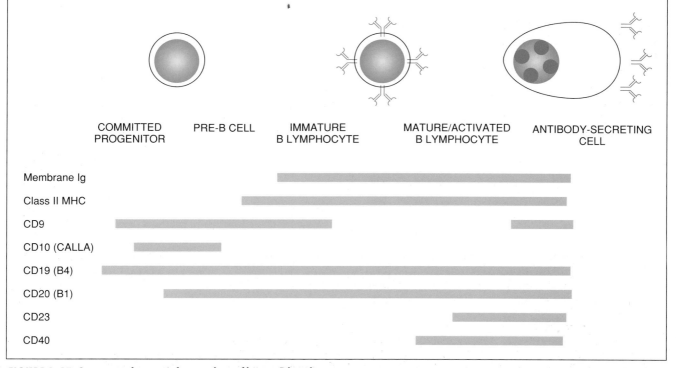

FIGURE 4–17. Ontogeny of some surface markers of human B lymphocytes. *Different surface molecules are expressed at distinct stages during the maturation and differentiation of B lymphocytes. (Adapted with permission from Zola, H. The surface antigens of human B lymphocytes. Immunology Today 8:308–315, 1987.)*

cyte growth and/or differentiation under different experimental conditions *in vitro*. Receptors for the Fc portions of IgG antibodies bind antigen-antibody complexes and inhibit B cell activation. This phenomenon of "antibody feedback" is an important regulatory mechanism that serves to control humoral immune responses (see Chapter 10). A protein called B7, expressed on activated B lymphocytes, binds to two T cell accessory molecules, CD28 and CTLA-4, and functions as a "costimulator" for T cells (see Chapter 7).

3. Antibodies against surface proteins can be used to localize and treat tumors derived from B lymphocytes. Some CD antigens are expressed at high levels on tumors of B cells, so that monoclonal antibodies specific for these antigens can be used to destroy or remove tumor cells. One recent application of such antibodies is in a treatment protocol for B cell–derived leukemias, which often express high levels of CD9 and CD10. Bone marrow is removed from patients with these leukemias and treated with antibodies to CD9 and CD10 conjugated to toxins; the patient is treated with high doses of radiation and/or chemotherapy; and the treated marrow devoid of leukemic cells is injected to reconstitute the hematopoietic system.

SUMMARY

The maturation of B lymphocytes is accompanied by specific changes in Ig gene structure and mRNA expression, which correspond to changes in the production of Ig molecules in different forms (Fig. 4–18). The earliest detectable change in Ig genes during B cell ontogeny is a somatic recombination of variable (V), joining (J), and, for heavy chains, diversity (D) gene segments so that one of each is assembled together on one chromosome. The recombination of Ig genes itself occurs in a precise sequence, with H chains being first, followed by κ and then λ. Functional rearrangement at each heavy or light chain locus inhibits rearrangement on the other allele (allelic exclusion). The constant (C) region heavy or light chain gene is attached to the VDJ or VJ complex by RNA splicing to generate a mature mRNA that is translated into heavy or light chain protein. The diverse repertoire of antibody specificities is generated by the presence of multiple germline V, D, and J genes; their combinatorial associations; junctional diversity; and, particularly in secondary antibody responses to protein antigens, somatic mutations in V genes. Co-expression of μ and δ heavy chains on the same B cell and the change from membrane to secreted Ig are mediated by alternative splicing of primary heavy chain RNA transcripts. Heavy chain class (isotype) switching results either from a process of switch recombination and deletion of C_H genes or from alternative splicing of long primary transcripts containing several or all of the C_H genes. Somatic mutations in V genes give rise to affinity maturation in antibody responses. Transcription and translation of Ig are controlled by numerous processes that are incompletely elucidated;

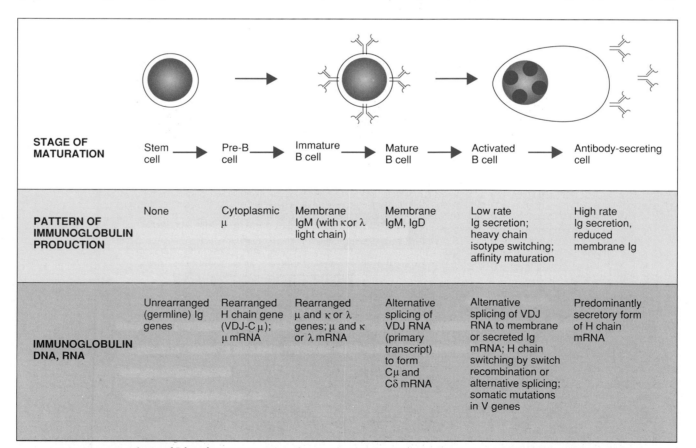

STAGE OF MATURATION	Stem cell	Pre-B cell	Immature B cell	Mature B cell	Activated B cell	Antibody-secreting cell
PATTERN OF IMMUNOGLOBULIN PRODUCTION	None	Cytoplasmic μ	Membrane IgM (with κ or λ light chain)	Membrane IgM, IgD	Low rate Ig secretion; heavy chain isotype switching; affinity maturation	High rate Ig secretion, reduced membrane Ig
IMMUNOGLOBULIN DNA, RNA	Unrearranged (germline) Ig genes	Rearranged H chain gene (VDJ-Cμ); μ mRNA	Rearranged μ and κ or λ genes; μ and κ or λ mRNA	Alternative splicing of VDJ RNA (primary transcript) to form Cμ and Cδ mRNA	Alternative splicing of VDJ RNA to membrane or secreted Ig mRNA; H chain switching by switch recombination or alternative splicing; somatic mutations in V genes	Predominantly secretory form of H chain mRNA

FIGURE 4–18. Scheme of B lymphocyte maturation, showing the patterns of Ig gene expression at different stages of maturation.

many of these processes are believed to be specific for B lymphocytes.

Analysis of these molecular events has provided a clear picture of the differentiation of B lymphocytes and the molecular basis of Ig expression. In addition, such studies form the basis of our rapidly increasing understanding of related fields, such as the evolution of B cell tumors, and are providing increasingly sophisticated tools for the diagnosis of diseases of B lymphocytes.

SELECTED READINGS

Alt, F. W., T. K. Blackwell, and G. D. Yancopoulos. Development of the primary antibody repertoire. Science 238:1079–1087, 1987.

Esser, C., and A. Radbruch. Immunoglobulin class switching: molecular and cellular analysis. Annual Review of Immunology, 8:717–735, 1990.

Kantor, A. B., and L. A. Herzenberg. Origin of murine B cell lineages. Annual Review of Immunology 11:501–538, 1993.

Kocks, C., and K. Rajwesky. Stable expression and somatic hypermutation of antibody V regions in B-cell developmental pathways. Annual Review of Immunology 7:537–559, 1989.

Koller, B. H., and O. Smithies. Altering genes in animals by gene targeting. Annual Review of Immunology 10:785–807, 1992.

Korsmeyer, S. J. Chromosomal translocations in lymphoid malignancies reveal novel proto-oncogenes. Annual Review of Immunology 10:785–807, 1992.

Pascual, V., and J. D. Capra. Human immunoglobulin heavy-chain variable region genes: organization, polymorphism, and expression. Advances in Immunology 49:1–74, 1991.

Pillai, S. Immunoglobulin transport in B cell development. International Review of Cytology 130:1–36, 1990.

Rajewsky, K. Early and late B cell development in the mouse. Current Opinion in Immunology 4:171–176, 1992.

Rolink, A., and F. Melchers. B lymphopoiesis in the mouse. Advances in Immunology 53:123–156, 1993.

Schatz, D. G., M. A. Oettinger, and M. S. Schlissel. V(D)J recombination: molecular biology and regulation. Annual Review of Immunology 10:359–383, 1992.

Staudt, L. M., and M. J. Lenardo. Immunoglobulin gene transcription. Annual Review of Immunology 9:373–398, 1991.

Tonegawa, S. Somatic generation of antibody diversity. Nature 302:575–581, 1983.

Waldmann, T. A. The arrangement of immunoglobulin and T cell receptor genes in human lymphoproliferative disorders. Advances in Immunology 40:247–321, 1987.

CHAPTER FIVE

THE MAJOR

HISTOCOMPATIBILITY

COMPLEX

The **major histocompatibility complex** (MHC) is a region of highly polymorphic genes whose products are expressed on the surfaces of a variety of cells. This locus was discovered in the 1940s in the artificial situation of transplantation of tissues from one individual to another. MHC-encoded proteins, which are commonly referred to as "MHC molecules" or "MHC antigens," are the principal determinants of graft rejection. Thus, individuals who express the same MHC molecules accept tissue grafts from one another, and individuals who differ at their MHC loci vigorously reject such grafts. Although the role of MHC molecules as the targets for immunologic rejection of transplants raised considerable interest, the importance of the MHC in physiologic immune responses was established almost 20 years after the discovery of these genetic loci. Baruj Benacerraf, Hugh McDevitt, and their colleagues showed in the 1960s that different inbred strains of guinea pigs and mice did or did not produce antibodies in response to immunization with simple polypeptide antigens and that this immune responsiveness was an autosomal dominant trait that mapped to the MHC region. The genes that controlled such immune responses were called **immune response (Ir) genes.** It was later shown that Ir genes controlled the activation of helper T lymphocytes, which were necessary for antibody responses to protein antigens. The central role of MHC genes in immune responses to protein antigens was explained in the late 1970s, with the demonstration that *antigen-specific T lymphocytes do not recognize antigens in free or soluble form but recognize portions of protein antigens* (i.e., peptides) *that are non-covalently bound to MHC gene products.* In other words, MHC molecules provide a system for displaying antigenic peptides to T cells. This allows T cells to survey the body for the presence of peptides derived from foreign proteins. There are two different types of MHC gene products, called **class I** and **class II MHC molecules,** and any given T cell recognizes foreign antigen bound to only one class I or class II MHC molecule. Furthermore, as we shall discuss in Chapter 6, in each individual the antigen receptors of mature T cells are specific for complexes of foreign protein antigens and self MHC molecules. Thus, MHC molecules are integral components of the ligands that T cells recognize.

Before we discuss the discovery and structure of MHC molecules, it is useful to summarize the principal physiologic importance of the specificity of T lymphocytes for self MHC-associated antigens.

1. Because MHC molecules are membrane-associated and not secreted, T lymphocytes can recognize foreign antigens only when bound to the surfaces of other cells. This limits T cell activation such that *T cells interact only with other cells that bear MHC-associated antigens and not with soluble antigens.* In fact, as we shall discuss in Chapter 7, *the T cell receptor for antigen interacts with amino acid side chains of both the bound peptide and the MHC molecule itself.* The cell that bears the MHC molecules is said to *present* the antigen to the T lymphocyte. The recognition of antigen on a cell surface also serves to localize the effector functions of the activated T cell to the anatomic site of antigen presentation. In contrast, antibodies can function in the circulation by binding to and neutralizing soluble antigens.

2. *The patterns of antigen association with class I or class II MHC molecules determine the kinds of T cells that are stimulated by different forms of antigens.* As we shall discuss later, the distinct pathways of biosynthesis and assembly of class I and class II MHC proteins determine the source of peptides associated with each class of MHC molecules. Peptide fragments derived from extracellular proteins usually bind to class II MHC molecules, whereas endogenously synthesized peptides, generated in the cytosol, generally associate with class I molecules. As a consequence, exogenously and endogenously synthesized proteins are, for the most part, recognized by functionally distinct T cell populations.

3. The immune response to a foreign protein is determined by the expression of specific MHC molecules that can bind and present peptide fragments of that protein to T cells. MHC genes are very polymorphic; i.e., many different alleles exist within the population, and these alleles differ in their ability to bind and present different antigenic determinants of proteins. This is one way in which *MHC genes control immune responses to protein antigens.*

4. Mature T cells in any individual recognize and respond to foreign antigens but are unresponsive to self proteins. The repertoire of antigen recognition by mature T cells is shaped by positive selection of developing thymic T cells specific for foreign peptides bound to self MHC molecules and elimination (negative selection) of T cells reactive with self peptides bound to self MHC molecules (see Chapter 8). Since the range of peptides that can be presented to developing T cells depends upon the ability of the inherited set of self MHC molecules to bind those peptides, *MHC molecules can influence immune responsiveness to particular antigens by shaping the repertoire of mature T cells.*

The functions of MHC gene products in T cell antigen recognition and in the development of the T cell repertoire are described in more detail in Chapters 6 to 8. However, these functional considerations make clear why our discussion of T cells must begin with a discussion of MHC molecules. The terminology and genetics of the MHC are best understood from a historical perspective, and we will begin our discussion with a description of how the MHC was discovered.

DISCOVERY OF THE MAJOR HISTOCOMPATIBILITY COMPLEX
Transplantation in Mice

The initial discovery of the murine MHC was made by George Snell and his colleagues, using classical genetic techniques to analyze the rejection of transplanted tumors and other tissues. In their simplest form, these experiments examined the outcome of skin grafts between individual animals. The key to the analysis was the use of inbred strains of laboratory mice.

In an animal population, some genes are represented by only one normal nucleic acid sequence; every variant nucleic acid sequence is an uncommon mutation and may result in a disease state. Such genes are said to be nonpolymorphic, and the normal, or wild type, gene sequence will usually be present on both chromosomes of a pair in each individual member of the species. (Recall that all chromosomes, except sex

chromosomes in the male, are present in pairs in a normal diploid animal.) In other genes, the nucleic acid sequences may vary at a relatively high frequency among normal individuals in the population; i.e., at least 1 per cent of individuals may express a gene that differs from the homologous gene in remaining members of the population. Such genes are said to be **polymorphic**. Each common variant of a polymorphic gene present in the population is called an **allele**. For polymorphic genes, any individual animal can have the

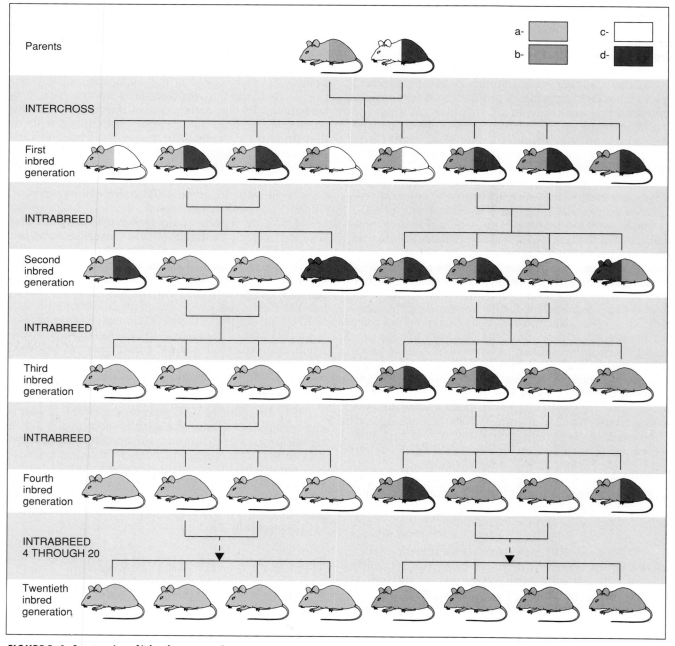

FIGURE 5–1. Construction of inbred mouse strains. *In this hypothetical breeding scheme, a particular genetic locus is represented in the outbred heterozygous parent animals by four different alleles: a, b, c, and d. Repetitive inbreeding leads to development of animal strains in which every individual is homozygous at this locus and expresses the same allele. Without selective pressure, which of the original parental alleles will be present in the inbred animals is random. In this example, two strains that preserve alleles a and b are generated; other strains that are homozygous for c or d could be derived from the same parents. Although only one locus is depicted, every other genetic locus in each inbred strain will also be homozygous and identical among all animals in the same strain.*

same allele at a genetic locus on both chromosomes of the pair (i.e., can be homozygous) or two different alleles, one on each chromosome (i.e., can be heterozygous).

Inbred mouse strains are produced by repetitive matings of siblings (Fig. 5–1). After about 20 generations, every individual animal of a given inbred mouse strain will have identical nucleic acid sequences at all locations on both members of each pair of chromosomes. In other words, *inbred mice are completely homozygous at every genetic locus. In addition, every mouse of an inbred strain is genetically completely identical (syngeneic) to every other mouse of the same strain.* In the case of polymorphic genes, each inbred strain, because it is completely homozygous, can express only one allele from the original population. However, the determination of which of four possible alleles (one on each member of the chromosome pairs in each of the two original parents) is preserved by inbreeding is random for any particular gene; different inbred strains derived from the same two parents may preserve different alleles (Fig. 5–1). Strains or individuals that express different alleles are said to be **allogeneic** to one another.

When a tissue or an organ, such as a patch of skin, is grafted from one animal to another, two possible outcomes may ensue. In some cases, the grafted skin survives and functions as normal skin. In others, the immune system destroys the graft, a process called **rejection.** By determining whether or not grafts exchanged among various inbred strains of mice were rejected, several key observations were made about the genetic basis of graft rejection.

1. Grafts of skin from one animal to itself (autologous grafts, or autografts) or grafts between animals of the same inbred strain (syngeneic grafts, or syngrafts) are usually not rejected.

2. Grafts between animals of different inbred strains or between outbred mice (allogeneic grafts, or allografts) are almost always rejected.

We will return to these experiments in Chapter 17, when we discuss transplantation. Suffice it to say here that the different outcomes of grafts between syngeneic animals and grafts between allogeneic animals established that there is a genetic basis for recognizing a graft as foreign. The genes responsible for causing a grafted tissue to be perceived as similar to one's own tissues or as foreign were called **histocompatibility genes,** and the differences between foreign and self were attributed to genetic polymorphisms among different histocompatibility alleles.

The tools of classical genetics, namely breeding and analysis of the offspring, were then applied to identify the relevant genes. The critical strategy in this effort was the breeding of **congenic mouse strains** (Box 5–1) that differed only by genes responsible for causing graft rejection. These studies indicated that although several different genes could contribute to rejection, *a single genetic region is responsible for most rejection phenomena.* The particular region identified in mice by Snell's group was linked to a gene encoding a polymorphic blood group antigen called Antigen II, and this region was subsequently called histocompatibility-2 or, simply, H-2. Initially, MHC congenic strains were thought to differ at a single gene locus. However, occa-

---

BOX 5–1. CONGENIC MOUSE STRAINS

A key development in defining the genes responsible for causing graft rejection was the development of congenic mouse strains that differ only by the relevant genes, now known as the MHC. The strategy for such breeding depends upon two circumstances. First, there must already exist a homozygous inbred mouse strain that will reproducibly reject transplanted grafts of another strain. Second, there must be a simple assay for graft rejection. Both of these conditions are met by transplanting skin between inbred strains that differ in alleles of MHC genes. The procedure is outlined in the accompanying figure.

A mouse of one inbred strain A is mated with a mouse from a second strain B. The MHC of a strain A mouse is referred to as being *aa* homozygous (with italics representing alleles) and that of a strain B mouse as being *bb* homozygous. All of the first filial (F1) generation will be *ab* heterozygotes. Next an F1 mouse is mated with a strain A mouse. This is called a backcross. Half of the offspring will be *aa* and half will be *ab*. Those mice that are *ab* can be identified by the fact that their skin will be rapidly rejected by strain A mice; in contrast, the skin of *aa* offspring will not be rapidly rejected by strain A mice. Step three is again to backcross one of the heterozygous *ab* mice with a strain A mouse. Once again, half of the offspring will be *aa* and half will be *ab*, and the heterozygous *ab* mice can be identified by the fact that strain A

mice will rapidly reject their skin. By continuing to carry out such backcrosses for multiple generations, two things occur. First, the *b* allele of the MHC will be indefinitely maintained in the offspring because its expression is necessary for skin graft rejection and this is the positive selection being imposed by the experimenter. Second, all other genetic loci from the strain B mice will disappear as a result of random backcrosses into strain A mice. This second effect can be thought of as serial dilution. The F1 mice will contain 50 per cent strain B genes; the offspring of the first backcross will contain, on average, 25 per cent; the offspring of the next backcross will contain, on average, 12.5 per cent, and so on, until by about 20 backcrosses no strain B genes except the MHC alleles will persist. At this point, a mouse strain has been bred that is identical to the strain A except that the MHC is heterozygous *ab*. If the new strain is allowed to interbreed, 25 per cent of the first generation offspring will be *aa* homozygous, 50 per cent will be *ab* heterozygous, and 25 per cent will be *bb* homozygous at the MHC. The *bb* MHC homozygotes can be identified as being the only mice that will rapidly reject strain A skin grafts. If the *bb* mice interbreed, a strain is produced that is identical to strain A at every locus except the MHC and is identical to strain B only at the MHC. These mice are congenic to strain A and are said to have the B MHC on an A background.

Continued

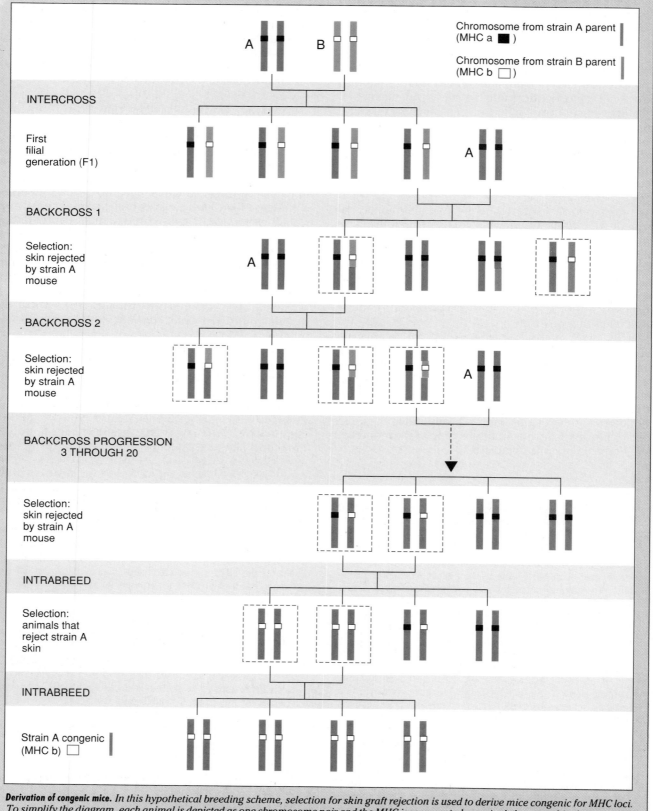

Derivation of congenic mice. *In this hypothetical breeding scheme, selection for skin graft rejection is used to derive mice congenic for MHC loci. To simplify the diagram, each animal is depicted as one chromosome pair and the MHC is represented as a single locus on this chromosome. Animals that are positively selected are indicated by dashed blue boxes around the chromosome pair. As described in the box, all non-MHC strain B genes are lost during progressive backcrosses with strain A animals; MHC b genes are preserved by selection, eventually allowing the breeding of a congenic strain that differs only at the MHC from parental strain A.*

sional recombination events occurred within the MHC during interbreeding of different strains, suggesting that the MHC actually contained several different but closely linked genes, each involved in graft rejection. The H-2 region in mice is now known to be homologous to genes that determine the fate of grafted tissues in other species, and all of these are grouped under the generic name, the "major histocompatibility complex."

The genetics of graft rejection indicated that the products of MHC genes are co-dominantly expressed; i.e., the alleles on both chromosomes of a pair are expressed. As a consequence, each parent of a genetic cross between two different strains can reject a graft from the offspring by recognizing MHC alleles inherited from the other parent.

In mice, the MHC alleles of particular inbred strains are designated by lower case letters (e.g., a, b, c). The individual genes within the MHC are named for the MHC type of the mouse strain in which they were first identified. The two independent MHC loci known to be most important for graft rejection in mice are called H-2K and H-2D. The K gene was first discovered in a strain whose MHC had been designated k, and the D gene was first discovered in a strain whose MHC had been designated d. In the parlance of mouse geneticists, the allele of the K gene in a strain with the k-type MHC is called K^k (pronounced K of k) whereas the allele of the K gene in a strain of MHC d is called K^d (pronounced K of d). A third locus similar to K and D was discovered later and called L.

Several other genes were subsequently mapped to the region between the K and D genes responsible for skin rejection. For example, S genes that code for polymorphic serum proteins, now known to be components of the complement system, were identified. Most importantly, *the polymorphic Ir genes mentioned earlier in the chapter were assigned to a region within the MHC called I* (the letter, not the Roman numeral). The I region, in turn, was further subdivided into I-A and I-E subregions on the basis of recombination events during breeding between congenic strains. The I region was

also found to code for certain cell surface antigens against which antibodies could be produced by interstrain immunizations. These antigens were called I region–associated or **Ia molecules.** As we shall discuss in Chapters 6 and 8, we now know that the I-A and I-E Ir genes are the structural genes that code for Ia antigens, which are called I-A and I-E molecules, respectively. The I-A molecule found in the inbred mouse strain with the K^k and D^k alleles is called I-A^k (pronounced I big A of k). Similar terminology is used for I-E molecules. The culmination of genetic analysis was the construction of a classical genetic map of the murine MHC, schematized in Figure 5–2.

MHC genes were initially identified by graft rejection and Ir gene phenomena, which are T cell–mediated immune responses. This is not unexpected because, as stated earlier and discussed in detail in Chapter 6, MHC molecules are crucial for T cell recognition of foreign antigens. Nevertheless, immunization of one congenic mouse strain with cells of another can be used to produce antibodies (i.e., B cell products) specific for MHC gene products. Such antibodies were important in the biochemical analysis of murine MHC molecules and played a central role in the discovery of the MHC in man.

Serologic Studies in Humans

The kinds of experiments used to discover and define MHC genes in mice, namely intentional inbreeding and skin graft rejection, obviously cannot be performed in humans. However, the development of allogeneic blood transfusion and especially allogeneic organ transplantation as methods of treatment in clinical medicine provided a strong impetus to detect and define genes that control rejection reactions in humans. Jean Dausset and others noted that patients who rejected kidneys or had transfusion reactions to white blood cells often developed circulating antibodies reactive with antigens on the white blood cells of the blood

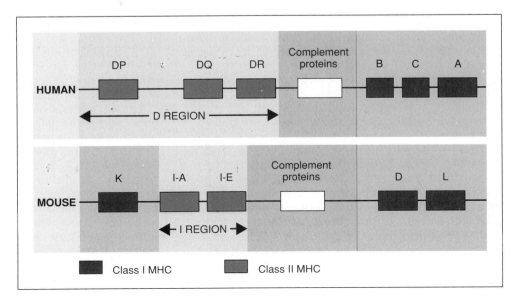

FIGURE 5–2. Schematic maps of human and mouse MHC loci. *Sizes of genes and intervening distances are not shown to scale. Each class II locus, e.g., DP and DQ, consists of multiple genes. HLA-DQ is much closer to HLA-DR than to HLA-DP; in fact, HLA-DQ is in strong "linkage disequilibrium" with HLA-DR; i.e., certain DQ alleles are inherited together with particular DR alleles, well out of proportion to their frequency in the population.*

or organ donor. In the presence of complement, the recipient's serum would lyse lymphocytes from the donor and also lyse lymphocytes obtained from some, but not all, third parties (i.e., individuals other than the blood or organ donor or the recipient). These sera, which react against the cells of allogeneic individuals, are called **alloantisera** (or allosera for short) and are said to contain **alloantibodies,** whose molecular targets are called **alloantigens.** It was presumed that these alloantigens are the products of polymorphic genes that distinguish foreign tissues from self. Panels of allosera from immunized donors, including multiparous women (who are immunized by paternal alloantigens expressed by the fetus during pregnancy) and actively immunized volunteers as well as transfusion or transplant recipients, were collected and compared for their ability to lyse panels of lymphocytes from different donors. Efforts at several international workshops, involving free exchanges of reagents among laboratories, led to the definition of at least six separate polymorphic genetic loci, clustered together in a single area of the genome, that can help to predict the strength of graft rejection. Because they are expressed on human leukocytes, the alloantigens recognized by these sera became known as **human leukocyte antigens (HLAs).** Family studies were then used to construct the map of these human genes (Fig. 5–2). The first three genes defined by purely serologic approaches were called HLA-A, HLA-B, and HLA-C. The second three to be identified mapped to an adjacent region, called HLA-D, which was originally detected by induction of proliferation of foreign T cells in the mixed leukocyte reaction (see below). The first gene product detected by alloantibodies that mapped to the HLA-D region was called "HLA-D related" or HLA-DR. The final two genes were subsequently called HLA-DQ and HLA-DP, with Q and P chosen for their proximity in the alphabet to R. *The HLA region is now known as the human MHC and is equivalent to the H-2 region of mice* (Fig. 5–2). The various HLA and H-2 loci are structurally and functionally homologous. *Specifically, human HLA-A, -B, and -C resemble mouse H-2K, D, and L and are called class I MHC molecules, whereas human HLA-DP, -DQ, and -DR resemble mouse I-A and I-E and are called class II MHC molecules.* Indeed, similar polymorphic genes and protein products have been found in every vertebrate species examined!

The studies of the mouse MHC were accomplished with a limited number of inbred and congenic strains. Although it was appreciated that mouse MHC genes were polymorphic, only 10 to 20 alleles were defined at each locus. The human serologic studies were conducted on outbred human populations. The most remarkable feature to emerge from the studies of the human MHC genes is the unprecedented and unanticipated extent of their polymorphism. More than 40 separate alleles have been identified to date for some of the HLA loci, and this is undoubtedly an underestimate resulting from the limited resolution of serology. *MHC genes are by far the most polymorphic genes present in the genome of every species analyzed.* The significance

of this polymorphism will become evident when we turn to the structure and functions of MHC molecules.

The use of antibodies to study alloantigenic differences between donors and recipients in human transplantation was complemented by the mixed leukocyte reaction (MLR), a test for T cell recognition of foreign MHC molecules. The MLR is also an *in vitro* model for allograft rejection and will be discussed more fully in the context of transplantation (see Chapter 17). Analysis of the allogeneic MLR led to the conclusion that two distinct classes of T lymphocytes recognize and respond to different types of MHC gene products. CD4+ T cells, most of which are cytokine-producing helper cells, are specific for class II MHC molecules, i.e., HLA-DR, -DQ, and -DP in man and I-A and I-E in mice. CD8+ T cells, most of which are cytolytic T lymphocytes (CTLs), are specific for class I MHC molecules, namely HLA-A, -B, and -C or H-2K, D, and L. As we shall see in Chapter 6, these MHC recognition specificities of CD4+ and CD8+ T cells apply not only to recognition of allogeneic MHC molecules but also to recognition of foreign protein, e.g., microbial antigens, in every individual. In other words, *CD4+ T cells recognize foreign antigens bound to self class II MHC molecules, and CD8+ T cells recognize foreign antigens bound to self class I molecules.*

The total set of MHC alleles present on each chromosome is also called an **MHC haplotype.** In humans, each HLA allele is given a numerical designation. For instance, an HLA haplotype of an individual could be HLA-A2, -B5, -DR3, and so on. All heterozygous individuals, of course, have two HLA haplotypes. Inbred mice, being homozygous, have a single haplotype. Thus, the haplotype of an H-2^k mouse is H-2K^k I-A^k I-E^k D^k L^k. In humans, certain HLA alleles at different loci are inherited together, a phenomenon called linkage disequilibrium. Such haplotypes, in which multiple HLA genes remain linked, are associated with certain autoimmune disease (see Chapter 19).

STRUCTURE OF MHC MOLECULES

The realization that MHC molecules play an essential part in the recognition of all protein antigens by T cells has led to an enormous effort in many laboratories to elucidate the structure of these molecules. The biochemical analysis of MHC molecules has been highly successful, especially with the solution of the crystal structures for the extracellular portions of human class I molecules, and, more recently, of human class II molecules, by Don Wiley, Jack Strominger, and colleagues. On the basis of this new knowledge, we can now address two interrelated structural issues that are important for understanding the functions of MHC molecules:

First, how do MHC molecules bind foreign peptide antigens, and how does the genetic polymorphism of MHC molecules contribute to the specificity of peptide binding?

Second, what structural features of MHC molecules underlie the specificity of CD8$^+$ T cells for class I molecules and of CD4$^+$ T cells for class II molecules?

We will initially consider class I and class II molecules separately, but, as we shall see, many features of these molecules now point to their fundamental similarity.

Class I MHC Molecules

All class I molecules contain two separate polypeptide chains: an MHC-encoded α or heavy chain of about 44 kilodaltons (kD) in humans, or about 47 kD in mice, and a non–MHC-encoded β chain of 12 kD in both species (Fig. 5–3). The α chain is formed by a core polypeptide of about 40 kD and contains one (human) or two (mouse) N-linked oligosaccharides. Each α chain is oriented so that about three quarters of the complete polypeptide, including the amino terminus and oligosaccharide group(s), extends into the extracellular milieu, a short hydrophobic segment spans the membrane, and the carboxy terminal 30 amino acid residues are located in the cytoplasm. The β chain interacts non-covalently with the extracellular portion of the heavy chain and has no direct attachment to the cell. Based upon primary amino acid sequences of many class I molecules and upon the crystal structure of the extracellular portions of several class I molecules, we can now divide class I molecules into four separate regions (Fig. 5–3): an amino terminal extracel-

lular peptide-binding region; an extracellular immunoglobulin (Ig)-like region; a transmembrane region; and a cytoplasmic region.

THE PEPTIDE-BINDING REGION

As we noted in the introductory section of this chapter, the principal function of MHC molecules is to bind fragments of foreign proteins, thereby forming complexes that can be recognized by T lymphocytes. The portion of class I molecules that interacts with protein antigens consists of approximately 180 amino acid residues at the amino terminus of the class I α chain. Analysis of amino acid sequences has indicated that this region is formed of two homologous segments of about 90 amino acid residues each, referred to as α1 and α2. Each human class I MHC molecule has a single N-linked oligosaccharide attached near the junction of α1 and α2. Murine class I MHC molecules contain a second oligosaccharide attached near the carboxy terminal side of α2. The α2 segment contains a disulfide bond, forming a loop of about 63 amino acid residues. Despite initial reports to the contrary, there is no evidence that the α1 or α2 segments of MHC molecules are structurally or evolutionarily related to Ig domains. Instead, α1 and α2 interact to form a platform of an eight-stranded, β-pleated sheet supporting two parallel strands of α-helix (Fig. 5–4 and Color Plate II, opposite page 51). Four strands of the β-pleated sheet and one of the α-helices are formed from amino acid residues of α1; the remaining four strands of the β-pleated sheet

FIGURE 5-3. Schematic diagram of a class I MHC molecule. *Different segments are not shown to scale. N and C refer to amino and carboxy termini of the polypeptide chains, respectively; S--S, to intrachain disulfide bonds; ¶, to carbohydrate; and P, to phosphorylation sites.*

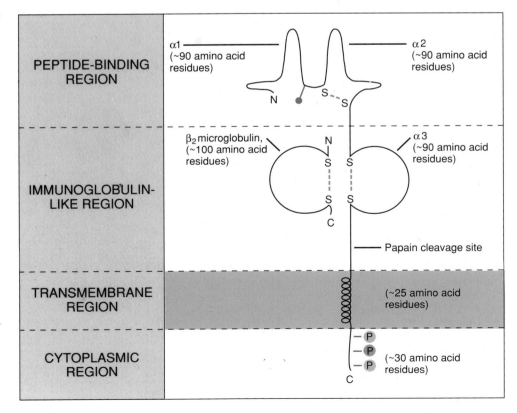

PEPTIDE-BINDING REGION

IMMUNOGLOBULIN-LIKE REGION

TRANSMEMBRANE REGION

CYTOPLASMIC REGION

α1 (~90 amino acid residues)

α2 (~90 amino acid residues)

N   S---S

β_2 microglobulin, (~100 amino acid residues)

α3 (~90 amino acid residues)

N   S   S

S   S

C

Papain cleavage site

(~25 amino acid residues)

P
P
P   (~30 amino acid residues)

C

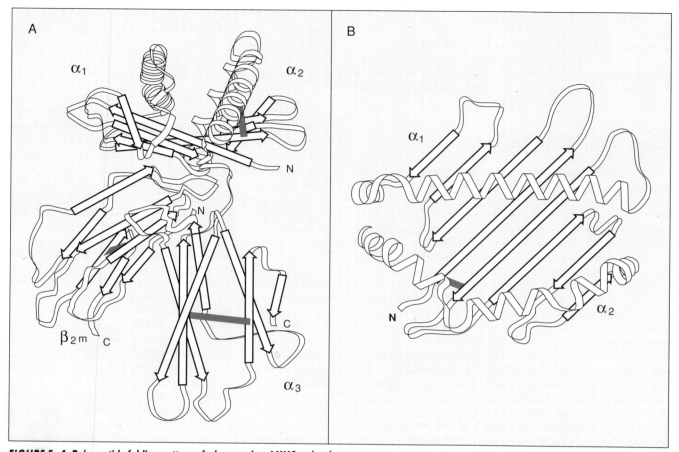

FIGURE 5–4. Polypeptide folding pattern of a human class I MHC molecule. *Panel A shows a side view and Panel B depicts a top view, revealing the peptide-binding cleft. The white arrows represent polypeptide folded as β-pleated sheet, the white coils represent polypeptide folded as α-helix, and the blue bars represent disulfide bonds. (Adapted with permission from Bjorkman, P. J., M. A. Saper, B. Samraoui, W. S. Bennet, J. L. Strominger, and D. C. Wiley. Structure of the human class I histocompatibility antigen HLA-A2. Nature 329:506–512, 1987. Copyright © 1987, Macmillan Magazines Ltd.)*

and the other α-helix are formed from amino acid residues of α2. The two α-helices form the sides of a cleft whose floor is formed by the strands of the β-pleated sheet. The cleft is of appropriate size (25Å × 10Å × 11Å) to bind a 9 to 11 amino acid fragment of a protein in a flexible, extended conformation and is the site where foreign peptides bind to MHC molecules for presentation to T cells. The ends of the clefts in class I MHC molecules are closed by interactions among the side chains of amino acid residues of the α-helices and the outermost β strands. Significantly, the cleft is too small to bind an intact globular protein and thus differs from the more planar binding site of antibody molecules (see Chapter 3). The small size of the cleft in MHC molecules requires that native globular proteins be "processed," to produce smaller fragments that can bind to MHC molecules and be recognized by T lymphocytes (see Chapter 6).

Comparisons of amino acid and nucleotide sequences of a large number of human and murine class I heavy chains have indicated that almost all of the polymorphic residues, i.e., those amino acids found to vary among different allelic forms, are located either in the α-helical sides of the cleft or on the β strands that form

the floor of the cleft and are oriented such that the amino acid side chains point into the cleft or toward the top of the helices. This finding suggested that *polymorphism among class I MHC alleles serves to create variation in the chemical surface of the peptide-binding cleft.* Other polymorphic residues of MHC molecules form contacts with T cell antigen receptors, further suggesting that *T cells specifically interact both with MHC-associated foreign antigens and with the MHC molecules themselves* (see Chapters 6 and 7). The N-linked oligosaccharides, although located in one peptide-binding region, do not contribute to the structure of the cleft or to peptide binding.

Each MHC molecule contains only a single site for peptide binding, and each MHC molecule may bind only one peptide at a time. MHC molecules purified from cells contain mixtures of peptides. Amino acid sequencing of the peptides recovered from purified class I MHC molecules established three important features.

1. The bound peptides range from 9 to 11 amino acid residues in length. Eleven amino acids appears to be the maximum size that can be accommodated within the cleft of a class I molecule.

2. All of the peptides isolated from a single allelic form of a class I molecule share common structural features. For example, peptides from HLA-Aw68 share conserved amino and carboxy termini but vary widely in the middle of their sequence.

3. The shared features of peptides isolated from one allelic form of a class I molecule are different from the shared features of peptides isolated from another allelic form.

Further details of peptides that bind to MHC molecules will be discussed in Chapter 6. Recent technical advances have allowed purified class I molecules to be reassembled *in vitro* with a single bound peptide. Crystallographic analyses of such artificially loaded class I molecules have revealed that the MHC peptide-binding site contains indentations ("pockets") that differ among alleles of class I molecules and are complementary to the conserved features of the peptides that bind to that allele, providing the basis of peptide specificity.

It has been proposed that the extraordinary polymorphism of MHC molecules has evolved and is maintained in each species by positive natural selection, so that members of the species express different alleles capable of binding many distinct foreign peptide antigens. Otherwise, if the number of variant MHC molecules in the population were limited, a microbe could simply mutate its antigens until they attained structures incapable of binding to MHC molecules. This would prevent T cell recognition of the antigens, and the microbe would evade specific immunity. However, with so many possible MHC molecules available within the gene pool, such microbial peptides unable to bind to all MHC molecules in the population are unlikely to emerge.

THE IMMUNOGLOBULIN-LIKE REGION

The $\alpha 3$ segment of the heavy chain is composed of about 90 extracellular amino acid residues between the carboxy terminal end of the $\alpha 2$ segment and the insertion into the plasma membrane. The amino acid sequence in this region is highly conserved among all class I molecules examined and by sequence analysis is homologous to Ig constant domains. The $\alpha 3$ segment contains an Ig-like disulfide-linked loop.

The β chain of class I molecules, which is encoded by a gene outside the MHC, is absolutely invariant among all human class I molecules examined. (In the mouse, there are two common alleles.) This polypeptide is identical to a protein previously identified in human urine, called β_2 **microglobulin** for its electrophoretic mobility (β_2), size (micro), and solubility (globulin). The β chain of class I molecules is usually called β_2 microglobulin even when attached to the cell surface. Like the $\alpha 3$ segment, β_2 microglobulin is structurally homologous to an Ig constant domain and contains a disulfide-linked loop. Indeed, the HLA-A2 crystal structure has confirmed that both $\alpha 3$ and β_2 microglobulin are folded to form Ig-like domains, and thus class I MHC molecules are considered to be part of the Ig superfamily (see Chapter 7, Box 7–2). These two domains interact with each other, and β_2 microglobulin also interacts with the β-pleated sheet platform of the peptide-binding region, forming extensive contacts with amino acid residues in $\alpha 1$ and $\alpha 2$. The interaction of β_2 microglobulin with heavy chain $\alpha 1$ and $\alpha 2$ is strengthened when $\alpha 1$ and $\alpha 2$ are interacting with peptide; similarly, the energetically favorable interaction of β_2 microglobulin with class I heavy chain stabilizes the binding of peptide. The native class I molecule is best thought of as a heterotrimer, consisting of heavy chain, light chain, and peptide.

The strong correlation of CD8 expression on T cells with specificity for class I MHC–associated peptides led to the simple proposal that CD8 might function by binding to a nonpolymorphic portion of a class I molecule. This hypothesis has now been proved by a variety of experiments (see Chapter 7). The nonpolymorphic $\alpha 3$ region contains the binding sites for CD8, based on mutational analysis of MHC molecules.

THE TRANSMEMBRANE REGION

The polypeptide of the α chain extends from the $\alpha 3$ segment into a short connecting region and then into a stretch of approximately 25 hydrophobic amino acid residues. This region is believed to form an α-helix that passes through the hydrophobic region of the plasma membrane lipid bilayer and anchors the MHC molecule in the membrane. As with all known transmembrane proteins, the hydrophobic sequence is immediately terminated at its carboxy terminal end with a cluster of basic amino acid residues that are believed to interact with the phospholipid head groups of the inner leaflet of the membrane bilayer. Some, but not all, class I heavy chains contain a cysteine residue within the hydrophobic sequence that may be modified by esterification with myristic acid. The significance of this covalent attachment of a fatty acid is unknown.

The hydrophobic segment of the class I molecule does not affect the conformation of the extracellular portions of the molecule, but several specific features are highly conserved. For example, no alterations in structure or in the spectroscopic properties of class I molecules have been found when the enzyme papain is used to cleave the transmembrane region from the extracellular portion. Papain treatment does affect the solubility of the molecule; after removal of the transmembrane region, the extracellular portions of class I molecules are soluble in aqueous buffers without detergents. The form of class I molecules used to solve the crystal structure was actually prepared by papain treatment to remove the transmembrane region.

THE CYTOPLASMIC REGION

The extreme carboxy terminal portion of class I α chains contains approximately 30 amino acids. This region is believed to be located in the cytoplasm. The overall sequence of this region is not conserved among different class I MHC molecules, but several specific features are highly conserved. For example, all class I α chains contain amino acid residues that form consensus phosphorylation sites for cyclic adenosine monophosphate (cAMP)–dependent protein kinase (protein kinase A) and for *src* tyrosine kinase. The extreme carboxy terminal region of all known class I molecules undergoes endogenous phosphorylation at yet a third conserved site. In addition, all class I heavy chains contain in their carboxy termini a glutamine residue that is a suitable substrate for transpeptidation by the enzyme transglutaminase. The functional significance of these structural features is unknown, but they may play a role in regulating the interaction of class I MHC molecules with other membrane proteins or with cytoskeletal elements. Furthermore, deletion of portions of the carboxy terminus has been found to inhibit internalization of class I molecules, directly implicating the carboxy terminal region in intracellular trafficking.

Class II MHC Molecules

All class II MHC molecules are composed of two non-covalently associated polypeptide chains (Fig. 5–5). In general, the two class II chains are similar to each other in overall structure. The α chain (32 to 34 kD) is slightly larger than the β chain (29 to 32 kD) as a result of more extensive glycosylation. In class II molecules, both polypeptide chains contain N-linked oligosaccharide groups, both polypeptide chains have extracellular amino termini and intracellular carboxy termini, and over two thirds of each chain is located in the extracellular space. The two chains of class II molecules are encoded by different MHC genes, and, with few exceptions, both class II chains are polymorphic.

The three-dimensional structure of class II molecules has recently been solved by x-ray crystallography. In addition, the nucleotide and amino acid sequences of many class II molecules are known. Both types of analyses reveal fundamental structural similarities between class I and class II molecules, especially in the peptide-binding cleft (Fig. 5–6). In parallel with the structural features of the class I molecules, it is useful to divide class II MHC molecules into a peptide-binding region, an Ig-like region, a transmembrane region, and a cytoplasmic region.

THE PEPTIDE-BINDING REGION

The extracellular portions of both the α and β chains have been subdivided into two segments of about 90 amino acid residues each, called $\alpha 1$ and $\alpha 2$ or $\beta 1$ and $\beta 2$, respectively. The peptide-binding region of the class II molecule is formed by an interaction of both chains involving the $\alpha 1$ and $\beta 1$ segments. This is different from class I MHC molecules, in which only the α chain is involved in forming the peptide-binding cleft. More specifically, $\alpha 1$ and $\beta 1$ fold to form an eight-stranded, β-pleated sheet platform supporting two α-helices; four strands of the β-pleated sheet and one of the α-helices are formed by $\alpha 1$, whereas the other four strands and the other α-helix are formed by $\beta 1$. Class II $\alpha 1$ (like class I $\alpha 1$) does not contain a disulfide-linked loop, whereas class II $\beta 1$ (like class I $\alpha 2$) does; the class II $\beta 1$ disulfide-linked loop is in the same position as the

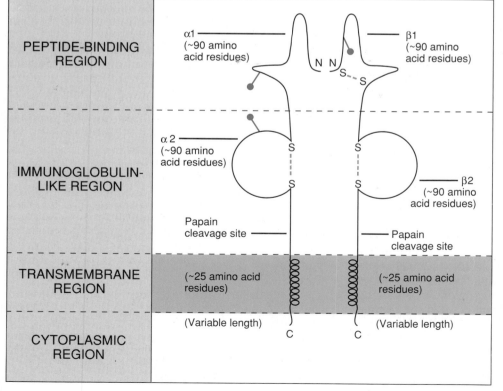

PEPTIDE-BINDING REGION	$\alpha 1$ (~90 amino acid residues) ... $\beta 1$ (~90 amino acid residues)
IMMUNOGLOBULIN-LIKE REGION	$\alpha 2$ (~90 amino acid residues) ... $\beta 2$ (~90 amino acid residues) Papain cleavage site ... Papain cleavage site
TRANSMEMBRANE REGION	(~25 amino acid residues) ... (~25 amino acid residues)
CYTOPLASMIC REGION	(Variable length) ... (Variable length)

FIGURE 5–5. Schematic diagram of a class II MHC molecule. *Different segments are not shown to scale. N and C, amino and carboxy termini of the polypeptide chains; S--S, intrachain disulfide bonds; and ↑, carbohydrate.*

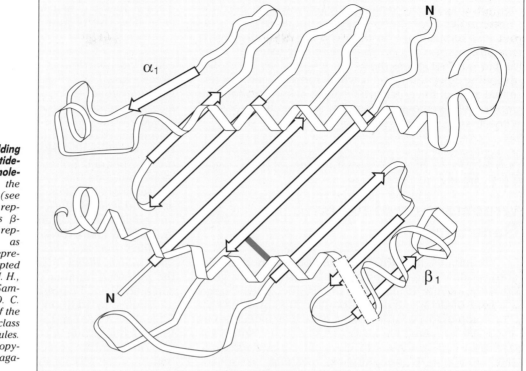

FIGURE 5–6. Polypeptide folding pattern proposed for the peptide-binding cleft of class II MHC molecule. *Note the similarities to the class I peptide-binding cleft (see Fig. 5–4B). The white arrows represent polypeptide folded as β-pleated sheet, the white coils represent polypeptide folded as α-helix, and the blue bar represents a disulfide bond. (Adapted with permission from Brown, J. H., T. Jardetzky, M. A. Saper, B. Samraoui, P. J. Bjorkman, and D. C. Wiley. A hypothetical model of the foreign antigen binding site of class II histocompatibility molecules. Nature 332:845–850, 1988. Copyright © 1988, Macmillan Magazines Ltd.)*

class I α2 disulfide-linked loop. As in the class I structure, the class II structure uses α-helices and β strands to form the sides and floor, respectively, of the peptide-binding cleft. In contrast to class I, the ends of the class II binding cleft are open, allowing bound peptides to extend out from the cleft. Indeed, peptides recovered from purified class II molecules have ranged from 10 to 30 or more amino acids in length, with a mean size of about 14 amino acids.

As in the case of class I molecules, the polymorphic residues of class II molecules are concentrated in α1 and β1 in locations such that they lie in the α-helical sides or β-pleated sheet floor of the peptide-binding cleft, with their side chains pointing into the cleft or toward the top of the helices. *Thus, as for class I molecules, genetic polymorphism of class II MHC molecules determine the chemical surface of the cleft and the principal determinant of the specificity and affinity of peptide binding and T cell recognition.* Bound peptides can interact with polymorphic outpockets in the floor of the cleft, but the structural details of peptide binding to class II MHC molecules are not yet known with the degree of precision established for peptide binding to class I MHC molecules (see Chapter 6). Again, both specificity and affinity for foreign antigens are much lower for class II molecules than for antibodies. As with class I, the use of inherited polymorphisms to determine antigen binding provides an explanation for the evolutionary drive to generate and maintain such polymorphism: a high level of polymorphism ensures that some MHC molecules are likely to be present in the population to bind any microbial antigenic peptides that may arise.

THE IMMUNOGLOBULIN-LIKE REGION

Both the α2 and β2 segments of class II molecules contain internal disulfide bonds and by amino acid sequence belong to the Ig superfamily. It is now known that these segments, like class I α3 and β2 microglobulin, are actually folded into Ig domains within the native MHC molecule. The class II α2 and β2 segments are essentially nonpolymorphic among various alleles of a particular class II gene but show some differences among the different genetic loci. Thus, the α2 regions of all DR alleles are similar, but DRα2 differs from DPα2 and DQα2. The correlation of CD4 expression on T cells with specificity for class II MHC molecules has been proposed to arise from binding of the CD4 molecule with the Ig-like nonpolymorphic β2 domain of the class II molecules.

The Ig-like regions of the class II molecules are probably important for non-covalent interactions between the two chains, although other portions of the polypeptide chains no doubt contribute as well. These interactions are quite strong and can be disrupted only by harsh denaturing conditions. In general, α chains of one locus (e.g., DR) pair best with β chains of the same locus and less commonly with β chains of other loci (e.g., DQ or DP).

THE TRANSMEMBRANE AND CYTOPLASMIC REGIONS

The carboxy terminal sides of the α2 and β2 segments extend into short connecting regions followed by approximately 25 amino acid stretches of hydrophobic residues, likely to span the membrane. Extended cleavage with papain can separate the extracellular portions of the molecule from the transmembrane region without loss of structure. In both chains, the hydrophobic transmembrane region ends with a cluster of basic amino acid residues; these are followed by short, hydrophilic cytoplasmic tails, which form the carboxy terminal ends of the polypeptides. Less is known about the intracellular regions of class II molecules than those of class I.

GENOMIC ORGANIZATION OF THE MHC

Organization of the MHC Gene Loci

In humans, the MHC is located on the short arm of chromosome 6. β_2 microglobulin is encoded by a gene on chromosome 15. The human MHC occupies a large segment of DNA, extending about 3500 kilobases (kb). (For comparison, a large human gene may extend up to 50 to 100 kb, and 3500 kb is the size of the entire *Escherichia coli* genome!) In classical genetic terms, it extends about 4 centimorgans, meaning crossovers within the MHC occur with a frequency of over 4 per cent at each meiosis. A recent molecular map of the human MHC is shown in Figure 5–7. Many of the genes found within the MHC code for proteins whose function is not yet known. The class II genes are located closest to the centromere in the order DP, DQ, and DR. A surprise from these gene-mapping studies is that there

may be two or three functional β chain genes for some class II loci but usually only one functional α chain gene. The use of more than one β chain gene allows some class II gene products, especially HLA-DR, to be expressed in more than two "allelic" forms on a single cell. This contributes to an important difference between class I and class II loci. For class I, *a heterozygous individual expresses six different polymorphic alleles (three from each parent) and six class I MHC molecules per cell.* For class II, although the individual also inherits only six different polymorphic loci, more than six class II MHC $\alpha\beta$ heterodimers can be expressed per cell. Some class II molecules are formed by more than one functional polymorphic β chain within the same allelic locus. Additional class II heterodimers are produced by the combination of the α chain from one allele and the β chain of the other allele. *Usually, individuals can express 10 to 20 different class II gene products per cell; the variation in number depends upon which alleles have been inherited.* This increases the potential number of foreign protein antigens that can bind to and be presented in association with class II molecules. In addition, there are several pseudogenes (defective genes) and additional class II–like sequences that encode proteins of unknown function.

An important recent discovery is that the class II region of the MHC also contains genes whose expression is necessary for efficient assembly of class I molecules. Two of these genes, called **transporter in antigen processing (TAP) 1 and 2,** are believed to encode subunits of a heterodimeric protein pump that transports peptides from the cytosol into the endoplasmic reticulum, where they can associate with newly translated class I MHC heavy chains. Other genes in this

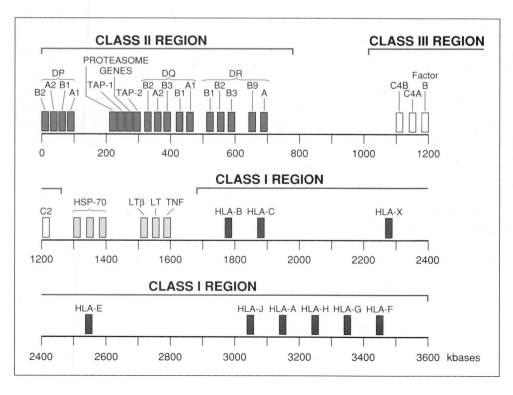

FIGURE 5–7. Molecular map of the human major histocompatibility complex. *HLA-F, G, H, J, and X are class I–like molecules. This map is simplified to exclude other class I– and class II–like genes, genes not of immunologic interest, and numerous genes of unknown function. The pattern of class II genes may vary with the inherited allele. C2, C4A, C4B, and Factor B are complement proteins; HSP-70 is a heat shock protein; lymphotoxin (LT), lymphotoxin β (LT-β), and tumor necrosis factor (TNF) are cytokine genes.*

cluster encode subunits of a cytosolic protease complex (the **proteasome**) that may be involved in generating peptides from cytosolic proteins. The functions of these proteins will be discussed later in this chapter and in Chapter 6.

The complement or so-called "class III" region is telomeric to the class II region and encodes components of the complement system (C2, C4A, C4B, and Factor B, which are homologous to the S or serum proteins of the mouse MHC) as well as the enzyme steroid 21-hydroxylase. The most telomeric portion of the MHC contains the class I α chain genes in the sequence B, C, and A. The genes for heat shock proteins and for the cytokines, tumor necrosis factor (TNF), lymphotoxin (LT), and lymphotoxin β (LT β), map between the complement and class I regions (see Chapter 12). Some heat shock proteins also map to these regions; these molecules normally bind to denatured proteins and may be involved in delivery of denatured cytosolic proteins to the proteasome for degradation. The large space located between the C and A genes contains additional genes that are class I–like. Many more class I–like genes have been found telomeric to HLA-A outside of the true MHC; these genes occupy another 11 centimorgans! Some of these class I–like sequences are pseudogenes, but some encode nonpolymorphic proteins that are expressed in association with β_2 microglobulin.

The function of the nonpolymorphic class I–like genes and their products is largely unknown. In mice, one such gene, called Tla, is expressed on thymocytes and leukemic T cells. Recently, another class I–like product has been described to function as an Fc receptor, binding and transporting IgG molecules across an epithelial barrier; however, the gene for this product has not yet been mapped. Rare T cells may recognize variant class I molecules instead of the conventional polymorphic class I molecules. (This has been shown most convincingly for a subset of T cells, discussed in Chapter 7, that recognizes CD1 molecules, class I–like proteins that are encoded on a different chromosome from the HLA complex.) An alternative proposal for the function of the nonpolymorphic class I–like genes and pseudogenes is that these genes serve as a repository of alternative nucleic acid sequences to be used for generating polymorphic sequences in the true class I molecules. According to this hypothesis, the process of **gene conversion** (i.e., incorporation of variant sequences into the true class I and class II genes without reciprocal crossing over) has occurred during evolution to generate the extraordinary polymorphism of the MHC alleles. Moreover, ongoing gene conversion events would provide a source of new mutations, constantly introducing new alleles into the population. Gene conversion would be far more efficient than point mutations because (1) several changes can be introduced at once, and (2) amino acids necessary for maintaining structure can remain unchanged if identical amino acids at those positions are encoded by both the genes involved in the conversion event.

The murine MHC, located on chromosome 17, occupies a somewhat smaller region than the human MHC, and the genes are organized in a slightly different order. Specifically, one of the class I genes (H2-K) is located centromeric to the class II region, but the other class I genes and the nonpolymorphic genes are telomeric to the class II region. A possible interpretation of this variant arrangement is that the basic form of the MHC, namely class II, complement, cytokines, and class I, arose prior to speciation between mouse and man. Subsequent to speciation, the murine MHC is presumed to have undergone a rearrangement, which resulted in dividing the class I genes. The molecular structure of the murine class II region has also revealed some surprises not fully anticipated by classical genetics. The I-A subregion, originally defined by classical genetics, codes for the α and β chains of the I-A molecule as well as the highly polymorphic β chain of the I-E molecule. The I-E subregion of classical genetics codes only for the less polymorphic α chain of the I-E molecule. As in the human, β_2 microglobulin is not coded for by the MHC, but is located on a separate chromosome (chromosome 2).

Organization of Individual Class I and Class II MHC Genes

The general patterns of intron-exon organization of the individual class I and class II genes are similar to each other. Schematic examples of class Iα and class IIα genes are depicted in Figure 5–8. In all MHC genes, the first exon encodes the leader or signal sequences that target the nascent proteins to the endoplasmic reticulum. These amino acid residues are not found in mature, cell surface MHC molecules (see the discussion of biosynthesis later in this chapter). Each of the approximately 90 amino acid residue extracellular segments (e.g., class I α1, α2, and α3 or class II α1, α2, β1, and β2) is coded for by a separate large exon. Since polymorphisms are localized to these protein domains, the polymorphic regions are contained within one or two exons per gene. Consequently, the polymorphisms of different alleles can be studied by sequencing a small portion of each gene, for example with the polymerase chain reaction (PCR) (Box 5–2). The transmembrane and cytoplasmic regions are encoded by several small exons. For class I α chains, each of the intracellular conserved phosphorylation sites is encoded by a separate small exon, emphasizing the probable importance these sites play in the intracellular trafficking of class I molecules.

EXPRESSION OF MHC MOLECULES

The expression of MHC molecules on different cell types determines whether or not T lymphocytes can interact with foreign antigens present on the surface of these cells. CD8$^+$ cytolytic T lymphocytes (CTLs) recognize foreign antigens such as viral polypeptides when they are bound to class I MHC molecules. The ability of

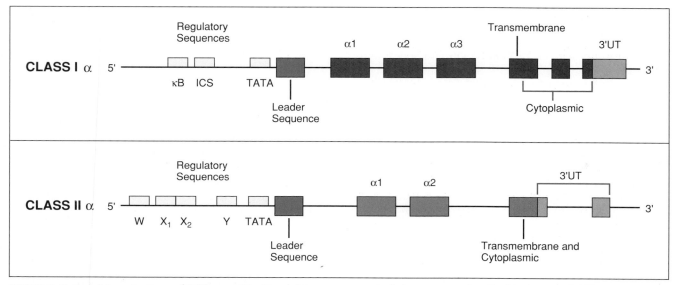

FIGURE 5–8. *Exon-intron structures of MHC genes.* *The 5' regulatory sequences include sequences described in the text. 3' UT indicates the 3' untranslated sequence. Note that exons and introns are not shown to scale.*

BOX 5–2. POLYMERASE CHAIN REACTION

The polymerase chain reaction (PCR) is a rapid and simple method for copying and amplifying specific DNA sequences up to about 1 kilobase in length. In order to use this method, it is necessary to know the sequence of a short region of DNA on each end of the larger sequence that is to be copied; these short sequences are used to specify oligonucleotide primers. The method consists of repetitive cycles of DNA melting, DNA annealing, and DNA synthesis (see figure). Double-stranded DNA containing the sequence to be copied and amplified is mixed with a large molar excess of two single-stranded DNA oligonucleotides (the primers). The first primer is identical to the 5' end of the sense strand of the DNA to be copied, and the second primer is identical to the anti–sense strand at the 3' end of the sequence. (Since double-stranded DNA is antiparallel, the second primer is also the inverted complement of the sense strand.) The PCR reaction is initiated by melting the double-stranded DNA at high temperature and cooling the mixture to allow DNA annealing. During annealing, the first primer (present in large molar excess) will hybridize to the 3' end of the anti–sense strand, and the second primer (also present in large molar excess) will hybridize to the 3' end of the sense strand. The annealed mixture is incubated with DNA polymerase I and all four deoxynucleotide triphosphates (A, T, G, and C), allowing new DNA to be synthesized. DNA polymerase I will extend the 3' end of each bound primer, synthesizing the complement of the single-stranded DNA templates. Specifically, the original sense strand is used as a template to make a new anti–sense strand and the original anti–sense strand is used as a template to make a new sense strand. This ends cycle one. Cycle two is initiated when the reaction mixture is remelted and then allowed to reanneal with the primers. In the DNA synthetic step of the second cycle, each strand synthesized in the first cycle serves as an additional template, having hybridized with the appropriate primers. (It follows that the number of templates in the reaction doubles with each cycle, hence the name "chain reaction.") The second cycle is completed when DNA polymerase I extends the primers to synthesize the complement of the templates. PCR reactions can be conducted for 20 or more cycles, doubling the sequence flanked by the primers at each step. These reactions are routinely automated by using temperature controlled cyclers to regulate melting, annealing, and DNA synthesis, and by using a DNA polymerase I enzyme isolated from thermostable bacteria that can withstand the temperatures used for melting of DNA.

PCR has many uses. For example, by choosing suitable primers, exon 2 of an unknown HLA-DR β allele (i.e., the exon that encodes the polymorphic $\beta1$ protein domain) can be amplified, the amplified DNA ligated into a suitable vector, and the DNA sequence determined without ever isolating the original gene from genomic DNA. This was the original purpose for which PCR was invented. PCR is also widely used for the cloning of known genes or genes related to known genes (e.g., by choosing primers from highly conserved regions of a gene family). PCR can be used to detect, or in some cases even quantify, the presence of particular DNA sequences in a sample (e.g., the presence of viral sequences in a clinical specimen). Levels of mRNA can also be quantified by using reverse transcriptase to make a cDNA copy of the mRNA prior to PCR amplification. Finally, since PCR can amplify DNA only when the two primers are near each other (i.e., within about 1 kilobase), PCR can be used to assay for specific gene rearrangements by choosing primers complementary to sequences that are brought together only when the gene is rearranged (e.g., with specific V and J segment sequences in the Ig genes, see Box 4–2).

Continued

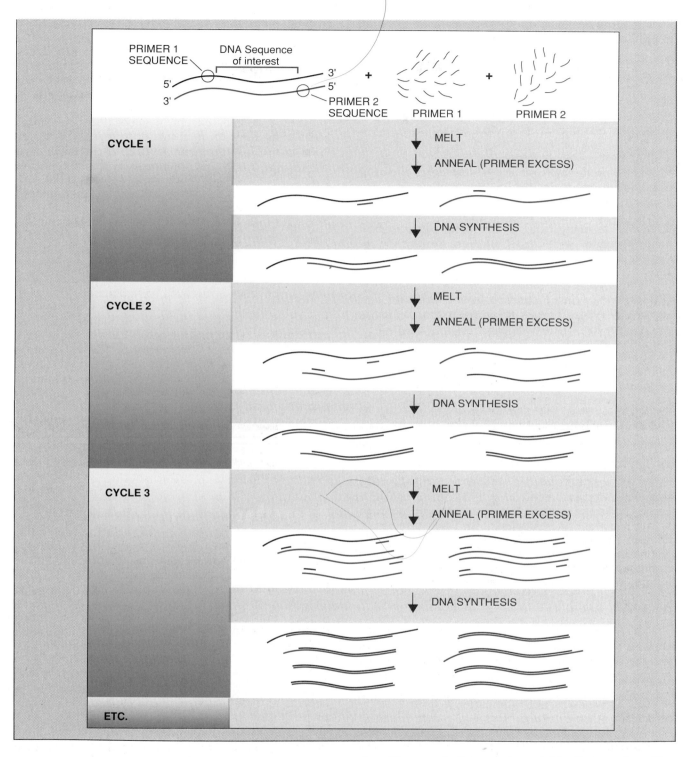

CTLs to lyse a virally infected cell is a direct function of the quantity of class I molecules expressed. In contrast, CD4$^+$ helper T lymphocytes recognize antigens bound to class II MHC molecules. Class II MHC molecules are expressed by fewer cell types than class I MHC molecules and are under different regulation. As a consequence, fewer cell types can present antigens to helper T cells (see Chapter 6). Furthermore, the ability to present antigen to helper T cells is, in large part, a function of the level of class II MHC molecule expres-

sion. The concluding portion of this chapter describes the regulation and biosynthesis of MHC molecule expression.

Regulation of MHC Molecule Expression

The expression of class I and class II MHC molecules is regulated both by differentiation, in a cell- and tissue-specific manner, and by extrinsic immune and inflammatory stimuli. There are four important features of MHC molecule expression:

1. *The constitutive expression of class I molecules is distinct from that of class II molecules.* In general, class I molecules are present on virtually all nucleated cells, whereas class II molecules are normally expressed only on B lymphocytes, macrophages, dendritic cells, endothelial cells, and a few other cell types.

2. *The rate of transcription is the major determinant of MHC molecule expression on the cell surface.*

3. *Transcription and expression of the various class I genes and molecules are coordinately regulated; similarly, the transcription and expression of different class II genes and their products are also coordinately regulated.* In many cells, β_2 microglobulin is coordinately regulated with class I α chains, despite the fact that the β_2 microglobulin gene is not located within the MHC.

4. *Cytokines can modulate the rate of constitutive transcription of class I and class II genes in a wide variety of cell types.* This is an important amplification mechanism for T cell responses, because most of the cytokines that enhance MHC expression are secreted by T cells, and MHC molecules are components of the ligands that T cells recognize and respond to. On almost all cell types examined, interferons (IFNs) -α, -β, and -γ markedly increase the level of expression of class I molecules. TNF and lymphotoxin can also increase class I molecule expression. (The biologic activities of cytokines are discussed in detail in Chapter 12.) These cytokine effects are mediated by increased levels of gene transcription that result from cytokine-activated transcription factors binding to regulatory DNA sequences in class I genes (Fig. 5–8). Specifically, IFNs cause binding of nuclear factors to an interferon consensus sequence (ICS) located in the flanking regions of all class I genes. (The ICS is structurally related to but distinct from the interferon sequence response element discussed in Chapter 12, Box 12–2). TNF and LT cause binding of factors related to NF-κB, first described as transcriptional activators of immunoglobulin genes (Chapter 4, Box 4–4).

In contrast to class I molecules, class II molecules showed marked differences in cell expression among various cell types and in their responses to cytokines. Among the cells that commonly present antigen to T cells, mononuclear phagocytes express only low levels of class II molecules, until stimulated to do so by IFN-γ or certain other cytokines. This expression is antagonized by interleukin-10. Epidermal Langerhans cells and vascular endothelial cells, like mononuclear phagocytes, increase class II expression in response to IFN-γ, whereas lymphoid dendritic cells are constitutively positive for class II expression and do not appear to respond to cytokines. B lymphocytes constitutively express class II molecules and can also respond to cytokines. However, resting B cells in mice increase expression of class II molecules in response to interleukin-4 and decrease expression in response to IFN-γ. Although most human cells express HLA-DR and HLA-DP at considerably higher levels than they express HLA-DQ molecules, B cells express HLA-DQ at greater levels than they express HLA-DP.

Most non-immune cell types express little if any class II MHC molecules unless exposed to high levels of IFN-γ. In some cells, such as pancreatic islet cells, additional cytokines like TNF may be necessary as cosignals for induction. These cells are unlikely to present antigens to T cells except in unusual circumstances. Some cells, such as neurons, do not respond to any known cytokine treatment and remain class II–negative. Finally, human but not mouse T cells express class II molecules upon activation; however, no cytokine has been identified in this response, and its functional significance is unknown.

Most information about transcriptional control of class II molecules has come from analyses of the HLA-DR α chain gene promoter region (Fig. 5–8). This promoter contains three conserved sequences necessary for expression of HLA-DR as a transfected gene or transgene. These sequences have been designated as the W, X, and Y boxes, and the X box is now known to consist of two tandem regulatory sequences called X1 and X2. The protein that binds to X2 is a member of the AP-1 family of transcription factors. The W, X, and Y boxes are occupied by proteins in all cells that express class II molecules; congenital deficiency in some of these binding proteins will prevent class II expression, a condition known as the "bare lymphocyte syndrome." No unique regulatory sequence has been identified as an IFN-γ responsive element in class II promoters. It seems more likely that IFN-γ increases the level and changes the composition of proteins that bind to the X box.

Biosynthesis of MHC Molecules

MHC molecules are translated from messenger RNA (mRNA) molecules on membrane-bound ribosomes and co-translationally inserted into the membrane of the endoplasmic reticulum. The signal sequence is removed from the nascent polypeptide during translation. N-linked high-mannose oligosaccharides are added in the endoplasmic reticulum, either during or immediately after translation. The MHC molecules then pass through to the Golgi apparatus, where the oligosaccharides are converted from high mannose to complex form. A protein called either calnexin or IP88/90 may act as a molecular chaperone to facilitate this transport process. Finally, the mature glycoproteins are translocated to the plasma membrane by vesicular transport. For class I molecules, association of the α chain with β_2 microglobulin occurs intracellularly, probably within the endoplasmic reticulum. Studies of a human B cell line called Daudi have been particularly informative about the importance of β_2 microglobulin for class I MHC molecule expression. Daudi lacks the genetic information for synthesizing β_2 microglobulin, and although it transcribes class I genes and translates class I mRNA, only unstable intracellular translation products appear. Upon transfection of a functional β_2 microglobulin gene into Daudi cells or fusion with a β_2 microglobulin–expressing partner, class I products derived from the Daudi line are "rescued" and appear on the cell surface. Similarly, as discussed in Chapter 8, transgenic mice that lack β_2 microglobulin fail to express class I molecules.

The surface expression of class I molecules is dependent on the binding of the newly synthesized molecules to peptides being produced within the cell. Association of such peptides with the peptide-binding cleft promotes association of the α chain with β_2 microglobulin and correct folding of the complete class I molecule. Again, examination of mutant cell lines has been helpful in elucidating this process. Several cell lines with deletion of the TAP-1 and/or TAP-2 genes are unable to efficiently express class I molecules. The expression of class I molecules can be "rescued" in such cells by addition of large quantities of peptides that bind to the class I molecules or by reintroduction of the TAP genes. The TAP proteins are subunits of a heterodimeric membrane protein that belongs to a family of ATP-dependent pump proteins. By analogy, it has been proposed that the TAP proteins function to transport peptides from the cytosol into the lumen of the endoplasmic reticulum where class I folding occurs. The expression of the TAP genes is regulated by the same cytokines as the class I structural genes. It is of interest that the class II region of the MHC contains genes that also encode subunits of the proteasome that could contribute to the generation of immunogenic peptides from cytoplasmic proteins. Although the MHC-encoded proteasome subunits are also regulated by cytokines, it is not yet clear that these gene products contribute to class I expression.

For class II molecules, the α and β chains must also be coordinately synthesized and presumably must associate within the endoplasmic reticulum. Certain inbred mouse strains lack functional I-E α chains, and I-E β products appear only as unstable intracellular proteins because cell surface expression requires covalently linked α and β chains. Upon interstrain breeding, a functional I-E α chain synthesized from the gene of the other parent can "rescue" these I-E β products, leading to cell surface expression of I-E from both parental alleles.

Within a cell, recently synthesized class II gene products are associated with a third, nonpolymorphic chain not encoded by the MHC. This peptide has been called either γ or **invariant,** because upon migration in two-dimensional gels it is "invariant" among different individuals and inbred strains, a reflection of nonpolymorphism. The invariant chain is about 30 kD in size and is a member of the Ig superfamily. Its orientation is reversed, in contrast to most transmembrane proteins, so that the amino terminus is intracytoplasmic and the carboxy terminus is intraluminal. The native invariant chain appears to be a homotrimer. Each subunit binds one newly synthesized class II $\alpha\beta$ heterodimer, forming a nine polypeptide chain complex (i.e., three $\alpha\beta$ heterodimers bound to one invariant chain homotrimer). The invariant chain separates from the mature class II $\alpha\beta$ heterodimer before it reaches the cell surface. The invariant chain may be required for proper folding of

class II molecules, similar to the role of peptide in catalyzing the folding of class I molecules. Furthermore, peptides are not able to associate with class II molecules until the invariant chain has dissociated in an acidic compartment beyond the Golgi apparatus. This phenomenon will be discussed in greater detail in Chapter 6.

SUMMARY

The MHC is a large genetic region coding for the class I and class II MHC molecules as well as other proteins. MHC molecules are extremely polymorphic, with more than 40 common alleles for each individual gene. Both class I and class II molecules were originally recognized for their role in triggering T cell responses that caused the rejection of transplanted tissue. It is now appreciated that MHC-encoded class I and class II molecules bind foreign protein antigens and form complexes that are recognized by antigen-specific T lymphocytes. Antigens associated with class I molecules are recognized by CD8+ CTLs, whereas class II–associated antigens are recognized by CD4+ helper T cells. The class I products are composed of a 44 kD transmembrane glycoprotein in a non-covalent complex with a nonpolymorphic 12 kD polypeptide (β_2 microglobulin). The class II products contain two MHC-encoded polymorphic chains (about 31 to 34 kD and 29 to 32 kD). It has been found that the three-dimensional structures of both classes of MHC molecules are similar and may be divided into an amino terminal extracellular peptide-binding region, an extracellular nonpolymorphic immunoglobulin-like region, a transmembrane region, and a cytoplasmic region. The peptide-binding region of class I molecules is formed by the α1 and the α2 segments of the heavy chain. It consists of a cleft measuring approximately 25Å $\times$ 10Å $\times$ 11Å with α-helical sides and an eight-strand β-pleated sheet floor. The cleft can accommodate a peptide of about 9 to 11 amino acid residues. Peptides bind to class I molecules largely through allele-specific motifs, which fit into complementary pockets formed by polymorphic residues of the class I molecule. The analogous cleft of class II molecules is formed by the α1 and β1 domains of the two chains. The cleft in class II molecules is open at the ends so that class II molecules can accommodate larger peptides of 10 to 30 or more amino acid residues. In both class I and class II molecules, the polymorphic amino acid residues located in the peptide-binding region determine the specificity of peptide binding and T cell antigen recognition.

The human MHC is very large (about 3500 kb) and is organized as follows: (1) class II genes (HLA-DP, HLA-DQ, HLA-DR), (2) complement genes, (3) heat shock protein and cytokine (TNF, LT, and LT-β) genes, and (4) class I genes (HLA-B, HLA-C, and HLA-A). The mouse MHC is smaller, and the sequence of genes is (1) class I (H-2K), (2) class II (I-A, I-E), (3) complement genes, (4) cytokine genes, and (5) class I (H-2D, H-2L). All MHC genes have similar exon-intron structure, and most regulatory sequences have been located in the 5' flanking region. The expression of the MHC gene products is highly regulated at the level of transcription both by cell type–specific factors and by inflammatory and immune stimuli, including cytokines like IFN-γ. In general, class I genes are expressed more widely, i.e., on more diverse cell types, than are class II genes. Different cell types have distinct patterns of expression of class II MHC molecules. Some cells, such as mononuclear phagocytes, can be induced to express class II molecules by cytokines, especially IFN-γ. Other cells, such as dendritic cells and B lymphocytes, constitutively express class II molecules.

Class I MHC molecules bind peptides during folding and assembly of newly synthesized chains in the endoplasmic reticulum, and peptides serve to catalyze efficient assembly and expression. The class II region–encoded TAP-1 and TAP-2 gene products are believed to form a heterodimeric transmembrane pump that transports peptides from the cytosol to the endoplasmic reticulum. The assembly of class II MHC molecules occurs in association with a nonpolymorphic invariant chain that may play a role similar to that of peptides for class I molecule folding. The invariant chain dissociates from class II molecules in a post-Golgi compartment.

SELECTED READINGS

Bjorkman, P. J., and P. Parham. Structure, function and diversity of class I major histocompatibility complex molecules. Annual Review of Biochemistry 59:253–288, 1990.

Bjorkman, P. J., M. A. Saper, B. Samraoui, W. S. Bennett, J. L. Strominger, and D. C. Wiley. Structure of the human class I histocompatibility antigen HLA-A2. Nature 329:506–512, 1987.

Brown, J. H., T. S. Jardetzky, J. C. Gorga, L. J. Stern, R. G. Urban, J. L. Strominger, and D. C. Wiley. Three-dimensional structure of the class II histocompatibility antigen HLA-DR1. Nature 364:33–39, 1993.

Campbell, R. D., and J. Trowsdale. Map of the human MHC. Immunology Today 14:349–352, 1993.

David-Watine, B., A. Israel, and P. Kourilsky. The regulation and expression of MHC class I genes. Immunology Today 11:286–292, 1990.

Glimcher, L. H., and C. J. Kara. Sequences and factors: a guide to MHC class II transcription. Annual Review of Immunology 10:13–49, 1992.

Parham, P. Antigen processing. Transporters of delight. Nature 348:674–675, 1990.

Robertson, M. Proteasomes in the pathway. Nature 353:300–301, 1991.

Silver, M. L., H.-C. Guo, J. L. Strominger, and D. C. Wiley. Atomic structure of a human MHC molecule presenting an influenza virus peptide. Nature 360:367–369, 1992.

ANTIGEN PROCESSING AND PRESENTATION TO T LYMPHOCYTES

T lymphocytes play a central role in specific immune responses to protein antigens. In Chapter 5, we introduced the concept that the physical forms of antigens recognized by T cells are actually peptide fragments that are derived from protein antigens and are bound to cell surface proteins encoded by genes of the major histocompatibility complex (MHC). Peptides bound to class I MHC molecules are typically derived from proteins synthesized in the cell that displays them (i.e., "endogenous antigens") and are recognized by CD8$^+$ T cells, which are usually cytolytic T lymphocytes (CTLs). CTLs provide a major host defense mechanism against intracellular microbes. In contrast, peptides derived from proteins in the extracellular environment ("exogenous antigens") are displayed in association with class II MHC molecules and are recognized by CD4$^+$ T cells, which are usually helper T lymphocytes. Helper T cells are required for the induction of humoral and cell-mediated responses, which are most effective in eliminating extracellular pathogens. In this chapter, we will describe in greater detail the characteristics of the peptide-MHC molecule complexes, the nature of the cells that form and display these complexes, and the mechanisms by which cells convert endogenous and exogenous protein antigens to peptides that can bind to MHC molecules. The activation and effector mechanisms of T cell subsets that occur subsequent to recognition of peptide-MHC complexes will be discussed in later chapters.

CHARACTERISTICS OF ANTIGEN RECOGNITION BY T LYMPHOCYTES

Our current understanding of T cell antigen recognition is the culmination of a vast amount of work that began with studies of the physicochemical forms of antigens that stimulated cell-mediated immunity. These studies led to the discovery that cells other than T lymphocytes play an obligatory role in T cell activation by foreign antigens, and later to the elucidation of the function of MHC molecules in T cell antigen recognition.

The Forms of Antigens Recognized by T Lymphocytes

The specificity of T lymphocytes for complexes of peptides and MHC molecules determines several characteristics of T cell antigen recognition, which differ in fundamental ways from antigen recognition by antibody molecules.

1. *T lymphocytes recognize only peptides*, whereas B cells can specifically recognize peptides, proteins, nucleic acids, polysaccharides, lipids, and small chemicals. As a result, T cell–mediated immune responses are induced only by protein antigens (the natural source of foreign peptides), whereas humoral immune responses are seen with protein and non-protein antigens. Some T cells are specific for chemically reactive forms of haptens such as dinitrophenol. In these situations, it is likely that the haptens bind to cell surface proteins, including MHC molecules, and peptides containing these hapten conjugates are recognized by T cells.

2. *T cells recognize only linear determinants of peptides defined predominantly by primary amino acid sequences* that assume extended conformations within the peptide-binding clefts of MHC molecules. In contrast, B cells specific for protein antigens may recognize conformational determinants that exist when proteins are in their native tertiary (folded) configuration or determinants that are exposed by denaturation or proteolysis. Thus, when an animal is immunized with a native protein, the antigen-specific T cells that are stimulated will respond to denatured or even proteolytically digested forms of that protein. In contrast, antibodies produced by B cells after immunization with the native protein react only with the native protein (Table

TABLE 6–1. Qualitative Differences in Antigen Recognition by T and B Lymphocytes

Immunizing Antigen	Secondary Antigen Exposure	Secondary Immune Response	
		B Cell–Mediated (Antibody Production)	T Cell–Mediated (Delayed-Type) Hypersensitivity
Native protein	Native protein	+	+
Denatured protein	Native protein	−	+
Native protein	Denatured protein	−	+
Denatured protein	Denatured protein	+	+

Antigen recognition by T and B lymphocytes is qualitatively different. In an immunized animal, B cells are specific for conformational determinants of the immunogen and, therefore, distinguish between native and denatured protein antigens. T cells, however, do not distinguish between native and denatured protein antigens because T cells recognize linear epitopes on short peptides derived from the intact proteins by proteolysis.

6–1). Consistent with this difference in the nature of antigenic determinants for T and B cell recognition is the finding that T cell responses to a soluble antigen cannot be inhibited using antibodies specific for conformational determinants of that antigen, whereas antigen recognition by B cells can be competitively inhibited by such antibodies.

3. *T cells recognize and respond to foreign peptide antigens only when the antigen is attached to the surfaces of other cells*, whereas B cells and secreted antibodies bind soluble antigens in body fluids or cell surface antigens. This is because MHC molecules form part of the complex that T cells recognize, and these molecules are cell surface–bound integral membrane proteins. The display of peptide-MHC complexes in a form that can be recognized by T cells is called **antigen presentation.** Cells that display antigens in this form are called **antigen-presenting cells (APCs).** The properties and functions of APCs are discussed later in the chapter. Although historically the term APC has most often been used to describe cells that present antigen to CD4$^+$ helper T lymphocytes, it is now appropriate to describe target cells of CTL lysis as APCs as well, since CTLs also recognize peptide-MHC complexes on the surface of these target cells.

Physicochemical Features of Peptide-MHC Complexes

In order to stimulate T cell responses, peptides derived from protein antigens must bind to MHC molecules and must remain stably bound long enough to allow specific T cells to engage the complex. We will first describe the characteristics of the peptide-MHC complexes that T cells recognize, and later we will describe how these complexes are formed. The structural basis for peptide binding to both class I and class II MHC molecules has been analyzed by three approaches: (1) binding assays of peptides to purified MHC molecules in cell-free solutions; (2) x-ray crystallographic analyses of purified MHC molecules with bound peptides; and (3) amino acid analysis of peptides eluted from MHC molecules purified from cell membranes. The following are the main features of MHC-peptide interactions elucidated by these approaches:

1. *The association of antigenic peptides and MHC molecules is a saturable, low-affinity interaction ($K_d = 10^{-6} M$) with a slow "on rate" and a very slow "off rate."* These features were determined first by the techniques of equilibrium dialysis (see Chapter 3 and Fig. 6–1) and

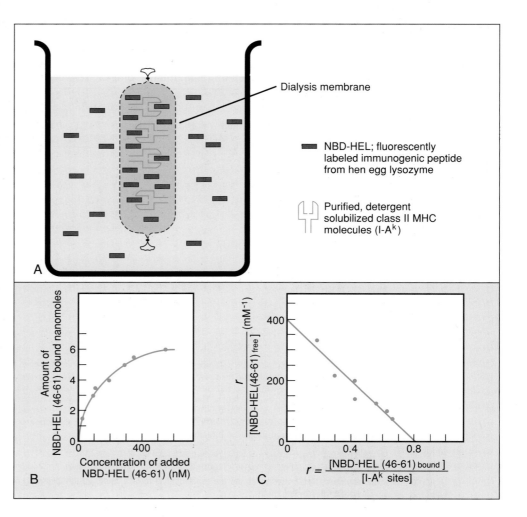

FIGURE 6–1. Demonstration of peptide binding to MHC molecules by equilibrium dialysis. *Purified I-A^k class II MHC molecules bind a peptide fragment of hen egg lysozyme (HEL), HEL(46–61), that is labeled with a fluorescent marker (NBD), which allows the concentration of the peptide to be determined (A). Analysis of the amount of HEL bound (i.e., the concentration within the dialysis membrane minus the concentration outside) at varying concentrations of peptide shows that the binding is saturable (B). Scatchard analysis shows that each I-A^k molecule has approximately one binding site (X-axis intercept), and the dissociation constant (K_d) is approximately $1 \times 10^{-6} M$ (calculated from the slope of the line). In this plot, r represents the number of peptide molecules bound to each MHC molecule when there is an excess of peptide (C). Note that HEL(46–61) is known to be presented in association with I-A^k molecules. (Modified with permission from Babbitt, B. P., P. M. Allen, G. Matsueda, E. Haber, and E. R Unanue. Binding of immunogenic peptides to Ia histocompatibility molecules. Nature 317:359–361, 1985. Copyright © 1985, Macmillan Magazines Ltd.)*

Dialysis membrane

NBD-HEL; fluorescently labeled immunogenic peptide from hen egg lysozyme

Purified, detergent solubilized class II MHC molecules (I-A^k)

A

B Amount of NBD-HEL (46-61) bound nanomoles

Concentration of added NBD-HEL (46-61) (nM)

C $\frac{r}{[\text{NBD-HEL (46-61)}_{\text{free}}]}$ (mM^{-1})

$r = \frac{[\text{NBD-HEL (46-61)}_{\text{bound}}]}{[\text{I-A}^k \text{ sites}]}$

gel filtration using purified class II MHC molecules and fluorescently or radioactively labeled peptides. The affinity of peptide-MHC interaction is much lower than that of antigen-antibody binding, which usually has a K_d of 10^{-7} to 10^{-11} M. In a solution, saturation of peptide binding to class II MHC molecules takes 15 to 30 minutes. Once bound, peptides may stay associated with either class I or class II MHC molecules for hours to many weeks! The slow on rate of association of peptides with class II MHC molecules suggests that conformational changes in both peptide and MHC molecule are required before stable binding occurs. The extraordinarily slow off rates make up for the low affinity by ensuring that the peptide-MHC complexes persist long enough to interact with T cells.

2. *Each class I or class II MHC molecule binds a single peptide* within a specialized cleft at the surface of the MHC molecule. This was apparent from the analysis of peptide binding to MHC molecules in solution, and was confirmed by the solution of the x-ray crystallographic structure of both class I and class II MHC molecules, which show a single binding cleft (see Chapter 5).

3. *Multiple different peptides can bind to the same MHC molecule.* This was first suggested by functional assays in which recognition of one peptide-MHC complex to a T cell could be inhibited by the addition of another structurally similar peptide. In these experiments, the MHC molecule apparently could bind different peptides, but the T cell recognized only one pep-tide-MHC complex. Definitive evidence for the ability of a single MHC molecule to bind different peptides came from direct binding studies with purified MHC molecules in solution (Table 6–2) as well as the analyses of peptides eluted from MHC molecules derived from intact cells. It is clear that a wide variety of peptides with divergent amino acid sequences are capable of binding to each MHC molecule, but there are certain constraints (discussed below) that prohibit all peptides from binding to an individual MHC molecule indiscriminately. These observations, together with the limited number of MHC alleles expressed in each individual, support the hypothesis that *MHC molecules show a broad specificity for peptide binding, and the fine specificity of antigen recognition resides largely in the antigen receptors of T lymphocytes.*

4. *The association of peptides with MHC molecules is determined by the primary and secondary structures of both molecules.* The crystal structures of class I and class II MHC molecules were described in Chapter 5 (Figs. 5–4 and 5–6). The single peptide-binding cleft of both molecules has a β-pleated sheet floor and α-helical sides. Polymorphic amino acid residues are concentrated in this peptide-binding region. Antigenic peptides lie within the cleft in molecular contact with the floor and the α-helical sides. All immunogenic peptides contain some amino acids that form contacts with the MHC molecule and other amino acids that point away from the cleft and are apparently recognized by T cells.

TABLE 6–2. Binding of Unrelated Peptides to an MHC Molecule: Correlation with Inhibition of Antigen Presentation

Competing Peptide	Ability of Peptide to Compete with OVA(323–339) for Binding to I-A^d	Ability of Peptide to Inhibit Presentation of OVA(323–339) by I-A^d–Expressing APC to T Cells Specific For OVA plus I-A^d
Ovalbumin OVA(323–339)	++++	NA
Influenza virus hemagglutinin Ha(130–142)	++++	++++
Hen egg lysozyme HEL(74–86)	++	+++
λ-repressor protein λ-(12–26)	++	++
Sperm whale myoglobin Myo(132–153)	±	±
Herpes simplex virus glycoprotein HSV(8–23)	±	±

Peptide binding to purified MHC molecules correlates with MHC-restricted presentation of peptide to T cells. Binding of ^{125}I-labeled ovalbumin-derived peptide, OVA(323–339), to purified, detergent solubilized murine I-A^d was measured by gel filtration in the presence of varying concentrations of unlabeled peptides. Presentation of OVA(323–339) by paraformaldehyde fixed, I-A^d–expressing APCs to an OVA(323–339)–specific, I-A^d–restricted T cell line, in the presence of varying concentrations of competing peptides, was assayed by measuring antigen-induced T cell cytokine secretion. The results indicate that the ability of a competing peptide to block OVA(323–339) binding to purified I-A^d correlates well with the ability of the same competing peptide to block I-A^d–restricted presentation of OVA(323–339) to T cells. Numbers following abbreviations of proteins refer to the amino acid residues of the native protein.

Abbreviations: MHC, major histocompatibility complex; NA, not applicable.

Adapted from Buus, S., A. Sette, S. M. Colon, C. Miles, and H. M. Grey. The relationship between major histocompatibility (MHC) restriction and the capacity of Ia to bind immunogenic peptides. Science 235:1353–1358, 1987. Copyright 1987 by the AAAS.

TABLE 6–3. Identification of MHC-Binding and T Cell Receptor–Binding Residues in Peptide Antigens

	HEL Peptide										Stimulation of HEL-Specific T Cells	Binding to Purified I-A^k	Competition with Native HEL for T Cell Stimulation
	Amino Acid Residue Position No.												
	52	*53*	*54*	*55*	*56*	*57*	*58*	*59*	*60*	*61*			
1	Asp	Tyr	Gly	Ile	Leu	Gln	Ile	Asn	Ser	Arg	+	+	NA
2	Asp	Tyr	Gly	Ile	Ala	Gln	Ile	Asn	Ser	Arg	–	+	+
3	Asp	Ala	Gly	Ile	Leu	Gln	Ile	Asn	Ser	Arg	–	+	+
4	Asp	Tyr	Gly	Ala	Leu	Gln	Ile	Asn	Ser	Arg	–	–	–
5	Asp	Tyr	Ala	Ile	Leu	Gln	Ile	Asn	Ser	Arg	+	+	NA

Synthetic peptides were produced that differed from the native hen egg lysozyme peptide HEL(52–61) (peptide 1) by substitutions for single residues, and the functional consequences of these engineered mutations were analyzed. Substitutions at positions 56 and 53 (peptides 2 and 3) result in loss of T cell stimulation, but retain I-A^k binding. The amino acids at these positions in the native peptide are part of the epitope recognized by the T cell receptor. Substitution of residue 55 (peptide 4) results in loss of T cell stimulation and I-A^k binding. This residue is in part of the peptide that binds to the class II MHC molecule. A substitution at position 54 (peptide 5) has no effect, and therefore this residue is not essential for binding of the peptide to either the MHC or T cell receptor molecules.

Abbreviations: MHC, major histocompatibility complex; HEL, hen egg lysozyme; NA, not applicable.

Adapted from Unanue, E. R., and P. M. Allen. The basis for the immunoregulatory role of macrophages and other accessory cells. Science 236:551–557, 1987. Copyright 1987 by the AAAS.

Mutational analysis of antigenic peptides is a useful method for defining which residues bind to MHC molecules and therefore compete with other peptides for binding, and which residues are recognized by T cells (Table 6–3). Amino acid analysis of the mixture of different peptides eluted from a particular class I or class II MHC molecule can also indicate which residues of a peptide contact the MHC molecule, because these residues will be conserved among many or all of the eluted peptides (Fig. 6–2). Such studies indicate that in order to stimulate T cells, peptides must be capable of forming non-covalent bonds with MHC molecules. This binding, however, is not sufficient for immunogenicity, because each peptide must contain residues that are recognized by specific T cells as well. Mutational analyses of MHC molecules have also indicated the requirements for certain polymorphic residues in the binding of peptides.

5. *There are distinct differences in the nature of peptides that bind to class I or class II MHC molecules,*

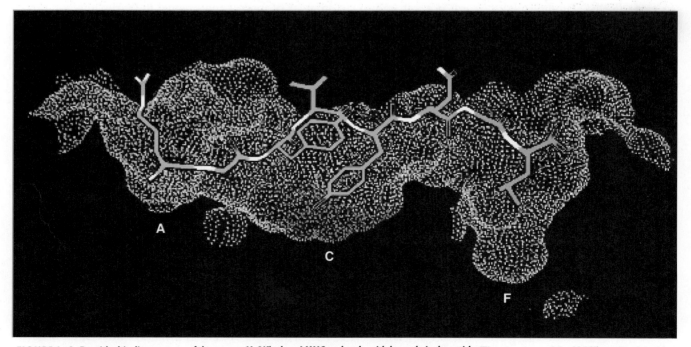

FIGURE 6–2. Peptide-binding groove of the mouse H-2K^b class I MHC molecule with bound viral peptide. *The structure of the H-2K^b molecule with a bound peptide derived from a vesicular stomatitis virus nucleoprotein was elucidated by x-ray crystallography. Pockets in the MHC-binding cleft are labeled A, C, and F. Note that side chains of the peptide, including the NH$_2$ terminus on the left, a tyrosine side chain in the middle, and the COOH terminal residue on the right are within pockets of the MHC-binding cleft. (Modified with permission from Matsumura, M., D. H. Fremont, P. A. Peterson, and I. A. Wilson. Emerging principles for the recognition of peptide antigens by MHC class I molecules. Science 257:927–934, 1992. Copyright 1992 by the AAAS.)*

and these are due to differences in the binding clefts of class I and class II MHC molecules. As described in Chapter 5, the cleft of the class I MHC molecule has closed ends, and the floor has one or more pockets into which fit the side chains of certain amino acid residues of the peptide (Fig. 6–2). These contact residues that bind to the pockets are often at the amino and carboxy terminal ends of the peptide. A peptide will bind to a particular class I MHC molecule only if it is the proper length to fit in the groove (9 to 11 amino acids) and only if it has terminal amino acid side chains that can bind non-covalently with the class I MHC amino acid residues that form the pockets. The many different peptides eluted from a particular allelic form of a class I MHC molecule all have conserved residues whose side chains fit into these pockets. The other residues of peptides that bind a class I MHC molecule are variable and form few close contacts with the cleft. In fact, in cases where the pocket-binding residues of the peptide are at the amino and carboxy termini, the center of the peptide can bow up from its tethered ends, allowing the cleft to accommodate peptides up to 11 amino acid residues in length. These observations suggest that the ability of a peptide to bind to a particular MHC molecule is determined largely by one or two residues of the peptide and that the other residues are displayed for recognition by the antigen receptor of the T cell (see Chapter 7). In contrast, the class II MHC cleft is open ended. This is reflected in the fact that there is a wider range of sizes of peptides that can bind to class II MHC molecules, ranging from 10 to 30 amino acids, and there is no requirement for the presence of certain amino acids at either end. Requisite structural motifs common to class II MHC–binding peptides are not yet known. Nonetheless, class II MHC molecules do show selectivity in peptide binding, with each allelic form of MHC molecule capable of binding different sets of peptides.

6. The association of antigenic peptides with MHC molecules is stabilized by the interaction of antigen-specific, MHC-restricted T cells with the peptide-MHC complexes. This has been directly demonstrated by measuring the strength of interactions between antigenic peptides and MHC molecules in the presence and absence of specific T cells. For instance, a peptide fragment of ovalbumin (OVA) binds to the mouse class II molecule, I-A^d, incorporated in synthetic lipid membranes. The proximity of the two can be estimated by attaching fluorescent labels to each and measuring resonance energy transfer. The resonance energy transfer is markedly increased if an OVA-specific, I-A^d–restricted T cell population is added.

The Phenomenon of MHC-Restricted Antigen Recognition by T Lymphocytes

A fundamental aspect of antigen recognition by helper T cells and CTLs is that any one T lymphocyte is restricted to recognizing a peptide antigen only when it is complexed to a single allelic form of an MHC molecule. This phenomenon is called **MHC restriction.** It was first discovered in the 1970s when investigators mixed T cells and APCs from different inbred strains of animals and measured various kinds of T cell responses. In these experiments, T cells from an animal immunized with an antigen would subsequently recognize and respond to that antigen *in vitro* only if the APCs came from the same animal (or from another that shared MHC alleles with the first animal). In other words, *T cells are self-MHC restricted; they recognize and respond to antigen presented by an APC only if that APC expresses MHC molecules that the T cell recognizes as self.* The MHC molecules that T cells recognize as self are those that the T cells encountered during their maturation from precursors (discussed in Chapter 8). Therefore, "self MHC" does not refer to MHC molecules expressed by the T cells themselves but to MHC molecules on the APCs or target cells. In the normal situation, T cells would only be exposed to self APCs, and therefore the phenomenon of self MHC restriction may seem physiologically irrelevant. The importance of self MHC restriction, however, is twofold. First, its discovery provided the initial evidence that T cell recognition of antigen involves MHC molecules and, furthermore, that T cells recognize polymorphic residues of MHC molecules, i.e., residues that distinguish self and non-self MHC alleles. Second, the phenomenon of self MHC restriction provided important insights into the process of T cell maturation (discussed in Chapter 8).

One of the earliest and clearest demonstrations of MHC restriction involved assays of virus-specific CTL-mediated lysis of virally infected target cells (Fig. 6–3). In most of these experiments, the virus-infected target cells are lysed by the CTLs only if they express allelic forms of MHC molecules that are expressed in the animal from which the CTLs were derived. Furthermore, by using congenic strains of mice, it could be shown that the CTLs and the target cell APC must be derived from mice that share a particular class I MHC allele. Thus, *CTL recognition of antigen is both self MHC– and class I MHC–restricted.* Essentially similar experiments demonstrated that *helper T lymphocyte responses to antigen are also self MHC–restricted, and usually class II MHC–restricted.* For instance, helper T cells will respond to antigens presented by macrophages or B cells that express self class II MHC molecules, and this form of recognition is critical for cell-mediated and humoral immune reactions. In fact, the class I or class II MHC restriction of T cells correlates more strongly with their expression of CD8 or CD4 than with the functional capabilities of the cells. Thus, *all CD8$^+$ T cells are class I–restricted,* because, as we will discuss in Chapter 7, the CD8 molecule binds to class I MHC molecules. Most of these cells are CTLs, although some may function mainly as cytokine-producing cells. Similarly, *all CD4$^+$ T cells are restricted by class II MHC molecules,* because CD4 binds to class II MHC molecules. Most CD4$^+$ cells are helper cells, although CD4$^+$ CTLs (again class II MHC–restricted) also exist.

The molecular basis of MHC-restricted antigen recognition by T cells was elucidated by parallel studies of

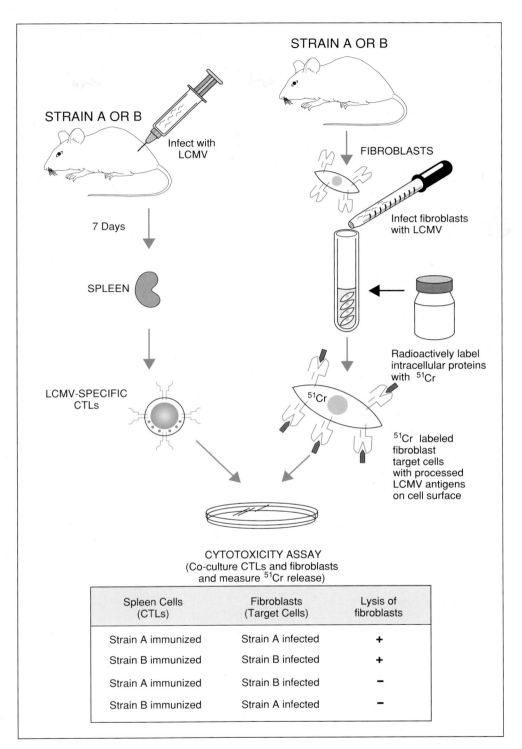

STRAIN A OR B

STRAIN A OR B

Infect with LCMV

FIBROBLASTS

Infect fibroblasts with LCMV

7 Days

SPLEEN

Radioactively label intracellular proteins with ^{51}Cr

LCMV-SPECIFIC CTLs

^{51}Cr

^{51}Cr labeled fibroblast target cells with processed LCMV antigens on cell surface

CYTOTOXICITY ASSAY
(Co-culture CTLs and fibroblasts and measure ^{51}Cr release)

Spleen Cells (CTLs)	Fibroblasts (Target Cells)	Lysis of fibroblasts
Strain A immunized	Strain A infected	+
Strain B immunized	Strain B infected	+
Strain A immunized	Strain B infected	−
Strain B immunized	Strain A infected	−

FIGURE 6–3. MHC restriction of cytolytic T lymphocytes (CTLs). Virus-specific CTLs from a strain A or strain B mouse lyse only syngeneic target cells infected with the specific virus. The CTLs do not lyse uninfected targets and are not alloreactive. Further analysis has shown that the CTLs and target cells must come from animals that share class I MHC alleles in order for the target cell to present viral antigens to the CTLs. Thus, CTL recognition of antigen is self class I MHC–restricted. LCMV, lymphocytic choriomeningitis virus.

the structure of the T cell receptor for antigen and of antigen presentation. As we shall see in Chapter 7, T cells express a single antigen receptor that simultaneously interacts with a peptide epitope of a protein antigen that is bound to MHC molecules and with polymorphic residues of MHC molecules (Fig. 6–4). In the remainder of this chapter, we will address the question of how large, complex proteins are converted to peptides that bind to MHC molecules and get displayed on APC surfaces.

MECHANISMS OF ANTIGEN PRESENTATION TO CLASS II MHC–RESTRICTED CD4$^+$ T CELLS

The activation of CD4$^+$ helper T cells by antigen requires the participation of cells other than T lymphocytes; these cells are often called **accessory cells.** The obligatory role of accessory cells in lymphocyte activa-

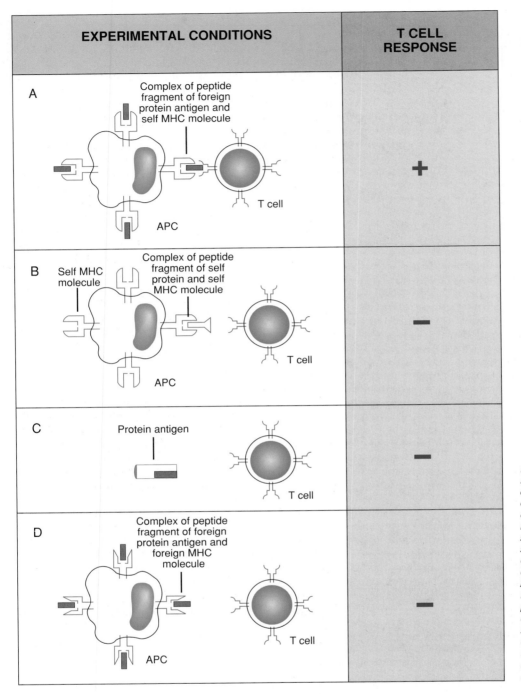

EXPERIMENTAL CONDITIONS	T CELL RESPONSE
A — Complex of peptide fragment of foreign protein antigen and self MHC molecule; APC; T cell	+
B — Self MHC molecule; Complex of peptide fragment of self protein and self MHC molecule; APC; T cell	−
C — Protein antigen; T cell	−
D — Complex of peptide fragment of foreign protein antigen and foreign MHC molecule; APC; T cell	−

FIGURE 6–4. Specificity of MHC-restricted T cells. Helper T cells and cytolytic T lymphocytes (CTLs) recognize complexes of self MHC molecules and peptide fragments of foreign antigens (A). MHC-restricted T cells do not recognize self MHC with self peptide (B), foreign antigens without MHC molecules (C), or complexes of foreign MHC molecules and peptide fragment of antigen (D). APC, antigen-presenting cell; MHC, major histocompatibility complex. (Note that some MHC molecules in this and other figures are depicted without bound peptides for the sake of clarity. Most MHC molecules actually do have bound self peptides.)

tion was formally established when techniques for stimulating immune responses *in vitro* were developed. For example, T cells isolated from the blood, spleen, or lymph nodes of individuals immunized with a protein antigen can be restimulated in tissue culture by that antigen. Stimulation may be measured by assaying the production of cytokines by the T cells or by the proliferation of the T cells. When contaminating macrophages and dendritic cells are removed from the cultures, the purified T lymphocytes no longer respond to antigen, and responsiveness can be restored by adding back the macrophages or dendritic cells. Such experimental approaches provide the basis for defining the

accessory functions of various cell types in T lymphocyte activation. The importance of accessory cells in immune responses *in vivo* is suggested by the observation that adjuvants often need to be administered in addition to antigen in order to elicit an immune response to the antigen. These adjuvants are usually insoluble or undegradable substances that promote nonspecific inflammation, with recruitment of mononuclear phagocytes at the site of immunization.

Accessory cells serve two important functions in the activation of CD4⁺ T cells. First, accessory cells are APCs, i.e., they convert protein antigens to peptides and they present peptide-MHC complexes in a form that can be recognized by CD4$^+$ T cells. The conversion of native proteins to MHC-associated peptide fragments by APCs is called **antigen processing.** As early as the 1950s, it was demonstrated that radioactively or fluorescently labeled antigens injected into animals were found in mononuclear phagocytes or follicular dendritic cells and not in lymphocytes. Later studies showed that an antigen that was taken up by macrophages *in vitro* and then injected into mice was up to 1000 times more immunogenic on a molar basis than the same antigen administered by itself, in a cell-free form. The explanation for this finding is that T cells respond only to antigen associated with macrophages or other APCs, and only a small fraction of an injected soluble antigen ends up in this processed, immunogenic cell-associated form.

The second function of accessory cells is to provide stimuli to the T cell, beyond those initiated by peptide-MHC complexes binding to the T cell antigen receptor. These stimuli, referred to as **costimulator activities,** are required for full physiologic activation of the T cells and are provided by membrane-bound or secreted products of accessory cells. In fact, adjuvants may enhance immune responses *in vivo* in part by inducing the expression of costimulator molecules on accessory cells. The antigen-presenting functions of accessory cells are discussed in more detail in this portion of the chapter, and their costimulator functions are discussed in Chapter 7.

Types of Antigen-Presenting Cells

The two requisite properties that allow a cell to function as an APC for class II MHC–restricted helper T lymphocytes are the ability to process endocytosed antigens and the expression of class II MHC gene products. Most mammalian cells appear to be capable of endocytosing and processing protein antigens, so that the critical property that enables a particular cell to function as an APC is the expression of class II MHC molecules (Table 6–4).

The best-defined APCs for helper T lymphocytes include: (1) mononuclear phagocytes, (2) B lymphocytes, (3) dendritic cells, (4) Langerhans cells of the skin, and (5) in humans, endothelial cells (Table 6–5).

Macrophages and other cells of the **mononuclear phagocyte system** actively phagocytose large particles. Therefore, they probably play an important role in presenting antigens derived from infectious organisms such as bacteria and parasites. Macrophages not only serve as APCs for antigens derived from certain microorganisms, but they also are important effector cells for the killing of these microorganisms. Macrophage presentation of microbial antigens to some CD4$^+$ T lymphocytes results in the secretion of the cytokine interferon-γ (IFN-γ) by the T cells. IFN-γ then activates the macrophages to become more effective killers of microorganisms. (The biologic activities of IFN-γ are described in Chapter 12.) This ability of macrophages to both stimulate and respond to T cells provides an amplification mechanism that increases the ability of the specific immune system to deal with infections.

B lymphocytes specific for a protein antigen are very efficient at presenting that antigen to helper T lymphocytes *in vitro* and may serve as APCs *in vivo*, particularly when the concentration of available antigen is low. The reason why antigen-specific B cells are highly efficient APCs is that their membrane Ig molecules can bind the antigen with high affinity and, therefore, at low concentrations. Ig-bound antigen is also efficiently endocytosed and delivered to intracellular sites of processing (discussed below). The antigen-presenting function of B cells is particularly important in helper T cell–dependent antibody production (see Chapter 9).

Dendritic cells of the spleen and lymph nodes are irregularly shaped, nonphagocytic cells making up a small fraction (<1 per cent) of the total cell population of these organs. They are derived from the bone marrow and may be related to the mononuclear phagocytic lineage (see Chapter 2). Dendritic cells are competent at presenting protein antigens to helper T cells, including naive T cells that have not previously been exposed to antigen. It is also believed that dendritic cells are important for inducing T cell responses to foreign (allo-

TABLE 6–4.   Requirement for Class II MHC Expression in Antigen Presentation to CD4$^+$ Antigen-Specific T Cells

APCs	Genes Transfected Into APCs	Surface Class II MHC	Surface Class I MHC	Antigen	Response of Cytochrome c–Specific, I-E^k–Restricted T Cell Line (Cytokine Secretion)
3T3 (murine fibroblast)	None	None	K^k, D^k	Cytochrome c	−
3T3 (murine fibroblast)	Murine class II Eα^k and Eβ^k	I-E^k	K^k, D^k	None	−
3T3 (murine fibroblast)	Murine class II Eα^k and Eβ^k	I-E^k	K^k, D^k	Cytochrome c	+

Class II MHC expression is required for antigen presentation to CD4$^+$ antigen-specific T cells. In this experiment, a murine fibroblast cell line, 3T3, derived from an H-2^k mouse, which expresses class I, but not class II, MHC molecules, does not present cytochrome c to a cytochrome c–specific, I-E^k–restricted, T cell hybridoma line. When functional genes encoding the α and β chains of the I-E^k molecule are transfected into 3T3 cells, they become competent at presenting antigen to the T cell line.

Abbreviations: MHC, major histocompatibility complex; APC, antigen-presenting cell.

TABLE 6–5. Properties and Functions of Antigen-Presenting Cells

Cell Type	Expression of:		Principal Function
	Class II MHC	*Costimulators*	
Dendritic cells (Langerhans cells, lymphoid dendritic cells)	Constitutive	Constitutive	Initiation of CD4⁺ T cell responses (priming); allograft rejection
Macrophages	Inducible by IFN-γ	Inducible by LPS, IFN-γ	Development of CD4⁺ effector T cells
B lymphocytes	Constitutive; increased by IL-4	Inducible by T cells	Stimulation of CD4⁺ helper T cells in humoral immune responses (cognate T cell–B cell interactions)
Vascular endothelial cells	Inducible by IFN-γ	Constitutive	Recruitment of antigen-specific T cells to site of antigen exposure or inflammation
Various epithelial and mesenchymal cells	Inducible by IFN-γ	Probably none	No known physiologic function; ? role in exacerbation of autoimmune reactions in tissues

Abbreviations: LPS, lipopolysaccharide; IFN-γ, interferon-γ; IL-4, interleukin-4.

geneic) MHC molecules in tissue allografts. Consistent with this hypothesis is the observation that dendritic cells are potent stimulators of mixed lymphocyte reactions (see Chapter 17).

Langerhans cells are specialized epidermal cells with a dendritic morphology. They are derived from bone marrow progenitors, express the CD1 marker, and contain an unusual cytoplasmic organelle called the Birbeck granule. Langerhans cells may be related in lineage to the dendritic cells of spleen and lymph nodes. In fact, they are capable of migrating from skin to lymph nodes and are likely to be the origin of dendritic cells in lymph nodes that drain cutaneous sites. They are the only resident epidermal cells known to be capable of antigen presentation and, therefore, may be important in presenting the antigens responsible for cutaneous contact sensitivity reactions (see Chapter 11).

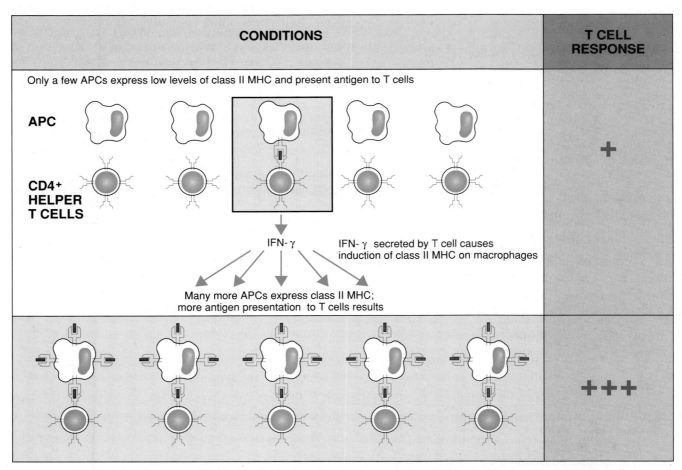

FIGURE 6–5. Interferon-γ amplifies T cell activation by enhancing the expression of MHC molecules on antigen-presenting cells.

In humans, *venular endothelial cells* express class II MHC molecules and may also interact with T cells. This may be particularly important in cell-mediated immune reactions, such as delayed-type hypersensitivity reactions in peripheral tissues (see Chapter 13).

In addition to cells that express class II MHC molecules constitutively, many cell types can be induced to express their class II MHC genes by the T lymphocyte–derived cytokine IFN-γ (Fig. 6–5). The induction of MHC genes in macrophages and endothelial cells may provide an amplification mechanism for enhancing the growth and differentiation of CD4⁺ T cells, and for recruiting and activating T cells at peripheral sites of antigen exposure. Epithelial and mesenchymal cells also express class II MHC molecules in response to IFN-γ. The physiologic significance of antigen presentation by these "non-professional APCs" is unclear. Since they generally do not provide costimulators, it is unlikely that they play an important role in most T cell responses.

Different types of APCs may be involved at different stages of a T cell–mediated immune response to protein antigens. During the cognitive phase of a primary immune response to a protein antigen, one population of APCs, e.g., dendritic cells, may be the predominant cell type involved in stimulating naive T cells that have never before been exposed to that antigen. Subsequent exposure to the same antigen may lead to a differentiation phase of the immune response in which the activated T cells may develop into effector cells in response to stimulation by other types of APCs, such as macrophages or B cells. APCs may determine not only the magnitude of T cell–mediated immune responses but also the relative expansion of subsets of CD4⁺ T cells that produce different cytokines and perform distinct effector functions. This role of APCs in regulating immune responses is discussed in Chapter 10.

Uptake and Processing of Extracellular Protein Antigens by Class II MHC–Expressing Antigen-Presenting Cells

Whether a peptide fragment of a protein antigen is presented by class I or class II MHC molecules is largely determined by the way the protein has come to be present in the cell. Processing of antigens that enter an APC from the extracellular environment usually results in peptide fragments of those proteins associating with class II MHC molecules. These exogenous antigens include the proteins synthesized by extracellular bacteria, fungi, and parasites as well as proteins administered during immunizations.

The initial step in the presentation of an exogenous protein antigen is the binding of the native antigen to an APC. Different APCs can bind protein antigens in several ways and with varying efficiencies and specificities. Macrophages and dendritic cells bind many different antigens, with little or no specificity, to surface mol-

ecules that are undefined. There are, however, special cases in which the surface molecule on the APC that mediates binding and subsequent internalization of the antigen is identified. For example, specific receptors for the Fc portions of immunoglobulins and receptors for the complement protein C3b, which are present on the surface of macrophages, can efficiently bind opsonized antigens and enhance their internalization. This may partially explain why secondary immune responses require lower doses of antigen than primary responses, since at the time of secondary immunization pre-existing specific antibody may augment binding of the antigen to APCs. Another example of specific receptors on APCs is the surface Ig on B cells.

Within minutes after antigens bind to APCs, they enter the cells, usually by phagocytosis or by receptor-mediated endocytosis in clathrin-coated vesicles. Soluble protein antigens may also be internalized into APCs by fluid phage pinocytosis, without actually binding to the cell surface. Such internalized antigens become localized in intracellular membrane–bound vesicles called **endosomes.** The precise ultrastructural and biochemical characteristics of endosomes are not well described. Rather, these organelles are defined mostly by their function, which is intracellular transport and degradation of internalized proteins. The endosomal pathway of protein traffic in the cell is continuous with and ends up at the lysosome, an organelle with well-defined ultrastructural features and enzyme content. Both endosomes and lysosomes may provide intracellular sites for processing of internalized antigens.

The next step in antigen presentation is the processing of the antigen that was internalized in its native form. Several characteristics of the processing of protein antigens are known:

1. *Antigen processing is a time- and metabolism-dependent phenomenon that takes place subsequent to internalization of antigen by APCs.* If macrophages (or other APCs) are incubated briefly ("pulsed") with a protein antigen such as ovalbumin (OVA), rendered metabolically inert by chemical fixation at various times thereafter, and tested for their ability to stimulate OVA-specific T cells, functional antigen presentation occurs only if 1 to 3 hours elapse between the antigen pulse and fixation (Fig. 6–6). This time is required for the APCs to process the antigen and present it in association with class II MHC molecules on the cell surface. Processing of antigen is inhibited by maintaining the APCs below physiologic temperatures, by adding metabolic inhibitors such as azide, or by fixation earlier than 1 hour after the antigen pulse.

2. *The endosomes and lysosomes where antigen processing takes place have an acidic pH, which is required for the processing.* Chemical agents that increase the pH of intracellular acid vesicles, such as chloroquine and ammonium chloride, are potent inhibitors of antigen processing.

3. *Cellular proteases are required for the processing of many protein antigens.* Protease inhibitors with specificities for cathepsin-like enzymes, such as leupeptin, block the presentation of protein antigens by

APCs. The function of proteases is to cleave native protein antigens into small peptides. These proteases also probably act on the invariant chain, promoting its dissociation from class II MHC molecules, as discussed later. Many cellular proteases function optimally at acid pH, and this is the likely reason why antigen processing occurs best in acidic compartments.

4. *The processed forms of most protein antigens that T cells recognize can be artificially generated by proteolysis in the test tube.* Macrophages that are fixed or that are treated with chloroquine before exposure to antigen can effectively present pre-digested peptide fragments of that antigen, but not the intact protein, to specific T cells (Fig. 6–6). Peptides generated by the *in vitro* proteolysis of a complex globular protein or produced synthetically that are capable of stimulating antigen-specific T cells in the presence of fixed APCs can be analyzed for amino acid sequence and secondary structure. Immunogenic peptides derived from many complex globular proteins, such as cytochrome c, ovalbumin, myoglobin, and lysozyme, have been characterized in detail in this way. More recently, as described earlier, naturally generated peptides have been eluted off class II MHC molecules from APCs and analyzed for common structural characteristics.

The net result of processing of a protein antigen is the generation of peptides, many of which are 10 to 30 amino acids long and capable of binding to the peptide-binding clefts of class II MHC molecules. The requirement for antigen processing prior to T cell stimulation explains why T cells recognize linear but not conformational determinants of protein and why T cells cannot distinguish between native and denatured forms of a protein antigen (see Table 6–1). Moreover, in mammalian cells, polysaccharides and lipids cannot be processed to a form that can associate with MHC molecules. This is the reason why polysaccharides and lipids are not recognized by MHC-restricted T lymphocytes and fail to stimulate cell-mediated immunity. It is also likely that most types of APCs, including macrophages, B cells, and dendritic cells, are qualitatively similar in their ability to process endocytosed antigens; however, there may be quantitative differences. For in-

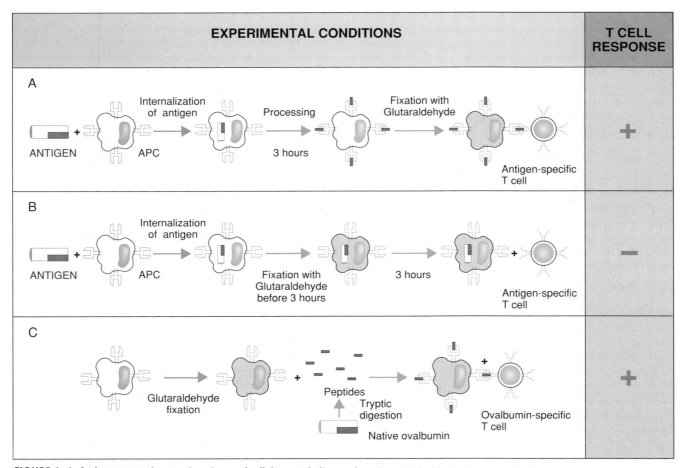

FIGURE 6–6. Antigen processing requires time and cellular metabolism and can be mimicked by in vitro proteolysis. *If an antigen-presenting cell (APC) is allowed to process antigen and is then chemically fixed (rendered metabolically inert) 3 hours or more after antigen internalization, it is capable of presenting antigen to T cells (A). Antigen is not processed or presented if APCs are fixed less than 1 to 3 hours after antigen uptake (B). Fixed APCs bind and present proteolytic fragments of antigens to specific T cells (C). The artificial proteolysis, therefore, mimics physiologic antigen processing by APCs. Effective antigen presentation is assayed by measuring a T cell response, such as cytokine secretion. (Note that T cell hybridomas respond to processed antigens on fixed APCs, but growth factor–dependent T cells may require costimulators that are destroyed by fixation. This is discussed fully in Chapter 10.)*

stance, macrophages contain many more proteases than do B cells and are more actively phagocytic, so that macrophages may be more efficient than B cells at internalizing and processing large particulate antigens and presenting peptide fragments of these antigens. It is also possible that different APCs generate distinct sets of peptides from the same native protein because of differences in their endosomal proteases. Furthermore, different APCs may present different peptides because the set of class II MHC molecules expressed by one APC may not be identical to those expressed by another. Therefore, it is possible that the APCs involved in presenting a particular protein antigen can influence which T cells are activated by that antigen.

Association of Processed Peptides with Class II MHC Molecules

After protein antigens are processed, they remain sequestered in membrane-bound vesicles and bind to class II MHC molecules within APCs. The exact site of this association is not known, although a variety of experimental data indicate that it occurs within an organelle of the endocytic pathway. As we discussed in Chapter 5, class II MHC molecules are synthesized and assembled in the endoplasmic reticulum (ER). The invariant chain also non-covalently associates with the class II MHC $\alpha\beta$ heterodimers in the ER, and is thought to perform at least two important functions. First, the presence of the associated invariant chain can effectively block the peptide-binding cleft of the class II MHC molecule, thereby preventing binding of any endogenous peptides that may be present in the ER. Second, by virtue of certain amino acid sequences in its amino terminal cytoplasmic tail, the invariant chain targets the movement of the class II MHC molecule through the Golgi complex to the membrane-bound organelles of the endocytic pathway. Studies employing immunoelectron microscopy and a variety of enzyme markers for organellar transport of proteins indicate that internalization and export pathways of membrane-bound subcellular organelles are interconnected. As the class II MHC molecules move through the exocytic pathway, they encounter endocytic vesicles containing peptides derived from exogenous protein antigens. During transport or after delivery to the endosome, proteolytic enzymes and low pH cause the invariant chain to dissociate from the class II $\alpha\beta$ heterodimer. This permits the class II MHC molecules to bind peptides that are present in the same compartment. The complexes of peptides and class II MHC molecules are then transported to and expressed on the surface of the APCs (Fig. 6–7).

One prediction from this model of class II–restricted antigen presentation is that self or autologous proteins should enter this antigen processing pathway as readily as foreign proteins. In fact, there are two types of experimental evidence that *autologous peptides bind to self class II MHC molecules in vivo*. First,

CD4$^+$ T cells can be generated that are specific for allelic forms of a self protein. Such T cells can respond to freshly isolated APCs presenting the self protein, indicating that self peptide–class II MHC complexes are present on the surface of those APCs. Second, a direct demonstration of autologous peptide–class II MHC association came from the amino acid analysis of peptides eluted from class II MHC molecules purified from B cells grown in tissue culture. Most of these peptides were derived from self proteins (discussed below). These findings raise two important questions. First, if individuals process their own proteins and present them in association with their own class II MHC molecules, why do we normally not develop immune responses against self proteins? It is likely that self-tolerance is mainly due to the absence of lymphocytes capable of recognizing and responding to self antigens, and this is why self peptide–MHC complexes do not normally induce autoimmunity (see Chapters 8 and 19). Second, if MHC molecules are constantly exposed to a great excess of processed autologous proteins, how can they efficiently bind and present enough foreign antigenic peptides to elicit immune responses? In part, this may be explained by the extraordinary sensitivity of T cells for specific peptide-MHC complexes. It has been estimated that as few as 100 to 200 complexes of a particular peptide with a particular class II MHC molecule on the surface of an APC can lead to activation of a T cell specific for that complex. This represents less than 0.1 per cent of the total number of class II molecules likely to be present on the surface of the APC, most of which would be occupied with self peptides. In fact, the indiscriminate ability of the APC to internalize, process, and present the heterogeneous mix of self and foreign extracellular proteins ensures that the immune system will not miss transient or quantitatively small exposures to foreign antigens.

There are many unresolved aspects of the model of antigen processing described above. It is not known how a protein antigen endocytosed by an APC avoids complete proteolytic degradation to amino acids, as is likely to occur in the lysosomal compartment of the cell. One possibility is that binding of a peptide to an MHC molecule prevents further enzymatic hydrolysis of the peptide. Purified peptides bound to MHC molecules are resistant to destruction by proteases *in vitro*, whereas the same peptides in the absence of MHC molecules are readily hydrolyzed into amino acids by proteolytic enzymes. The complex interactions of invariant chain, peptide, and class II MHC molecules are still not fully understood. For example, although peptide is not required for initial assembly of class II MHC heterodimers, there is evidence that peptide binding changes the conformation and stabilizes the heterodimer. In addition, there may be a role for accessory proteins called **chaperones,** which regulate the delivery and binding of some peptides to class II MHC molecules.

Although the bulk of experimental evidence supports the model described above for the generation of most class II MHC–peptide complexes, there are potentially important alternate intracellular pathways for the generation of these complexes that may be immunolog-

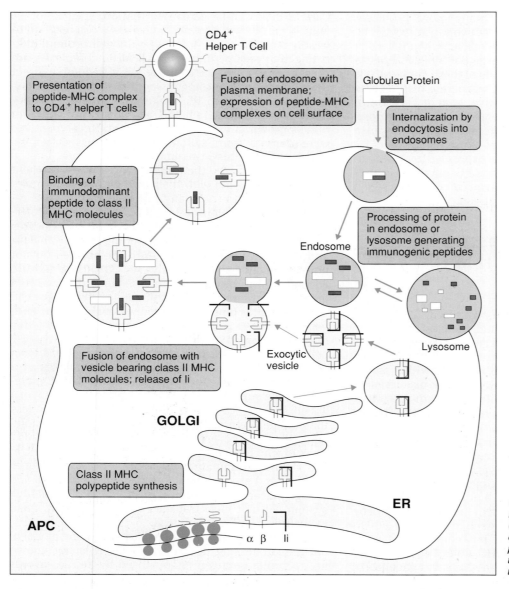

FIGURE 6–7. Pathway of class II MHC–restricted presentation of an exogenous protein antigen. *Vesicles of the endocytic-lysosomal pathway are shaded. Ii refers to the invariant chain; ER refers to the endoplasmic reticulum.*

ically significant. First, it is possible that cell surface class II molecules may be recycled by internalization into endosomes, where they bind newly generated peptide fragments of internalized protein. This process would likely require an exchange of previously bound peptides with the new ones. Second, there are exceptions to the general case that class II MHC molecules bind peptides derived from internalized exogenous proteins. Cell surface complexes of class II MHC molecules with peptides derived from endogenously synthesized proteins have been detected by both T cell responses to such proteins and by direct analysis of eluted peptides from cell surface–derived class II MHC. In some cases, this may result from a normal cellular pathway for the turnover of cytoplasmic contents, referred to as autophagy. In this pathway, cytoplasmic contents are entrapped within ER-derived membrane vesicles called autophagosomes, these vesicles fuse with lysosomes,

and the cytoplasmic proteins are proteolytically degraded. The association of the peptides generated by this route would require movement of the peptides to a class II–bearing compartment, as described previously for trafficking of exogenously derived peptides. In addition, some peptides that associate with class II MHC are derived from endogenously synthesized membrane proteins. Before they are expressed on the surface, these proteins may have ready access to class II MHC molecules because they would be synthesized and transported through the same ER-Golgi compartments as the membrane-bound class II MHC molecules themselves. How such membrane proteins are processed is currently unknown. Alternatively, it is possible that after cell surface expression, membrane proteins may reenter the cell by the same endocytic pathway as exogenous proteins. The ability to generate peptide–class II complexes with membrane-derived proteins is theoretically important in stimulating CD4$^+$-dependent immune responses to membrane proteins synthesized by intracellular microbes.

In summary, the principal steps in class II MHC–associated antigen presentation (see Fig. 6–7) are the following:

1. Internalization of native protein antigens from the extracellular environment into APCs.

2. Processing of the antigen in acidic endosomes or lysosomes, leading to the generation of peptide fragments.

3. Binding of peptides to class II MHC molecules within the exocytic vesicles.

4. Expression of peptide-MHC complexes on the cell surface.

5. Recognition of the complexes by T cells that are specific for the foreign peptide and the self MHC molecule.

MECHANISMS OF ANTIGEN PRESENTATION TO CLASS I MHC–RESTRICTED CD8$^+$ T CELLS

As we have mentioned previously, CD8$^+$ T cells, most of which are CTLs, recognize peptides that are usually derived from protein antigens that are synthesized within APCs, processed and subsequently expressed on the APC surface in association with class I MHC molecules. Examples of endogenously synthesized foreign proteins are viral proteins and tumor antigens. CTLs are the principal immunologic defense mechanisms against viruses and may be important in the immune destruction of tumors. In contrast to the restricted expression of class II MHC molecules, almost all cells express class I MHC molecules and have the ability to display peptide antigens in association with these MHC molecules on the cell surface. This ensures that any cell synthesizing viral or mutant proteins can be marked for recognition and killing by CD8$^+$ CTLs. As is the case with class II MHC–restricted antigen presentation, generation of peptide–class I MHC complexes is a continuous normal function of cells, which does not discriminate between foreign and self proteins. This portion of the chapter describes the known features of the generation of peptide–class I MHC complexes on the surface of cells.

Cytosolic Processing of Endogenous Proteins

The prerequisite for entry of a protein into the processing pathway leading to peptide–class I MHC association is simply location in the cytosol. Several lines of evidence support this.

1. If a viral protein, such as influenza nucleoprotein, or a protein like ovalbumin, is added in soluble form to a cell that expresses class I and class II MHC molecules, the antigen is internalized, processed, and presented only in association with class II MHC molecules. Such exogenously added antigens will be recognized by class II–restricted, antigen-specific CD4$^+$ T cells but will not sensitize the APC to lysis by CD8$^+$ cells. On the other hand, if the gene encoding the viral protein or ovalbumin is transfected into the APCs so that the antigen is synthesized endogenously, the cell becomes sensitive to lysis by specific class I–restricted CD8$^+$ cells (Fig. 6–8).

2. If an antigen is introduced into the cytoplasm of a cell by making the plasma membrane transiently permeable to macromolecules or by membrane fusion of an APC with lipid vesicles containing the protein, the antigen is subsequently processed and peptides associate only with class I MHC molecules (Fig. 6–8). This further supports the concept that the traffic patterns of intracellular and endocytosed proteins are different.

The intracellular mechanisms that generate complexes of antigenic peptides with class I MHC molecules are distinctly different from the mechanisms described earlier for peptide–class II MHC associations. This is evident from the observations that the agents that raise endosomal and lysosomal pH, or direct inhibitors of endosomal proteases, block class II– but not class I–restricted antigen presentation.

Peptides that bind to class I MHC molecules are proteolytically generated in the cytoplasm prior to entry into the exocytic pathway that delivers the peptide-MHC protein complex to the cell surface. This conclusion is supported by a variety of experimental observations.

1. Cells infected with a virus become sensitized to lysis by virus-specific CTLs; this is because the cell displays peptides derived from viral proteins in association with class I MHC on the cell surface. Some of these proteins, such as influenza nucleoprotein, are neither membrane bound nor secreted, i.e., they do not gain access to exocytic pathways in their intact form. Furthermore, the genes encoding viral membrane proteins can be altered to eliminate the membrane insertion sequences. When these genes are transfected into cells, the encoded proteins cannot gain access to the endoplasmic reticulum and exocytic pathway, yet peptides from these proteins are still presented to CD8$^+$ CTL.

2. When peptide epitopes for CTL recognition are synthesized directly in the cytoplasm of a cell as products of transfected minigenes, the cell becomes sensitized for lysis. This implies that peptides generated in the cytoplasm have direct access to the exocytic pathway for cell surface expression of class I MHC molecules.

If proteins are first broken down into peptides in the cytosol and then delivered to the exocytic pathway where class I MHC molecules are located, there must be mechanisms for cytosolic proteolysis and for movement of the peptides through the limiting membranes

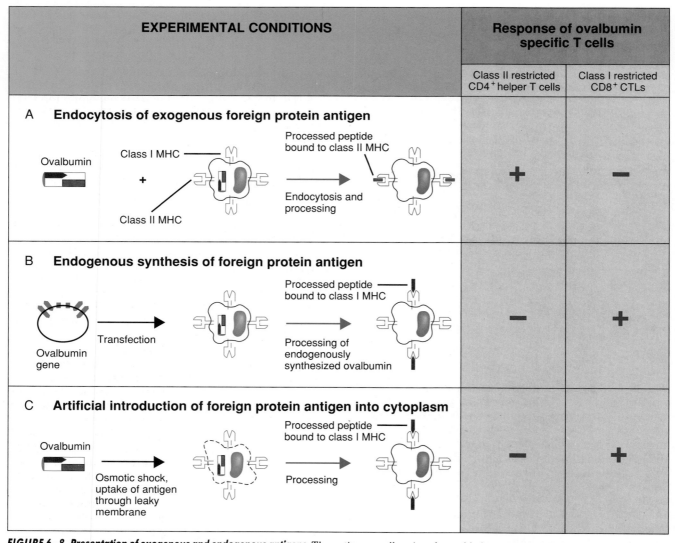

EXPERIMENTAL CONDITIONS	Response of ovalbumin specific T cells	
	Class II restricted CD4+ helper T cells	Class I restricted CD8+ CTLs
A Endocytosis of exogenous foreign protein antigen	+	−
B Endogenous synthesis of foreign protein antigen	−	+
C Artificial introduction of foreign protein antigen into cytoplasm	−	+

FIGURE 6–8. Presentation of exogenous and endogenous antigens. *The antigen, ovalbumin, when added to an antigen-presenting cell (APC) that expresses class I and class II MHC molecules, is presented only in association with class II (A). The same ovalbumin synthesized intracellularly as a result of transfection of its gene (B) or introduced into the cytoplasm through membranes made leaky by osmotic shock (C) is presented in association with class I MHC molecules. The measured response of class II–restricted helper T cells is cytokine secretion, and the measured response of class I–restricted cytolytic T lymphocytes (CTLs) is killing of the APCs.*

of exocytic organelles. Likely explanations for the cytosolic proteolysis of protein antigens and delivery of peptides into the exocytic pathway have come from the elucidation of the structure and function of certain proteins that are encoded by genes in the class II region of the MHC. These genes, which were mentioned in Chapter 5, are the **proteasome** and **transporter in antigen processing (TAP)** genes. There are two proteasome genes in the MHC that encode for two subunits of a large (650 kD) cytoplasmic organelle called the low molecular mass polypeptide complex or proteasome. The proteasome is composed of up to 24 protein subunits that form a cylindrical complex. A major function previously attributed to the proteasome is the degradation of cytosolic proteins that are tagged for turnover by covalent linkage to a small protein called ubiquitin. When a cytosolic protein becomes "ubiquinated," it apparently gains access to the proteasomal enzymatic ac-

tivity. There is preliminary evidence that certain protein antigens require ubiquination before they can be presented to class I–restricted T cells. Furthermore, proteasomes do not always include the subunits encoded by the genes in the MHC, but those proteasomes that do are particularly capable of generating class I MHC–binding peptides. The general importance of the proteasome in generating antigenic peptides remains to be established. The *TAP-1* and *TAP-2* genes are homologous to a family of genes that encode proteins that mediate ATP-dependent transport of low molecular weight compounds across intracellular membranes. The products of the *TAP-1* and *TAP-2* genes are believed to form a heterodimer that functions to transport peptides from the cytoplasm into the ER. Cell lines with mutations in the *TAP* genes fail to present cytosolic proteins in association with class I MHC molecules (Fig. 6–9). It is, therefore, likely that *the proteasome de-*

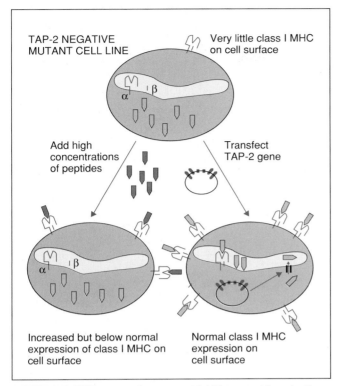

sized proteins including class I and class II MHC and foreign viral proteins, and inhibits the class I–restricted presentation of endogenously synthesized viral protein more than the class II–restricted presentation of exogenously encountered proteins. Second, the adenovirus E19 protein specifically binds to and prevents transport of class I MHC molecules out of the ER. The ability of E19 to block nascent class I transport correlates with its ability to block class I–restricted antigen presentation.

Further evidence for the requirement of peptides in the ER for assembly and surface expression of class I MHC molecules has come from analysis of the effects of defective *TAP* genes. In both mutant cell lines and cells from *TAP* gene knockout mice, class I MHC expression on the cell surface is significantly reduced. Those class I MHC molecules that do get expressed have bound peptides that are mostly derived from signal sequences of proteins destined for secretion or membrane expression. These signal sequences are cleaved off and degraded to peptides within the ER during translation, without a requirement for TAP-1:TAP-2.

Thus, the association of peptide antigens with class I versus class II MHC molecules is due to the trafficking of the antigens through different intracellular compartments (Fig. 6–10). In most cases, the commitment to one or another traffic pattern is determined by where the antigen comes from: cytosolic, usually endogenously synthesized antigens end up associated with class I MHC, and exogenously synthesized and endocytosed antigens end up associated with class II MHC. There are exceptions, however, when exogenous antigens do end up being presented in association with class I MHC molecules. These are usually protein antigens made by bacteria or protozoa, which enter the cell by phagocytosis and then become intracellular parasites. There is some evidence that proteins made by these organisms escape from phagolysosomes and gain access to the cytosolic antigen processing pathway, which handles endogenously synthesized proteins. Such antigens stimulate CD8$^+$ T cells, which play an important role in killing host cells infected with these microbes.

FIGURE 6–9. TAP gene products are required for assembly and cell surface expression of peptide–class I MHC complexes. *A cell line with a nonfunctional TAP-2 gene expresses very few surface class I MHC molecules. The peptides bound to these few surface class I MHC molecules are predominantly derived from the signal sequences of membrane or secreted proteins. The addition of high doses of peptides can induce some class I MHC molecule assembly and expression. In this case, it is not known if the assembly of the peptide–class I complexes occurs at the cell surface or intracellularly. When a functional TAP-2 gene is transfected into the cell line, normal assembly and expression of peptide-class I MHC molecules is restored.*

grades cytosolic proteins into peptides, and the TAP-1:TAP-2 heterodimer delivers the peptides to the exocytic pathway where they can associate with class I MHC molecules (Fig. 6–10).

Association of Processed Peptides with Class I MHC Molecules

The actual assembly and surface expression of stable class I MHC molecules requires the presence of peptides. Peptides generated in the cytoplasm and delivered to the ER bind to newly synthesized class I MHC heavy chains and stabilize their association with newly synthesized β_2-microglobulin. The association of peptides with newly synthesized MHC molecules in the ER was first suggested by the molecular actions of two agents that block class I–restricted antigen presentation. The first is Brefeldin A, which causes dissolution of the Golgi apparatus and therefore blocks protein transport out of the ER. This drug inhibits the post-translational modification and transport of all newly synthe-

PHYSIOLOGIC SIGNIFICANCE OF MHC-ASSOCIATED ANTIGEN PRESENTATION

So far we have discussed the specificity of CD4$^+$ and CD8$^+$ T lymphocytes for MHC-associated foreign protein antigens and the mechanisms by which complexes of peptides and MHC molecules are produced. *Both the class I and class II MHC pathways of antigen presentation sample pools of predominantly normal self proteins for display to the T cell repertoire, which surveys these samples for the rare foreign or mutant peptide.* In addition, the central role of MHC molecules in T cell antigen recognition influences the immunogenicity of different protein antigens and the response patterns of the T cells.

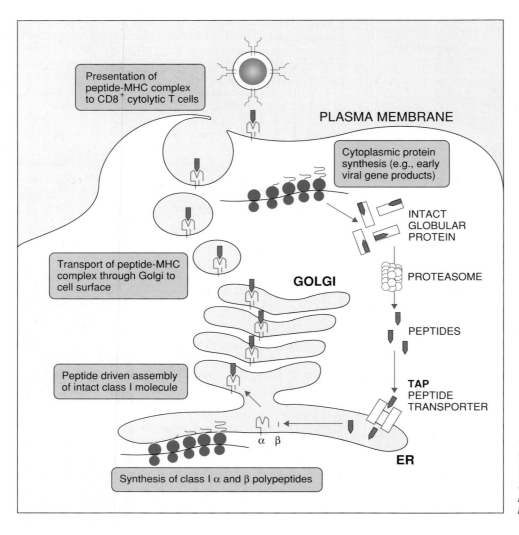

Presentation of peptide-MHC complex to CD8$^+$ cytolytic T cells

PLASMA MEMBRANE

Cytoplasmic protein synthesis (e.g., early viral gene products)

Transport of peptide-MHC complex through Golgi to cell surface

INTACT GLOBULAR PROTEIN

GOLGI

PROTEASOME

PEPTIDES

Peptide driven assembly of intact class I molecule

TAP PEPTIDE TRANSPORTER

α   β

ER

Synthesis of class I α and β polypeptides

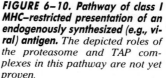

FIGURE 6–10. Pathway of class I MHC–restricted presentation of an endogenously synthesized (e.g., viral) antigen. *The depicted roles of the proteasome and TAP complexes in this pathway are not yet proven.*

Immunogenicity of Protein Antigens

MHC molecules may determine the immunogenicity of protein antigens in two related ways:

1. *The immunodominant epitopes of complex proteins are often the peptides that bind most avidly to MHC molecules.* If an individual is immunized with a multideterminant protein antigen, in many instances the majority of the responding T cells are specific for one or a few linear amino acid sequences of the antigen. These are called the "immunodominant" determinants or epitopes. For instance, in H-2^k mice immunized with hen egg lysozyme (HEL), more than half the HEL-specific T cells are specific for the epitope formed by residues 46 to 61 of HEL in association with the I-A^k but not the I-E^k molecule. This is because HEL(46–61) binds to I-A^k better than do other HEL peptides and does not bind to I-E^k. However, it is not yet known exactly which structural features of a peptide determine immunodominance. As mentioned earlier, for class I–restricted antigen presentation, immunodominant peptides are

required to have amino residues whose side chains fit into pockets of the MHC molecule peptide-binding cleft. Common features of immunodominant peptides for class II MHC–restricted antigen presentation have not yet been defined. The question is an important one because an understanding of these features may permit the efficient manipulation of the immune system with synthetic peptides. An obvious application of such knowledge is the design of vaccines. For example, a protein encoded by a viral gene could be analyzed for the presence of amino acid sequences that would form a typical immunodominant secondary structure capable of binding to MHC molecules with high affinity. Vaccines composed of synthetic peptides mimicking this region of the protein theoretically would be effective in eliciting T cell responses against the viral peptide expressed on an infected cell, thereby establishing protective immunity against the virus.

2. *The expression of particular class II MHC alleles in an individual determines the ability of that individual to respond to particular antigens.* The phenomenon of immune response (Ir) gene–controlled immune responsiveness was mentioned in Chapter 5. We now know that Ir genes that control antibody responses are

class II MHC genes. They influence immune responsiveness in part because various allelic class II MHC molecules differ in their ability to bind different antigenic peptides and, therefore, to stimulate specific helper T cells. For instance, H-2^k mice are responders to HEL(46–61), but H-2^d mice are non-responders to this epitope. Equilibrium dialysis experiments have shown that HEL(46–61) binds to I-A^k but not to I-A^d molecules (see Fig. 6–1). A possible molecular basis for this difference in MHC association is suggested from the model of the class II molecule and the known amino acid sequences of I-A^k and I-A^d proteins. If the HEL(46–61) peptide is hypothetically placed in the predicted binding cleft of the I-A^k molecule, charged residues of the HEL peptide become aligned with oppositely charged residues of the MHC molecule. This would presumably stabilize the bimolecular interaction. In contrast, the I-A^d molecule has different amino acids in the binding cleft that would result in the aligning of similarly charged residues with the HEL peptide. Therefore, HEL(46–61) would not bind to or be presented in association with I-A^d, and the H-2^d mouse would be a non-responder. Similar results have been obtained with numerous other peptides. MHC-linked immune responsiveness may also be important in humans. For instance, Caucasians who are homozygous for an extended HLA haplotype containing HLA-B8,DR3,DQw2a are low responders to hepatitis B virus surface antigen. Individuals who are heterozygous at this locus are high responders, presumably because the other alleles contain one or more HLA genes that confer responsiveness to this antigen. Thus, HLA typing may prove to be valuable for predicting the success of vaccination. These findings support the **determinant selection model** of MHC-linked immune responses. This model, which was proposed many years before the demonstration of peptide-MHC binding, states that the products of MHC genes in each individual select which determinants of protein antigens will be immunogenic in that individual. We now understand the structural basis of determinant selection and Ir gene function in antigen presentation. Most Ir gene phenomena have been studied by measuring helper T cell function, but the same principles apply to CTLs. Individuals with certain MHC alleles may be incapable of generating CTLs against some viruses. In this situation, of course, the Ir genes may map to one of the class I MHC loci.

Although these concepts are based largely on studies with simple peptide antigens and inbred strains of mice, they are also relevant to the understanding of immune responses to complex multideterminant protein antigens in outbred species. It is likely that all individuals will express at least one MHC molecule capable of binding at least one determinant of a complex protein, so that all individuals will be responders to such antigens. As stated in Chapter 5, this may be the evolutionary pressure for maintaining MHC polymorphism.

This discussion of the influence of MHC gene products on the immunogenicity of protein antigens has focused on antigen presentation and has not considered the role of the T cells. We have mentioned earlier that the exquisite specificity and diversity of antigen recognition are attributable to antigen receptors on T cells. MHC-linked immune responsiveness is also dependent, in part, on the presence and absence of specific T cells. In fact, some peptides bind to MHC molecules in a particular inbred mouse strain but do not activate T cells in that strain (see Table 6–3). It is likely that these mice lack T cells capable of recognizing the particular peptide-MHC complexes. *Thus, Ir genes may function by determining antigen presentation or by shaping the repertoire of antigen-responsive T cells* (Fig. 6–11). The development of the T cell repertoire and the role of the MHC in T cell maturation are discussed in Chapter 8.

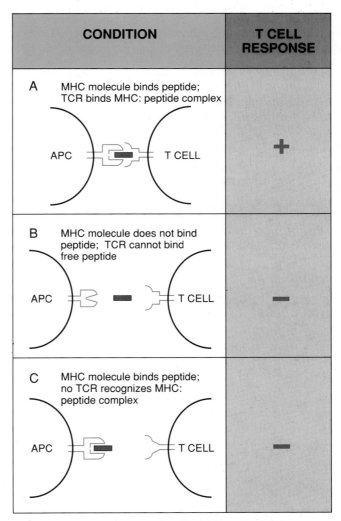

CONDITION	T CELL RESPONSE
A MHC molecule binds peptide; TCR binds MHC: peptide complex	+
B MHC molecule does not bind peptide; TCR cannot bind free peptide	−
C MHC molecule binds peptide; no TCR recognizes MHC: peptide complex	−

FIGURE 6–11. Mechanisms of MHC-linked immune response (Ir) gene function. Antigen presentation and T cell activation occur when an individual expresses MHC molecules that can bind peptides derived from the processed antigen and T cells are present that specifically recognize complexes of these MHC molecules with the peptides (A). If an individual does not inherit genes encoding MHC molecules that can bind the peptides, no T cell response occurs (B). Alternatively, if no T cells are present that recognize the MHC molecules as self, no T cell response occurs (C). The development of self-restricted T cells is discussed in Chapter 8.

Nature of T Cell Responses

Based on this knowledge of antigen presentation to T cells, we can now explain other physiologic consequences of MHC-restricted antigen recognition that were introduced in Chapter 5.

1. Because T cells recognize only MHC-associated protein antigens, they can respond only to antigens associated with other cells (the APCs) and are unresponsive to soluble or circulating proteins. *This unique specificity for cell-bound antigens may be essential for the functions of T lymphocytes, which are largely mediated by cell-cell interactions and by cytokines that act at short distances.* For instance, helper T cells help B lymphocytes and activate macrophages. Not surprisingly, B lymphocytes and macrophages are two of the principal cell types that express class II MHC genes, function as APCs for CD4+ helper T cells, and focus helper T cell effects to their immediate vicinity. Similarly, CTLs can lyse any nucleated cell producing a foreign antigen, and all nucleated cells express class I MHC molecules, which are the restricting elements for antigen recognition by CD8+ CTLs.

2. The patterns of MHC association of different forms of antigens determine which subset of T cells is preferentially or selectively activated (Fig. 6–12). Extracellular antigens usually activate class II–restricted CD4+ T cells, which function as helpers to stimulate effector mechanisms such as antibodies and phagocytes that serve to eliminate extracellular antigens. Conversely, endogenous antigens usually activate class I–restricted CD8+ CTLs, which lyse cells producing these intracellular antigens. *Thus, different forms of antigens selectively stimulate the T cell population that is most effective at eliminating that type of antigen.* This is particularly significant because neither the antigen receptors of helper T cells and CTLs nor class I and class II MHC molecules themselves have the ability to distinguish between extracellular (e.g., bacterial) and intracellular (e.g., viral) protein determinants.

SUMMARY

T cells recognize antigens only on the surface of accessory cells in association with the product of a self MHC gene. CD4+ helper T lymphocytes recognize antigens in association with class II MHC gene products (class II MHC–restricted recognition), and CD8+ CTLs recognize antigens in association with class I gene products (class I MHC–restricted recognition). Exoge-

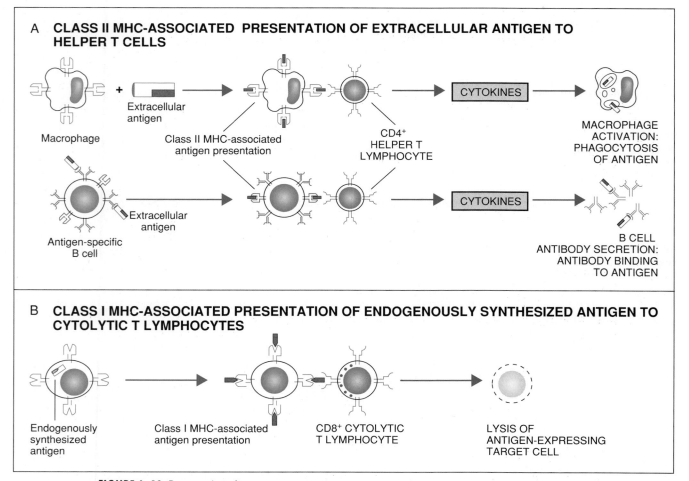

A **CLASS II MHC-ASSOCIATED PRESENTATION OF EXTRACELLULAR ANTIGEN TO HELPER T CELLS**

Macrophage

+ Extracellular antigen

Class II MHC-associated antigen presentation

CD4+ HELPER T LYMPHOCYTE

CYTOKINES

MACROPHAGE ACTIVATION: PHAGOCYTOSIS OF ANTIGEN

Antigen-specific B cell

Extracellular antigen

CYTOKINES

B CELL ANTIBODY SECRETION: ANTIBODY BINDING TO ANTIGEN

B **CLASS I MHC-ASSOCIATED PRESENTATION OF ENDOGENOUSLY SYNTHESIZED ANTIGEN TO CYTOLYTIC T LYMPHOCYTES**

Endogenously synthesized antigen

Class I MHC-associated antigen presentation

CD8+ CYTOLYTIC T LYMPHOCYTE

LYSIS OF ANTIGEN-EXPRESSING TARGET CELL

FIGURE 6–12. Presentation of exogenous and endogenous protein antigens to different subsets of T cells.

nous foreign proteins are internalized in APCs, where they undergo processing in an acidic vesicular compartment. Processing ensures that portions of a protein (the immunodominant peptides) will bind to class II MHC molecules and form immunogenic complexes. These complexes are expressed on the surface of APCs, where they are recognized by CD4$^+$ T cells. Many cell types have the capacity to present antigens to CD4$^+$ helper T cells; a minimal requirement is the expression of class II MHC genes. The regulation of class II MHC gene expression is an important control point for immune responses.

The target antigens for CD8$^+$ CTLs are endogenously synthesized proteins, such as viral antigens, which are processed and associate with class I MHC molecules. Peptides are generated from endogenously synthesized antigens in the cytosol and are delivered to the ER for association with newly synthesized chains of class I MHC molecules.

SELECTED READINGS

Allen, P. M. Antigen processing at the molecular level. Immunology Today 8:270–273, 1987.

Babbitt, B. P., P. M. Allen, G. Matsueda, E. Haber, and E. R. Unanue. Binding of immunogenic peptides to Ia histocompatibility molecules. Nature 317:359–361, 1985.

Benacerraf, B. A hypothesis to relate the specificity of T lymphocytes and the activity of I-region–specific Ir genes in macrophages and B lymphocytes. Journal of Immunology 120:1809–1812, 1978.

Buus, S., A. Sette, S. M. Colon, C. Miles, and H. M. Grey. The relationship between major histocompatibility complex (MHC) restriction and the capacity of Ia to bind immunogenic peptides. Science 235:1353–1358, 1987.

Germain, R. H., and D. M. Marguiles. The biochemistry and cell biology of antigen processing and presentation. Annual Review of Immunology 11:403–450, 1993.

Monaco, J. J. A molecular model of MHC class I–restricted antigen processing. Immunology Today 13:173–179, 1992.

Moore, M. W., F. R. Carbone, and M. J. Bevan. Introduction of soluble protein into the class I pathway of antigen processing and presentation. Cell 54:777–785, 1988.

Neefjes, J. J., and H. L. Ploegh. Intracellular transport of MHC class II molecules. Immunology Today 13:179–189, 1992.

Unanue, E. R., and P. M. Allen. The basis for the immunoregulatory role of macrophages and other accessory cells. Science 236:551–557, 1987.

Yewdell, J. W., and J. R. Resnick. Cell biology of antigen processing and presentation to major histocompatibility complex class I molecule-restricted T lymphocytes. Advances in Immunology 52:1–23, 1992.

Zinkernagel, R. M., and P. C. Doherty. Activity of sensitized thymus-derived lymphocytes in lymphocytic choriomeningitis reflects immunological surveillance against altered self components. Nature 251:547–548, 1974.

CHAPTER SEVEN

MOLECULAR BASIS OF T CELL ANTIGEN RECOGNITION AND ACTIVATION

In Chapter 6 we introduced the concept that helper and cytolytic T lymphocytes (CTLs), unlike B cells, recognize peptides derived from foreign protein antigens that are physically associated with self major histocompatibility complex (MHC) molecules on the surfaces of antigen-presenting cells (APCs) or target cells. Antigen recognition by T cells is the initiating stimulus for T cell activation. In different T cells, activation leads to the secretion of cytokines, proliferation, and the performance of regulatory or cytolytic effector functions. The elucidation of the structure and function of the molecules involved in T cell antigen recognition is one of the most important advances in immunology in the last decade. This relatively new knowledge has provided a molecular basis for the study of normal and pathologic immune responses in which the T cell plays a central role.

The receptors on T cells that are responsible for the specific recognition of and response to antigen plus MHC are composed of a complex of several integral plasma membrane proteins. Some of the proteins in this complex mediate specific binding to peptide-MHC complexes on the surface of APCs or target cells. As would be expected, the subunits of this complex that are involved in antigen binding differ among T cells with different antigen specificities. Other proteins in the complex are invariant among all T cells, and they probably function in signal transduction into the interior of the T cell. In addition to the receptor for peptide plus MHC, T cells express a number of other cell surface proteins, which are collectively called **accessory molecules.** These molecules are important in the cognitive, activation, and effector phases of T cell responses. Several of these accessory molecules function to strengthen the

adhesion of the T cells to other cells, thereby promoting maximally effective interactions between helper T cells and APCs or between CTLs and their targets. Several of these same accessory molecules may transduce signals in addition to signals transduced by the antigen receptor complex that are important for activation of the T cells.

In this chapter, we describe the structure of the T cell antigen receptor proteins as well as the structure and function of the accessory molecules on T cells and how they may act coordinately with the antigen receptor to ensure a functional T cell response to antigen. In addition, we describe the intracellular events that occur in response to antigen binding to the T cell surface. The early biochemical changes inside the T cell are considered to be the "second messengers" that link the binding of antigen to the transcriptional regulation of certain genes and subsequent functional responses of the T cell. Later biochemical events, such as cytokine synthesis, mark the beginning of the effector phase of the T cell response to antigen.

THE $\alpha\beta$ T CELL RECEPTOR FOR PEPTIDE ANTIGEN AND MHC MOLECULES

Identification of the T Cell Antigen Receptor

The molecular nature of the T cell receptor (TCR) responsible for MHC-restricted antigen recognition was

---

BOX 7–1.   MONOCLONAL T CELL POPULATIONS

The development of techniques for propagating monoclonal T cell populations *in vitro* has been crucial to many of the recent advances in our understanding of T cell recognition of antigen and T cell activation. By definition, all the T cells in a monoclonal population are genetically identical to one another (except for rare spontaneous mutants) and therefore express identical TCR. This provides a homogenous population of cells for functional, biochemical, and molecular analyses. Three types of monoclonal T cell populations have been frequently utilized in experimental immunology.

1. *Antigen-specific T cell clones* are derived by *in vivo* immunization of an individual with a particular antigen, isolation of T cells from either blood or lymphoid tissue, repetitive *in vitro* stimulation with the immunizing antigen plus MHC–matched APCs (which drive proliferation of T cells only with the appropriate specificities), and cloning single antigen-MHC–responsive cells in semisolid media or in liquid media by limiting dilution. Permanent lines can be expanded and maintained by periodic *in vitro* restimulation with antigen and MHC-matched APCs. Antigen-specific responses can be easily measured in these populations, since all the cells in a cloned line have the same receptors and have been selected for growth in response to a known antigen-MHC complex. The full range of activation events, including early signal transduction, proliferation, and differentiation to ef-

fector function, can be observed in T cell clones. Both helper and CTL clones have been established from mice and humans.

2. *Antigen-specific T-T hybridomas* are created in a way similar to that for B cell hybridomas (see Box 3–1, Chapter 3). Mice are immunized with the antigen of interest, lymph nodes draining the site of immunization are removed, and T cells are purified. These cells are fused with an autonomously growing T cell tumor line, and metabolic selection is applied so that only the fused cells grow. From the resultant hybridomas, cells responding to the desired antigen:APC combination are selected and cloned. TCR-mediated activation events ranging from early signal transduction to cytokine secretion can be measured in T-T hybridomas. Since hybridomas are already autonomously growing, stimulation of proliferative responses cannot be observed. Murine T-T hybridomas can be easily made, including those derived from both mature T cells and thymocytes. Human T-T hybridomas have also been made recently.

3. *Tumor lines derived from T cells* have been established *in vitro* after removal of malignant T cells from animals or humans with T cell leukemias or lymphomas. Some tumor-derived lines express functional cell surface TCR molecules. Even though the antigen specificities of these lines are not known, they can be activated via their TCRs in other ways, e.g., with anti-TCR antibodies or lectins, leading to early signal events, gene transcription, and cytokine secretion.

elucidated in the 1980s, several years after immunoglobulin (Ig) molecules and their genes were described. After the phenomenon of MHC restriction of antigen-specific T cells was discovered, two alternative theories about the structure of the T cell antigen receptor were proposed. One hypothesis was that T cell antigen recognition required the simultaneous binding of two independent receptors, one to foreign antigen and the other to self MHC. The alternative postulate, which we now know to be correct, was that *a single T cell receptor specifically recognizes MHC-associated antigen.* The evidence that processed antigen and MHC molecules

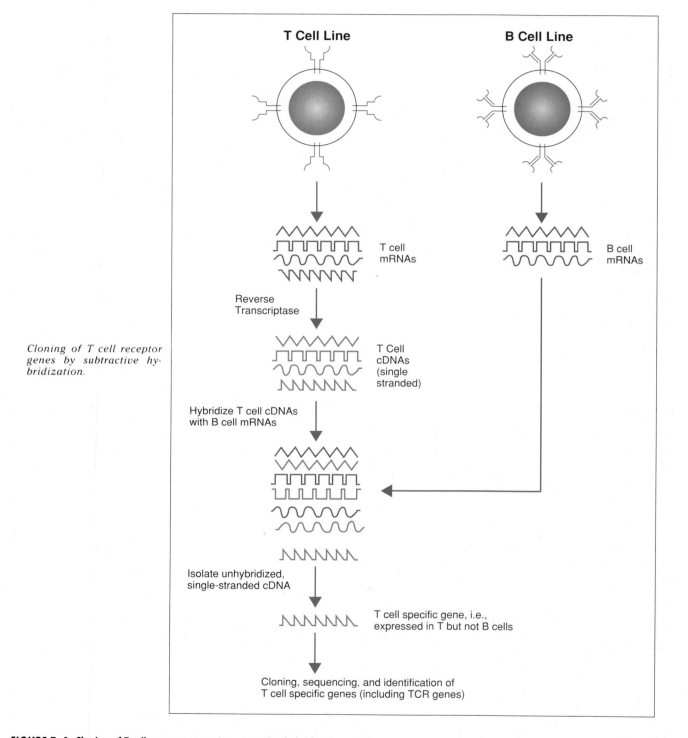

Cloning of T cell receptor genes by subtractive hybridization.

FIGURE 7–1. Cloning of T cell receptor genes by subtractive hybridization. *cDNAs prepared from a T cell line will include a few genes uniquely expressed in T cells, such as the TCR genes, as well as many other genes expressed in other cells. By mixing T cell cDNAs with messenger RNA (mRNA) from B cells and discarding the heteroduplexes formed by hybridization of complementary sequences, T cell–specific cDNAs can be greatly enriched and then characterized.*

are expressed as complexes on the APC surface, prior to involvement of the T cell (see Chapter 6), is most consistent with a single receptor model. A more complete understanding of T cell recognition required analysis of the structure and specificity of the relevant molecules on the T cell surface.

An important advance in the study of T cell receptors was the development of technologies for propagating monoclonal T cell populations *in vitro*, including T-T hybridomas and antigen-specific T cell clones (Box 7–1). All the cells in a clonal T cell population are derived from a single cell, are genetically identical, and therefore express identical TCRs that are different from the receptors produced by all other clones. Antibodies specific for unique (idiotypic) determinants on the antigen receptors of individual T cell clones or tumor lines were used to immunoprecipitate, purify, and biochemically characterize TCR molecules. These anti-TCR antibodies have also been used to induce functional effects when they bind to the antigen receptors on T cells, either mimicking or blocking the activation of T cells by peptide-MHC complexes on APCs.

A seminal accomplishment of modern molecular immunology was the isolation and characterization of TCR genes at a time when the biochemical analysis of the proteins was largely incomplete. In fact, most of the fine details of the structure of TCR molecules discussed below are predicted from the nucleotide sequences of the cloned genes. The strategy behind the first successful identification of TCR genes was based on the following three assumptions:

1. The TCR genes would be uniquely expressed in T cells.
2. Like immunoglobulin genes (see Chapter 4), the functional TCR genes would undergo somatic rearrangement during T cell development and would therefore appear different, by Southern analysis, in mature T cells compared with the germline configuration seen in non-T cells.
3. The TCR genes would have some homology to Ig genes.

T cell receptor genes were first identified by preparing complementary DNA (cDNA) clones of messenger RNA (mRNA) from clonal T cell populations and testing these cDNAs for the properties listed above. One approach used to isolate cDNAs encoding TCR genes was **subtractive hybridization,** by which irrelevant cDNAs not unique to T cells were removed by complementary binding to mRNA from B cells (Fig. 7–1). The TCR genes were then identified among the pool of subtracted, T cell–specific cDNAs. The predicted amino acid sequences from the cloned TCR genes matched the limited amino acid sequence data that had been obtained from purified TCR proteins. The characteristics of TCR proteins are discussed in the following sections. The genomic organization of TCR genes and the mechanisms of their rearrangements leading to TCR diversity are discussed in detail in Chapter 8, in the context of development of T cells from bone marrow–derived precursors.

Biochemical Characteristics of the $\alpha\beta$ T Cell Receptor

The receptor for peptide-MHC complexes on the majority of T cells, including MHC-restricted helper T cells and CTLs, is a heterodimer consisting of two polypeptide chains, designated α and β, covalently linked to each other by disulfide bonds (Fig. 7–2). (Another less common type of TCR, found on a small subset of T cells, is composed of γ and δ chains and is discussed later.) The **α chain** is a 40 to 60 kilodalton (kD) acidic glycoprotein, and the **β chain** is a 40 to 50 kD uncharged or basic glycoprotein. There are striking structural similarities between the α and β chains of the TCR and Ig polypeptides. Both α and β chains have variable (V) and constant (C) regions. The carboxy-terminal end of the V region, i.e., the junction between V and C regions, is encoded by a joining (J) segment gene, and, in the case of the β chain only, a diversity (D) segment gene (Fig. 7–3). The presence of V, D, J, and C regions is also characteristic of Ig (see Chapter 4).

The V regions of α and β chains are 102 to 119 amino acids long and contain two cysteine residues spaced appropriately to allow the formation of an intrachain disulfide bonded loop. Furthermore, there are

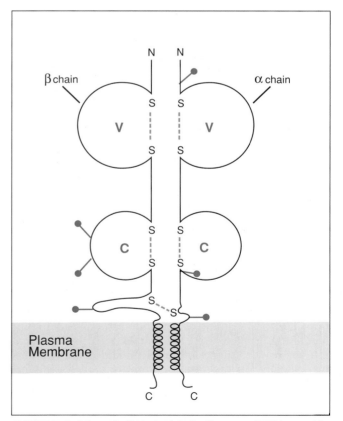

FIGURE 7–2. Schematic diagram of the T cell receptor (TCR) for peptide-MHC complexes. *V and C refer to Ig-like variable and constant domains, respectively, of the α and β chains; N and C refer to the amino and carboxy termini of the polypeptides, respectively. S--S indicates a disulfide bond, and ——• indicates approximate location of carbohydrate groups.*

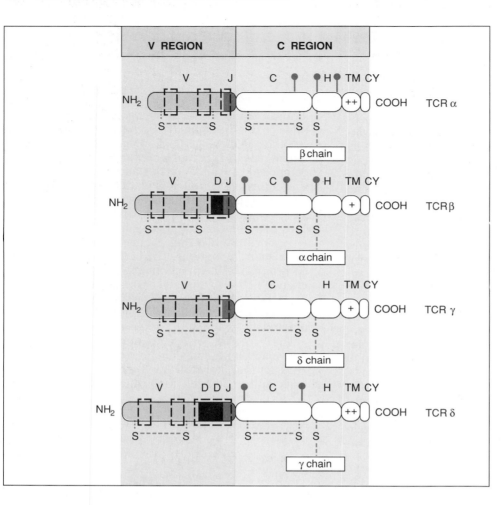

FIGURE 7-3. *Relation of T cell receptor (TCR) gene segments to domains of polypeptide chains. The V region is encoded by variable (V), diversity (D), and joining (J) gene segments. Locations of disulfide bonds (S--S) and carbohydrates (——•) are approximate. Areas in dashed boxes are hypervariable (complementarity-determining) regions; "+" refers to positively charged amino acids in the transmembrane region. H, hinge region; TM, transmembrane domain; CY, cytoplasmic domain. Compare with Figure 4–5 for Ig. (Modified with permission from Davis, M., and P. J. Bjorkman. T cell antigen receptor genes and T cell recognition. Nature 334:395–402, 1988. Copyright © 1988, Macmillan Magazines Ltd.)*

many amino acid residues that are conserved between the V regions of TCR and Ig molecules. These residues in the TCR V region may contribute to the formation of a tertiary structure like the Ig V domain. The similarities in amino acid sequences and conformation between TCR and Ig V regions probably reflect the fact that both molecules have the similar function of binding extremely diverse foreign antigens. In Chapters 3 and 4 we introduced the concept that membrane proteins that contain domains that are structurally homologous to Ig V and C domains are members of a family of molecules that constitute the **Ig superfamily** (Box 7–2). Proteins belonging to this family are thought to have evolved from one ancestral gene. Many of these proteins play important roles in cell-cell interactions.

The C regions of the α and β chains range in length from 138 to 179 amino acids, and each consists of four functional domains that are usually encoded by separate exons. The most amino terminal domain contains two cysteine residues spaced appropriately for the formation of an intrachain disulfide bonded loop, which also probably folds into a tertiary structure similar to an Ig constant region domain. A short hinge region or connecting peptide constitutes the second part of the C region and contains a cysteine residue that is involved in the disulfide linkage of the two chains. The third part of the C region of both α and β chains is the transmembrane domain, composed of 20 to 24 predominantly

hydrophobic amino acid residues. An unusual feature of these transmembrane portions is the presence of a lysine residue (β chain) or a lysine and an arginine residue (α chain), the positively charged side chains of which may be crucial for interactions with negatively charged residues found in the transmembrane portions of the CD3 polypeptides (see below). The carboxy terminal part of the C region of both α and β chains forms a 5 to 12 amino acid long cytoplasmic tail. These cytoplasmic regions are thought to be too small to have intrinsic signal transducing properties, and other molecules physically associated with the TCR are needed to provide signal-transducing functions. Unlike Ig, the TCR α and β chains do not undergo changes in C region expression, i.e., "isotype switching," during T cell differentiation. Also, the C regions of TCR molecules are not known to participate in effector functions as do the C regions of antibodies.

Since the x-ray crystallographic structure of the TCR has not yet been solved, the three-dimensional structure of the binding site for peptide-MHC complexes can only be inferred from sequence homologies with antibody molecules and the known three-dimensional structure of Ig and MHC molecules. Although amino acid variability from one receptor to another appears to be more spread out over the TCR molecule compared with Ig, there are at least three highly diverse regions in both the α and β chains of the TCR that

BOX 7–2. THE Ig SUPERFAMILY

Many of the cell surface and soluble molecules that mediate recognition, adhesion, or binding functions in the vertebrate immune system share partial amino acid sequence homology and tertiary structural features that were originally identified in Ig heavy and light chains. In addition, the same features are found in many molecules outside the immune system that also perform similar functions. These diverse proteins are members of the **Ig superfamily.** A superfamily is broadly defined as a group of proteins that share a certain degree of sequence homology, usually at least 15 per cent. These conserved sequences contribute to the formation of a compact tertiary structure referred to as a domain, and most often the entire sequence of a domain characteristic of

a particular superfamily is encoded by a single exon. Members of a superfamily likely derive from a common precursor gene by divergent evolution, and multidomain proteins may belong to more than one superfamily.

The criterion for inclusion of a protein in the Ig superfamily is the presence of one or more Ig domains (also called Ig homology units), which are regions of 70 to 110 amino acid residues homologous to either Ig V or C domains. The Ig domain contains conserved residues that permit the polypeptide to assume a globular tertiary structure called an **antibody (Ig) fold** (see Chapter 3), composed of a sandwich arrangement of two β-sheets, each made up of three to five antiparallel β-strands of five to ten amino acid

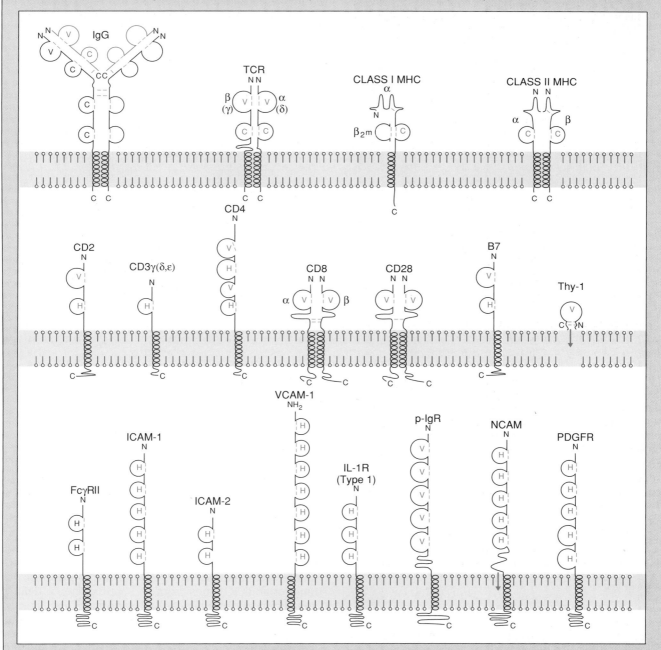

Examples of proteins in the Ig superfamily. V, Ig variable-like domain; C, Ig constant–like domain; H, primordial (C2) Ig-like domain; FcγRII, Fc receptor II; ICAM-1, intercellular adhesion molecule–1 (CD54); ICAM-2, intercellular adhesion molecule–2; VCAM-1, vascular cell adhesion molecule–1; IL-1R, interleukin-1 receptor; p-IgR, poly-Ig receptor (transports antibodies across epithelial cells); NCAM, neural cell adhesion molecule; PDGFR, platelet-derived growth factor receptor. (Modified from Hunkapiller, T., and L. Hood. Diversity of the immunoglobulin gene/superfamily. Advances in Immunology 44:1–63, 1989.)

Continued

residues. The sandwich-like structure is stabilized by hydrophobic amino acid residues on the β-strands pointing inward, which alternate with hydrophilic residues pointing out. Since the inwardly pointing residues are essential for the stability of the tertiary structure, they are the major contributors to the regions that are conserved between Ig superfamily members. In addition, there are usually conserved cysteine residues that contribute to the formation of an intrachain disulfide-bonded loop of 55 to 75 amino acids (approximately 90 kD). Ig domains are classified as V-like or C-like on the basis of closest homology to either Ig V or C domains. V domains are formed from a longer polypeptide than C domains and contain an extra pair of β-strands within the β-sheet sandwich. A third type of Ig domain, called C2 or H, has a similar length to C domains but has sequences typical of both V and C domains.

Using several criteria of evolutionary relatedness, such as primary sequence, intron-exon structure, and ability to undergo DNA rearrangements, molecular biologists have postulated a scheme, or family tree, depicting the evolution of members of the Ig superfamily. In this scheme, a very early event was the duplication of a gene for a primordial surface receptor followed by divergence of V and C exons. Modern members of the superfamily contain different numbers of V and/or C domains. The early divergence is reflected by the lack of significant sequence homology in Ig and TCR V and C units, although they share similar tertiary structures. A second early event in the evolution of this family was the acquisition of the ability to undergo DNA rearrangements, which has remained a unique feature of the antigen receptor gene members of the family.

Members of the Ig superfamily (shown in the accompanying figure) are for the most part unlinked, being present on many different chromosomes. This is true even for different members that form functional complexes with one another, such as the CD3 γ, δ, and ϵ protein genes (on human chromosome 11) and the TCR α and β chain genes (on human chromosomes 14 and 7, respectively). There are, however, important exceptions in which groups of genes encoding Ig homology units are closely linked. These include the linkage of the rearranging V, D, and J gene segments of all the antigen receptors to C domain genes on the same chromosome, the linkage of the members of the MHC, the linkage of the two CD8 chain genes and the V_κ locus, and the linkage of the CD3, NCAM, and Thy-1 genes.

Most identified members of the Ig superfamily are integral plasma membrane proteins with Ig domains in the extracellular portions, transmembrane domains composed of hydrophobic amino acids, and widely divergent cytoplasmic tails with no homology to one another or to previously identified signal-transducing structures. There are exceptions to these generalizations. For example, the platelet-derived growth factor receptors have cytoplasmic tails with tyrosine kinase activity, and the Thy-1 molecule has no cytoplasmic tail but, rather, is anchored to the membrane by a phosphatidyl inositol linkage.

One recurrent characteristic of the Ig superfamily members is that interactions between Ig domains on different polypeptide chains are essential for the function of the molecules. These interactions can be homophilic, occurring between identical domains on opposing polypeptide chains of a multimeric protein, as in the case of C_H:C_H pairing to form functional Fc regions of Ig molecules. Alternatively, they can be heterophilic, as occurs in the case of V_H:V_L or V_β:V_α pairing to form the antigen-binding sites of Ig or TCR molecules, respectively. Heterophilic interactions can also occur between Ig domains on entirely distinct molecules expressed on the surfaces of different cells. Such interactions provide adhesive forces that stabilize immunologically significant cell-cell interactions. For example, the presentation of an antigen to a helper T cell by an APC probably involves heterophilic intercellular Ig domain interactions between at least four pairs of Ig superfamily molecules, including TCR:class II MHC, CD4:class II MHC, CD2:LFA-3, and CD28:B7. The importance of all these interactions is demonstrated by the observation that antibodies that block the binding of these molecules to one another also block antigen plus APC–induced T cell activation. Several Ig superfamily members have been identified on cells of the developing and mature nervous system, consistent with the functional importance of highly regulated cell-cell interactions in these sites.

correspond to the antigen-binding complementarity-determining regions (CDRs) of Ig. These hypervariable regions are presumed to form the contact points for the binding of complexes of foreign antigen and self MHC molecules. Two of these TCR hypervariable regions are encoded by V gene segments, and one is composed of sequences encoded by V and J gene segments (in the α chain) or V, D, and J segments (in the β chain) (Fig. 7–3).

Role of the $\alpha\beta$ Receptor in Recognition of MHC-Associated Antigen

The $\alpha\beta$ heterodimer recognizes complexes of processed peptides, generated from foreign protein antigens, bound to self MHC molecules. This has been demonstrated by several experimental approaches:

1. Anti-idiotypic antibodies generated against clones of antigen-specific, MHC-restricted T cells immunoprecipitate only the $\alpha\beta$ heterodimer.

2. The key features of T cell specificity, namely self MHC restriction and foreign antigen recognition, are always linked and do not segregate independently. For example, when two T cells with different antigen specificities and MHC restrictions are fused, the hybrid cell line recognizes each of the antigens recognized by the two parent T cell fusion partners, but only with the same independent MHC restrictions as the parent T cells. Therefore, a single receptor confers specificity for both antigen and MHC.

3. Definitive proof that the $\alpha\beta$ heterodimer is responsible for both the antigen (peptide) specificity and the self MHC restriction of a T cell came from experiments with isolated TCR genes. In these experiments, functional TCR genes from a T cell clone of defined specificity were transfected into another T cell. For example, when the α and β genes isolated from a cytochrome c-specific, I-E^k–restricted murine T cell clone were transfected into a T cell with an unknown specificity, the transfectants began to respond to cytochrome c plus I-E^k (Fig. 7–4). Neither the TCR α gene nor the TCR β gene alone confers antigenic specificity or MHC restriction upon a cell.

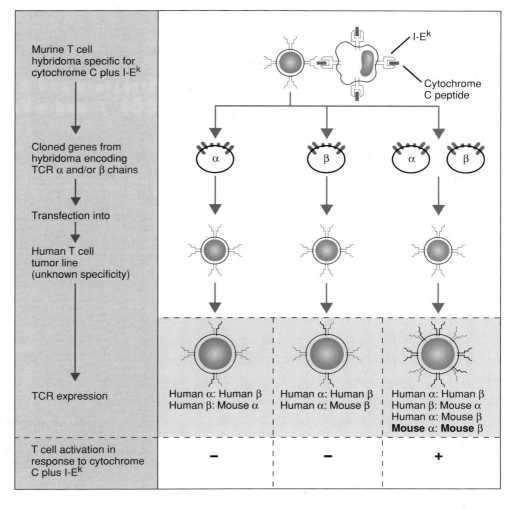

FIGURE 7-4. T cell specificity for antigen and MHC is a function of TCR α and β chain gene products. *In this experiment, the α and β chain genes from a murine T cell hybridoma of defined specificity were transfected into a human T cell line of unknown specificity. Although murine α chains could pair with human β chains, and vice versa, only the co-transfection of both genes encoding murine α and β chains led to expression of a TCR with the specificity of the original T cell from which the genes were cloned. Furthermore, specificity for antigen alone or MHC alone could not be conferred upon the human T cell line by transfection of only one of the mouse TCR genes, indicating that the αβ heterodimer is responsible for recognizing both the antigen and MHC molecule.*

Based on the predicted tertiary structure of the TCR and the sequencing of TCR genes from a large number of monoclonal T cells, the following important features of TCR specificity have been established:

1. In most cases, both α and β chains are involved in binding both foreign peptide and self MHC molecules; i.e., neither chain is independently specific for antigen or MHC (Fig. 7–5).

2. Different portions of the hypervariable regions of α and β chains, i.e., V, D, or J segments, may interact with the helical sides of the peptide-binding cleft of MHC molecules or with amino acid residues of the foreign peptide protruding out of this cleft. These fine structural details can be definitively resolved only by crystallographic analyses of isolated TCR molecules bound to peptide-MHC complexes. Such analyses have not been done yet.

3. Whether a particular T cell is class I or class II MHC–restricted is not determined by the V, D, J, or C genes used by the α or β chain of the antigen receptor of that cell. In other words, the same sets of TCR genes can be expressed in class I– and class II–restricted T cells, and no TCR genes are exclusive for one subpopulation. As we mentioned in Chapter 6 and will discuss in more detail later in this chapter, the ability of a particular T cell to respond to either class I– or class II–associated antigen is determined mainly by the expression of CD8 or CD4, respectively.

THE CD3, ζ, AND η PROTEINS ASSOCIATED WITH THE T CELL RECEPTOR COMPLEX

The TCR αβ heterodimer provides T cells the ability to recognize peptide antigens bound to MHC molecules, but both the cell-surface expression of TCR molecules and their function in activating T cells are dependent on four or five other proteins that non-covalently associate with the αβ heterodimer. Together, these proteins form the functional **TCR complex** (Fig. 7–6 and Table 7–1). Three members of the complex are called **CD3 proteins,** and include a 25 to 28 kD glycosylated **γ chain,** a 20 kD glycosylated **δ chain,** and a 20 kD nonglycosylated **ε chain.** These CD3 chains most likely exist as monomers in the TCR complex. In addition, 90 per cent of TCR complexes contain a homodimer of 16 kD nonglycosylated **ζ chains,** and the remaining 10 per cent contain a heterodimer of a ζ chain

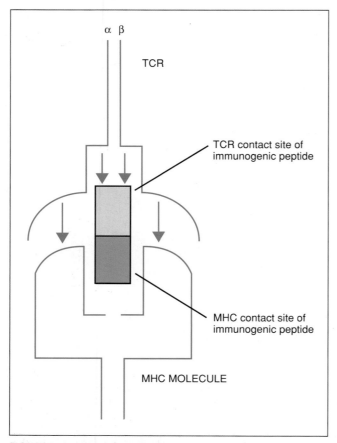

FIGURE 7–5. Contacts between the T cell receptor (TCR) and MHC-associated peptide. *Every immunogenic peptide contains sites that bind to MHC molecules and other sites that are recognized by the T cell. The TCR molecule has regions that contact the foreign peptide and other regions that recognize polymorphic determinants of the MHC molecules (both shown by bold arrows).*

with a 22 kD nonglycosylated **η chain.** Thus, the minimal stoichiometry of the most common TCRs is $\alpha\beta{:}\gamma\delta\epsilon\zeta_2$.

Structure and Association of CD3, ζ, and η Proteins

The CD3 proteins were first identified, before the $\alpha\beta$ heterodimer, by the use of monoclonal antibodies raised against T cells, and the ζ and η chains were identified later by co-immunoprecipitation with $\alpha\beta$ and CD3 proteins. The structures of these proteins associated with the TCR $\alpha\beta$ heterodimer have been elucidated by biochemical analysis and sequencing of cDNA clones that encode the molecules. The γ, δ, and ϵ chain genes are highly homologous to each other, are located on human chromosome 11, and probably all arose from a common ancestral gene by gene duplication. Each γ, δ, and ϵ chain protein includes an N-terminal extracellular region, a short connecting peptide, a transmembrane segment, and a cytoplasmic tail. The extracellular regions of γ, δ, and ϵ chains each contains a single Ig-like domain, and therefore these three proteins are members of the Ig superfamily. There is no variability or polymorphism identified in the extracellular domains of the CD3 proteins or their genes, and therefore it is not likely that these proteins contribute to the specificity of antigen recognition. The transmembrane segments of all three chains contain a negatively charged aspartic acid residue. This unusual feature may be important for the physical association or functional interactions of the CD3 proteins with the TCR α and β chains, since each of the latter polypeptides contains at least one positively charged residue in its trans-

TABLE 7–1. Proteins in T Cell Antigen Receptor Complexes

Name	Function	Size (kD) Human	Size (kD) Mouse	Multimeric Form	Comments
TCR α	One chain of receptor for recognition of antigen-MHC complexes	40–60	44–55	$\alpha\beta$	Ig superfamily member; rearranging genes; on CD4$^+$ or CD8$^+$ T cells
TCR β	One chain of receptor for recognition of antigen-MHC complexes	40–50	40–55	$\alpha\beta$	Ig superfamily member; rearranging genes; on CD4$^+$ or CD8$^+$ T cells
TCR γ	One chain of receptor for unknown forms of antigen	45–60	45–60	$\gamma\delta$ or $\gamma\gamma$	Ig superfamily member; rearranging genes, predominantly on CD4$^-$CD8$^-$ T cells
TCR δ	One chain of receptor for unknown forms of antigen	40–60	40–60	$\gamma\delta$	Ig superfamily member; rearranging genes, predominantly on CD4$^-$CD8$^-$ T cells
CD3 γ	Signal transduction for $\alpha\beta$ and $\gamma\delta$ TCR Cell surface expression of TCR complex	25–28	21		Ig superfamily member; phosphorylated on serine and tyrosine residues
CD3 δ	Signal transduction for $\alpha\beta$ and $\gamma\delta$ TCR Cell surface expression of TCR complex	20	28		Ig superfamily member; phosphorylated on serine and tyrosine residues
CD3 ϵ	Signal transduction for $\alpha\beta$ and $\gamma\delta$ TCR Cell surface expression of TCR complex	20	25		Ig superfamily member; phosphorylated on serine and tyrosine residues
CD3 ζ	Signal transduction for $\alpha\beta$ and $\gamma\delta$ TCR Cell surface expression of TCR complex	16	16	$\zeta\zeta$ or $\zeta\eta$	Phosphorylated on tyrosine residues
CD3 η	Signal transduction for $\alpha\beta$ and $\gamma\delta$ TCR Cell surface expression of TCR complex	22	22	$\zeta\eta$	

Abbreviation: TCR, T cell receptor.

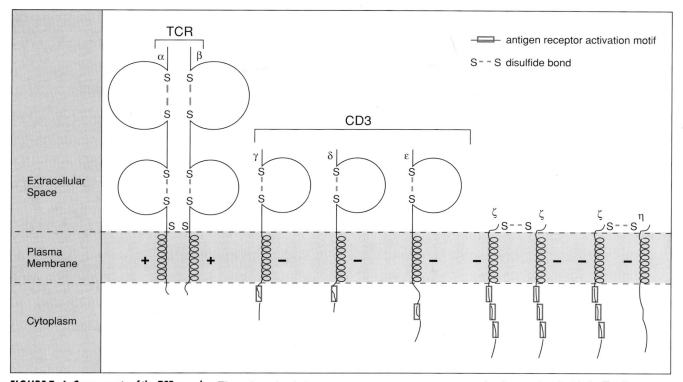

FIGURE 7–6. Components of the TCR complex. *The γ, δ, and ε chains are present as monomers, non-covalently associated with the T cell receptor αβ heterodimer and with one another. ζ and η chains are present as ζζ homodimers or as ζη heterodimers, and these chains may also physically associate with the TCR or with other CD3 chains. Disulfide-bonded loops of Ig-like domains are indicated in the extracellular regions of the TCR α and β chains and the CD3 γ, δ, and ε chains. The + and − symbols refer to charged residues in the transmembrane regions that probably mediate association of chains. Antigen receptor activation motifs in cytoplasmic tails are conserved sequences that include sites of tyrosine phosphorylation (see text).*

membrane domain. The cytoplasmic domains of the CD3 γ, δ, and ε proteins range from 44 to 81 amino residues long and, therefore, are of sufficient size to transduce signals to the cell interior. In fact, the cytoplasmic tail of each of the CD3 proteins contains a sequence motif also found in the cytoplasmic tails of several other membrane proteins involved in signal transduction, including the Igα and Igβ proteins associated with membrane IgM and IgD (see Chapter 9), the FcεRI-β and -γ chains (see Chapter 14), and the TCR complex ζ and η chains (see below). This motif, called the **antigen recognition activation motif,** is composed of 17 amino acid residues in which the sequence tyrosine-X-X-leucine occurs twice, where X is an unspecified amino acid. The motif occurs once in the cytoplasmic tails of each of the CD3 chains, and is likely to be important in mediating signal transduction functions, as we will discuss later.

The ζ and η chains are encoded by alternatively spliced RNA transcripts of the same gene located on chromosome 1 in humans. Both ζ and η chains have identical amino acids in their extracellular and transmembrane domains, but differ in their cytoplasmic tails. The extracellular domains are short (nine amino acids), the transmembrane domains contain a negatively charged aspartic acid residue (similar to the CD3 γ, δ, and ε chains), and the cytoplasmic domains are long (113 and 155 amino acids for ζ and η chains, re-

spectively). The cytoplasmic tail of the ζ chain contains three of the antigen recognition activation motifs found in the cytoplasmic tails of the CD3 chains. As we will discuss in Chapter 13, the ζ chain is associated with other receptors such as the Fcγ receptor (FcγRIII) of natural killer (NK) cells.

The physical association of the αβ heterodimer, CD3, and ζ/η chains has been demonstrated in two ways.

1. Antibodies against the TCR αβ heterodimer or the CD3 proteins co-precipitate both the heterodimer and the associated proteins from solubilized cell membrane preparations.

2. When intact T cells are treated with either anti-CD3 or anti-αβ heterodimer antibodies, the entire TCR complex is endocytosed and disappears from the cell surface; i.e., the proteins are co-modulated.

The Role of CD3, ζ, and η Proteins in Assembly of the TCR Complex

A major function of the CD3, ζ, and η proteins is the facilitation of expression of the entire TCR complex. In fact, the TCR αβ heterodimer and the associated CD3 and ζ/η proteins are mutually dependent upon one another for cell surface expression. T cell tumor lines that have lost cell surface expression of the TCR heterodimer because of mutations in α or β chain genes also do not express CD3 molecules on their surface. When functional TCR genes are transfected into these cells to replace the mutated genes, expression of both the TCR heterodimer and associated proteins is restored (Fig. 7–7).

The synthesis of the components of the TCR complex, their assembly, and their surface expression are tightly regulated and coordinated phenomena that occur during the maturation of T cells in the thymus (see Chapter 8). The genes encoding the CD3 γ, δ, ϵ and ζ/η proteins are expressed by very immature thymocytes, before TCR α or β chain genes are expressed. Furthermore, the protein products of the CD3 genes are post-translationally modified and form $\gamma\delta\epsilon$ core structures in the absence of TCR α or β chains. The association of the TCR $\alpha\beta$ heterodimer with the CD3$\gamma\delta\epsilon$ complex takes place in the endoplasmic reticulum (ER), after which the complex is transported to the Golgi, where

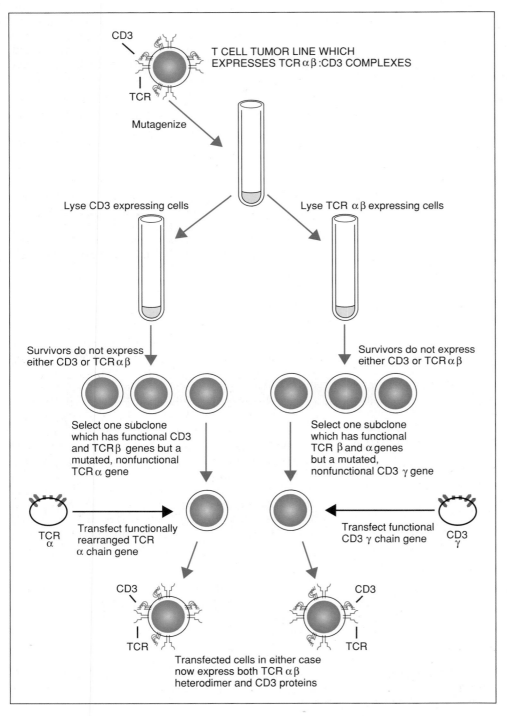

FIGURE 7–7. Co-expression of T cell receptor (TCR) and CD3 molecules. *If T cell mutants are selected for loss of either TCR or CD3, the surviving cells do not express either. In individual mutants lacking one functional TCR or CD3 chain gene, transfection of a normal gene encoding this chain restores expression of the entire TCR:CD3 complex.*

CD3

T CELL TUMOR LINE WHICH
EXPRESSES TCR $\alpha\beta$:CD3 COMPLEXES

TCR

Mutagenize

Lyse CD3 expressing cells

Lyse TCR $\alpha\beta$ expressing cells

Survivors do not express
either CD3 or TCR $\alpha\beta$

Survivors do not express
either CD3 or TCR $\alpha\beta$

Select one subclone
which has functional CD3
and TCR β genes but a
mutated, nonfunctional
TCR α gene

Select one subclone
which has functional
TCR β and α genes
but a mutated,
nonfunctional CD3 γ gene

TCR
α

Transfect functionally
rearranged TCR
α chain gene

Transfect functional
CD3 γ chain gene

CD3
γ

CD3

CD3

TCR

TCR

Transfected cells in either case
now express both TCR $\alpha\beta$
heterodimer and CD3 proteins

further modification of N-linked oligosaccharides takes place. Incomplete complexes do not make their way to the plasma membrane, probably because some mechanism inhibits transport of these proteins out of the Golgi to the plasma membrane until they all are physically associated with one another. TCR-α, TCR-β, CD3-γ, CD3-δ, and CD3-ϵ chains are all synthesized in great excess over the quantity that is expressed on the cell surface, whereas the ζ chain, in contrast, is synthesized in limiting amounts. There is evidence that $\zeta\zeta$ homodimers must associate with a TCR$\alpha\beta$–CD3$\gamma\delta\epsilon$ complex in order for the entire assembly of proteins to be routed to the plasma membrane. *Thus, ζ chain synthesis and association with the other proteins are the rate-limiting steps in the assembly and surface expression of the TCR complex.* The key role of the ζ chain in expression of the TCR complexes has been confirmed in mice with homologous recombination-mediated disruption of the ζ chain gene (see Box 4–1). These ζ chain gene knockout mice have markedly reduced TCR expression in developing T cells in the thymus, and as a consequence, few mature T cells in the periphery. A 90 kD phosphoprotein called **calnexin** associates transiently with partially complete TCR complexes within the ER. Calnexin plays a role in assembly of the TCR as well as other multichain protein complexes including membrane Ig and class I MHC molecules (see Chapter 5), and may function to retain individual members of the TCR complex within the ER before they are assembled together. In addition, there is evidence that another 28 kD cytoplasmic protein called ω or T cell receptor–associated protein (TRAP) associates with incompletely assembled components of the TCR:CD3 complex but is not present as part of the mature complex on the surface of T cells. This protein is hypothesized to control assembly and transport of the TCR:CD3 complex, but its mechanism of action is not yet defined.

Signaling Functions of the CD3, ζ, and η Proteins

When antigen binds to the TCR, the associated CD3 and ζ/η chains transduce the signals to the cytoplasm of the T cell, which lead to functional activation. Several lines of evidence support this concept.

1. Antibodies against CD3 proteins can often stimulate T cell functional responses that are identical to antigen-induced responses. However, unlike antigens, which stimulate only specific T cells, anti-CD3 antibodies stimulate all T cells in a mixed population, regardless of antigen specificity. Thus, anti-CD3 antibodies are polyclonal activators of T cells.

2. The cytoplasmic tails of either the CD3 ϵ or ζ chain can transduce the necessary signals for T cell activation in the absence of the other components of the TCR complex. This was shown by expressing genetically engineered chimeric molecules containing the cytoplasmic portions of the CD3 ϵ or the ζ protein fused

to the extracellular and transmembrane domains of other cell surface receptors for soluble ligands, such as the interleukin-2 receptor. Ligand binding to these chimeric molecules expressed in T cell tumor lines resulted in activation responses identical to those induced by stimulation through a normal T cell receptor complex.

3. The CD3 and ζ proteins are substrates of and may bind tyrosine kinases, which are rapidly activated after ligand binding to the TCR. Tyrosine residues within the shared motifs in the cytoplasmic tails of the CD3 and ζ proteins become phosphorylated soon after T cells are stimulated, and cytosolic tyrosine kinases physically associate with these cytoplasmic tails. Tyrosine kinase activities are considered to be key in the signaling cascade that leads to gene transcription and functional responses of T cells. These signaling events will be discussed in detail later in the chapter.

In the subsequent discussion we will refer to T cell antigen recognition or activation being mediated by the "TCR complex." It should be noted, however, that recognition of antigen is due to the TCR $\alpha\beta$ heterodimer only, and the signals that initiate activation are transduced not by the antigen-binding heterodimer but by the associated proteins in the complex. It should also be noted that although the signals transduced by the TCR complex are necessary for initiating the activation of normal T cells, they are usually not sufficient. Additional costimulators, which interact with T cell surface molecules other than the TCR complex, are also required, as we will discuss later.

THE $\gamma\delta$ T CELL RECEPTOR

The $\gamma\delta$ TCR is a second type of diverse, CD3-associated disulfide-linked heterodimer expressed on a small subset of $\alpha\beta$-negative peripheral T cells and immature thymocytes. (It is completely distinct from the γ and δ components of the CD3 complex.) Its existence was first suggested when the γ chain gene was cloned and characterized as an Ig-like gene that is somatically rearranged and expressed only in T cells, but with no sequences compatible with the N-linked glycosylation sites that were known to exist on TCR α and β chains. Subsequent cloning of the Ig-like δ chain gene, and concurrent immunochemical identification of a CD3-associated heterodimeric protein on cells not expressing α or β chains, confirmed the existence of the $\gamma\delta$ receptor. As is the case with the $\alpha\beta$ receptor, much of the information available about the protein structure of the $\gamma\delta$ receptor is predicted from the sequences of the cloned genes. Although the function of this receptor is not known, there are several interesting properties of the genes encoding it and the cells on which it is expressed that are areas of active investigation. The protein structure, specificity, and postulated function of $\gamma\delta$ receptors are discussed below. The genomic organization, rearrangement, and generation of diversity of $\gamma\delta$ receptor genes are described in Chapter 8.

Biochemical Characteristics of the $\gamma\delta$ T Cell Receptor

The γ and δ proteins are present on T cells that express the CD3 proteins but do not produce $\alpha\beta$ receptors. γ and δ chains are transmembrane glycoproteins with structures similar to the α and β chains. Both γ and δ chains include extracellular Ig-like V and C regions, short connecting or hinge regions, hydrophobic transmembrane segments, and short cytoplasmic tails (see Fig. 7–3). The hinge regions usually contain cysteines involved in interchain disulfide linkages. In humans, the $\gamma\delta$ heterodimer may be disulfide linked or non-covalently linked, depending on the use of different exons encoding the constant region of the γ chain (see Chapter 8). The transmembrane regions of γ and δ chains, similar to α and β chains, contain positively charged lysine residues that may be important in interacting with the negatively charged aspartic acid residues found in the transmembrane regions of the CD3 polypeptides. In addition, the transmembrane region of the δ chain (like the α chain) contains a second positively charged arginine residue. The amino acid sequence of γ chains is most like that of TCR β chains, and δ chains are most like α chains. The human γ chain is a glycoprotein with a size varying from 36 to 55 kD glycoprotein, depending on differences in both polypeptide backbone length and extent of glycosylation. The human δ chain is a 40 to 60 kD glycoprotein. In the mouse, only disulfide-linked $\gamma\delta$ heterodimers have been identified.

Specificity and Function of $\gamma\delta$ Receptors

Our current understanding of the structure of the $\gamma\delta$ receptor is a tribute to modern molecular biology, in that the information about the genes encoding the molecule is available well before any thorough understanding of the molecule's function. Two interrelated approaches to analyzing the function of the $\gamma\delta$ receptor have been (1) characterization of the location and function of cells that express the receptor, and (2) determination of what $\gamma\delta$ receptors recognize.

The percentages of T cells expressing the $\gamma\delta$ TCRs vary widely, depending on tissue and species, but overall, less than 5 per cent of T cells express this form of receptor. Studies of the rearrangements of the γ and δ genes in $\alpha\beta$ TCR–expressing cells, as well as studies of T cell development in mice expressing γ and δ transgenes, indicate that $\gamma\delta$ T cells are of distinct lineage from $\alpha\beta$ T cells (see Chapter 8). Furthermore, there are subsets of $\gamma\delta$ T cells that can be distinguished from one another on the basis of when they develop during ontogeny, which genes they use to encode their V regions, their sites of development, and the tissues they populate. Studies in mice indicate that some $\gamma\delta$ T cells using particular V genes are generated at different times during fetal or postnatal life, and these cells eventually populate different tissues. Several of these populations express identical $\gamma\delta$ TCRs with the same VDJ and C sequences and virtually no junctional diversity. For example, many mouse $\gamma\delta$ T cells in the skin express one particular TCR, whereas many of the $\gamma\delta$ T cells in the vagina, uterus, and tongue express another. These monospecific populations of $\gamma\delta$ T cells arise in the thymus. There is evidence that their lack of diversity results from both molecular constraints on germline rearrangements of γ and δ TCR genes and selection pressures based on their specificities (see Chapter 8). Some $\gamma\delta$ T cells develop in athymic mice, perhaps in the intestinal mucosa.

One intriguing feature about $\gamma\delta$ T cells is their predominance in various epithelial tissues of certain species. For example, greater than 50 per cent of lymphocytes within the small bowel mucosa of mice and chickens, called **intraepithelial lymphocytes,** are $\gamma\delta$-expressing T cells. In the mouse epidermis, there is a population of intraepidermal T cells most of which express the $\gamma\delta$ receptor. Equivalent cell populations are not as abundant in humans; only 10 per cent of human intestinal T cells express the $\gamma\delta$ receptor, compared with less than 5 per cent of blood T cells.

The $\gamma\delta$ heterodimer apparently associates with the same CD3 and ζ/η proteins as do $\alpha\beta$ receptors. Furthermore, the signaling events and activation responses typical of $\alpha\beta$-expressing T cells discussed later in this chapter are also observed in $\gamma\delta$ T cells. Most of the other cell surface molecules found on $\alpha\beta$ T cells are also found on $\gamma\delta$ T cells. Two notable exceptions are CD4 and CD8, neither of which is found on the majority of $\gamma\delta$ T cells. A variety of biologic activities have been ascribed to different $\gamma\delta$ T cells that are also characteristic of $\alpha\beta$ T cells, including secretion of various cytokines and lysis of target cells.

The question of what the $\gamma\delta$ TCR recognizes remains unresolved. There are rare examples of cloned $\gamma\delta$ T cells that recognize peptides associated with classical MHC molecules, just like other T cells. There is evidence that some $\gamma\delta$ T cells recognize nonpolymorphic MHC-like molecules described in Chapter 5, perhaps in association with low molecular weight ligands. The limited diversity of the $\gamma\delta$ TCRs in many tissues suggests that the physiologic ligand for these receptors is not polymorphic. Consistent with this idea is the finding that many $\gamma\delta$ T cells may be stimulated by microbial products called superantigens, which bind to multiple different TCRs. (Superantigens will be discussed later in this chapter.) Stimulation of $\gamma\delta$ T cells by heat shock proteins is also commonly observed. A working hypothesis for the function and specificity of $\gamma\delta$ receptor–expressing T cells is that they may recognize frequently encountered antigens at epithelial boundaries between the host and external environment. Thus, they may initiate immune responses to a small number of common microbes at these sites prior to recruitment of more specific $\alpha\beta$ T cells.

ACCESSORY MOLECULES ON T CELLS

The proteins in the TCR complex are the key molecules involved in specific antigen recognition by and antigen-induced activation of MHC-restricted helper T lymphocytes and CTLs. In addition, T cells express several other integral membrane proteins that play significant roles in the functional responses to antigen presentation (Table 7–2). These proteins, often collectively called **accessory molecules,** were initially discovered and characterized by the use of monoclonal antibodies raised against T cells. The antibodies were first used to identify T cell surface molecules by immunofluorescence and immunoprecipitation techniques. These antibodies were also used to block or initiate functional responses of T cells and thus served as probes for studying the physiologic roles of accessory molecules. There are several common properties shared by these accessory molecules:

1. *Accessory molecules on T cells specifically bind other molecules (ligands) present on the surface of* other cells, such as APCs, target cells or vascular endothelium, or molecules in the extracellular matrix including proteins and proteoglycans.

2. *Accessory molecules are nonpolymorphic and invariant.* Thus, unlike the TCR or MHC molecules, accessory molecules are essentially identical on all T cells in all individuals of a species. This implies that these molecules have no capacity to specifically recognize many different, variable ligands, such as antigens.

3. As a consequence of binding their specific ligands on the surfaces of other cells, *many accessory molecules increase the strength of adhesion between a T cell and an APC or target cell.* This property helps to ensure that the T cell and APC remain attached to one another long enough to allow functional interactions to occur between the TCRs and the rare peptide-MHC molecules to which they bind on the APC. In addition, accessory cell–dependent intercellular adhesion may ensure that the APC is bound long enough to be influenced by the effector functions of the T cell.

4. *Accessory molecule binding to endothelial cell surfaces and extracellular matrix ligands contributes to T cell recirculation and retention in tissues* (see Chapter 11).

TABLE 7–2. T Cell Surface Accessory Molecules

Name	Synonyms	Biochemical Characteristics	Gene Family	Cellular Distribution	Ligand	Function in T Cells	
						Adhesion	*Signal Transduction*
CD4	T4 (human), L3T4 (mouse)	55 kD monomer	Ig	TCR α/β positive class II MHC–restricted T cells; macrophages	Class II MHC molecules	+	+
CD8	T8 (human), Lyt-2 (mouse)	α/α homodimer with 78 kD α chain or α/β heterodimer	Ig	TCR α/β positive class I MHC–restricted T cells	Class I MHC molecules	+	+
CD11aCD18	LFA-1	α/β heterodimer with 180 kD α chain, 95 kD β chain	Integrin	All bone marrow–derived cells	ICAM-1, ICAM-2	+	+
CD49CD29	VLA-4,5,6	α/β heterodimer	Integrin	Leukocytes, other cells	Matrix molecules, VCAM-1	+	+
CD28	Tp44	80–90 kD homodimer	Ig	All CD4 positive T cells; 50% CD8 positive T cells	B7	?	+
CD2	T11, LFA-2, Leu-5, SRBC receptor	50 kD monomer	Ig	>90% mature human T cells, >70% human thymocytes	LFA-3	+	+
CD45R	T200; leukocyte common antigen; B220 (on B cells)	180–220 kD monomers; cytoplasmic tyrosine phosphatase domain	?	All immature and mature leukocytes	?	+	+
CD5	T1, Leu-1 (humans), Lyt-1 (mice)	67 kD monomer	—	All T cells and thymocytes	?	?	+
Ly6	—	10–18 kD monomers; glycophospholipid membrane anchor	—	Immature and mature T and B cells; various other tissues	?	?	+
CD44	PgP-1	80–200 kD monomer; variably glycosylated, chondroitin sulfated	Cartilage link proteins	Thymocytes, T cells, granulocytes, macrophages, erythrocytes, fibroblasts	Collagen fibronectin, hyaluronate	+	?

Abbreviations: HEV, high endothelial venule; ICAM, intercellular adhesion molecule; kD, kilodalton; LFA, lymphocyte function-associated antigen; MHC, major histocompatibility complex; TCR, T cell receptor; VCAM, vascular cell adhesion molecule; VLA, very late activation.

5. *Many accessory molecules may transduce biochemical signals* to the interior of the T cell that are important in regulating functional responses. Signal transduction presumably occurs as a consequence of ligand binding and may act in concert with other signals generated by the TCR complex.

6. *Many T cell accessory molecules are members of the Ig superfamily or the integrin family.*

7. *T cell accessory molecules are useful cell surface "markers" that facilitate immunocytochemical identification of T cells in pathologic lesions, such as T cell lymphomas and leukemias.* In addition, antibodies against these markers can be used to physically isolate T cells for experimental or diagnostic procedures.

Accessory molecules contribute to the regulation of immune responses in various ways. First, different accessory molecules are expressed on T cells depending on their stage of differentiation and prior encounter with antigen. The ligands for these molecules may be differentially expressed on endothelium in different tissues. Thus, the variable expression of these molecules influences the way the T cells recirculate from blood to sites of antigen in either lymphoid or peripheral tissues (see Chapter 11). Second, cells that express ligands for accessory molecules may function more efficiently as APCs or CTL targets than cells that do not express these ligands. Several different accessory cell interactions with ligands on APCs or CTL target cells have

been defined (Fig. 7–8). Therefore, variations in the expression of either the T cell accessory molecules or their ligands on APCs may influence the ability of the T cell to respond to antigen presentation. It is possible that T cell accessory molecule–dependent adhesion to APCs may precede TCR binding of peptide-MHC complexes. Once the TCR does bind its ligand, however, signals are generated within the T cell that increase the avidity of certain accessory molecules for their ligands (discussed in more detail later in the chapter). This may serve as a positive amplification step that promotes the tight adhesion of T cells to APCs only if the T cells recognize foreign antigen presented by the APC. The importance of accessory molecules in antigen presentation is suggested by many experiments showing that antibodies against one or more of these molecules can block T cell responses to antigens.

CD4 and CD8: Accessory Molecules Involved in MHC-Restricted T Cell Activation

CD4 and CD8 are T cell surface glycoproteins that are expressed on mutually exclusive subsets of mature T cells with distinct patterns of MHC restriction. CD4 and

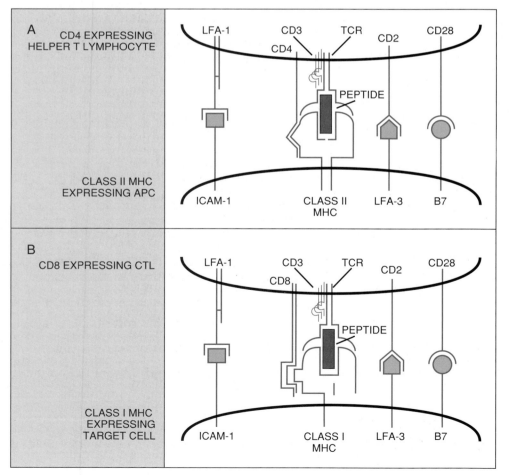

FIGURE 7–8. T lymphocyte surface molecules and their ligands involved in antigen recognition and T cell responses. *Interactions between a CD4+ T cell and an antigen-presenting cell (APC) (A) or a CD8+ cytolytic T lymphocyte (CTL) and a target cell (B) involve multiple T cell surface proteins that recognize different ligands on the APC or target cell.*

CD8 serve as accessory molecules by facilitating interactions of T cells with APCs or CTL target cells. The functions of CD4 and CD8 are intricately associated with TCR function, and therefore these accessory molecules are often called *coreceptors.* Both molecules are members of the Ig superfamily, but they are no more related to one another than to other members of the family. Nonetheless they have very similar functions. Approximately 65 per cent of peripheral $\alpha\beta$-positive T cells express CD4, and 35 per cent express CD8. (Altered ratios of CD4$^+$:CD8$^+$ peripheral T cells are often used as a clinical parameter for immune dysfunction, although the informational value of this parameter is very limited.)

STRUCTURE OF CD4

CD4 is a transmembrane glycoprotein, approximately 55 kD in size, which is expressed as a monomer on the surface of both peripheral T cells and thymocytes. In humans, it is also present on monocytes and macrophages. The three-dimensional structure of the CD4 molecule has been in part predicted from the sequences of cDNA clones and in part determined by x-ray crystallography. There are four extracellular Ig-like domains, including two V-like domains and two domains that are neither C- nor V-like. In addition, there is a hydrophobic transmembrane region, and a highly basic cytoplasmic tail 38 amino acids long. The CD4 gene is located on human chromosome 12.

FUNCTIONS OF CD4

The role of CD4 in T cell function was initially demonstrated by the ability of anti-CD4 antibodies to block class II MHC–restricted antigen stimulation of CD4+ T cells *in vitro* and *in vivo.* The CD4 molecule is thought to have two important functions in the activation of T cells.

First, *CD4 serves as a cell-cell adhesion molecule,* by virtue of its specific affinity for class II MHC molecules (Fig. 7–8). Experiments have shown that the binding of CD4 to class II MHC molecules stabilizes the interaction of a class II MHC–restricted T cell with an APC bearing class II MHC-associated antigen. For example, class II MHC–expressing cell lines bind to monolayers of fibroblasts that express transfected CD4 genes, but no such binding occurs with untransfected fibroblasts or with mutant cell lines not expressing class II MHC (Fig. 7–9).

The invariant CD4 molecule binds via its two N-terminal Ig-like domains to the nonpolymorphic β_2 domain of the class II MHC molecule. It is clear that there is a wide spectrum of affinities of TCRs for their specific antigen-MHC molecule ligands. The adhesive role of CD4 may be most critical when the TCR affinity is low.

Second, *the CD4 molecule may transduce signals* or facilitate TCR complex–mediated signal transduction upon binding class II MHC molecules, thereby promoting the subsequent functional responses of class II–restricted T cells. The signal transducing role of CD4

has been suggested by a variety of experimental observations.

1. Monoclonal antibodies against CD4 have stimulatory or inhibitory effects on MHC-independent T cell activation induced by binding of anti-TCR or anti-CD3 antibodies. Such activation is independent of recognition of MHC molecules.

2. Phosphorylation of serine residues in the cytoplasmic tail of the CD4 molecule occurs rapidly upon stimulation of T cells by antigen plus MHC or by anti-TCR antibodies. Furthermore, a lymphocyte-specific protein tyrosine kinase, called lck (or p56^{lck}), is physically associated with the cytoplasmic tail of the CD4 molecule. Transfection studies using various mutant forms of the CD4 molecule with altered cytoplasmic tails indicate that lck binding to CD4 may be required for full T cell activation. The possible role of such protein kinases in T cell activation is discussed later in this chapter.

3. CD4 becomes associated with the TCR soon after the TCR binds peptide-MHC complexes or activating anti-TCR antibodies. Furthermore, bifunctional antibodies that simultaneously bind CD4 and CD3 are more potent activators of T cell responses than are antibodies reactive with CD3 alone. Thus, a CD4 molecule may act as a coreceptor with the TCR, both molecules binding to different parts of a single peptide-bearing class II MHC molecule.

CD4 expression on immature T cells in the thymus is critical for development of mature class II MHC–restricted T cells, as will be discussed in Chapter 8.

In addition to its physiologic roles, CD4 is the receptor for the human immunodeficiency virus (see Chapter 21).

STRUCTURE OF CD8

The structure of the CD8 molecule varies among species and at different stages of T cell maturation. On human blood T cells, the CD8 molecule consists of either a disulfide-linked heterodimer of two distinct 32- to 34-kD glycoproteins called CD8α and CD8β, respectively, or as a homodimer of CD8α chains. Most of the commonly used antibodies against human CD8 recognize epitopes on CD8α. Soluble forms of both the CD8 α and β chains without transmembrane segments are produced by alternative splicing of RNA transcripts. On human T cells in the thymus, CD8α may associate with the nonpolymorphic class I MHC–like molecule CD1. In mice, most, if not all, CD8 molecules are composed of heterodimers homologous to the human CD8$\alpha\beta$ heterodimers. CD8α and CD8β are members of the Ig superfamily with N-terminal extracellular Ig V-like domains (confirmed by x-ray crystallography), connecting peptides, hydrophobic transmembrane regions, and highly basic cytoplasmic tails that are 25 to 27 amino acid residues long.

FUNCTIONS OF CD8

The functional significance of CD8 was first demonstrated by experiments showing that anti-CD8 anti-

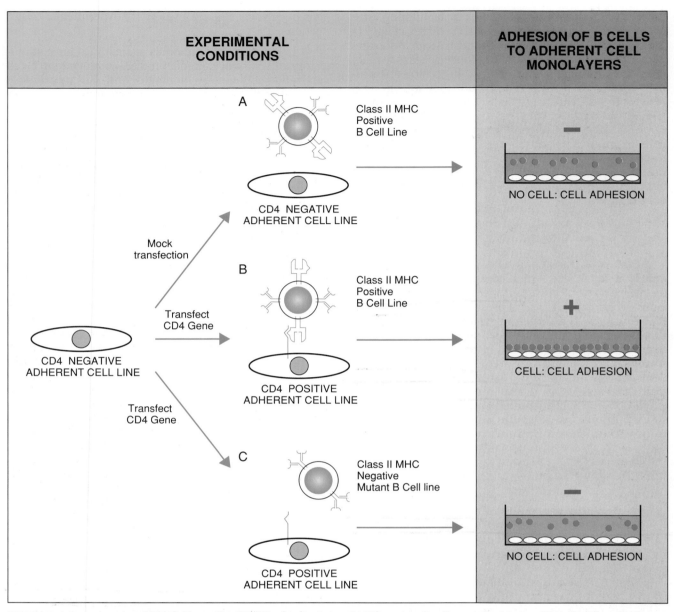

FIGURE 7–9. *Demonstration of CD4 binding to class II MHC molecules. A class II MHC–positive B cell tumor line binds to CD4⁺ fibroblasts (B) but not to CD4⁻ fibroblasts (A). A mutant B cell line that does not express class II molecules also fails to bind to CD4⁺ fibroblasts (C).*

bodies blocked class I–restricted killing of target cells by CTLs. The CD8 molecule is thought to have the same two general roles as CD4, namely in cell-cell adhesion and in signal transduction.

First, *CD8 serves as a cell-cell adhesion molecule*, by binding to nonpolymorphic immunoglobulin-like α3 domains of class I MHC molecules, thereby stabilizing the interaction of a class I MHC–restricted T cell (usually a CTL) with a target cell bearing class I MHC–associated antigen (see Fig. 7–8). This has been established by experiments similar to the ones described above for CD4.

1. Anti-CD8 antibodies can block the formation of conjugates between class I MHC–restricted CTLs and class I MHC–expressing target cells, thereby inhibiting cytolytic activity.

2. Fibroblast monolayers expressing transfected CD8α genes tightly bind class I MHC–expressing cells, whereas untransfected fibroblast monolayers do not.

3. If the TCR α and β genes are isolated from a CD8⁺ CTL clone and transfected into another T cell line that does not express CD8, the transfected line will not kill target cells bearing the relevant MHC-associated antigen. Cytolytic activity against such targets is restored, however, if the CD8α gene is co-transfected along with the TCR genes.

Experiments utilizing α3 domain mutant class I MHC molecules demonstrate that in order for a CTL to recognize its specific target, the TCR and CD8 molecules must bind to the same class I MHC molecules. Cotransfection studies with CD8 α and β chain genes indicate that the heterodimeric form of CD8 is more effective in performing adhesive functions than is the homodimer. Furthermore, signaling through the TCR increases the avidity of CD8 for class I MHC molecules. As with CD4, the adhesive role of CD8 is probably most important when T cells express antigen receptors with low affinity for specific peptide-MHC complexes or when the concentration of these complexes expressed on the surface of target cells is low.

Second, *the CD8 molecule may transduce signals* or may facilitate TCR:CD3–mediated signal transduction upon binding class I MHC molecules, thereby promoting subsequent functional responses of class I–restricted T cells. The signal-transducing role of CD8 has been suggested by a variety of experimental observations.

1. Coaggregation of CD8 and TCR complexes by bifunctional monoclonal antibodies enhances the ability of T cells to be activated, whereas segregation of CD8 from the TCR complex inhibits T cell activation.

2. Antibodies specific for CD8 block CTL killing of target cells, and this occurs even when the antibodies are added after the CTLs bind to their targets. This is consistent with a role of the CD8 molecule in CTL activation beyond target cell adhesion.

3. The cytoplasmic domain of the CD8 molecule becomes rapidly phosphorylated upon ligand binding to the TCR. Furthermore, as with the CD4 molecule, the tyrosine kinase called lck is physically associated with the CD8 molecule, and this association is required for full T cell activation responses.

CD8 also plays an essential role in the thymic development of mature class I–restricted T cells, as discussed in Chapter 8.

Other Accessory Molecules Involved in T Cell Activation and Cell-Cell Interactions

In addition to CD4 and CD8, several other T cell integral membrane proteins can influence T cell activation and/or the functional interactions of T cells with other cells. The precise roles of these accessory molecules in antigen-driven activation of T cells are not completely understood, and in several cases the ligands to which they bind are not known. Nonetheless natural ligand or antibody binding to these proteins has profound effects on T cells, raising the possibility that these T cell surface molecules may serve significant physiologic functions. We will order our discussion of these molecules based on the superfamilies to which they belong. Additional accessory molecules with poorly defined functions will be mentioned briefly. Characteristics of all these molecules are listed in Table 7–2.

THE T CELL INTEGRINS, LFA-1 (CD11aCD18) AND VLA MOLECULES

The integrin family of heterodimeric leukocyte proteins functions primarily as adhesion molecules, although they may serve signaling functions as well (Box 7–3). We will discuss two subfamilies of lymphocyte integrins, the β_2 integrins represented by LFA-1, and the β_1 integrins represented by the VLA molecules.

LFA-1, a member of the β_2 integrin family, is expressed on more than 90 per cent of thymocytes and mature T cells, B cells, granulocytes, and monocytes.

Anti–LFA-1 antibodies inhibit a wide variety of adhesion-dependent lymphocyte functions, including antigen and APC-induced helper T cell stimulation, CTL-mediated killing of target cells, and lymphocyte adhesion to endothelium (see Chapters 11 and 13). This effect is in part due to the ability of these antibodies to block conjugate formation between the T lymphocyte and other cells. The avidity of LFA-1 binding to its ligands is increased shortly after stimulation of T cells through the TCR, although the precise mechanism for this phenomenon is not known. This ensures that antigen recognition and integrin-mediated intercellular adhesion function coordinately to optimize T cell–APC interactions.

One specific ligand for LFA-1 is **intercellular adhesion molecule–1** (ICAM-1), an 80 to 114 kD integral membrane glycoprotein that contains five extracellular Ig-like domains and is thus a member of the Ig superfamily. ICAM-1 is expressed on a variety of hematopoietic and nonhematopoietic cells, including B and T cells, fibroblasts, keratinocytes, and endothelial cells, and the level of expression on these cells can be upregulated by various cytokines. Soluble recombinant forms of ICAM-1 can enhance TCR-complex–mediated activation of T cells, suggesting that LFA-1 may deliver costimulatory signals to T cells. ICAM-1 has been shown to be a specific receptor for rhinoviruses, the etiologic agents of many cases of the common cold.

Some LFA-1–dependent cell adhesion phenomena cannot be blocked by anti–ICAM-1 antibody or by soluble ICAM-1; in fact, another LFA-1–binding molecule called ICAM-2 has been identified. ICAM-2 is also an Ig superfamily member, with two extracellular Ig-like domains; it has a similar tissue distribution to ICAM-1, but is apparently expressed constitutively and is not regulated by cytokines. A third ligand for LFA-1, called ICAM-3, is expressed on lymphoid cells. ICAM-1, but not ICAM-2 or ICAM-3, can also bind to the β_2 integrin CD11bCD18 (Mac-1).

The VLA (very late activation) molecules, or β_1 integrins, all share the same β chain (CD29), as described in Box 7–3. Three members of this family, VLA-4, VLA-5, and VLA-6, are expressed on resting T cells. Like LFA-1, these molecules are increased in number, and their affinity for specific ligands also increases, upon T cell activation. VLA-4 mediates binding of lymphocytes to endothelium at inflammatory sites by interacting with a protein called vascular cell adhesion molecule–I (VCAM-1) expressed on activated endothelium.

BOX 7-3. THE INTEGRIN SUPERFAMILY OF ADHESION PROTEINS

The specific (nonrandom) adhesion of cells to other cells or to extracellular matrices is a basic component of cell migration and recognition and underlies many biologic processes, including embryogenesis, tissue repair, and immune and inflammatory responses. It is, therefore, not surprising that many different genes have evolved that encode proteins with specific adhesive functions. These genes display homologies indicative of a common ancestral gene. *The integrin superfamily consists of about 30 structurally homologous proteins that promote cell-cell or cell-matrix interactions.* The Ig superfamily, which is described in Box 7-2, is another set of homologous genes encoding proteins with adhesive and recognition functions.

All integrins are heterodimeric cell surface proteins composed of two non-covalently linked polypeptide chains, α and β. The α chain varies from 120 to 200 kD, and the β chain varies from 90 to 110 kD. The N-terminus of each chain forms a globular head that contributes to the interchain linking and to ligand binding. The globular heads of the α subunits contain divalent cation-binding domains; divalent cations are essential for integrin receptor function. Stalks extend from the globular heads to the plasma membrane, followed by transmembrane segments and cytoplasmic tails, which are usually less than 50 amino acid residues long. The extracellular domains of the two chains bind to various ligands, including extracellular matrix glycoproteins, complement components, and proteins on the surface of other cells. Several integrins bind to Arg-Gly-Asp (RGD) sequences in the fibronectin and vitronectin molecules, but most do not. Some integrins may bind Asp-Gly-Glu-Ala (DGEA) in type I collagen, and Glu-Ile-Leu-Asp-Val (EILDV) in fibronectin. The cytoplasmic domains of the integrins interact with cytoskeletal components (including vinculin, talin, actin, α-actinin, and tropomyosin), and it is hypothesized that the integrins coordinate (i.e., "integrate") the binding of cells to extracellular proteins with cytoskeleton-dependent motility, shape change, and phagocytic responses.

Three integrin subfamilies were originally defined on the basis of which of three β subunits were used to form the heterodimers. This led to a simplified organizational scheme because it was thought that each of these β chains could pair with a distinct and non-overlapping set of α chains. More recently, five additional β chains have been identified, and many examples have

The Integrins

Subunits		Name	Ligands/Counter Receptors	Functions
β_1	α_1	VLA-1 (CD49aCD29)	Collagens, laminin	Cell-matrix adhesion
	α_2	VLA-2 (CD49bCD29)	Collagens, laminin	Cell-matrix adhesion
	α_3	VLA-3 (CD49cCD29)	Fibronectin, collagens laminin	Cell-matrix adhesion
	α_4	VLA-4 (CD49dCD29)	Fibronectin, VCAM-1	Cell-matrix adhesion; T cell homing; ? T cell costimulation
	α_5	VLA-5 (CD49eCD29)	Fibronectin	Cell-matrix adhesion
	α_6	VLA-6 (CD49fCD29)	Laminin	Cell-matrix adhesion
	α_7	CD49gCD29	Laminin	Cell-matrix adhesion
	α_8	CD49hCD29	?	?
	α_v		Vitronectin, fibronectin	Cell-matrix adhesion
β_2	α_L	CD11aCD18 (LFA-1)	ICAM-1, ICAM-2, ICAM-3	Leukocyte adhesion to endothelium; T cell–APC adhesion; ? T cell costimulation
	α_M	CD11bCD18 (MAC-1, CR3)	iC3b, fibrinogen, factor X, ICAM-1	Leukocyte adhesion and phagocytosis; cell-matrix adhesion
	α_x	CD11cCD18 (p150,95; CR4)	iC3b; fibrinogen	Leukocyte adhesion and phagocytosis; cell-matrix adhesion
β_3	α_{iib}		Fibrinogen, fibronectin, von Willebrand factor, vitronectin, thrombospondin	Platelet adhesion and aggregation
	α_V	Vitronectin receptor (CD51CD61)	Vitronectin, fibrinogen, von Willebrand factor, thrombospondin, fibronectin, osteopontin, collagen	Cell-matrix adhesion
β_4	α_6		Laminin (?)	
β_5	α_V		Vitronectin	Cell-matrix adhesion
β_6	α_V		Fibronectin	Cell-matrix adhesion
β_7	α_4		Fibronectin, VCAM-1, mucosal addressin	
	α_{HML}		?	
β_8	α_V		?	

Abbreviations: VLA, very late antigen; LFA, leukocyte function–associated antigen; ICAM, intercellular adhesion molecule; iC3b, C3b inactivated.
Adapted from Hynes, R.O. Integrins: versatility, modulation, and signaling in cell adhesion. Cell 69:11–25, 1992. Copyright by Cell Press.

Continued

been found of a single α chain pairing with more than one kind of β chain. Nonetheless, the subfamily designation is still useful for consideration of integrins relevant to the immune system; the major members of these subfamilies are listed in the table.

The β_1-containing integrins are also called VLA molecules, referring to "very late activation" antigens, because $\alpha_1\beta_1$ and $\alpha_2\beta_1$ were first shown to be expressed on T cells 2 to 4 weeks after repetitive stimulation *in vitro*. In fact, other VLA integrins, including VLA-4, are constitutively expressed on some T cells or rapidly induced on others. The β_1 integrins are also called CD49a-fCD29, CD49a-f referring to different α chains (α_1-α_6) and CD29 to the common β_1 subunit. Most of the β_1 integrins are widely expressed on leukocytes and non-blood cells and mediate attachment of cells to extracellular matrices. VLA-4 ($\alpha_4\beta_1$ or CD49dCD29) is expressed only on leukocytes and can mediate attachment of these cells to endothelium by interacting with VCAM-1. VLA-4 may be one of the principal surface proteins that mediate homing of lymphocytes to endothelium at peripheral sites of inflammation. The β_2 integrins, also known as the LFA-1 (leukocyte function-associated antigen-1) family, were identified by monoclonal antibodies that blocked adhesion-dependent lymphocyte functions such as killing of target cells by CTLs. LFA-1 plays an important role in the adhesion of lymphocytes with other cells, such as accessory cells and vascular endothelium. This family is also called CD11CD18, CD11 referring to different α chains and CD18 to the common β_2 subunit. LFA-1 itself is termed CD11aCD18. Other membranes of the family include CD11bCD18 (Mac-1 or CR3) and CD11cCD18 (p150,95 or CR4), both of which have the same β subunit as LFA-1. CD11bCD18 and CD11cCD18 both mediate leukocyte attachment to endothelial cells and subsequent extravasation. CD11bCD18 also functions as a complement receptor on phagocytic cells, binding particles opsonized with a by-product of complement activation called the inactivated C3b (iC3b) fragment. An autosomal recessive inherited deficiency in LFA-1, Mac-1, and p150,95 proteins, called leukocyte adhesion deficiency, type 1 has been identified in a few

families and is characterized by recurrent bacterial and fungal infections, lack of polymorphonuclear leukocyte accumulations, and profound defects in adherence-dependent lymphocyte functions. The disease is a result of mutations in the CD18 gene, which encodes the β chain of LFA-1 subfamily molecules, and it demonstrates the physiologic importance of the LFA-1–related proteins.

A general characteristic of integrins is their ability to be functionally modulated by physiologic activation of the cell on which they are expressed. The activation of cells that leads to integrin modulation is mediated by other cell surface receptors, e.g., the TCR complex in T cells. The functional modulation of the integrins may include changes in ligand specificity or, more commonly, affinity. For example, in T cells, the affinity of LFA-1 ($\alpha_L\beta_2$) for its ligand ICAM-1 increases rapidly and transiently in response to TCR signaling. Similarly, neutrophil LFA-1 affinity for ICAM-1 increases when the cell is stimulated with cytokines (e.g., chemokines such as interleukin-8) or complement system mediators (e.g., C5a). The increase in affinity is thought to be due to conformational changes in the extracellular domains, but the exact mechanism for these changes is unknown. It has been proposed that changes in affinity are initiated by intracellular biochemical events such as phosphorylation of cytoplasmic tails of the integrins or associated proteins. The significance of this activation-dependent increase in ligand binding activity is that the adhesive functions of the integrins can be turned on specifically at sites where leukocyte adhesion to other cells or extracellular matrix is physiologically needed, e.g., at sites of inflammation. This may be particularly relevant to lymphocyte trafficking out of blood vessels (see Chapter 11). In addition to adhesion, integrins deliver stimulatory signals to cells upon ligand binding. The mechanism of signaling may involve tyrosine phosphorylation of different substrates. Furthermore, ligand binding to the β_1 integrins on T lymphocytes enhances activation responses, including cytokine gene expression.

Thus VLA-4:VCAM-1 interactions, like LFA-1:ICAM-1 interactions, may regulate the movement of lymphocytes out of blood vessels to inflammatory sites (see Chapters 11 and 13). In addition, T cell VLA molecules bind to extracellular matrix ligands (fibronectin for VLA-4 and VLA-5, laminin for VLA-6), and these adhesive interactions may be important for the retention of T cells in tissues. VLA-4 binding to both VCAM-1 and extracellular matrix proteins has also been demonstrated to provide costimulatory signals for T cell activation.

CD28 AND CTLA-4

CD28 is an Ig superfamily member that serves an important role in T cell activation responses. It is expressed as a disulfide-linked homodimer of 44 kD polypeptide chains, each of which includes a single extracellular Ig V domain, a transmembrane domain, and a cytoplasmic tail with no intrinsic kinase activity. A homologous molecule, CTLA-4 is expressed on activated T cells. Both CD28 and CTLA-4 genes are closely linked on human chromosome 2. One identified ligand for both CD28 and CTLA-4 is the B7 molecule, a 60 kD Ig superfamily member constitutively expressed on dendritic cells and inducibly expressed on B cells and

monocytes/macrophages. The binding of B7 to CD28 is important for the delivery of costimulatory signals required for full activation responses of T cells to antigens. A second CD28/CTLA-4–binding molecule expressed on APCs has been identified and named B7-2. We will discuss this costimulation pathway later in the chapter.

CD2

The CD2 protein, also called LFA-2, or sheep red blood cell (SRBC) receptor, is an Ig superfamily member expressed as a 45 to 58 kD glycoprotein on more than 90 per cent of mature T cells and on 50 to 70 per cent of thymocytes. CD2 is also present on natural killer (NK) cells. The molecule contains two extracellular Ig domains including an N-terminal V domain and a membrane proximal C2 domain, followed by a hydrophobic transmembrane region and a long (116 amino acid residue) cytoplasmic tail.

CD2 functions as an intercellular adhesion molecule. The principal human ligand for CD2 is the structurally similar molecule called **leukocyte function-associated antigen-3** (LFA-3, CD58). LFA-3 is a 55 to 70 kD surface glycoprotein expressed on a wide variety of hematopoietic and nonhematopoietic cells. It has a

CD_2 or LFA = $LFA3$ or $CD58$.

similar extracellular domain structure to CD2; but in contrast to CD2, it can be expressed either as a typical transmembrane protein or as a phosphatidyl inositol–anchored surface molecule. The genes encoding CD2 and LFA-3 are closely linked on human chromosome 1. CD2 binding to LFA-3 promotes cell-cell adhesion. This may be critical for the functional binding of helper T cells to APCs, CTLs to their target cells, and maturing thymocytes to thymic epithelial cells (see Fig. 7–8). Consistent with this hypothesis is the finding that anti-CD2 antibodies can block conjugate formation between T cells and other LFA-3–expressing cells, and perhaps, as a consequence of diminishing cell-cell adhesion, these antibodies can block both CTL activity and antigen-stimulated helper T cell responses. In mice, the principal ligand for CD2 is CD48, which is distinct from but structurally similar to LFA-3.

Mature human T lymphocytes form rosettes with SRBCs, and SRBC rosetting is used as a technique to purify T cells from other leukocytes in the blood. *It is now known that CD2 is the SRBC receptor* and binds to an LFA-3 homolog on the surface of SRBC.

In addition to its adhesive function, CD2 is also a signal-transducing molecule. Certain combinations of anti-CD2 antibodies can activate T cells to secrete cytokines and to proliferate. CD2–LFA-3 interactions may also provide costimulatory signals to T cells *in vitro*. This pathway of activation is dependent on expression of TCR complexes in T cells or CD16 in NK cells. It is unclear if CD2–LFA-3 interactions influence T cell activation *in vivo*. CD2 gene knockout mice do not show detectable defects in T cell development or immune function.

CD45

CD45 (T-200, leukocyte common antigen) consists of a group of integral membrane glycoproteins, ranging in molecular weight from 180 to 240 kD, which are expressed only on immature and mature leukocytes, including T and B cells, thymocytes, mononuclear phagocytes, and polymorphonuclear leukocytes. The CD45 family consists of multiple members that are all products of a single complex gene on chromosome 1 of mice and humans. This gene contains 34 exons, three of which (called A, B, and C) are alternatively spliced at the primary RNA transcript level to generate up to eight different mRNAs and eight different protein products. The predicted amino acid sequences of the protein products include external domains varying in length from 391 to 552 amino acids, a transmembrane region, and a 705 amino acid, highly conserved cytoplasmic domain, which is one of the largest yet identified among all membrane proteins. Different glycosylation patterns of the same peptide backbone also contribute to heterogeneity of the members of this protein family. Several different monoclonal antibodies that recognize individual members have been useful for studying the distribution and functions of CD45 proteins. Isoforms of CD45 proteins that are expressed on a restricted group of cell types are designated CD45R (see Chapter 2).

CD45R expression on T cells is of interest for several reasons. First, the expression of different forms of CD45R is regulated during the process of maturation and activation of T cells. As discussed in Chapter 2, naive T cells express a form of CD45R called CD45RA, and memory T cells induced by prior exposure to antigen express a different isoform called CD45RO. Second, the large *cytoplasmic domain of CD45 contains an intrinsic tyrosine phosphatase activity*, which is important in the regulation of various activation pathways that involve tyrosine kinase activity (discussed later in this chapter). CD45 gene knockout mice show a block in T cell maturation and a defect in B cell activation.

OTHER T CELL ACCESSORY MOLECULES (CD5, Ly-6, CD44)

Immunologists have identified several additional T cell surface proteins that may perform adhesive and/or signaling functions. Like the accessory molecules already discussed, these molecules were also initially discovered by raising antibodies against T cells. In many cases, these antibodies could augment or interfere with functional responses of the T cells. Since the roles of these molecules in physiologic T cell activation are still poorly defined, they are described only briefly here, and in Table 7–2.

CD5 is a 67 kD protein expressed on all mature T cells, thymocytes, and a subset of B cells. The B cell–specific molecule CD72 is a natural ligand for CD5. Antibodies specific for CD5 can enhance TCR-mediated T cell activation.

Ly6 molecules and **Thy-1** are phosphatidylinositol-linked membrane proteins found on T cells as well as other cells. Monoclonal antibody binding to these proteins on mouse T cells can induce activation responses that are dependent on the expression of the TCR complex.

CD44 (PgP-1, Ly-24) is an acidic sulfated integral membrane glycoprotein expressed in several alternatively spliced and variably glycosylated forms on a wide variety of cell types, including mature T cells, thymocytes, B cells, granulocytes, macrophages, erythrocytes, and fibroblasts. A soluble form of CD44 also circulates in the plasma. CD44 binds hyaluronate, and this property is partially responsible for T cell binding to endothelium at sites of peripheral inflammation and maybe Peyer's patch HEV (see Chapter 11). CD44 may also play a role in retention of T cells in extravascular tissues. Antibodies against CD44 can alter T cell activation responses by as yet unknown mechanisms.

T CELL ACTIVATION

So far in this chapter, we have discussed the cell surface proteins that are involved in T lymphocyte antigen recognition. The consequence of T cell antigen recognition is the generation of biologic responses of the T cell, including the following (Fig. 7–10):

1. *Proliferation of T cells*, in response to antigen recognition, is mediated primarily by an **autocrine growth** pathway, in which the responding T cell secretes its own growth-promoting cytokines and also

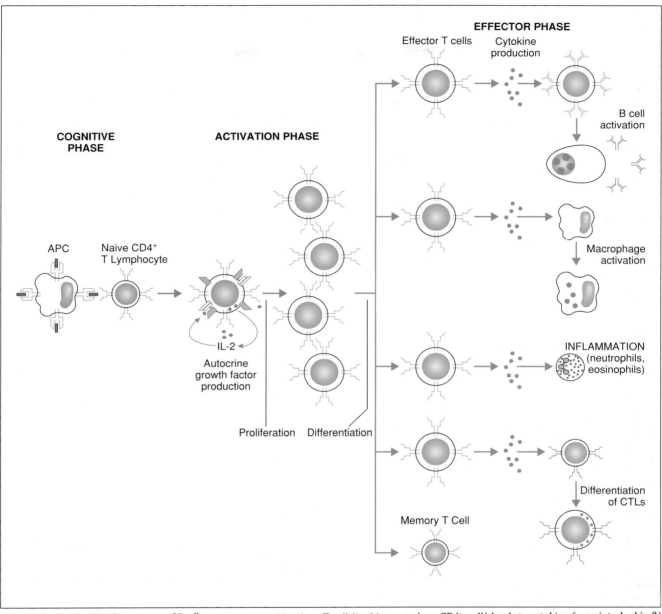

FIGURE 7–10. Functional responses of T cells. *Antigen recognition by a T cell (in this example, a CD4⁺ cell) leads to cytokine (e.g., interleukin-2) production, proliferation as a result of autocrine stimulation, and effector functions (e.g., B cell stimulation, macrophage activation, and promotion of inflammation and help for CTL differentiation). CD8⁺ cytolytic T lymphocytes (CTLs) show less autocrine growth, and their principal effector function is cytolysis mediated by discharge of granule contents. APC, antigen-presenting cell.*

expresses cell surface receptors for these cytokines. The principal autocrine growth factor for most T cells is IL-2. Some T cells may exclusively use a different autocrine growth factor, interleukin-4 (IL-4); the properties and functions of these subsets of T cells are discussed in Chapter 10. The result of the proliferative response is **clonal expansion** of antigen-specific T cells, which are necessary in large numbers to handle foreign antigen. Some of the progeny of antigen-responsive cells develop into **antigen-specific memory T cells,** which initiate larger secondary immune responses upon subsequent exposures to the antigen.

2. *Effector functions of T cells* initiated by antigen recognition are the biologic activities that enable T

cells to mount a useful immune response to foreign antigen. *The major effector function of CD4-expressing helper T cells is the secretion of cytokines,* which act on the same T cells and on other cells, including B cells, macrophages, other T cells, inflammatory leukocytes, and vascular endothelium. These cytokines exert various effects that promote and regulate humoral and cell-mediated immune responses and inflammation. Activation of helper T cells also induces the expression of a membrane protein called gp39, which binds to CD40 on other cells and mediates cell contact–dependent helper functions for B cells (see Chapter 9) and macrophages (see Chapter 13). The major effector function of CTLs is to lyse antigen-bearing target cells; in addition,

CTLs secrete some cytokines. The details of these various effector functions of helper and cytolytic T cells are discussed in Chapters 9 and 13.

The response of T cells to peptide antigen plus MHC consists of a series of cellular events collectively called **T cell activation.** The binding of peptide-MHC complexes to the TCR complex generates intracellular signals that transiently increase the transcription of several genes that are quiescent in unstimulated T cells. This, in turn, leads to the transient production of proteins that are essential for T cell mitosis and function. (In contrast, some cell types, including CTLs and mast cells, show transient responses to external stimuli by releasing pre-formed molecules; this is a fundamentally different type of response from cytokine secretion by T cells.) Thus, T cell activation includes the following interrelated steps:

1. Early signal transduction events.
2. Transcriptional activation of a variety of genes.
3. Expression of new cell surface molecules.
4. Secretion of effector cytokines and/or performance of cytolytic functions.
5. Induction of mitotic activity.

Functional and mitotic responses of T cells to antigenic stimulation last only for brief periods, and the responses quickly wane as the antigen is eliminated.

The early events of T cell activation have largely been defined by *in vitro* models, often using monoclonal T cell populations, in which the molecular consequences of ligand binding to TCR complexes are analyzed (see Box 7–4). Recent research has been directed at understanding how stimulation of the TCR complex is linked to transcriptional activation of genes. After the TCR binds a peptide-MHC complex, a cascade of events ensues that leads to new gene transcription. The phosphorylation status of tyrosine, threonine, and serine residues on a variety of proteins plays a critical role at several steps in the cascade. The addition of phosphate groups to proteins, catalyzed by **protein kinases,** and the removal of phosphate groups by **phosphatases** are key events that allow the cascade to proceed. The proteins that undergo these phosphorylation changes include membrane-bound enzymes involved in the earliest steps. Furthermore, the addition or removal of phosphates from trans-acting DNA-binding proteins (nuclear factors, see Box 4–4, Chapter 4) appears to be critical in regulating the transcription of T cell genes. In the remainder of this chapter, we will discuss some of the intracellular events in T cell activation, concentrating mainly on cytokine-secreting CD4+ helper T cells. The activation of CTLs, leading to granule discharge and cytolytic activity, may be basically similar but is not as well understood (see Chapter 13).

Early Membrane/Intracellular Signal Events in T Cell Activation

When antigen is presented to a T cell or when the TCR is bound by an activating antibody or a lectin (Box 7–4), a series of membrane and cytoplasmic events rapidly occur. These early "signal" events are similar to those that cell biologists have described in the stimulus-response physiology of a variety of non-lymphoid cells, such as mast cells, platelets, endocrine secretory epithelium, and muscle (Fig. 7–11). Four major, interrelated early activation events are (1) tyrosine phosphorylation of membrane and cytoplasmic proteins, (2) plasma membrane inositol phospholipid hydrolysis, (3) increases in cytoplasmic calcium concentrations, and (4) increases in protein kinase C activity.

BOX 7–4. METHODS OF ANALYSIS OF T CELL ACTIVATION

Most of our current knowledge of the cellular events in T cell activation is based on *in vitro* experiments in which T cells can be stimulated in a controlled manner and their responses can be measured accurately. The T cell responses in these experiments are believed to be the same as those that occur normally *in vivo* when antigen-MHC complexes on the surface of APCs or target cells bind to the TCR. For studying the mechanisms of T cell activation *in vitro*, immunologists have employed several kinds of T cell populations and several kinds of stimuli.

Polyclonal populations of normal T cells with a wide variety of different antigen specificities can be derived from the blood and peripheral lymphoid organs of specifically immunized individuals. The immunization serves to expand the number of antigen-specific T cells, which can then be restimulated *in vitro* by adding antigen and MHC-matched APCs to the T cells. In T cell populations from unimmunized animals or people, however, the number of individual cells with a particular antigen plus MHC specificity represents a very small fraction of the total cell number, and thus it is not possible to measure antigen-specific responses. Functional responses of these cells can be more easily studied by the use of **polyclonal activators,** which bind to many or all TCR complexes regardless of specificity and mimic antigen plus MHC–induced perturbations of the TCR complex. For example, polymeric plant proteins called **lectins** bind specifically to certain sugar residues on T cell surface glycoproteins, including the TCR and CD3 proteins, and thereby stimulate the T cells. Commonly used T cell activating lectins include **concanavalin-A (Con-A)** and **phytohemagglutinin (PHA).** Alternatively, polyclonal T cell populations can be stimulated by binding antibodies specific for invariant framework epitopes on TCR or CD3 proteins. Often, these antibodies need to be immobilized on solid surfaces or beads or cross-linked with secondary anti-antibodies in order to induce an optimal activation response. More recently, mice expressing transgenic TCRs have provided a means of stimulating large numbers of uncloned T cells with specific antigen.

Monoclonal populations of T cells, such as **antigen-specific T cell clones** and **antigen-specific T-T hybridomas** (see Box 7–1), can also be used to study functional responses to specific antigen plus MHC. (These monoclonal populations, of course, can also be activated by lectins and anti-TCR/CD3 antibodies.) The results of T cell activation experiments must always be qualified by defining what type of T cell population is being used, since the signals required for mitogenesis or development of effector function may be quite different among these different types of T cells.

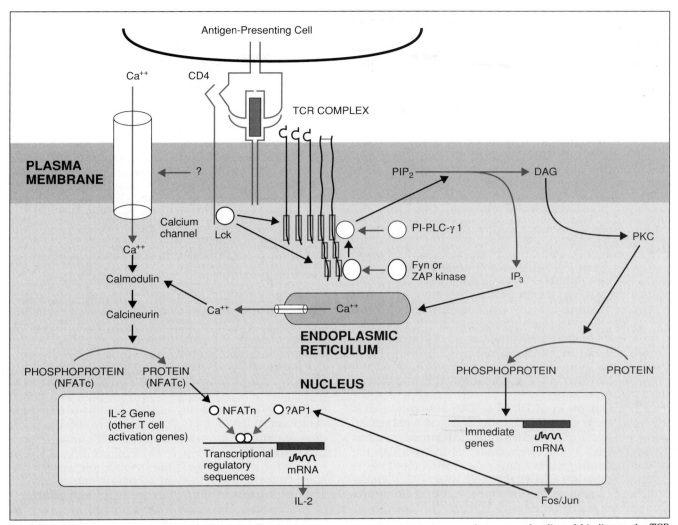

FIGURE 7–11. Intracellular signaling pathways in T cell activation. *The principal biochemical events that occur after ligand binding to the TCR complex are depicted. Association of enzymes with the cytoplasmic tails of the ζ chain is depicted, but the CD3 chains may also be involved.*

TYROSINE PHOSPHORYLATION AND TYROSINE KINASES IN T CELL ACTIVATION

Phosphorylation of tyrosine residues of proteins has previously been shown to be an essential component of signal transduction by many growth factor receptors in various cell types. In fact, the earliest measurable biochemical changes that occur after ligand binding to the TCR are the appearance of newly phosphorylated tyrosine residues on a variety of cytoplasmic and membrane proteins, only some of which have been clearly identified. These phosphorylation events, mediated by **phosphotyrosine kinases (PTKs)** are detectable within the first minute after ligand binding to the TCR. Phosphorylation of tyrosine residues on a protein has two general consequences. First, it allows other proteins that contain specific tyrosine phosphate binding sites to bind to the phosphorylated protein. These binding sites are structurally conserved and are called src-homology-2 (SH2) domains because they were first identified in the src protein. Therefore, phos-

phorylation of tyrosine residues in the cytoplasmic tail of a membrane protein may lead to binding of SH2-containing proteins to that site. Different SH2 domains may bind to different amino acid sequences containing tyrosine phosphate, and phosphorylation of multiple tyrosines in the same membrane protein can lead to assembly of multiprotein complexes. Second, certain enzymes may be activated by phosphorylation of tyrosine residues. Many of these enzymes, such as src, contain SH2 domains, and activation occurs after the enzyme "docks" at a phosphotyrosine-containing membrane receptor.

In the case of the T cell, the antigen recognition activation motifs of the CD3 and ζ chains in the TCR complex are tyrosine phosphorylated after TCR stimulation. This leads to docking of the enzyme **phosphatidylinositol phospholipase C-γ1 (PI-PLC-γ1)** which is then rapidly tyrosine phosphorylated, causing activation of enzymatic activity. PI-PLC-γ1 plays a significant role in subsequent events of T cell activation, as discussed below. The precise PTK that phosphorylates PI-

PLC-γ1 is not known, but there are three different PTKs that have been implicated in these early phosphorylation events of T cell activation. Two of these, **lck** and **fyn,** are members of the src family of PTKs. Lck is expressed primarily in T cells, and as we mentioned earlier in the chapter, it is physically associated with the cytoplasmic tails of CD4 and CD8. A variety of genetic studies indicate the importance of lck in T cell activation, including a lack of T cell development in mice with *lck* null mutations, and an inability to stimulate T cells through the TCR in cells expressing only mutant forms of CD4 that cannot bind lck. It is likely that upon TCR and CD4 or CD8 recognition of peptide-MHC complexes at the cell surface, CD4- or CD8-associated lck is brought closer to a variety of potential substrates, including the cytoplasmic tails of the TCR complex proteins. Fyn is expressed in many hematopoietic cells and can be weakly associated with the antigen recognition activation motif of ζ chain of the TCR complex. Fyn kinase activity increases rapidly after TCR stimulation, and overexpression of fyn in transfected cells or transgenic mice results in enhanced TCR-induced activation responses. However, homologous recombination-mediated deletion of the *fyn* gene in mice did not result in significant effects on T cell development, although there were defects in activation of a subset of thymic T cells and peripheral T cells. The third PTK that is implicated in TCR signaling is the ζ **associated protein of 70 Kd** or **ZAP kinase,** which is homologous to a B cell PTK called syk, but is expressed exclusively in T cells and NK cells. ZAP kinase contains SH2 domains and becomes tightly associated with the cytoplasmic antigen recognition activation motif of the ζ and perhaps the CD3 chains only after TCR stimulation. ZAP kinase enzymatic activity is apparently dependent on this association. The substrates for ZAP kinase are poorly defined.

Another key regulatory element in early T cell activation events is the CD45 molecule, which carries an intrinsic tyrosine phosphatase activity in its cytoplasmic tail. It is clear that CD45 expression is required for optimal T cell activation, and that it can catalyze the removal of phosphates from tyrosine molecules on several potentially important substrates, including lck and fyn. It is also known that certain tyrosine residues on lck and fyn serve as negative regulators of these enzymes in that phosphorylation at these sites turns off PTK activity. One likely way CD45 may regulate T cell activation is to mediate the removal of phosphates from the negative regulatory tyrosine residues on lck or fyn, thereby facilitating tyrosine phosphorylation of other substrates. It is also possible that CD45 may down-regulate T cell activation at later steps by removing phosphates from other tyrosine residues. Ligands for the extracellular domain of CD45 have not been identified, and the way CD45 may be inducibly engaged into the T cell activation pathway is not known.

In a current simplified model for the role of these PTKs in the early events of T cell activation, TCR recognition of peptide-MHC complexes induces CD4 or CD8 to associate with the TCR complex, bringing lck into close proximity to the cytoplasmic tails of the TCR complex proteins. Lck or other tyrosine kinases then phosphorylate tyrosine residues on the antigen recognition activation motifs of CD3 and ζ chains, which allows docking, phosphorylation, and enzymatic activation of Zap kinase. PI-PLC-γ1 is also "docked" to the TCR complex and is phosphorylated by a PTK, perhaps by ZAP kinase. Activated PI-PLC-γ1 and perhaps other ZAP kinase substrates are responsible for later events in the signaling cascade discussed below. The redundancy of the antigen recognition activation motifs on the cytoplasmic tails of the TCR complex proteins may serve to amplify the effect of antigen binding by allowing several effector molecules, such as ZAP kinase, to bind. Alternatively, it is possible that different effector molecules bind to the different copies of the motif.

INOSITOL PHOSPHOLIPID HYDROLYSIS AND INCREASED CALCIUM

Within minutes of binding of ligands to the TCR, there is an increased rate of PI-PLC-γ1 catalyzed hydrolysis of a plasma membrane phospholipid called phosphatidylinositol 4,5-bisphosphate (PtdInsP$_2$). As discussed above, this probably is a result of SH2 domain–dependent binding of the PI-PLC-γ1 to newly phosphorylated tyrosines on TCR complex protein cytoplasmic tails. Subsequent tyrosine phosphorylation of PI-PLC-γ1 activates this enzyme, leading to increased cytoplasmic levels of two PtdInsP$_2$ breakdown products: **inositol 1,4,5-trisphosphate (IP$_3$)** and **diacylglycerol (DAG)** (see Fig. 7–11). PtdInsP$_2$ breakdown is followed by a rapid rise in the cytoplasmic ionized calcium concentration, thought to be a result of the IP$_3$-stimulated release of membrane sequestered intracellular calcium stores. A sustained increase in cytoplasmic calcium is often maintained for over an hour, and this is dependent on influx of extracellular calcium. In addition, certain isoforms of **protein kinase C (PKC),** a serine/threonine protein phosphokinase, are activated as a result of the increases in DAG and calcium. Elevated calcium concentrations also favor the formation of complexes of this ion with the ubiquitous calcium-dependent regulatory protein called **calmodulin.** Calcium-calmodulin complexes can activate several enzymes, including kinases (which have substrates distinct from those of PKC) and, importantly, phosphatases such as **calcineurin.** The relevance of these biochemical changes to the functional activation of T cells is supported by the fact that PKC activators such as phorbol myristate acetate (PMA) and calcium ionophores such as ionomycin, which raise cytoplasmic calcium concentrations, act synergistically to promote the later differentiative and mitotic events normally seen in T cells in response to TCR binding ligands. The way calcium and PKC signals may be directly linked to gene transcription events is discussed later. Our understanding of signaling pathways in T cell activation is incomplete, and several additional components that are likely to be involved soon after early tyrosine phosphorylation are under active investigation. These include the other serine/threonine kinases including mitogen activated kinase (MAP kinase) and the ref protein, as well as GTP-binding proteins such as ras.

Transcriptional Activation and Expression of T Cell Genes

Within minutes of the binding of ligands to the TCR complex, T cells begin transcribing a variety of genes whose protein products are assumed or known to be essential for functional activation to proceed. These genes, which number more than 70, have been categorized as immediate, early, and late on the basis of the time course of their activation (Table 7–3). Transcription of immediate genes does not require protein synthesis, whereas early and late gene transcription does. The distinction probably arises because some transcription factors, i.e., those responsible for immediate gene expression, are preformed and can be activated independently from new protein synthesis (e.g., NF-κB, see Box 4–4, Chapter 4). Other transcription factors, i.e., those responsible for early gene expression, need to be synthesized. Immediate and early genes are transcribed prior to mitosis, and late genes are transcribed after mitosis. The genes transcribed in activated T cells can also be categorized on the basis of the functions of their protein products. Three main functional categories of genes that are expressed early during T cell activation are (1) cellular proto-oncogenes/transcription factor genes, (2) cytokine genes, and (3) cytokine receptor genes.

CELLULAR PROTO-ONCOGENES/ TRANSCRIPTION FACTOR GENES

Cellular proto-oncogenes are normal cellular genes whose products are involved at various cellular sites in the regulation of cell growth and differentiation. Many act as transcription factors regulating the expression of other genes. They are so named because overexpression of these genes, or expression of mutated forms of these genes or their viral homologs, leads to malignant transformation of cells. Several cellular proto-oncogene transcripts are significantly elevated in T cells after TCR-mediated stimuli, as they are in many non-lymphoid cell types that are stimulated by external ligands. Two of the most frequently studied genes are c-fos and c-myc. Both are in the immediate gene category; transcripts are first detectable within 15 minutes and 1 hour, respectively, after T cell stimulation, and peak levels of transcription are present within 1 hour for fos and 6 hours for myc. The products of these two cellular oncogenes act within the nucleus as trans-acting transcriptional regulatory proteins. The fos protein is a component of the AP-1 and NFAT complexes that regulate IL-2 gene transcription (Box 7–5). The myc protein may be required for the initiation of DNA synthesis, probably by transcriptional regulation of other genes. Other cellular proto-oncogenes are transcriptionally activated at later stages of T cell activation and require prior expression of other genes. For example, c-myb is transcribed only after autocrine IL-2 stimulation of T cells; the myb protein is found in the nucleus, but its function is not known.

TABLE 7–3. Representative Genes Expressed by Activated T Lymphocytes

Name	Functional Category	Time of Earliest Defection of mRNA After T Cell Stimulation	Location	Fold Increase After Activation
		Immediate		
c-fos	Nuclear-binding protein	15 min	Nucleus	<100
c-myc	Cellular oncogene	30 min	Nucleus	20
		Early		
IFN-γ	Cytokine	30 min	Secreted	>100
IL-2	Cytokine	45 min	Secreted	>1000
TGF-β	Cytokine	≤2 hr	Secreted	>10
IL-2 receptor (p55)	Cytokine receptor	2 hr	Plasma membrane	>50
IL-3	Cytokine	1–2 hr	Secreted	>100
Lymphotoxin	Cytokine	1–3 hr	Secreted	>100
IL-4	Cytokine	<6 hr	Secreted	>100
IL-5	Cytokine	<6 hr	Secreted	>100
IL-6	Cytokine	<6 hr	Secreted	>100
c-myb	Cellular oncogene	16 hr	Nucleus	100
Transferrin receptor	Receptor	14 hr	Plasma membrane	5
GM-CSF	Cytokine	<20 hr	Secreted	?
		Late		
HLA-DR	Class II MHC molecule	3–5 days	Plasma membrane	10
VLA–1	Adhesion molecule	7–14 days	Plasma membrane	?

Abbreviations: GM-CSF, granulocyte-monocyte colony-stimulating factor; HLA, human leukocyte antigen; IFN-γ, interferon-γ; IL, interleukin; mRNA, messenger RNA; NF-AT, nuclear factor of activated cell; TGF, transforming growth factor; VLA, very late activation.
Modified from Crabtree, G. R. Contingent genetic regulatory events in T lymphocyte activation. Science 243:355–361, 1989. Copyright 1989 by the AAAS.

BOX 7-5. TRANSCRIPTIONAL REGULATION OF THE INTERLEUKIN-2 GENE

The induction of cytokine production in response to antigen recognition is a hallmark of T cell activation. In particular, the mechanisms of TCR-mediated induction of interleukin-2 gene transcription has become a paradigm for T cell activation physiology. There is an extensive body of experimental work on the transcription of the IL-2 gene. The IL-2 gene promoter comprises a region of approximately 300 bp 5' of the transcriptional initiation site, which is required for responsiveness to TCR signaling. Within this regulatory region are multiple short stretches of DNA that play a role in enhancing transcription of the IL-2 gene or responding to signals generated by the TCR complex and accessory molecules. This information was obtained by creating DNA constructs that included different parts of the enhancer region linked to a reporter gene whose protein product is not normally made by T cells and can be easily detected. Examples of reporter genes used in these sorts of analyses include the enzymes bacterial chloramphenicol acetyltransferase (CAT) and firefly luciferase. T cells are transfected with constructs including different 5' sequences of the IL-2 gene linked to a reporter gene, and the transfected T cells are stimulated with TCR-binding ligands or pharmacologic agents such as phorbol myristate acetate (PMA) and ionomycin. The presence of reporter gene product under these conditions indicates that the IL-2 gene sequences in the construct respond to the activating stimuli applied to the transfected cell. These types of analyses, together with mobility shift and DNA footprinting analyses of protein-DNA interactions (see Box 4–4, Chapter 4), have yielded a functional map of the regulatory region of the IL-2 gene (see figure). Within this region there are sequence motifs that bind ubiquitous (non–T cell-specific) and constitutively expressed nuclear factors (e.g., Oct1). Other sequences bind ubiquitous factors that are induced in T cells by TCR stimulation such as AP-1 and NF-κB. AP-1 is composed of fos and jun proteins, both of which are products of cellular proto-oncogenes, and is necessary for induction of IL-2 gene transcription. Protein kinase C activation can lead to fos synthesis and AP-1 generation, thus establishing one link between early biochemical changes in the T cell activation cascade and regulation of gene transcription. NF-κB is constitutively present but sequestered in the cytoplasm by association with an inhibitor called IκB. PKC-mediated phosphorylation of IκB results in its dissociation from NF-κB, allowing the nuclear factor to move to the nucleus, bind to the IL-2 promoter, and enhance transcription of the gene.

Two sequences in the IL-2 promoter bind factors that are uniquely expressed in T cells only after TCR stimulation. The factors have been named nuclear factor of activated T cells (NFAT) and NFIL-2A. The induction of NFAT and NFIL-2A DNA-binding activity is dependent on increases in cytoplasmic calcium and is inhibitable by the immunosuppressive drugs, cyclosporin A (CsA) and FK506. These drugs, which are natural products of fungi, are the main therapeutic agents used to block allograft rejection (see Chapter 17) and they function largely by blocking T cell cytokine gene transcription. Studies on the way these drugs work in the T cell have provided insight into the link between calcium signals and IL-2 gene transcription. CsA binds to a protein called cyclophilin in the cytoplasm of the T cell, and FK506 binds to a distinct protein called FK506 binding protein (FKBP). Cyclophilin and FKBP are also called **immunophilins.** Their natural functions are not well understood; they both possess an enzymatic activity that catalyzes the rotation of certain peptide bonds, but this activity is not related to their effects on cytokine gene transcription. Importantly, both CsA-cyclophilin complexes and FK506-FKBP complexes bind to and inhibit a cytoplasmic calcium-calmodulin–dependent serine-threonine phosphatase called **calcineurin.** Furthermore, it has been shown that both CsA and FK506 block translocation of a constitutively expressed cytoplasmic component of NFAT, called NFATc, to the nucleus. These observations are consistent with a model of TCR-inducible IL-2 gene transcription in which increased calcium promotes the dephosphorylation of NFATc by calcineurin, which in turn permits NFATc to enter the nucleus. Once in the nucleus, NFATc combines with newly induced AP-1 proteins, and the complex then binds to the NFAT binding sequence of the IL-2 promoter. NFIL-2A is composed of two proteins, including a ubiquitously expressed factor called Oct1, and an inducible, T cell–specific protein called Oct1 activating protein (OAP). It is not known if activation of NFIL-2A occurs by a similar mechanism as NFAT.

There is also a sequence in the regulatory region of the IL-2 gene that is required for CD28-mediated costimulation of IL-2 promoter activity. The nuclear factor(s) that bind to this CD28 response element (CD28RE) are not well defined, although there is some evidence that NF-κB–related proteins may be involved. The signals initiated by CD28 that lead to the generation or activation of this factor are also not yet clear.

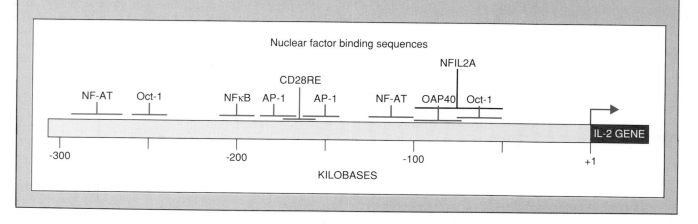

CYTOKINE GENES

T cell cytokine gene transcripts are significantly elevated within 4 hours of TCR:CD3–mediated stimulation. The IL-2 gene has served as a paradigm for the regulation of cytokine gene transcription during T cell activation. IL-2 is the autocrine growth factor for the majority of normal T cells, and therefore the transcriptional regulation of its gene is essential for the mitotic component of functional T cell activation. The transcription of the IL-2 gene (and other cytokine genes such as interferon-γ) begins within 1 hour following TCR-mediated stimulation of normal human lymphocytes. The elevation in RNA transcripts of cytokine genes is largely due to increased transcription as opposed to decreased RNA degradation.

The IL-2 gene contains an enhancer located 5′ of the transcriptional initiation site, which operates in a tissue-specific manner to direct IL-2 gene transcription only in T cells. Several DNA-binding proteins that bind to the IL-2 gene enhancer region are believed to be important links between antigen plus MHC binding to the TCR and transcriptional regulation of the IL-2 gene (Box 7–5).

CYTOKINE (AUTOCRINE GROWTH FACTOR) RECEPTOR GENES

The transcription of **IL-2 receptor** genes is another component of the T cell activation process that is necessary for the autocrine growth of the T cell in response to the IL-2 that it secretes. IL-2–induced growth of T cells requires the formation of a complex composed of the cytokine and three integral membrane receptor proteins, called α, β, and γ (see Chapter 12). TCR-mediated stimulation of T cells leads to increased expression of the α subunit of the IL-2 receptor. This response is due, in part, to increased gene transcription. The gene encoding the IL-2 receptor α chain has a 5′ enhancer region that can bind PMA-inducible nuclear factors such as NF-κB. The genes encoding the β and γ chains of the IL-2 receptor have been recently cloned, but analysis of transcriptional regulation is not yet available. Production and association of the α chain with the pre-existing $\beta\gamma$ chains lead to the formation of a high-affinity IL-2 receptor that binds IL-2 and stimulates mitosis. The interaction of IL-2 with its receptor is discussed in more detail in Chapter 12. Genes encoding receptors for other cytokines, e.g., IL-4 are also transcriptionally activated upon T cell stimulation and may be regulated in a similar manner to the IL-2 receptor gene.

Proliferation of T Cells

Mitotic division of activated T cells results in the expansion of clones of cells with the same antigen specificity and thereby augments the immune response to a particular antigen. Along with cytokine assays, the measurement of mitotic activity by ^{3}H-thymidine incorporation into newly synthesized DNA is one of the most frequently used assays for T cell activation. When T cells are stimulated through the TCR complex, mitotic activity can be measured within 48 to 72 hours *in vitro*. Depending on the T cell population, this induction of mitosis reflects cell cycle transition from either G_0 or G_1 to the S phase of the cell cycle. The binding of T cell growth factors, particularly IL-2 or IL-4, to their receptors initiates a series of poorly understood events that culminate in mitotic activity. No rapid change in cytoplasmic ionized calcium has been observed after IL-2 or IL-4 binding, and there are no clear indications that membrane phospholipid hydrolysis or PKC activation occurs in response to IL-2 or IL-4 binding to cells. By analogy with studies of fibroblast growth physiology, ligands that bind the TCR complex have been referred to as competence factors, meaning they allow cells to enter the cell cycle but not to progress through G_1 to S phase. In contrast, IL-2 has been called a progression factor, because it does allow cells to reach S phase.

Requirement for Costimulators in TCR-Mediated T Cell Activation

The functional activation of helper T cell populations, particularly normal resting T cells, requires more than binding of a ligand (anti-TCR antibody or MHC-associated peptide antigen) to the TCR complex. For example, highly purified normal T cells do not respond to lectins or antibodies that cross-link TCR complexes. Additional signals are required, and they can be provided in several ways. Accessory cells, such as monocytes, macrophages, dendritic cells, and B lymphocytes, can provide such signals in addition to serving as APCs. This has been shown *in vitro* by thoroughly depleting contaminating accessory cells from T cell populations. These purified populations show markedly reduced proliferative responses to lectins or anti-TCR antibodies, and normal responses can be restored by adding back macrophages or B cells. Since lectins or anti-TCR antibodies provide MHC-independent stimuli, it is clear that the role of accessory cells goes beyond antigen presentation. The ability of accessory cells to complement TCR-mediated signals for the induction of T cell activation is attributed to **costimulator molecules** produced by the accessory cell, which bind to receptors on T cells. Upon specific ligand binding, the receptors deliver signals that act synergistically with TCR-induced signals to enhance T cell activation. The requirement for adjuvants in eliciting a primary immune response to a protein antigen may be a reflection of the requirement for costimulators as well as antigen-presenting function, since adjuvants promote the migration of macrophages to the site of antigen administration and enhance the expression of costimulators on these macrophages.

Costimulators may also be important in determining whether the interaction of T cells with MHC-associated antigens leads to activation or tolerance. For example, the absence of costimulators at the time of TCR binding of antigen can lead to unresponsiveness of a T cell either to growth factors or to subsequent antigen presentation (see Chapter 10). This has been demonstrated *in vitro* by exposing T cells to antigen plus MHC on artificial membranes or by the use of anti-TCR antibodies in the absence of costimulators. This may be an important mechanism of self-tolerance, because T cells that see a self antigen presented by resident tissue APCs that lack costimulators may be rendered unresponsive to that antigen (see Chapter 19).

Perhaps the best defined costimulator-costimulator receptor pair is B7 and CD28. As mentioned previously, B7 is expressed on several "professional" APCs, including B lymphocytes, dendritic cells, and macrophages. When B7 binds to the CD28 molecule on T cells that are concurrently stimulated by TCR ligands, signals are generated that enhance IL-2 gene transcription and perhaps stabilize IL-2 messenger RNA. A sequence in the 5' regulatory region of the IL-2 gene has been identified as a response element for CD28-mediated signals, and presumably binds a transcription factor generated in response to those signals. B7 expression on some APCs may be up-regulated by a variety of stimuli, and therefore immune responses may be dependent in part on these stimuli. For example, interferon-γ treatment of monocytes, endotoxin treatment of mouse B cells, and B cell class II MHC binding to the TCR during the course of antigen presentation all lead to increased expression of B7. Besides CD28, B7 binds to CTLA-4 on activated T cells, but the role of this interaction is unknown. Furthermore, there are other ligands on APCs that bind to CD28 and act as costimulators including B7-2. The administration of soluble agents that bind CD28 ligands can block T cell–dependent immune responses in mice, including T cell help for antibody production and acute xenograft rejection. These effects are presumably due to a blockade of the interaction of B7 or B7-2 on APCs with CD28 on T cells.

Costimulators may act at different steps in T cell activation besides IL-2 gene expression. For example, some costimulators may enhance TCR-mediated T cell activation by prolonging elevations in cytoplasmic calcium, or other intracellular biochemical signals.

Other cell surface molecules that may act as costimulators for T cell cytokine expression and proliferation are VCAM-1, ICAM-1, and LFA-3, which bind to VLA-4, LFA-1 and CD2, respectively, on T cells. In addition, costimulatory activities for both T cell cytokine expression and proliferation have been attributed to some cytokines, including IL-1 and IL-6, largely based on *in vitro* experiments; the role of these cytokines as costimulators *in vivo* is uncertain.

SUMMARY

MHC-restricted T cells express clonally distributed, disulfide-linked heterodimeric protein receptors (αβ TCR) that are homologous to Ig molecules. These receptors specifically bind processed peptide antigen complexed to MHC molecules as well as polymorphic determinants of self MHC molecules on the surface of APCs. The αβ heterodimer is non-covalently associated with a complex of up to five distinct, invariant membrane proteins, including the CD3 ζ/η proteins. The assembly of TCR αβ and associated proteins is called the TCR complex. The CD3 and ζ/η proteins function as the signal-transducing component for the TCR complex. The γδ receptor is another clonally distributed, CD3-associated heterodimer that is expressed on a small subset of αβ-negative T cells. The nature of the ligand of the γδ receptor and the functions of γδ-expressing cells are unknown. In addition to the TCR complex, several accessory molecules are important in antigen-induced T cell activation. Some of these molecules bind ligands on APCs or target cells and thereby provide stabilizing adhesive forces. In addition, accessory molecules may transduce activating or regulatory signals. CD4 and CD8 are accessory molecules expressed on mutually exclusive subsets of mature T cells and bind nonpolymorphic determinants of class II and class I MHC molecules, respectively. CD4 is expressed on class II–restricted T cells, and CD8 is expressed on class I–restricted CTLs. Other T cell accessory molecules include the integrins LFA-1 and VLA-4, which bind ICAMs and VCAM-1, respectively, on the surface of other cells; the Ig superfamily members CD28 and CD2, which bind B7 and LFA-3, respectively; and CD45, a tyrosine phosphatase. The result of antigen-MHC binding to T cells is a series of intracellular events, collectively called T cell activation, beginning with second messenger generation and ending with T cell proliferation and the development of effector functions. The earliest events in this cascade include tyrosine kinase activation, membrane phospholipid breakdown, elevated protein kinase C activity, and rises in cytoplasmic calcium. These second messengers stimulate the transcription of genes required for the proliferative and effector responses of the T cell.

SELECTED READINGS

Ashwell, J. D., and R. D. Klausner. Genetic and mutational analysis of the T-cell antigen receptor. Annual Review of Immunology 8:139–167, 1990.

Bierer, B. E., B. P. Sleckman, S. E. Ratnofsky, and S. J. Burakoff. The biologic roles of CD2, CD4 and CD8 in T-cell activation. Annual Review of Immunology 7:579–600, 1989.

Crabtree, G. R. Contingent genetic regulatory events in T lymphocyte activation. Science 243:355–361, 1989.

Haas W., P. Pereira, and S. Tonegawa. Gamma/delta cells. Annual Review of Immunology 11:637–686, 1993.

Hemler, M. E. VLA proteins in the integrin family: structure, functions, and their role on leukocytes. Annual Review of Immunology 8:365–400, 1990.

Hunkapillar, T., and L. Hood. Diversity of the immunoglobulin gene superfamily. Advances in Immunology 44:1–63, 1989.

Hynes, R. O. Integrins: Versatility, modulation, and signaling in cell adhesion. Cell 69:11–25, 1992.

Jorgensen, J. L., P. A. Reay, E. W. Ehrich, and M. Davis. Molecular components of T-cell recognition. Annual Review of Immunology 10:835–873, 1992.

Keegan, A. D., and W. E. Paul. Multichain immune recognition receptors: similarities in structure and signaling pathways. Immunology Today 13:63–68, 1992

Linsley, P. S., and J. L. Ledbetter. The role of the CD28 receptor during T cell responses to antigen. Annual Review of Immunology 11:191–212, 1993.

Marrack, P., and J. W. Kappler. The antigen-specific, major histocompatibility complex–restricted receptor on T cells. Advances in Immunology 38:1–30, 1986.

Miceli, M. C., and J. R. Parnes. The role of CD4 and CD8 in T cell activation and differentiation. Advances in Immunology 53:59–122, 1993.

Perlmutter, R. M., S. D. Levin, M. W. Appleby, S. J. Anderson, and J. Alberola-Ila. Regulation of lymphocyte function by protein tyrosine phosphorylation. Annual Review of Immunology 11:451–500, 1993.

Raulet, D. H. The structure, function, and molecular genetics of the γ/δ T cell receptor. Annual Review of Immunology 7:175–208, 1989.

Schreiber, S. L., and G. R. Crabtree. The mechanism of action of cyclosporin A and FK506. Immunology Today 13:136–142, 1992.

Weiss, A. T cell antigen receptor signal transduction: a tale of tails and cytoplasmic protein-tyrosine kinases. Cell 73:209–212, 1993.

CHAPTER EIGHT

T CELL
MATURATION IN
THE THYMUS

The total number of T lymphocyte specificities for different antigens in an individual is called the **T cell repertoire.** Any individual's repertoire of mature helper and cytolytic T lymphocytes (CTLs) has two fundamental properties. First, as discussed in Chapter 6, *antigen recognition by T cells is self MHC restricted;* i.e., T cells in each individual can recognize and respond to peptide fragments of foreign antigens only in association with self major histocompatibility complex (MHC) molecules. Second, *the mature T cell repertoire is self-tolerant;* i.e., T cells in each individual do not respond to self antigens in association with self MHC molecules. Failure to maintain self-tolerance leads to immune responses against one's own tissue antigens and autoimmune diseases. Therefore, understanding how the mature T cell repertoire develops is important for understanding the specificity of T cells and may help us unravel the pathogenesis of autoimmune diseases.

The thymus is the major site of maturation of both helper T cells and CTLs. This was first suspected because of immunologic deficiencies associated with the lack of a thymus. If the thymus is removed from a neonatal mouse, this animal does not develop a normal T cell repertoire and remains deficient in T cells throughout its life. The congenital absence of the thymus, as occurs in the DiGeorge syndrome in humans or in the "nude" mouse strain, is characterized by low numbers of mature T cells in the circulation and peripheral lymphoid tissues and severe functional deficiencies in T cell–mediated immunity. The fact that some functional T cells with a mature phenotype do exist in athymic individuals suggests that extrathymic sites of T cell maturation may exist, but the location of these sites is unknown and their contribution to the development of T cell immunity is apparently minor. Furthermore, although the thymus is clearly the principal site of T cell maturation, the organ involutes with age and is virtually undetectable in postpubertal humans. Nevertheless, at least some maturation of T cells continues throughout adult life. It may be that the remnant of the involuted thymus is adequate for some T cell maturation or that other tissues can assume the role of the thymus. Since memory T cells have a long life span (perhaps longer than 20 years in humans), the need for generating new T cells decreases with age.

This chapter describes the development of the mature T cell repertoire. T cell maturation consists of three closely related processes.

1. Migration and proliferation: *Pre–T cell populations originating from the bone marrow migrate through the thymus, where some cells are stimulated to grow and others die.* Immature T cells that have recently arisen from precursors in the bone marrow are committed to the T lymphocyte lineage but do not express TCR or accessory molecules, and they have no capacity to recognize antigens or perform effector functions. These precursors leave the bone marrow, circulate in the blood, and enter the thymic cortex. Within the cortex, many of the cells proliferate and many die. Cell death is selective so that only MHC-restricted, self-tolerant T cells survive. The surviving cells migrate from the thymic cortex to the medulla and are finally released as mature T cells into the periphery.

2. Differentiation: *The mature phenotype of T cells develops in the thymus.* TCR complexes are expressed early during intrathymic T cell maturation, after the formation of functional TCR genes by somatic rearrangement of different gene segments. In addition to the TCR complex, surface expression of a variety of accessory molecules occurs during thymic maturation, some of which—including CD4 and CD8—play important roles in antigen recognition and T cell activation. Functional maturation, which is the ability to perform helper or cytolytic functions, occurs simultaneously with, and in large part depends on, the expression of these T cell surface molecules.

3. Selection: *The mature repertoire of foreign antigen–specific, self MHC–restricted T cells is selected in the thymus from the larger set of possible specificities encoded in the germline.* All individuals contain essentially the same full sets of T cell receptor (TCR) genes in their genomes. These TCR genes code for many receptors that can recognize many different peptides in association with many MHC molecules. Therefore, in every individual, as T cells arise from bone marrow precursors, they have the potential of expressing receptors that can recognize peptides derived from virtually any protein (self or foreign) in association with any MHC molecule (also self or foreign). After different receptors are expressed on the surface of different clones of developing T cells, the repertoire is modified or shaped by two related selection processes (Fig. 8–1). **Positive selection** is the process by which the T cell repertoire becomes self MHC–restricted. A second **negative selection** process eliminates or inactivates potentially autoreactive clones, ensuring that mature T cells are self-tolerant. The selective growth or death of different cells results in the self MHC–restricted, self antigen–tolerant mature T cell repertoire.

MIGRATION AND PROLIFERATION OF MATURING T CELLS IN THE THYMUS

T lymphocytes, like B lymphocytes, originate from precursors in the bone marrow. At present, little is known about the marrow stem cells that give rise to T or B lymphocytes or when and why they become committed to mature along a particular lineage. We also do not know why T cell precursors selectively migrate to the thymus. It is likely that these precursors express surface molecules, as yet unidentified, that selectively bind to receptors on thymic vascular endothelial cells. This binding may be the first step in the recruitment of progenitors to the thymic cortex. In mice, immature lymphocytes are first detected in the thymus on the 11th day of a normal 21-day gestation. This corresponds to about week 7 or 8 of gestation in humans. The cells that first appear in the fetal thymus do not express TCR molecules, CD3, CD4, or CD8 and are inca-

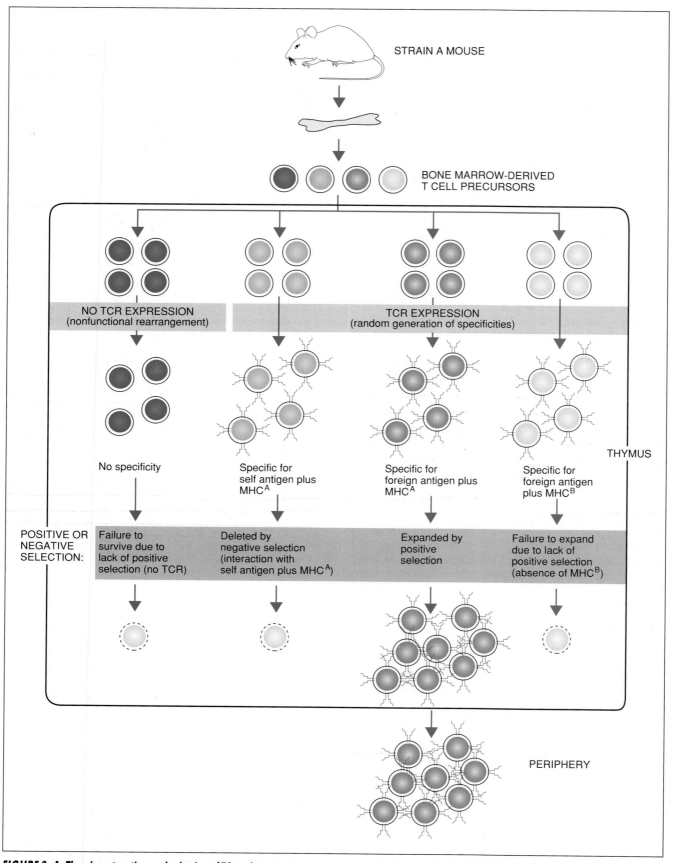

FIGURE 8–1. Thymic maturation and selection of T lymphocytes. *Bone marrow–derived precursors have unrearranged T cell receptor (TCR) genes and do not express TCRs. During intrathymic maturation, TCR gene rearrangements occur and maturing thymocytes express TCRs with random specificities. Only those clones specific for foreign antigen peptides bound to self MHC molecules are selected to mature and leave the thymus to populate peripheral lymphoid tissues.*

pable of recognizing or responding to antigen or performing effector functions. T cells in the thymus are also called **thymocytes.** The most immature thymocytes are found in the cortex, and the most mature thymocytes are detected in the medulla, from where they leave the thymus on their way to the peripheral lymphoid tissues. There is a high rate of mitosis in the cortex, with each bone marrow–derived precursor giving rise to multiple progeny. *Nonetheless, more than 95 per cent of the cortical thymocytes die before reaching the medulla.* This is probably due to the selection processes that preserve the minority of developing T cells that express self MHC–restricted, foreign antigen–specific TCRs, and eliminate the cells that express receptors of all other specificities. Consistent with this view that thymic selection processes occur in the cortex is the fact that TCR expression, as well as CD4 and CD8 expression, is first detected on cortical thymocytes. These selection processes are considered in more detail later in the chapter.

As they are maturing, thymocytes come into close physical contact with a variety of non-lymphoid cells in the thymus. These include thymic epithelial cells and bone marrow–derived cells, including macrophages and dendritic cells (see Fig. 2–9, Chapter 2). The superficial cortical thymic epithelial cells include **nurse cells,** which surround thymocytes within membrane invaginations. Deeper within the cortex, epithelial cells form a meshwork of long cytoplasmic processes, around which thymocytes must pass in order to reach the medulla. Epithelial cells are also present in the medulla. Bone marrow–derived dendritic cells are present at the corticomedullary junction and within the medulla, whereas macrophages are present primarily within the medulla. The migration through this anatomic arrangement allows sequential interactions between thymocytes and these other cells, and such interactions are necessary for the maturation of T lymphocytes.

Two types of molecules produced by the nonlymphoid thymic cells may be important for T cell maturation. The first are **MHC molecules,** which are expressed by many of the non-lymphoid cells in the thymus. Cortical macrophages, epithelial cells, and dendritic cells express high levels of class II MHC molecules; medullary epithelial and dendritic cells express both class I and class II MHC molecules; and medullary macrophages express high levels of class I MHC molecules. The interaction of maturing thymocytes with these MHC molecules within the thymus may be important for the selection of the mature T cell repertoire, as will be discussed in detail later. Second, thymic stromal cells, including epithelial cells, secrete thymic hormones and cytokines, which are postulated to promote T cell maturation. These hormones include a variety of proteins that have been well characterized biochemically but whose physiologic roles are largely unknown. They have been given various names, including thymosin, thymopoietin, thymulin, and thymic humoral factor. Thymic hormones have been shown to induce the appearance of some T lymphocyte lineage–specific surface molecules on bone marrow cells or immature thymocytes *in vitro* and to enhance T cell functional responses, such as proliferative responses to polyclonal activators. Some of these hormones have also been used in clinical trials for the treatment of immunodeficiency states in humans. Thymic stromal cells may also secrete interleukin-7 (IL-7), a cytokine that may stimulate the proliferation and maturation of developing T cells in the thymus. However, no combination of thymic hormones and cytokines has yet been shown to support the extrathymic development of immunocompetent, TCR-expressing T cells from bone marrow precursors or from immature cortical thymocytes *in vitro.*

T CELL RECEPTOR GENES: ORGANIZATION, REARRANGEMENTS, AND GENERATION OF DIVERSITY

The selection processes that shape the mature T cell repertoire begin only after developing T cells first express randomly generated TCR molecules with diverse specificities. The expression of TCRs is necessary for both positive and negative selection because both processes are dependent on specific recognition of self MHC and/or self antigens on the surfaces of thymic epithelial cells, dendritic cells, and macrophages. This portion of the chapter describes the organization of TCR genes and the mechanisms for generating the diverse repertoire of TCR specificities prior to selection.

Genomic Organization of T Cell Receptor α and β Genes

Functional TCR α and β chain genes, which are capable of being expressed as polypeptides, are normally present only in cells of the T lymphocyte lineage. *These functional TCR genes are formed by somatic rearrangement of germline gene segments,* by a process that is very similar to Ig gene rearrangements (see Chapter 4). The genomic organization of TCR α and β genes is fundamentally the same in all species studied (Figs. 8–2 and 8–3) and is similar to the organization of Ig genes. Each TCR locus consists of variable (V), joining (J), and constant (C) region genes, and the β chain locus also contains diversity (D) gene segments. Complete mapping of the unrearranged β chain locus has been achieved in mice; other TCR loci in mouse and man are still incompletely described. The β chain locus is on chromosome 7 in humans and on chromosome 6 in mice. In humans, there are two nearly identical C_β genes, each containing four exons. Each C_β gene is associated with a 5′ cluster of five J segments and one D

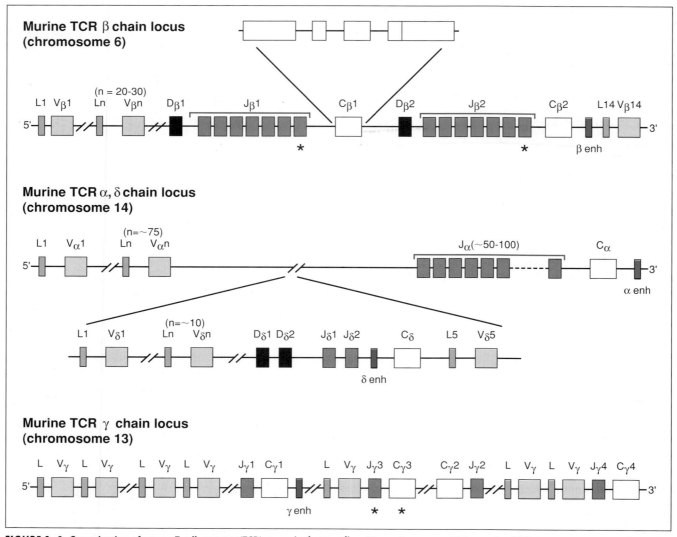

FIGURE 8–2. Organization of mouse T cell receptor (TCR) genes in the germline. *Sizes of exons and intervening DNA sequences are not shown to scale. The TCR β locus has been completely sequenced; other loci are incompletely defined. Note that the δ locus is located within the α chain locus. All of the C genes are actually composed of multiple exons, as shown for the $C_\beta 1$ gene. *indicates nonfunctional pseudogenes. The numbering of V_γ genes is not yet uniformly defined. Abbreviation: enh, enhancer.*

segment. In mice there are 20 to 30 V_β segments that can be grouped into 20 families, members of which are more than 75 per cent homologous in DNA sequence. Most V_β segments are located 5' of the two clusters of C and J segments. Interestingly, some strains of mice have deletions of up to half of the V_β segments or half of the D_β and J_β segments, and yet they are immunologically normal. The α chain locus is present on chromosome 14 in both humans and mice. There is a single C_α gene of four exons associated with a large 5' cluster of up to 50 different J segments. D segments have not been identified in the α locus. There are about 75 V_α gene segments, grouped into at least 12 families, all located 5' of the J and C regions. There is a very large region of intervening DNA between the V_α and J_α exons, which includes the entire TCR δ chain locus (discussed below).

Rearrangement and Expression of T Cell Receptor α and β Chain Genes

The TCR genes in the earliest T cell precursors are in the nonfunctional germline configuration, which is characterized by the spatial separation of V, D, J, and C gene segments on the chromosome. During maturation of T cells in the thymus, the TCR gene segments are rearranged in a defined order, resulting in the formation of functional TCR α and β genes in which V, D, J, and C segments are in close proximity to one another (Fig. 8–4). This process of somatic rearrangement is a prerequisite to TCR gene expression and is important for the generation of TCR diversity, as we will discuss below.

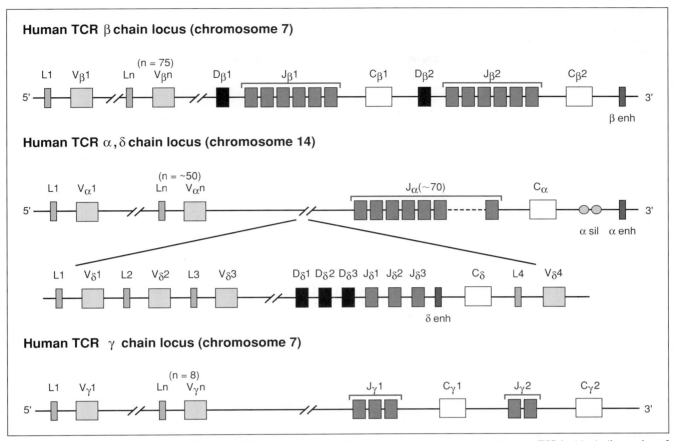

FIGURE 8–3. Organization of human T cell receptor (TCR) genes in the germline. *The genomic organization of human TCR loci is similar to that of the mouse (see Fig. 8–2); the human loci have not been completely sequenced. Abbreviations: enh, enhancer; sil, silencer.*

Somatic rearrangements of TCR V, D, and J genes are mediated by recombinases, which are thought to recognize specific sequences of nucleotides in the genome adjacent to each rearranging segment (see Chapter 4). These recognition sequences are essentially the same in Ig and TCR gene segments, and the same recombination mechanism mediates both types of receptor gene rearrangements. In fact, germline TCR genes transfected into immature B cell lines are efficiently rearranged. Furthermore, the products of the RAG-1 and RAG-2 genes (discussed in Chapter 4) are essential for both Ig and TCR gene rearrangements, and mice with null mutations in these genes do not develop mature B or T cells. The recognition sequences for TCR gene rearrangements include a conserved heptamer and nonamer separated by either a 12-base pair (bp) or 23-bp nonconserved spacer sequence. The locations of heptamer, nonamer, and spacer sequences flanking the V, D, and J gene segments in the β chain locus are such that either VDJ joining or (unlike Ig) direct VJ joining can occur. As a result, T cell receptor β transcripts do not always contain D sequences. The mechanisms that have been proposed for Ig DNA rearrangements, including excision and inversions, may all be operational in T cell receptor DNA rearrangements. Despite the fact that Ig and TCR genes use the same recombinases, Ig

genes are functionally rearranged only in B cells, and TCR genes in T cells. The basis for this lineage specificity of antigen receptor gene expression is still not well understood.

The β chain locus rearranges prior to the α locus, and the process begins with the joining of one D_β segment with one J_β segment. This is followed by a second rearrangement in which the newly formed DJ segment is joined to a V_β segment, resulting in a VDJ gene. The genomic sequences between the rearranging elements, including D, J, and possibly $C_\beta 1$ genes (if $C_\beta 2$ is used), are deleted during this rearrangement process.

The primary nuclear transcripts of the TCR β genes contain noncoding sequences (introns) between the VDJ and C genes. These are spliced out to form a mature messenger RNA (mRNA) in which VDJ segments are juxtaposed to either one of the two C_β genes. The two C_β genes may be thought of as structurally analogous to the Ig heavy chain isotype genes; but unlike Ig genes, the use of $C_\beta 1$ versus $C_\beta 2$ appears to be random, and there is no evidence that an individual T cell ever switches from one C_β gene to another. Furthermore, there is no known association of the use of either C_β gene segment with a particular function or specificity of the TCR.

β chain promoters have been identified in the 5′

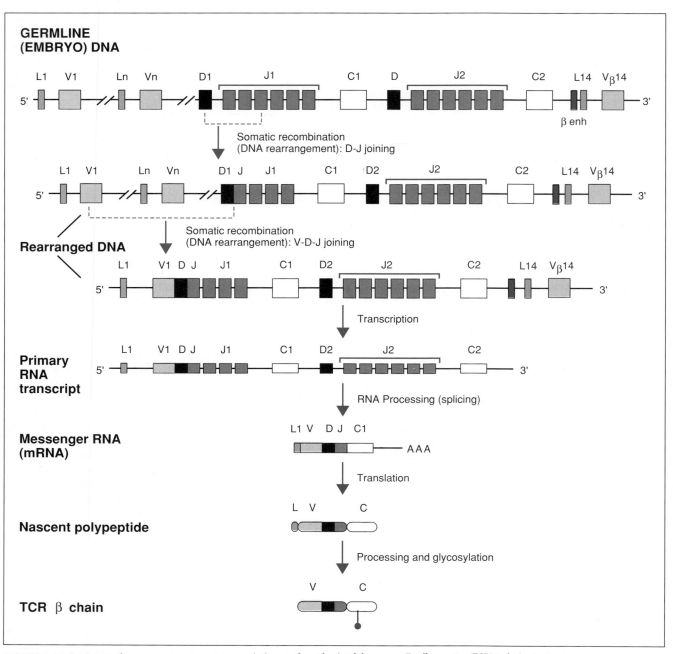

FIGURE 8–4. Sequence of gene rearrangement, transcription, and synthesis of the mouse T cell receptor (TCR) β chain. *In the example shown, the V region is encoded by exons V1, D1, and the third exon in the J1 cluster; the C region is encoded by C1. Each C gene consists of multiple exons that are not shown. Unused V and J segments located between rearranged V and J genes are deleted. Note that in this example the DNA rearrangement involves DJ, followed by V joining to DJ; but direct VJ joining may also occur in the β chain locus.*

flanking regions of V_β genes. These promoters are minimally active and not T cell specific. A powerful β chain enhancer is located 3′ of the $C_\beta2$ gene, which is responsible for high-level, T cell–specific activity of the V_β promoters. Several nuclear binding proteins associate with this enhancer, but most of these factors are not expressed uniquely in T lymphocytes. Nonetheless, TCR β chain transcription is T cell specific. In part, this may be due to T cell–specific rearrangements that bring β chain promoters in proximity to β chain enhancers. Other regulatory mechanisms that may impose T cell specificity on the promoter and enhancer activities have been postulated but not yet characterized.

Functional rearrangement, and probably transcription, of the β chain genes stimulates the rearrangement of the α chain locus. The rearrangement of the α chain gene segments is basically similar to the β chain gene rearrangements. Since there are no D segments in the α locus, rearrangement consists solely of the joining of V and J segments. Once VJ joining has occurred, transcription of the α chain gene ensues. Transcriptional regulation of the α chain gene is apparently similar to that of the β chain. There are promoters 5′ of each V_α gene that have low-level T cell–nonspecific activity but that are responsible for high-level T cell–specific transcription when brought in proximity to an α chain enhancer located 3′ of the C_α gene. Nuclear binding proteins and some consensus binding sequences have been shown to be functionally important for the α chain enhancer. Some of these factors are T cell specific but not yet well characterized, and others are expressed in other cell types as well. In addition, 5′ to the α chain enhancer, there are "silencer" sequences that can inhibit α chain transcription in non–T cells as well as in cells of the γδ lineage. Since there is only one C_α gene, RNA processing of the primary transcript gives rise to only one possible complete α chain mRNA.

Only one of the two inherited β chain loci are functionally rearranged and expressed in any one T cell. This is the phenomenon of **allelic exclusion,** and, as in Ig genes, it occurs because the productive rearrangement of a TCR locus on one chromosome inhibits the rearrangement of the corresponding allelic locus on the other chromosome. Allelic exclusion of TCR genes has been demonstrated by transfection and transgene experiments, in which the introduction of an exogenous, functionally rearranged TCR β chain gene into immature T cells inhibits the rearrangement and expression of the endogenous genes. In normal development, nonproductive rearrangements of one or both alleles of the α and β chain locus are quite common. When the β chain gene locus on one chromosome is nonfunctionally rearranged, such that it cannot be transcribed or its transcript cannot be translated, rearrangement of the other β chain locus proceeds. Successful rearrangement of the second locus does not shut off transcription of nonfunctional products at the first locus to have attempted rearrangement. Therefore, mature T cells often contain truncated, nonfunctional β chain transcripts as well as a functional, full-length mRNA. If both alleles of the β chain locus are nonproductively rearranged, the developing T cell will die. The rearrangement and expression of α chain loci proceed in a similar manner in those cells that have produced functional β chains except that functional rearrangement of α chains often occurs on both chromosomes.

Estimates of the potential size of the unselected immature T cell repertoire range from 10^{10} to 10^{15} specificities. As discussed in Chapter 7, homologies of the TCR to Ig molecules suggest that the peptide-MHC binding site of a TCR αβ heterodimer is formed by the V, D, and J regions of both chains. The structural diversity of the TCR heterodimers is generated by molecular mechanisms that are essentially similar to the mechanisms that generate antibody diversity (Table 8–1). These include the following:

1. *Multiple germline V, D, and J segments* can be used to create TCRs of different specificities. Although there are fewer V genes in TCR α and β loci than in Ig, the much greater number of J gene segments more than compensates for this. For instance, there are up to 50 J_α segments in mice compared with only 4 each in the IgH and κ chain loci.

2. During TCR gene rearrangements, *combinatorial associations of different V, D, and J gene segments generate TCR diversity.*

3. *Junctional diversity,* involving coding sequences at VJ, VD, and DJ junctions, contributes significantly more to TCR diversity than to Ig diversity. Several different mechanisms are involved in TCR junctional diversity. First, the random addition of nucleotides that are not part of the genomic sequence, at VD, DJ, and VJ

TABLE 8–1. Contribution of Different Mechanisms to Generation of Diversity of T Cell Receptor (TCR) and Immunoglobulin (Ig) Genes

Mechanism	Immunoglobulin		TCR αβ		TCR γδ	
	Heavy Chain	κ	α	β	γ	δ
Variable segments	250–1000	250	75	25	7	10
Diversity (D) segments	12	0	0	2	0	2
D segments read in all three reading frames	Rare	—	—	Often	—	Often
N-region diversification	V-D, D-J	None	V-J	V-D, D-J	V-J	V-D₁, D₁-D₂, D₁-J
Joining segments	4	4	50	12	2	2
Variable segment combinations	62,500–250,000		1875		70	
Total potential repertoire with junctional diversity	~10^{11}		~10^{16}		~10^{18}	

The mechanisms are described in the text. TCR loci have fewer V gene segments than Ig loci, but there is potentially much greater junctional diversity in TCR genes. The contribution of somatic mutation, which occurs in the Ig but not the TCR genes, is not included in the table, since these mutations tend to increase affinities of Ig molecules for antigen but may or may not change specificity. The numbers are representative of mouse Ig and TCR loci.

Adapted from Davis, M. M., and P. J. Bjorkman. T-cell receptor antigen genes and T-cell recognition. Nature 334:395–402, 1988. Copyright © 1988, Macmillan Magazines Ltd.

junctions, called **N-region diversification,** occurs in both α and β genes but only in Ig heavy chain and not light chain genes. N-region diversification is catalyzed by the enzyme terminal deoxyribonucleotidyl transferase (TdT). Second, the joining of TCR gene segments can be imprecise and still result in functionally rearranged genes, a phenomenon called "flexibility." For example, more than one 3' nucleotide of a V_α gene can join to J_α segments, and more than one 5' nucleotide of a J_β segment can join with D_β segments. Third, many D_β segments can be translated in all three possible reading frames, an uncommon feature for Ig heavy chain genes. Because of this, imprecise VD joining more often results in functional rearrangements.

4. The *pairing of α and β chains* serves to multiply the diversity generated for each chain. For example, there are up to 50 V_α and 75 V_β genes in the human genome, contributing up to 3750 potential $V_\alpha V_\beta$ region combinations.

In summary, TCR genes fundamentally resemble Ig genes in their mechanisms of diversity generation and expression, but they also differ from Ig genes in several respects. Although there are far fewer TCR V genes than Ig V genes, the potential diversity of TCR molecules has been estimated to be greater than that for Ig, largely because of the greater number of J segments and the greater junctional diversity in TCR genes (Table 8–1). Once a TCR gene is functionally rearranged, however, there are no further genetic alterations leading to changes in function or affinity of the protein receptor. Thus, unlike Ig genes, there is no isotype switching in TCR. Furthermore, *there is no evidence of somatic mutation in TCR genes;* consequently, affinity maturation of the TCR is not observed in secondary T cell immune responses as is observed in secondary antibody responses.

T Cell Receptor γ and δ Genes

The γ chain locus is located on the short arm of chromosome 7 in humans and on chromosome 13 in mice, distinct from either TCR α or β locus. The human γ locus is organized similarly to the TCR β chain locus (Figs. 8–2 and 8–3) with two JC clusters containing five J segments and two C segments in total, located 3' of multiple V_γ gene segments (up to 14 in total, including six nonfunctional "pseudogenes"). In mice, the arrangement is more complex, with up to seven V_γ gene segments interspersed with four JC clusters. (One of the murine V_γ gene segments and one of the JC_γ clusters are nonfunctional.) No D_γ segments have been identified. One striking difference in the γ chain locus compared with the TCR α and β chain loci is the variation among the multiple C_γ gene segments, including differences in sequence, length, and number of the exons encoding the hinge region (connecting peptide) of the protein. This variation results in different molecular weights and different N-linked glycosylation patterns of the expressed γ chain proteins on different cells as well

as the presence of both disulfide and non-covalent linkages of the γ chain with the δ chain.

The δ chain locus is unusual in that it is located entirely within the α chain locus between the V_α gene segments and the JC_α clusters (see Figs. 8–2 and 8–3). In humans, the δ locus consists of up to four V gene segments and one C gene segment associated with three J and two D segments. The arrangement in mice is fundamentally similar, but up to eight murine V_δ families (and more than ten individual V_δ gene segments) have been identified.

Rearrangements of γ and δ genes occur by the same mechanism as Ig and TCR α and β genes, utilizing the same recombinases and recognition signals as the other antigen receptor loci. Since the δ locus lies between the V_α and C_α genes, functional rearrangements of the α locus will delete the δ locus. Three different groups of V genes can be defined in this locus, based on which J segments they join to. One group only joins to J_δ segments, and a second group joins only to J_α segments. The molecular basis for these exclusive α or δ specific rearrangements is not understood. A third group of V genes, however, can pair with either J_δ or J_α segments. Thus, there are some V genes found in both $\alpha\beta$ and $\gamma\delta$ TCRs.

The small number of γ and δ V gene segments suggests a limited amount of combinatorial diversity among $\gamma\delta$ receptors. The limitations are even greater because of the selective use of certain V_γ segments during different stages of life (see below). There is, however, an enormous potential diversity of $\gamma\delta$ receptors as a result of variations in junctional sequences, especially in the δ chain. This potential junctional diversity is largely due to the unique feature that either one or both D_δ segments in tandem can be used within a single rearranged δ gene. Because imprecise joining of V, D, and J segments and N-region diversification also occur in rearranging δ and γ genes, there are theoretically more possible $\gamma\delta$ molecules than $\alpha\beta$ or Ig molecules (Table 8–1).

In the mouse, there are subsets of $\gamma\delta$ T cells that are distinguished both by their anatomic location and by the V_γ or V_δ gene segments they utilize (see Chapter 7). Two of the earliest $\gamma\delta$ T cell subsets to appear in mouse fetuses exhibit no TCR diversity, i.e., all their TCRs are identical (but of unknown specificity). For example, one of these $\gamma\delta$ T cell subsets populates mouse skin, and all the cells in this subset utilize the same rearranged V, J, and C segments, namely $V_\gamma 5J_\gamma 2C_\gamma 1$ and $V_\delta 1D_\delta 2J_\delta 1C_\delta$. In addition to these populations with identical $\gamma\delta$ TCRs, there is a limited use of other V_γ and V_δ genes in other human and mouse $\gamma\delta$ T cells, but these populations do incorporate different J and D segments and exhibit greater junctional diversity.

Transcription of rearranged γ and δ genes is apparently controlled by locus-specific enhancers, similar to those described for α and β loci. A γ chain enhancer has been identified 3' to the $C_\gamma 1$ gene segment, and a δ chain enhancer is located between $J_\delta 3$ and C_δ of the human locus. These enhancers are active only in T cells. A γ silencer analogous to the α silencer mentioned above has been identified 3' to the $C_\gamma 1$ gene segment that is likely to be partly responsible for keeping γ gene expression turned off in $\alpha\beta$-expressing T cells. This is especially pertinent since up to one third of $\alpha\beta$ T cells have undergone potentially functional γ gene rearrangements.

ONTOGENY OF T CELL RECEPTOR AND ACCESSORY MOLECULE EXPRESSION

The rearrangement and expression of TCR genes during intrathymic maturation are the necessary first steps in the development of the T cell repertoire. TCR gene expression occurs coordinately with the expression of other proteins, including CD3, CD4, and CD8, which are important for the selection of MHC-restricted helper T cells and CTLs. Subpopulations of thymocytes may be identified based on the expression of surface molecules, mainly TCR, CD4, and CD8, and these remain the most informative markers for stages of T cell maturation. The anatomic locations, sizes, and functional properties of these subpopulations—and changes induced in them by experimental manipulations—provide important insights into the mechanisms of thymic selection. We next discuss the ontogeny of T cell surface molecule expression and the characteristics of the best-defined thymocyte subsets.

Ontogeny of T Cell Receptor Expression

Most studies of T cell ontogeny have relied on fetal murine thymuses, in which distinct populations of developing T cells can be identified. The events that occur in these fetal organs are similar to what has been found in adult murine, fetal human, and adult human thymuses. As described above, T cell precursors are first detected in the fetal thymus on the 11th day of gestation in mice, and these cells do not express TCR complexes. Organ culture of embryonic thymuses, in which there is no ongoing influx of bone marrow precursors, has demonstrated that these CD3$^-$ cells are the precursors to all more mature forms. Surface molecules that are expressed on this immature population of thymocytes prior to or shortly after their entry into the thymus include CD44 (PgP-1), Thy-1 (in mice), and the CD1 class I MHC–like molecules. The functions of these molecules are not known; CD44 may play a role in the migration of T cell precursors to the thymus.

In mouse thymocytes, TCR genes are in the germline configuration until day 13 or 14 of fetal life (corresponding to about 8 to 9 weeks' gestation in humans). The first TCR gene rearrangements are detected at this time and involve the γ and δ genes (Figs. 8–5 and

8–6). Full-length mRNA transcripts of the γ and δ genes are detectable by day 14, and surface expression of a CD3-associated $\gamma\delta$ heterodimeric protein occurs by day 14 or 15. The genes encoding the CD3 polypeptides are first transcribed concomitantly with the $\gamma\delta$ genes and are expressed on the surface of thymocytes in association with $\gamma\delta$ heterodimers. *Thus, the $\gamma\delta$ receptor is the first TCR to be expressed during T cell development.*

Although nonfunctional DJ rearrangements at the β chain locus begin simultaneously with γ and δ chain rearrangements on day 13 or 14, functional β chain VDJ rearrangements and full-length 1.3 kb transcripts are first detectable on day 16. The α chain genes are the last to rearrange and to generate functional mRNA, on day 17 of fetal life. Surface expression of CD3-associated $\alpha\beta$ heterodimers is first detected on day 17, about 2 days after $\gamma\delta$ expression. Expression of $\alpha\beta$ receptors rapidly overtakes expression of $\gamma\delta$ receptors, so that by birth most TCR : CD3–expressing thymocytes have $\alpha\beta$ receptors. This is consistent with the fact that more than 90 per cent of mature peripheral T cells express only the $\alpha\beta$ form of antigen receptors.

There is strong evidence that $\gamma\delta$- and $\alpha\beta$-expressing thymocytes are separate lineages with a common precursor. Southern blot analysis of mature $\alpha\beta$-expressing T cells often show out-of-frame rearrangements of γ genes that are incapable of being transcribed, indicating that these cells could never have expressed $\gamma\delta$ receptors. The δ chain gene segments are located between the V_α and J_α gene segments (see Figs. 8–3 and 8–4), and they are deleted in a circle of DNA when the α chain gene rearranges. Analysis of these deleted DNA circles from murine thymuses shows that the δ chain gene is in the germline configuration in many cells that have rearranged their α chain genes. This finding also indicates that $\alpha\beta$-expressing T cells have never expressed $\gamma\delta$ receptors and that the two types of antigen receptors are produced by two distinct lineages of T cells. Consistent with this is the observation that mice expressing full-length rearranged γ and δ transgenes display normal $\alpha\beta$ T cell development, implying that rearranged γ or δ genes do not cause allelic exclusion of α or β genes. In addition, β gene knockout mice develop normal numbers of $\gamma\delta$ T cells, and δ gene knockout mice develop normal numbers of $\alpha\beta$ T cells. Interestingly, $\gamma\delta$ transgenic mice in which the γ silencer of the transgene has been deleted do not develop $\alpha\beta$ T cells, suggesting that at some early point in T cell development, silencing of γ transcription is required in order for α and β gene expression to proceed. A hypothetical scheme of these lineage relationships is shown in Figure 8–5.

This temporal pattern of early $\gamma\delta$ gene expression followed by $\alpha\beta$ expression is seen in chickens, mice, and humans. In human fetal thymuses, $\gamma\delta$ receptor expression begins at about 9 weeks of gestation, followed by TCR $\alpha\beta$ expression at 10 weeks. This evolutionary conservation of the sequence of receptor expression suggests that the presence of thymocytes expressing $\gamma\delta$ receptors prior to $\alpha\beta$-expressing cells may play a role in the normal development of T cells. We can only

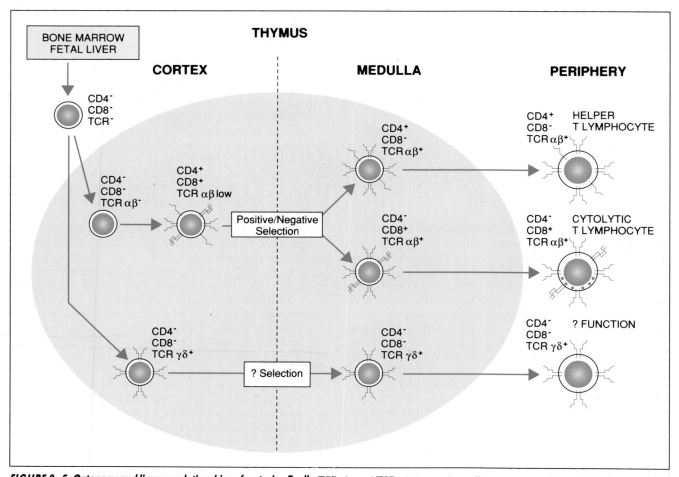

FIGURE 8–5. Ontogeny and lineage relationships of maturing T cells. *TCRγδ- and TCRαβ-expressing cells are separate lineages that develop from a common precursor. In the αβ lineage, the majority of thymocytes express both CD4 and CD8. TCR expression commences in this double-positive stage, beginning with low numbers of receptors on each cell and increasing as maturation proceeds. Single-positive, i.e., CD4+ or CD8+ TCRαβ-expressing mature cells are selected from this population. Some γδ cells express CD4 or CD8.*

speculate on that role, since the functions of mature γδ-bearing T cells and the nature of the ligand that the γδ receptor binds are as yet largely unknown.

The TCR gene rearrangements described above take place in a rapidly dividing population of cells. A single primitive T cell precursor that enters the thymus can generate multiple cells, each with a unique TCR conferring a distinct antigen-binding specificity. This has been demonstrated by an experiment in which a single precursor cell with unrearranged TCR genes was introduced into a thymus previously depleted of thymocytes. The progeny of this cell showed multiple, different β chain rearrangements after 12 days. As discussed in the previous section, N-region diversification significantly contributes to the diversity of TCR and is most likely catalyzed by the enzyme TdT. It is interesting to note that in murine fetal thymuses TdT is not expressed until after the earliest rearranged δ chain genes have already been transcribed; as a result, the first δ chains expressed show far less diversity than later ones. TdT activity was used as a marker of lymphocyte lineage in phenotypically immature cells, such as certain leukemias, long before the significance of this

enzyme in the generation of receptor diversity was understood.

Ontogeny of CD4 and CD8 Expression

CD4 and CD8 molecules are commonly used as markers to categorize subsets of thymocytes and to define the sequence of thymocyte maturation. Furthermore, recent experiments indicate that the expression of these molecules may be important in the selection processes that shape the T cell repertoire. Thymocytes can be divided into four main groups on the basis of CD4 and CD8 expression (Fig. 8–7). These groups include (1) CD4⁻CD8⁻ "double-negative" cells; (2) CD4⁺CD8⁺ "double-positive" cells; and (3 and 4) CD4⁺CD8⁻ or CD4⁻CD8⁺ "single-positive" cells.

In addition, several other surface molecules, including CD1, CD2, CD5, Thy1, peanut agglutinin receptor, and CD44, are used to further subdivide populations of thymocytes. The significance of these smaller

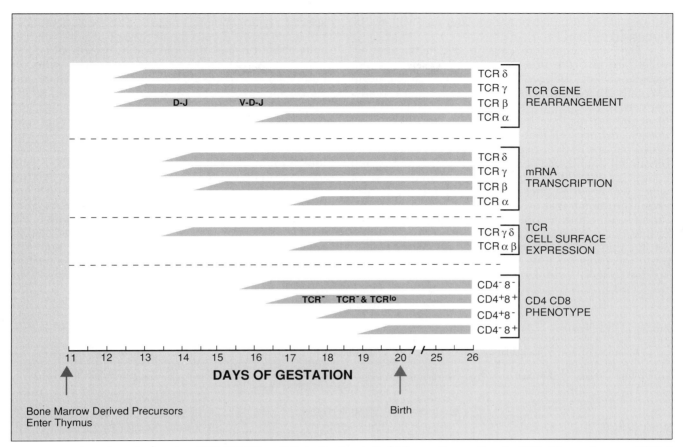

FIGURE 8–6. Chronology of expression of TCR, CD4, CD8, and effector functions in the fetal mouse thymus. *Note that TCRαβ heterodimers and TCRγδ heterodimers are expressed on different cells. (Modified with permission from Fowlkes, B. J., and D. M. Pardoll. Molecular events in T cell development. Advances in Immunology 44:207–264, 1989. Courtesy of Academic Press, Orlando, FL.)*

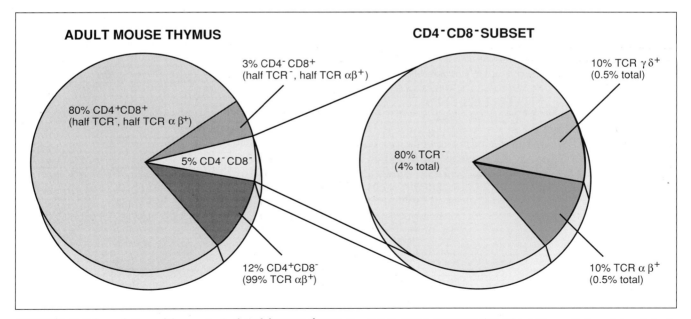

FIGURE 8–7. Subpopulations of thymocytes in the adult mouse thymus. *T cell maturation continues throughout life, so that even in adults the thymus contains different populations of thymocytes, which represent different stages in T cell development identified in the fetal thymus. (Modified with permission from Fowlkes, B. J., and D. M. Pardoll. Molecular events in T cell development. Advances in Immunology 44:207–264, 1989. Courtesy of Academic Press, Orlando, FL.)*

subsets is not completely known, and they will not be discussed further.

The most immature cells in the thymic cortex, which are also the precursors of all T cells, do not express CD4 or CD8 (see Fig. 8–5). These double-negative cells are a heterogeneous group making up about 5 per cent of the total thymocytes in an adult (Fig. 8–7). Most (80 per cent) of these cells are rapidly dividing cortical thymocytes that are actively rearranging TCR genes but are not yet expressing TCR complexes. The remaining double-negative cells are more mature and consist mainly of $\gamma\delta$-positive thymocytes (most of which will never express CD4 or CD8). Little is known about the stimuli that drive the proliferation and maturation of immature double-negative thymocytes. Many of these cells have been shown to express transcripts for IL-2 and IL-4. In addition, double-negative cells express receptors for IL-2 and proliferate *in vitro* in response to IL-7, a cytokine first identified as a B cell–

specific lymphopoietic factor. Therefore, cytokines produced by the T cells themselves or by non-lymphoid cells in the thymus may function as growth and differentiation factors for these immature thymocytes. To date, neither cytokine gene knockout mice nor transgenic cytokine–over-expressing mouse strains have revealed a critical role for any single factor, suggesting that these cytokines may have redundant roles in T cell development.

Many double-negative thymocytes eventually mature into TCR $\alpha\beta$-expressing, MHC-restricted T cells that express either CD4 or CD8, but not both. During this maturation pathway, the double-negative cells first go through a transient stage when low levels of either CD8 or CD4 alone are expressed (at gestation day 16–17 in the mouse), and then they become double-positive cells (at day 17–18), which express both CD4 and CD8 simultaneously (see Fig. 8–5). Double-positive cells constitute up to 80 per cent of the cells in an adult

TABLE 8–2. Genetic Approaches to the Study of T Cell Development in the Thymus

Molecule	Genetic Manipulation	Phenotypes	Mechanisms
Class II MHC α chain	Knockout	No surface class II MHC expression CD4$^+$CD8$^+$ thymocytes present; CD4$^+$CD8$^-$ thymocytes reduced Few mature CD4$^+$ T cells in periphery	Lack of positive selection of CD4$^+$ thymocytes
β_2 microglobulin	Knockout	No surface class I MHC expression CD4$^+$CD8$^+$ thymocytes present; CD4$^-$CD8$^+$ thymocytes reduced Few mature CD8$^+$ T cells in periphery	Lack of positive selection of CD8$^+$ thymocytes
CD4	Knockout	No surface CD4 expression No CD4$^-$CD8$^-$ TCR$^+$ thymocytes Few class II–restricted T cells in periphery	Lack of positive selection of class II–restricted thymocytes
CD8	Knockout	No surface CD8 expression No CD4$^-$CD8$^-$ TCR$^+$ thymocytes Few class I–restricted T cells in periphery	Lack of positive selection of class I–restricted thymocytes
RAG-2	Knockout	No $\alpha\beta$ TCR expression No CD4$^+$CD8$^+$ thymocytes No T cells in periphery	Lack of positive selection of any thymocyte Lack of β chain signaling for early maturation to CD4$^+$CD8$^+$ stage
TCR β chain	Knockout	No $\alpha\beta$ TCR expression No CD4$^+$CD8$^+$ thymocytes No $\alpha\beta$ T cells in periphery	Lack of positive selection of any thymocyte Lack of β chain signaling for early maturation to CD4$^+$CD8$^+$ stage
TCR α chain	Knockout	No $\alpha\beta$ TCR expression CD4$^+$CD8$^+$ thymocytes present No CD4$^+$CD8$^-$ or CD4$^-$CD8$^+$ thymocytes No $\alpha\beta$ T cells in periphery	Lack of positive selection of any thymocyte β chain signaling for early maturation to CD4$^+$CD8$^+$ stage
RAG-2/TCR β chain	*RAG-2* knockout TCR β transgene	No $\alpha\beta$ TCR expression CD4$^+$CD8$^+$ thymocytes present No CD4$^+$CD8$^-$ or CD4$^-$CD8$^+$ thymocytes No $\alpha\beta$ T cells in periphery	No endogenous recombinase activity, therefore no α chain expression Transgenic β chain signaling for early maturation to CD4$^+$CD8$^+$ stage
TAP-1	Knockout	No cellular TAP expression Very few class I MHC molecules expressed CD4$^+$CD8$^+$ thymocytes present Few CD4$^-$CD8$^+$ thymocytes Few CD8$^+$ T cells in periphery	No peptides delivered to ER for class I MHC assembly Lack of positive selection of class I–restricted thymocytes
Lck	Knockout	No cellular Lck expression Very few thymocytes (reduced CD4$^-$CD8$^-$ and CD4$^+$CD8$^+$ cells)	Defect in intracellular signaling required for early thymocyte growth and differentiation
$\alpha\beta$ TCR specific for peptide X plus MHC Y	Transgenes	Varies depending on mouse strain and presence or absence of antigen	See text

mouse thymus (Fig. 8–7). Rearrangement and expression of the TCR β chain genes occur during the double-negative stage. Transgenic and knockout mice have provided valuable information about these processes of T cell maturation and selection in the thymus (Table 8–2). For example, analysis of β chain and *RAG-2* gene knockout mice indicates that β (but not α) chain expression is required for maturation of double-negative cells to double-positive cells. It is possible that intracellular β chain proteins may serve a signaling function for maturation of the T cells, similar to the role of μ and surrogate light chains in pre–B cells (see Chapter 4). Furthermore, lck knockout mice show a profound block in the maturation of double-negative to double-positive thymocytes. Therefore, lck expression is likely to be required in this developmental step. Small numbers of double-negative cells remain CD4$^-$CD8$^-$, and this population includes many cells that will go on to express $\gamma\delta$ TCRs.

The rearrangement of the TCR α chain genes, and the expression of TCR $\alpha\beta$ heterodimers, occur in the double-positive population as these cells migrate from the cortex to medulla (see Fig. 8–5). By day 17 or 18 of gestation, the mouse thymus contains CD4$^+$CD8$^+$ cells that also express low levels of TCR complexes. In the adult thymus, about half the double-positive cells are TCR $\alpha\beta$: CD3–positive and half are TCR $\alpha\beta$: CD3–negative (see Fig. 8–7). The great majority of double-positive cells die *in vivo*, because selection processes act at this stage of maturation. As we will discuss in detail later, thymocytes need to be positively selected by TCR engagement with peptide-MHC complexes in order to escape programmed death. One reason for a lack of positive selection is unproductive TCR gene rearrangements that occur frequently, leading to failure to express TCR molecules, and therefore programmed cell death.

The CD4$^+$CD8$^+$ cells give rise to mature CD4$^+$ and CD8$^+$ (single-positive) peripheral T cells, which also express high levels of TCR complexes (see Fig. 8–5). This has been established by a variety of experiments. For instance, if neonatal mice are injected with anti-CD4 antibody, the number of both CD4$^+$ and CD8$^+$ cells in the periphery are reduced. This is interpreted to indicate that the antibody bound to and induced the complement-dependent lysis of double-positive thymocytes and inhibited the maturation of all single-positive cells. CD4$^+$CD8$^-$TCR $\alpha\beta$–expressing thymocytes are first detected at day 18 of gestation in mice and make up about 12 per cent of adult thymocytes (see Fig. 8–7). These cells display functional helper activity in *in vitro* assays and migrate to the circulation and peripheral lymphoid tissues to constitute the mature, class II MHC–restricted helper T cell subset. CD4$^-$CD8$^+$TCR $\alpha\beta$–expressing cells appear by day 19 of gestation and make up about 3 per cent of thymocytes in the adult. They can develop cytolytic activity *in vitro* and migrate out of the thymus to become mature, class I MHC–restricted CTLs in the periphery. We do not know the stimuli that induce a particular CD4$^+$CD8$^+$ cell to selectively express either CD4 or CD8 and to simultaneously acquire the functional capabilities of a helper or cyto-

lytic cell, respectively. It is clear that the specificity of the TCR on a given thymocyte determines if CD4 or CD8 will ultimately be expressed. Thus, thymocytes whose TCRs are specific for class I MHC and peptide will ultimately express only CD8, whereas thymocytes whose TCRs are class II MHC–restricted will mature into cells expressing only CD4. The possible mechanisms underlying this process will be discussed later in this chapter.

This sequence of T cell maturation—from CD4$^-$CD8$^-$TCR$^-$ to CD4$^+$CD8$^+$TCR$^-$, to CD4$^+$CD8$^+$TCR$^+$, and finally to CD4$^+$CD8$^-$TCR$^+$ or CD4$^-$CD8$^+$TCR$^+$ cells—has been most clearly established in mice. It is difficult to examine the maturation pathway of T cells during fetal life in humans because of many obvious limitations. The information that is available suggests that the same sequence of maturation events occurs in humans as in mice. It is clear that in both mice and humans, TCR $\alpha\beta$ receptors are first expressed on double-positive cortical thymocytes. This is when the selection processes that determine the specificities of the mature T cell repertoire begin to occur.

THYMIC SELECTION PROCESSES LEADING TO T CELL MHC RESTRICTION AND SELF-TOLERANCE

The next important event in intrathymic T cell maturation, after expression of the TCR, CD4, and CD8 molecules, is the selection of cells that will make up the repertoire of mature T cells in the periphery. Selection processes are responsible for the survival of T cells that express only "useful" TCRs, i.e., TCRs that recognize foreign antigens in association with self MHC molecules. Although the cellular and biochemical mechanisms of selection are not well understood, the current model of this process has the following general features (see Fig. 8–1).

1. Before selection can begin, TCRs must be expressed on the developing thymocytes. This is because thymocytes are selected to survive or to be eliminated on the basis of their specificities, determined by the binding of the TCRs to MHC molecules and peptide antigens expressed in the thymus.

2. Because of the random nature of the molecular events in TCR gene expression, all possible antigen and MHC specificities are represented in the TCR-expressing, preselected, immature thymocyte population.

3. **Positive selection** is the process in which thymocytes whose TCRs bind self MHC molecules complexed with self or foreign peptides are permitted to survive and all those that have no affinity for self MHC die. This step eliminates all non–self MHC–restricted T cells, which would be incapable of recognizing antigen in the periphery because the APCs obviously only express self MHC molecules. Positive selection leaves both useful foreign antigen–specific, self MHC–restricted T cells and potentially harmful self antigen–specific, self MHC–restricted T cells.

4. During **negative selection,** clones of thymocytes whose TCRs bind with high affinity to self peptide antigens in association with self MHC molecules are eliminated **(clonal deletion)** or inactivated **(clonal anergy).** After this step, the only functional thymocytes that are left are those whose TCRs bind self MHC molecules associated with non-self peptides, so that mature T cells are self MHC–restricted and self-tolerant. It is commonly assumed that positive selection precedes negative selection, but there is no clear evidence to prove this.

Positive Selection Processes in the Thymus: Development of the Self MHC–Restricted T Cell Repertoire

Positive selection is the process that results in mature peripheral T lymphocytes expressing only self MHC–restricted TCRs. Once a thymocyte expresses a T cell receptor, it cannot change its specificity. Therefore, *positive selection works by promoting the selective survival and expansion of thymocytes with self MHC–restricted TCRs and permitting thymocytes whose TCRs are not self MHC–restricted to die.* In this portion of the chapter, we will discuss the current understanding of the process of positive selection.

THE ROLES OF MHC MOLECULES, CD4, AND CD8 IN POSITIVE SELECTION

Well before T cell specificity for MHC-peptide complexes was understood, experiments had shown that T cells are self MHC–restricted because they encounter self MHC molecules during maturation. Bone marrow chimeras were used to first demonstrate that *MHC genes of the host animal in which T cells develop determine the MHC restriction pattern of the mature T cells.* In these experiments, chimeras were created by transferring the bone marrow–derived hematopoietic stem cells from a mouse with one MHC haplotype into a lethally irradiated mouse of a partially different MHC haplotype (Table 8–3.) By immunizing these mice and defining the MHC restriction of the CTLs and helper T cells, it was found that the T cells that matured in these chimeras recognized antigen only in association with MHC molecules of the host strain.

Further analysis showed that *the thymus is the critical host element for the development of the MHC restriction patterns of T cells.* This was accomplished by creating bone marrow plus thymic chimeras. These host animals were prepared by lethally irradiating adult mice of one MHC haplotype, removing their thymuses, and transplanting into them different combinations of bone marrow and thymuses from mice with other MHC haplotypes (Table 8–4). The transplanted thymuses were either irradiated or treated with cytotoxic drugs (such as deoxyguanosine) to kill all resident macrophages, dendritic cells, and lymphoid cells, leaving only the radioresistant **thymic epithelial cells.** Again, ma-

TABLE 8–3. Development of MHC Restriction in Bone Marrow Chimeric Mice

Marrow Donor Strain	Host	Specific Killing of Virus-Infected Targets From	
		Strain A	*Strain B*
(A × B)F1	(A × B)F1	+	+
(A × B)F1	A	+	−

Bone marrow chimeras are created as described in Figure 2–2. Strain A and B mice have different class I MHC alleles. The MHC restriction specificity of mature T cells in these mice is tested by assaying the ability of CTLs generated in response to viral infection to kill virus-infected target cells from different mouse strains *in vitro*. These experiments demonstrate that the host MHC type, and not the bone marrow donor type, determines the restriction specificity of the mature T cells.

Abbreviations: MHC, major histocompatibility complex; CTL, cytolytic T lymphocyte.

ture T cells developed in these mice, and their MHC restriction was examined after immunization and *in vitro* restimulation of T cells with antigen plus APCs. Antigen recognition by these T cells was always restricted by MHC gene products expressed on the transplanted thymic epithelial cells and not necessarily by MHC gene products expressed on extrathymic cells (Table 8–4).

TCR receptor transgenic mice have provided the clearest evidence that thymocytes are positively selected by recognition of self MHC molecules in the thymus. These mice are created by standard transgenic techniques (see Box 4–1, Chapter 4) using the functionally rearranged TCR α and β genes derived from a T cell clone of known antigen and MHC specificity (Fig. 8–8). It is relatively simple to study the selection and maturation of T cells in these transgenic mice, since virtually all developing T cells in these animals express the transgenically encoded TCR, and endogenous TCR gene rearrangements are blocked (by allelic exclusion). When the transgenic α and β TCR genes encode a TCR that recognizes a foreign peptide in association with a particular MHC molecule, the transgenic T cells will mature and populate peripheral lymphoid tissue only in mice expressing that MHC molecule. If the mouse is of another MHC haplotype and does not express the class I MHC molecule that the transgenic TCR recognizes, then very few transgenic TCR-expressing T cells mature. In the thymuses of these mice that cannot positively select T cells, there are normal numbers of CD4$^+$CD8$^+$ thymocytes but very few CD4$^+$ or CD8$^+$ single-positive cells. This result demonstrates that developing T cells must express TCRs that can bind self MHC molecules in order to survive. As we shall see later, the same experimental system has been used to study negative selection.

The requirement for thymocyte recognition of MHC molecules in the process of positive selection can be demonstrated using strains of mice that are deficient in either class I or class II MHC expression (see Table 8–2). These mouse strains are created using homologous recombination-targeted disruption of the appropriate genes (see Box 4–1, Chapter 4). Mice that lack

TABLE 8–4. Development of MHC Restriction Patterns in Bone Marrow Plus Thymic Chimeras

	Chimera			Stimulation of Mature T Cells	
Host	*Bone Marrow Donor*	*Thymus Donor*	*Antigen*	*Strain of APC*	*Response*
A	(A × B)F1	A	+	A	+
A	(A × B)F1	A	+	B	−
A	(A × B)F1	A	−	A	−
A	(A × B)F1	B	+	B	+
A	(A × B)F1	B	+	A	−
A	(A × B)F1	B	−	B	−

In the chimeric mice, the mature T cells that develop respond to foreign antigen in association with the MHC allele expressed on the thymic epithelial cells.

Abbreviations: APC, antigen-presenting cell; MHC, major histocompatibility complex.

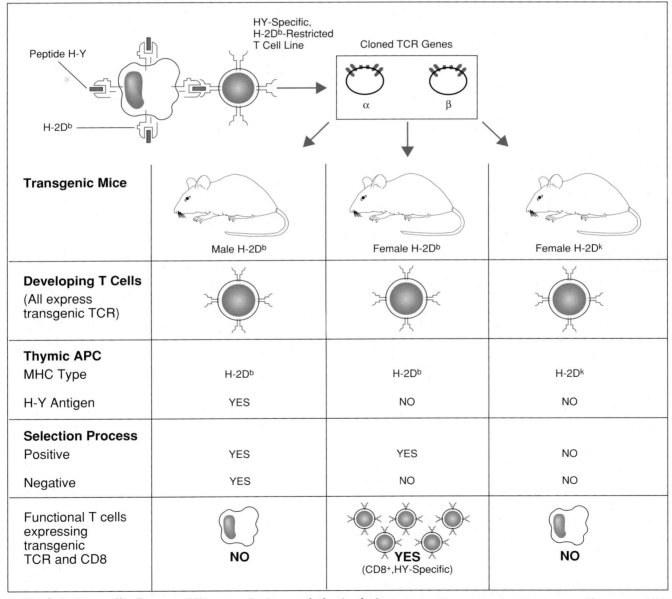

FIGURE 8–8. The use of T cell receptor (TCR) transgenic mice to study thymic selection processes. *The transgenic mice express a D^b-associated H-Y (male-specific) antigen, which is, in effect, a foreign antigen for a female mouse. Functional T cells expressing the transgene mature in female mice expressing the D^b allele, but not in H-Y^+ male mice (because of negative selection as a result of self antigen recognition), nor in female mice not expressing D^b (because of lack of positive selection of the D^b-restricted TCR-expressing cells).*

class I MHC expression because of disruption of the β_2 microglobulin gene do not develop mature CD8$^+$ T cells, but do develop CD4$^+$ T cells. Conversely, class II MHC–deficient mice do not develop CD4$^+$ T cells, but do develop CD8$^+$ cells. Since class I MHC–restricted T cells are CD8$^+$ and class II MHC–restricted T cells are CD4$^+$, the findings in these MHC gene knockout mice are entirely consistent with a need for TCR (and co-receptor) recognition of MHC molecules in positive selection.

Cell surface MHC molecules generally contain peptides within their binding clefts, and therefore these peptides are likely to play a role in the TCR recognition events that lead to positive selection of thymocytes. Analysis of the maturation of CD8$^+$ T cells in mice with class I MHC mutations provided the first evidence that peptides do indeed play a role in determining which T cells are positively selected. For example, mutations in the floor of K^b class I MHC–binding clefts, which are predicted to alter peptide binding significantly, reduce positive selection of T cells restricted by the wild type K^b MHC molecules. More recently, experiments with mice deficient in the TAP-1 peptide transporter protein have also demonstrated a role for peptides in determining which and how many thymocytes are positively selected. As discussed in Chapters 5 and 6, the TAP-1 and TAP-2 gene products are both required for delivery of cytosolic peptides into the ER for assembly with class I MHC proteins. Mice made deficient in the TAP-1 protein by gene disruption have significantly reduced levels of surface class I MHC molecules, consistent with the role of endogenous peptides in assembly and surface expression of class I MHC. As expected, maturation of CD8$^+$ cells is defective in these animals. The few MHC molecules which do get out to the surface of cells in these mice are unstable heavy (α) chain monomers that can be stabilized by addition of exogenous peptides and β_2 microglobulin. Thus, TAP-1– or TAP-2– deficient mice provide an experimental system in which the peptides bound to surface class I MHC molecules can be manipulated without contributions from endogenously synthesized proteins. When thymus organ cultures from TAP-1–deficient mice are supplemented with 9 amino acid long peptides and β_2 microglobulin, both class I MHC expression and CD8$^+$ T cell development increase, consistent with previous demonstrations of the need for class I MHC molecules in positive selection of CD8$^+$ T cells. The key finding in this experiment is that some mixtures of peptides are particularly good at inducing positive selection, whereas others are not, and these differences do not correlate with the relative abilities of the different peptide mixtures to induce stable cell surface class I MHC expression. Thus, the nature of the peptide itself contributes to positive selection, presumably because of direct recognition by T cells. In fact, in this system, complex mixtures of peptides extracted from thymuses are the most effective inducers of positive selection. These experiments suggest that thymocyte recognition of both self MHC molecules and some subset of self peptides is responsible for positive selection.

These experiments have led to a theory on how positive selection proceeds. According to this theory, thymic epithelial cells may present to thymocytes a special set of self peptides not ubiquitously presented by other APCs. The recognition of these peptides in association with self MHC molecules would rescue thymocytes from programmed death (which will be discussed below). The nature of these peptides would permit them to be recognized by many different clones of thymocytes, but each positively selected clone would have a unique specificity for a foreign peptide with self MHC. There is, in fact, some experimental evidence that thymic epithelial cells do generate peptide-MHC complexes not found on other APC populations, but the role of these complexes in positive selection is not yet established.

CD4 and CD8 molecules are also intimately involved in thymic selection processes. The importance of CD4 and CD8 in positive selection has been unequivocally demonstrated by experiments with mice in which CD4–class II MHC interactions or CD8–class I MHC interactions have been eliminated. Blockade of CD8 or CD4 *in vivo* by noncytotoxic antibodies that do not deplete thymuses of double-positive cells results in a lack of development of CD8 or CD4 single-positive cells, respectively. Furthermore, in CD4 or CD8 gene knockout mice, there is no mature CD4$^-$CD8$^-$TCR–expressing population, implying that cells that normally would have matured from double-positive into either CD4$^+$ or CD8$^+$ single-positive T lymphocytes do not get positively selected in the absence of CD4 or CD8. It is not clear how CD4 and CD8 molecules promote positive selection, but it is likely that they function as coreceptors with TCRs, providing both adhesive interactions with MHC molecules and signaling functions. This would be analogous to the roles of CD4 and CD8 in the activation of mature T cells (see Chapter 7).

As we alluded to earlier, another important feature of positive selection is that during the transition from double-positive to single-positive thymocytes, cells with class I–restricted TCRs become CD8$^+$, and cells with class II–restricted TCRs become CD4$^+$. One possible way this may occur involves a **stochastic** mechanism by which there is a random loss of expression of either CD4 or CD8 in developing thymocytes with no relation to the specificity of the TCR. If, by chance, any developing T cell has the right combination of CD4 preservation with a class II MHC–restricted TCR, or CD8 with a class I–restricted TCR, then that cell will be effectively stimulated by MHC expressing thymic epithelium, and therefore will be positively selected. If the wrong combination exists, the cell will not be effectively stimulated and it will die by default, just like thymocytes with TCRs that have no affinity for any self MHC–peptide complex. An alternative model for the appropriate pairing of CD4 and CD8 with class I– and class II–restricted thymocytes is called the **instructive model.** It proposes that when the TCR and CD4 or CD8 coreceptor on a double-positive thymocyte bind to a peptide-MHC complex on a thymic epithelial cell, signals are generated that instruct the thymocyte and its progeny to turn off expression of the "wrong" accessory molecule. A variety of transgenic and knockout mouse strains have been used to address which model of subset differentiation is accurate, and to date the stochastic model appears more likely to be correct.

MECHANISMS OF POSITIVE SELECTION IN THE THYMUS

It is clear that a large proportion of $CD4^+CD8^+$ thymocytes in the thymic cortex undergo a process of biologically programmed death. It is hypothesized that the cellular basis of positive selection may be the rescue of a thymocyte from programmed death by signals generated after TCR binding to peptide-MHC complexes. Thus, thymocytes whose TCRs have no affinity for self MHC with any bound peptide will die by default, and the survivors will have TCRs with some affinity for self MHC. It is likely that the signals generated by the TCR complex that rescue a thymocyte from death during positive selection are similar to those involved in T cell activation in mature T cells, but it is not clear which signals may be critical. If a special set of self peptides expressed by thymic epithelial cells mediates positive selection, as described above, these peptides would have to stimulate the TCR to generate different signals than those stimulated by other peptides. There is, in fact, evidence that different peptides presented by the same MHC molecule can generate qualitatively distinct responses in identical mature T cells. The relevance of these findings to positive selection of immature thymocytes is not yet known.

Negative Selection Processes in the Thymus: Development of Self-Tolerance

The importance of self-tolerance to the health of all individuals has been mentioned previously, and the development of autoimmunity as a result of the breakdown of self-tolerance will be described in Chapter 19. Individuals may be tolerant to self antigens because they lack B and/or T lymphocytes specific for these antigens, or because such lymphocytes are present but cannot respond to self antigens. It is now clear that *tolerance to self proteins is largely because of T cell tolerance, and a principal mechanism for inducing T cell tolerance is the deletion of self-reactive clones of T cells during their maturation in the thymus.* This process, also called **negative selection,** is discussed here because it is closely related to positive selection of T cells.

THE PHENOMENON OF NEGATIVE SELECTION IN THE THYMUS

The possibility that self-reactive clones of T cells are deleted in the thymus was suggested many years ago, when the role of the thymus in the development of mature T cells was first appreciated. In addition to the lack of positive selection, much of the cell death that occurs in the thymic cortex is postulated to be due to deletion of self-reactive clones. Formal proof for clonal deletion of T cells in the thymus has come from two recently developed experimental approaches, both of which allow investigators to observe the effects of self antigen recognition by a large number of developing T cells in the thymus.

One approach that suggests that T cell tolerance results from intrathymic clonal deletion of self-reactive clones employs TCR transgenic mice mentioned above. In these studies, if the TCR transgenic mouse expresses the protein and MHC molecule that the transgenic TCR recognizes, there is a block in the development of mature T cells expressing this TCR. For example, in one such study, transgenic mice were made that expressed a class I MHC–restricted transgenic TCR specific for the sex associated H-Y molecule; H-Y is a self antigen abundantly expressed on many cell types in male mice, but not in female mice (Fig. 8–8). Female mice with this transgenic TCR had normal numbers of T cells in the periphery and normal numbers of thymocytes in the thymic medulla. In contrast, male transgenic mice had few mature peripheral T cells, and few TCR-expressing, single-positive thymocytes in the medulla. There was an apparent block of T cell maturation after the cortical double-positive stage, presumably because all the maturing transgenic TCRs recognized the self H-Y antigen on thymic epithelial cells, macrophages, or dendritic cells and were deleted before they could mature into single-positive cells. Clonal deletion of thymocytes has also been demonstrated by culturing intact fetal thymuses from TCR transgenic mice *in vitro* and adding the peptide for which the TCR is specific. This approach has shown that the concentration of antigens needed to cause elimination of self-reactive clones is similar or even lower than concentrations needed to stimulate mature T cells of the same specificity.

Another approach for analyzing negative selection is based on the observation that TCRs that utilize certain V_β genes specifically bind particular MHC-protein complexes, irrespective of which D_β and J_β gene segments are used, or which α chains are present. The proteins that bind to all TCRs that utilize a particular V_β gene segment, regardless of the nature of the other parts of the antigen receptor, have been called "super-antigens" and are discussed in Chapter 16. Some mouse super-antigens are proteins encoded by endogenous retroviruses. Super-antigens are presented to T cells by class II MHC molecules, and T cell responses to super-antigen–MHC complexes are apparently similar to responses to peptide-MHC complexes. Because super-antigens stimulate large numbers of cells, their effects on T cell development may be analyzed to study negative selection. For example, in mice, the use of the V_β17a gene segment imparts a TCR with specificity for a super-antigen that binds exclusively to an I-E class II MHC molecule. In strains of mice that express I-E class II MHC molecules, there are virtually no V_β17a-expressing T cells in the peripheral lymphoid organs, or in the thymic medulla, but there are $V_\beta17a$-expressing thymocytes in the cortex. In contrast, strains of mice that do not express I-E molecules, because of a genetic defect in the class II MHC locus, have readily detectable $V_\beta17a$-expressing T cells in the periphery (Table 8–5). This suggests that as T cells mature in the thymus of an I-E$^+$ mouse, all $V_\beta17a$-expressing thymocytes encounter the self super-antigen complexed with I-E molecules and are deleted. If they do not encounter this self antigen–I-E complex, as would be the case in the I-E–deficient mice, they may mature normally. It is not clear how $V_\beta17a$-expressing thymocytes are positively selected in I-E$^-$ mice, but it is possible that they may also be specific for complexes of foreign peptide bound to the other type of mouse class II MHC molecule, I-A.

The clonal deletion of self-reactive T cells presumably occurs when the TCR on a CD4$^+$CD8$^+$ thymocyte binds to a self antigen presented by another thymic cell. There is strong evidence that bone marrow–derived cells within the thymus, such as dendritic cells or macrophages, can present self antigens to and cause the deletion of self antigen–reactive T cell clones. The evidence that thymic epithelial cells can also mediate clonal deletion of self-reactive thymocytes is not as clear. As with positive selection, the CD4 and CD8 molecules likely play a role in negative selection because they promote effective interactions between the developing thymocytes and the "tolerizing" thymic APCs. For example, *in vivo* administration of anti-CD4 antibody to I-E–expressing mice blocks the elimination of $V_\beta17a$-expressing CD4$^+$CD8$^-$ thymocytes. Thus, the interaction of both CD4 and $V_\beta17a^+$ TCR with the I-E class II MHC molecule is necessary for deletion of the $V_\beta17a^+$-expressing cells.

Mechanisms of Negative Selection in the Thymus

The cellular basis of clonal deletion in the thymus is a particular form of programmed cell death called **apoptosis,** which is characterized by cell shrinkage, DNA fragmentation into nucleosomes, and nuclear frag-

mentation. When the DNA fragments from an apoptotic cell are separated by electrophoresis in a gel, and visualized by staining with ethidium bromide, they appear as a characteristic ladder of incrementally sized fragments reflecting cleavage of the DNA between nucleosomes. It is likely that a variety of enzymatic activities, including nucleases, mediate apoptotic cell death, and these activities are turned on by TCR-generated signals. For example, when intact antigen or specific peptide is administered to the thymus of TCR transgenic mice, many thymocytes undergo apoptosis. This process can be mimicked by anti-CD3 antibody treatment of immature thymocytes in tissue culture. Therefore, thymocyte apoptosis is sometimes called *activation-induced cell death.* (There is no evidence that the programmed cell death of thymocytes that occurs because of a lack of positive selection is apoptotic.) TCR $\alpha\beta$ heterodimers and the associated CD3 proteins appear not to be functionally coupled in immature thymocytes, since anti-$\alpha\beta$ antibodies induce increases in cytoplasmic calcium in mature T cells but not double-positive thymocytes, whereas anti-CD3 antibodies induce calcium fluxes in both thymocytes and mature T cells. This suggests that the qualitative signals generated by peptide-MHC binding to the TCR in an immature thymocyte may be distinctly different than those generated in a mature T cell, and these differences may be the basis for the differences in the outcome of antigen recognition in the two cell populations.

Unresolved Issues in Selection and Differentiation Processes in the Thymus

The phenomena of positive and negative selection discussed above raise several questions that are presently unresolved. One important question is how both positive and negative selection processes can occur if both are dependent on TCR binding of peptide-MHC complexes; i.e., a thymocyte can be rescued from pro-

TABLE 8–5.   Clonal Deletion of $V_\beta17a$-Positive T Cells in I-E–Expressing Mice

	Mouse Strain	I-E Expression	Peripheral T Cells Expressing TCRs Utilizing $V_\beta17a$ (Per Cent)
A.	SWR	None	14.2
	SJL	None	9.4
	SJA	None	8.5
B.	C57BR	Yes	0.1
	BALB/c	Yes	0
	AKR	Yes	0
	B10.TL	Yes	0

Mature T cells with $V_\beta17a$-containing TCRs are present in I-E$^-$(A) but not in I-E$^+$(B) inbred mouse strains, because these TCRs recognize an I-E–associated self antigen and are deleted in I-E$^+$ mice.

Abbreviations: TCR, T cell receptor; MHC, major histocompatibility complex.
Adapted from Kappler, J., N. Roehm, and P. Marrack. T cell tolerance by clonal elimination in the thymus. Cell 49:273, 1987. Copyright by Cell Press.

grammed death by recognition of peptide-MHC, but it can also be killed by apparently the same type of recognition event. Several theories have been proposed to explain this paradox. The first, called the **affinity model,** postulates that the affinity of the TCR for self MHC–peptide complexes determines the outcome of the recognition events, with low-affinity TCR binding leading to positive selection and high-affinity binding leading to negative selection. A TCR that binds to self peptide–MHC complexes with low affinity may bind to a foreign peptide–self MHC complex with high affinity. Therefore, positive selection of T cells that recognize self peptides plus self MHC weakly may result in mature T cells that recognize foreign peptides strongly and are activated by foreign antigens. This would be the basis for the creation of the self MHC–restricted, foreign antigen–specific T cell repertoire. Thymocytes whose TCRs have high affinity for self peptide–MHC complexes would be potentially harmful to the host, and are eliminated. This would ensure that the repertoire is self antigen–tolerant. This model implies that TCR-mediated signaling is different depending on the affinity of the TCR for peptide-MHC complexes. Studies of mice with transgenic class I–restricted TCRs and variable levels of expression of transgenic CD8 indicate that low CD8 levels on thymocytes correlate with positive selection and high levels correlate with negative selection. Since CD8 will contribute to the affinity of the T cell interaction with thymic APCs, these findings are consistent with the affinity model.

A second model of how both positive and negative selection can be operative highlights the importance of special peptides discussed previously, which may be differentially expressed on different thymic APCs. This **peptide model** postulates that when thymocytes recognize complexes of particular self peptides with MHC molecules on thymic epithelial cells, the thymocytes are saved from death, whereas recognition of ubiquitously expressed self peptide–MHC complexes on bone marrow–derived APCs in the thymus leads to clonal deletion. Many different clones of thymocytes would recognize and be positively selected by the limited number of peptide-MHC complexes uniquely expressed on the thymic epithelial cells. This would ensure the survival of thymocytes with TCRs that could potentially recognize complexes of foreign peptide and self MHC molecules, but such positively selected cells may include self peptide–reactive thymocytes as well. Those thymocytes that could recognize ubiquitously expressed self peptides would be eliminated, either before or after positive selection.

An obvious problem in this postulated peptide model of negative selection is that ubiquitous self proteins must be presented by negatively selecting thymic APCs while foreign antigens are not, otherwise the T cell repertoire would be devoid of useful foreign antigen–specific T cells as well as self-reactive T cells. It is possible that most self proteins are not tissue-specific and are present in thymic cells or thymic blood. Therefore, a majority of self proteins could be presented to thymocytes and lead to deletion of self-reactive clones. On the other hand, some T cells reactive with self anti-

gens not present in the thymus may mature and exit the thymus but may be rendered anergic to self antigens in the periphery (see Chapter 19). It is likely, also, that most foreign antigens are not continually present in the thymus, especially since the thymus lacks afferent lymphatics (see Chapter 11). Furthermore, even if foreign antigens do gain access to thymic APCs, their concentrations may be much lower than those of self proteins, and they may therefore not be presented frequently to the developing T cells. This would prevent negative selection of foreign antigen–specific T cells. Most immunologists favor the affinity model of thymic selection, but peptide-based selection may also occur.

The final stages in the maturation of T cells in the thymus, which occur after the selection processes, are also poorly understood. For example, we do not know what drives the differentiation of thymocytes into either helper T cells or CTLs, nor why these functional capabilities usually correlate with CD4 or CD8 expression, respectively. The mechanisms that promote the selective emigration of functionally mature T cells from the thymus into the blood are also not known.

SUMMARY

Stem cells committed to developing into T cells first arise in the bone marrow and migrate to the thymus during both fetal and adult life. The earliest T lineage immigrants to the thymus have unrearranged TCR genes and do not express CD4 or CD8 molecules. The developing T cells within the thymus, called thymocytes, initially populate the outer cortex, where they undergo population growth, rearrangement of TCR genes, and surface expression of CD3, TCR, CD4, and CD8 molecules. The TCR α and β polypeptides are encoded by functional genes that are created only in T cells by the somatic rearrangement of variable, diversity (β only), and joining gene segments, bringing them in the vicinity of C gene segments. Multiple combinatorial possibilities for the joining of the different gene segments, as well as several mechanisms that generate junctional diversity, result in the generation of a large repertoire of T cell specificities. Unlike Ig genes, there is no somatic mutation or affinity maturation in TCR genes. The functional genes encoding the TCR γ and δ polypeptides are also formed by somatic rearrangement of germline genes. The mechanisms of generation of TCR $\gamma\delta$ diversity are similar to those described for the $\alpha\beta$ receptor, except that there are fewer V genes in the γ and δ loci and significantly more potential junctional diversity. TCR $\gamma\delta$ receptors are the first receptors to be expressed on a small subset of cortical thymocytes, followed by the more abundant expression of TCR $\alpha\beta$ receptors on a distinct lineage of developing T cells. The TCR $\alpha\beta^+$,CD4$^+$CD8$^+$ cortical thymocytes interact with MHC-expressing cortical epithelial cells and bone marrow–derived, non-lymphoid cells and undergo selection processes that shape the T cell repertoire toward self MHC restriction and self-tolerance. Positive selection of self MHC–restricted T cells involves CD4$^+$CD8$^+$ thymocyte recognition of peptide-MHC complexes on thymic epithelial cells, leading to a rescue from programmed death. T cell tolerance is at least in part due to clonal deletion of self-reactive T cells during the TCR $\alpha\beta^+$, CD4$^+$CD8$^+$ stage of development. Clonal deletion involves apoptotic cell death of thymocytes that recognize self peptide–MHC complexes on thymic antigen-presenting cells. Most of the cortical thymocytes do not survive these selection processes. As the surviving TCR $\alpha\beta^+$ thymocytes mature, they move into the medulla and become either CD4$^+$CD8$^-$ or CD4$^-$CD8$^+$. Medullary thymocytes acquire helper or cytolytic functional capabilities and finally emigrate to peripheral lymphoid tissues, where they reside as self MHC–restricted, foreign antigen–responsive helper T cells and CTLs.

SELECTED READINGS

Adkins, B., C. Mueller, C. Y. Okada, R. Reichert, I. L. Weissman, and G. J. Spangrude. Early events in T-cell maturation. Annual Review of Immunology 5:325–365, 1987.

Ashton-Rickardt, P. G., L. V. Kaer, T. N. M. Schumacher, H. L. Ploegh, and S. Tonegawa. Peptide contributes to the specificity of positive selection of CD8$^+$ T cells in the thymus. Cell 73:1041–1049, 1993.

Blackman, M., J. Kappler, and P. Marrack. The role of the T cell receptor in positive and negative selection of developing T cells. Science 248:1335–1341, 1990.

Cohen, J. J., R. C. Duke, V. A. Fadok, and K. S. Sellins. Apoptosis and programmed cell death in immunity. Annual Review of Immunology 10:267–293, 1992.

Davis, M. M., and P. J. Bjorkman. T-cell antigen receptor genes and T-cell recognition. Nature 334:395–402, 1988.

Fink, P. J., and M. J. Bevan. H-2 antigens of the thymus determine lymphocyte specificity. Journal of Experimental Medicine 148:766–775, 1978.

Fowlkes, B. J., and D. M. Pardoll. Molecular and cellular events of T cell development. Advances in Immunology 44:207–264, 1989.

Kappler, J. W., N. Roehm, and P. Marrack. T cell tolerance by clonal elimination in the thymus. Cell 49:273–280, 1987.

Leider, J. M. Transcriptional regulation of T cell receptor genes. Annual Review of Immunology 11:539–570, 1993.

Moss, P. A. H., W. M. C. Rosenberg, and J. I. Bell. The human T cell receptor in health and disease. Annual Review of Immunology 10:71–96, 1992.

Ransdell, F., and B. J. Fowlkes. Clonal deletion versus clonal anergy: The role of the thymus in inducing self tolerance. Science 248:1342–1348, 1990.

Sprent, J., E.-K. Gao, and S. R. Webb. T cell reactivity to MHC molecules: immunity versus tolerance. Science 248:1357–1363, 1990.

Strominger, J. L. Developmental biology of T cell receptors. Science 244:943–950, 1989.

von Boehmer, H. Developmental biology of T cells in T cell–receptor transgenic mice. Annual Review of Immunology 8:531–556, 1990.

von Boehmer, H., and P. Kisielow. Self-nonself discrimination by T cells. Science 248:1369–1373, 1990.

B CELL ACTIVATION

AND ANTIBODY

PRODUCTION

Humoral immunity is mediated by antibodies, which are produced by cells of the B lymphocyte lineage. The physiologic function of antibodies is to neutralize and eliminate the antigen that induced their formation. The elimination of different antigens or microbes requires several effector mechanisms, which are dependent on distinct classes, or isotypes, of antibodies (see Chapter 3). The humoral immune system has the capacity to respond to different types of antigens by producing different classes of antibodies. The humoral immune response is also different at various anatomic sites. For instance, mucosal lymphoid tissues are uniquely adapted to produce high levels of IgA in response to the same antigens that stimulate other antibody isotypes in non-mucosal lymphoid tissues.

A fundamental feature of humoral immunity is that production of all these varied classes of antibodies is initiated by the interaction of antigens with a small number of mature IgM and IgD–expressing B lymphocytes specific for each antigen. Mature antigen-responsive B lymphocytes develop in the bone marrow prior to overt antigenic stimulation. Such cells enter peripheral lymphoid tissues, which are the sites of interaction with foreign antigens. An antigen binds to the membrane IgM and IgD on specific B cells and initiates a series of responses that lead to two principal changes

in that clone of B cells: **proliferation,** resulting in expansion of the clone, and **differentiation,** resulting in the progeny of the membrane Ig-expressing, antigen-responsive B cells actively secreting antibodies of different heavy chain isotypes or becoming memory cells (Fig. 9–1). Therefore, the analysis of humoral immune responses is, in essence, an analysis of the growth and differentiation of B lymphocytes that occur following specific antigenic stimulation. The molecular mechanisms that regulate the expression of immunoglobulin genes have been described in Chapter 4. This chapter describes the cellular basis of the humoral immune response, in particular the stimuli that induce B cell growth and differentiation and the patterns of responses of B lymphocytes.

GENERAL FEATURES OF HUMORAL IMMUNE RESPONSES

The earliest studies of specific immunity were devoted to analyses of antibody responses. As a result, until the 1960s, much of our knowledge of the immune system was based on our understanding of humoral immunity. The basic features of humoral immune re-

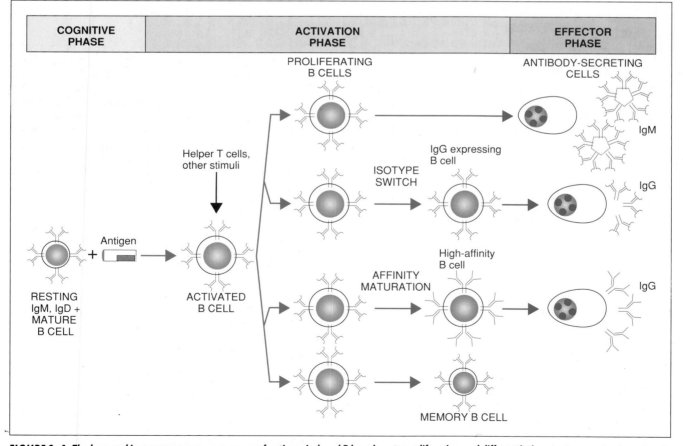

FIGURE 9–1. The humoral immune response: sequence of antigen-induced B lymphocyte proliferation and differentiation. *Antigen and other stimuli, including helper T cells, stimulate the proliferation and differentiation of a specific B cell clone. Progeny of the clone may produce IgM or other Ig isotypes (e.g., IgG), may undergo affinity maturation, or may persist as memory cells.*

sponses were established before it was known that B lymphocytes and their progeny were the only cells capable of producing antibodies. The most important general properties of antibody responses are the following:

1. Protein antigens do not induce antibody responses in the absence of T lymphocytes, for instance, in T cell–deficient individuals. For this reason, proteins are classified as "thymus-dependent" or "T-dependent" antigens. This observation led to the hypothesis that antibody production in response to protein antigens requires T cells, which are called **helper T cells,** as well as Ig-producing B cells. As we shall see later in this chapter, a great deal is now known about the specificity and functions of helper T cells. The demonstration of their role in antibody responses is the basis of the concept that *resting B cells, which have not been previously exposed to antigen, require two distinct types of signals or stimuli for their proliferation and differentiation.* One type of signal is provided by the antigen, which interacts with membrane Ig molecules on specific B cells. The second type of signal is provided by helper T lymphocytes and their secreted products. The "two-signal" theory of lymphocyte activation may apply to most or all lymphocytes, because antigen-specific helper and cytolytic T lymphocytes (CTLs) also need other stimuli, in addition to antigens, for their full growth and differentiation (see Chapters 7 and 13).

2. Non-protein antigens like polysaccharides and lipids induce antibody responses without a requirement for antigen-specific helper T lymphocytes, e.g., in T cell–deficient individuals. Therefore, polysaccharide and lipid antigens are called "thymus-independent" or "T-independent (TI)."

3. *Primary and secondary antibody responses differ qualitatively and quantitatively in several respects* (Table 9–1). First, the secondary response develops more rapidly than the primary response, and larger amounts of antibodies are produced in the secondary response. This is a clear example of immunologic

memory. Primary antibody responses result from the activation of previously unstimulated B cells, whereas secondary responses are due to stimulation of expanded clones of memory cells. Second, the dominant class of secreted antibody in the primary response is usually IgM because resting B cells express only IgM (and IgD, which is rarely secreted). In contrast, other Ig isotypes, such as IgG, IgA, and IgE, are relatively increased in secondary responses. This change results from **heavy chain class** or **isotype switching.** Third, the average affinity of specific antibodies produced in a secondary response is higher than in the primary response. This is called **affinity maturation,** and results from somatic mutations in Ig genes and selective activation by antigen of those B cells whose membrane Ig molecules have increased affinity for that antigen. Affinity maturation is seen in both the membrane Ig on specific memory B cells and in the secreted antibodies. The increased affinity of antibodies following antigenic stimulation makes an individual better able to combat microbes that cause recurrent infections. Affinity maturation of membrane Ig explains why the optimal antigen doses required for stimulating secondary antibody responses are lower than those for primary responses.

4. Memory cell generation, heavy chain class switching, and affinity maturation are typical of humoral immune responses to proteins, but generally do not occur following immunization with thymus-independent antigens. This finding suggests that these responses of B cells are induced by helper T cells and/or their secreted products.

Much of our understanding of the activation of B lymphocytes and the induction and regulation of antibody responses has evolved from attempts to explain these features of humoral immunity. Among the most useful analytical approaches are *in vitro* experiments, in which different stimuli are used to activate B cells, and their proliferation and differentiation can be measured accurately (Box 9–1). The current view of the mechanisms of B cell activation is based largely on these *in vitro* studies, and defining the cell interactions in humoral immune responses *in vivo* remains a challenge for immunologists.

EFFECTS OF ANTIGENS ON B LYMPHOCYTES

Foreign antigens that are introduced into an individual interact with specific B lymphocytes mostly in peripheral lymphoid tissues, such as the spleen for blood-borne antigens, lymph nodes for antigens collected in the lymph, mucosal lymphoid tissues for ingested or inhaled antigens, and, to a lesser extent, at other sites of antigen entry (e.g., the skin). *The binding of an antigen to membrane Ig on B cells is the initiating event in B lymphocyte activation* and, therefore, in humoral immune responses. Thymus-dependent protein antigens are thought to initiate two distinct types of responses in B cells. First, these antigens stimulate intracellular second messengers that stimulate the entry

---

TABLE 9–1.   Features of Primary and Secondary Antibody Responses

	Primary Response	Secondary Response
Lag after immunization	Usually 5–10 days	Usually 1–3 days
Peak response	Smaller	Larger
Antibody isotype	Usually IgM > IgG	Relative increase in IgG and, under certain situations, in IgA or IgE
Antibody affinity	Lower average affinity, more variable	Higher average affinity ("affinity maturation")
Induced by	All immunogens	Only protein antigens
Required immunization	Relatively high doses of antigens, optimally with adjuvants	Low doses of antigens, adjuvants usually not necessary

Abbreviation: Ig, immunoglobulin.

BOX 9–1.   ASSAYS FOR B LYMPHOCYTE ACTIVATION

The responses of B lymphocytes to antigens and other stimuli that are described in this chapter consist of the following:

1. Early intracellular alterations, including the generation of "second messengers."

2. Proliferation, leading to expansion of the stimulated clone(s) of B cells.

3. Differentiation from membrane Ig-expressing cells to cells that actively secrete Ig of different heavy chain classes.

The most frequently used assays for B cell responses measure cellular proliferation and antibody secretion.

ASSAYS FOR PROLIFERATION. The proliferation of B lymphocytes, like that of other cells, is measured *in vitro* by determining the amount of ^{3}H-labeled thymidine incorporated into the replicating DNA of cultured cells. Thymidine incorporation provides a quantitative measure of the rate of DNA synthesis, which is usually directly proportional to the rate of cell division. Cellular proliferation *in vivo* can be measured by injecting ^{3}H-thymidine into animals and determining the number of cells with radioactively labeled nuclei (called the "labeling index"), or by injecting bromodeoxyuridine (BrdU) and staining cells with anti-BrdU antibody to identify nuclei that have incorporated this thymidine analog.

ASSAYS FOR ANTIBODY PRODUCTION. Antibody production is measured in two different ways: assays for **cumulative Ig secretion**, which measure the amount of Ig that accumulates in the supernatant of cultured lymphocytes or in the serum of an immunized individual, and **single-cell assays**, which determine the number of cells in an immune population that secrete Ig of a particular specificity and/or isotype.

The most accurate, quantitative, and widely used techniques for measuring the total amount of Ig in a culture supernatant or serum sample are radioimmunoassay (RIA) and enzyme-linked immunosorbent assay (ELISA), described in Chapter 3. By using antigens bound to solid supports, it is possible to use RIA or ELISA to quantitate the amount of a specific antibody in a sample. In addition, the availability of anti-Ig antibodies that detect immunoglobulins of different heavy or light chain classes allows one to measure the quantities of different isotypes in a sample. Other techniques for measuring antibody levels include hemagglutina-

tion for anti-erythrocyte antibodies, and complement-dependent lysis for antibodies specific for known cell types. Both assays are based on the demonstration that if the amount of antigen (i.e., cells) is constant, the concentration of antibody determines the amount of antibody bound to cells, and this is reflected in the degree of cell agglutination or subsequent binding of complement and cell lysis. Results from these assays are usually expressed as antibody titers, which are the dilution of the sample giving half-maximal effects or the dilution at which the end-point of the assay is reached.

A widely used single-cell assay for antibody secretion is the **hemolytic plaque assay**, in which the antigen is either an erythrocyte protein(s) or a molecule covalently coupled to an erythrocyte surface. Such erythrocytes serve as "indicator cells." They are mixed with lymphocytes, among which are the specific antibody-producing cells, and incubated in a semisolid supporting medium to allow secreted antibody to bind to the erythrocyte surface. If the antibody binds complement avidly, the subsequent addition of complement leads to lysis of the indicator cells that are coated with specific antibody. As a result, clear zones of lysis, called **plaques**, are formed around individual B lymphocytes or plasma cells that secrete the specific antibody. These antibody-secreting cells are also called **plaque-forming cells** (PFCs). This assay can also be used to detect antibodies that do not fix complement by incorporating into the medium a complement-binding anti-Ig antibody that will coat indicator cells to which the specific Ig is bound first. In another refinement, the same basic method can be used to detect PFCs that secrete Ig of a particular isotype irrespective of antigenic specificity. Another technique for measuring the number of antibody-secreting cells is the **ELISPOT assay**. In this method, antigen is bound to the bottom of a well, antibody-secreting cells are added in a semisolid medium, and antibodies that have been secreted and are bound to the antigen are detected by an enzyme-linked anti-Ig antibody, as in an ELISA. Each spot represents the location of an antibody-secreting cell. Single-cell assays provide a measure of the numbers of Ig-secreting cells, but they cannot accurately quantitate the amount of Ig secreted by each cell or by the total population. These assays can be applied to B cells stimulated *in vitro* or isolated from animals immunized with particular antigens.

---

of resting B cells into the cell cycle. Interaction with antigen may also prepare the B cells for subsequent responses to helper T lymphocytes. Second, protein antigens are internalized and processed by the B cells and presented to antigen-specific helper T cells, which are thus activated at the sites of specific antigen–B cell interactions. The subsequent growth and differentiation of B cells in response to protein antigens are actually stimulated by helper T lymphocytes and their secreted products. Thymus-independent antigens stimulate B cell responses without specific T cell help; they are discussed at the end of the chapter.

It is technically difficult to study the effects of antigens on normal B cells because, as the clonal selection hypothesis predicted, very few lymphocytes in an individual are specific for any one antigen. In order to examine the effects of antigen binding to B cells, investigators have attempted to isolate antigen-specific B cells from complex populations of normal lymphocytes or to

produce cloned B cell lines with defined antigenic specificities. The latter effort has met with limited success, so far. Recently, transgenic mice have been developed in which virtually all B cells express the transgenic Ig. Thus, even though the B cells are derived from multiple progenitors (and are, therefore, polyclonal), they respond to the same antigen because they express the same Ig. Another approach to circumventing this problem is to use anti-Ig antibodies as analogs of antigens, with the assumption that anti-Ig will bind to constant regions of membrane Ig molecules on all B cells and have the same biologic effects as an antigen that binds to the hypervariable regions of membrane Ig molecules only on the antigen-specific B cells. To the extent that precise comparisons are feasible, this assumption appears generally correct, indicating that anti-Ig antibody is a valid model for antigens. Thus, anti-Ig antibody is frequently used as a polyclonal activator of B lymphocytes. The same concept underlies the use of antibodies against framework determinants of T cell receptors or against receptor-associated CD3 molecules as polyclonal activators of T lymphocytes (see Chapter 7). Much of our knowledge of the effects of antigens on B lymphocytes is actually deduced from experiments using anti-Ig antibodies.

Biochemical Effects of Antigen on B Lymphocytes

The interaction of a multivalent or bivalent antigen or anti-Ig antibody with membrane Ig on a B cell results in cross-linking of Ig molecules and the transduction of a series of biochemical signals to the cell interior. Membrane IgM and IgD, the antigen receptors of resting, mature B cells, have short cytoplasmic domains composed of only three amino acids, lysine, valine, and lysine. These cytoplasmic tails are insufficient to transduce signals generated by binding of antigen or anti-Ig. Both IgM and IgD are expressed on the cell surface in non-covalent associations with at least two other proteins, called Igα and Igβ (Fig. 9–2). These two proteins are required for the surface expression of IgM and IgD. In addition, Igα and Igβ link membrane Ig molecules to several tyrosine kinases, and are themselves phosphorylated upon binding of anti-Ig. Cross-linking of membrane Ig molecules serves to bring together intracellular proteins, e.g., kinases, that are involved in signaling. A similar function is attributed to the CD3 and ζ proteins of the T cell receptor (TCR) complex in T lymphocytes (see Chapter 7). Indeed, the cytoplasmic domains of Igα, Igβ, and several proteins of the TCR complex show significant sequence homologies.

The series of biochemical events triggered in B cells by cross-linking of membrane IgM and IgD are, in essence, similar to the events that occur in T lymphocytes following TCR-mediated stimulation (see Fig. 7–10, Chapter 7).

1. Within the first minute, tyrosine kinases are activated, leading to the tyrosine phosphorylation of a number of proteins. Although several kinases have been identified in B lymphocytes, and some of these appear to be B cell–specific, their relative roles in the functional responses of B cells are not yet clear.

2. One of the proteins that is phosphorylated is the γ1 isoform of the enzyme phosphatidyl inositol–specific phospholipase C (called PI-PLC-γ1). This enzyme becomes active, and cleaves membrane phosphatidylinositol bisphosphate to generate two main products, inositol triphosphate (IP$_3$) and diacylglycerol (DAG). IP$_3$ mobilizes ionic Ca^{++} from intracellular stores, leading to a rapid elevation of cytoplasmic Ca^{++}. DAG activates protein kinase C and translocates it to the cytoplasm, where the enzyme can phosphorylate other proteins on serine/threonine residues. All these changes are detectable in B cells within 1 to 5 minutes of stimulation by anti-Ig antibody.

3. The subsequent biochemical events in B cell activation are less well defined. Phosphoproteins may act as transcription factors to induce the transcription of particular genes. In fact, within 1 hour of stimulation,

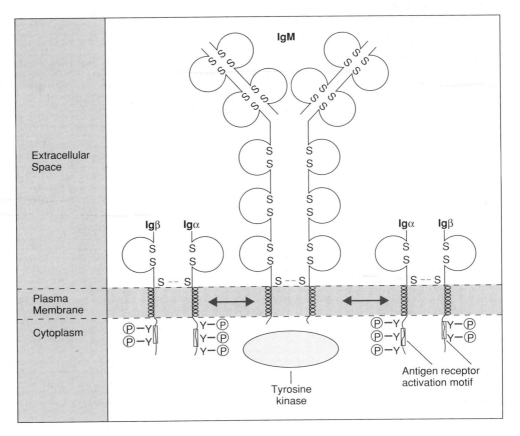

FIGURE 9–2. The B cell antigen receptor complex. *Membrane IgM (and IgD) on the surface of mature B cells are associated with Igα and Igβ, which link the complex to intracellular tyrosine kinases. Arrows indicate non-covalent associations of the μ heavy chain with Igα. Y-Ⓟ indicates the approximate locations of tyrosine residues that are phosphorylated upon cross-linking of the membrane Ig. Boxed areas represent conserved sequences found in antigen receptors in T and B lymphocytes. Note the similarity to the T cell receptor complex (see Fig. 7–5).*

Extracellular Space

Plasma Membrane

Cytoplasm

IgM

Igβ   Igα

Igα   Igβ

Tyrosine kinase

Antigen receptor activation motif

levels of messenger RNA (mRNA) for cellular proto-oncogenes, such as *c-fos* and *c-myc*, are increased. These genes code for components of DNA-binding proteins that regulate the transcription of other genes.

Beginning at about 12 hours after stimulation, the B cells become larger, contain increased amounts of cellular RNA, and are thought to move from the resting, or G$_0$, stage to the G$_1$ stage of the cell cycle. Thus, the cells are poised to proliferate once they receive additional signals. Activated B cells also express increased levels of class II MHC molecules, costimulators such as B7, and membrane receptors for helper T cell–derived cytokines. *Such changes make antigen-stimulated B cells better able to interact with and respond to helper T lymphocytes and their secreted mediators.*

The link between the initial biochemical changes detected in B cells after binding of antigen or anti-Ig antibody and the subsequent growth and differentiation of the B cells is not established. It is not even known which, if any, of these biochemical signals are required for the functional responses to be initiated. In fact, most natural protein antigens contain only one or a few epitopes and, therefore, cannot effectively cross-link Ig molecules on antigen-specific B cells. Furthermore, helper T cells and cytokines may be able to activate B cells without any antigen-mediated signals being transduced. Therefore, in antibody responses to protein antigens, the signaling function of membrane Ig may not be critical, and may be circumvented or replaced by T cell–mediated signals. In these situations, the principal function of membrane Ig may be to bind and internalize the protein antigen for subsequent presentation to helper T cells (discussed below). On the other hand, responses to thymus-independent antigens, which cannot stimulate specific T cell help, may require Ig-mediated signal transduction to initiate B cell growth and differentiation. Most thymus-independent antigens are polymeric, containing multiple identical epitopes, and are able to cross-link Ig molecules on individual B cells. Thus, *the importance of biochemical signals and second messengers induced by antigen binding to B cell Ig may vary, depending on the nature of the antigen and the presence and absence of helper T cells.*

Presentation of Antigens by B Cells to Helper T Lymphocytes

Following the binding of an antigen or anti-Ig antibody to a B cell, the complex of bound ligand and Ig molecules is internalized by receptor-mediated endocytosis (Fig. 9–3). If the ligand is a protein, it is subsequently processed as in other antigen-presenting cells (see Chapter 6). This results in the generation of peptide fragments of the antigen that are re-expressed on the cell surface non-covalently attached to class II MHC molecules. These peptide-MHC molecule complexes can subsequently be recognized by antigen-specific, MHC-restricted helper T lymphocytes. As we shall discuss in detail later, antigen-specific B cells are extremely efficient at presenting the antigen they recog-

nize, because membrane Ig molecules function as high-affinity receptors that enable the cells to bind, internalize, and present very low concentrations of antigens. Antigen processing and presentation occur within 1 to 6 hours of binding of a protein antigen to B cells *in vitro*. Over the next 8 to 24 hours, new membrane Ig molecules are synthesized and re-expressed, so that the B cell is able to bind more antigen molecules. Thymus-independent antigens such as polysaccharides and glycolipids may also be endocytosed following binding to Ig on specific B cells, but these antigens cannot be processed and associated with MHC molecules and, therefore, are not recognized by specific class II MHC–restricted helper T cells.

ROLE OF HELPER T LYMPHOCYTES IN ANTIBODY RESPONSES

The second signals for B lymphocyte activation that have been most thoroughly investigated are provided by contact with activated helper T cells and by cytokines secreted by these cells. A role for T lymphocytes in antibody responses was formally demonstrated by experiments done in the late 1960s, even before the classification of lymphocytes into T and B cell subsets was established. These experiments showed that if mouse bone marrow lymphocytes, which we now know contain mature B cells but few or no mature T cells, were adoptively transferred into irradiated syngeneic recipients, they would not produce specific antibody upon immunization with sheep red blood cells (SRBCs), a model protein antigen. If, however, mature thymocytes or thoracic duct lymphocytes (which contain T lymphocytes but few antibody-producing B cells) were transferred at the same time, antibody responses did develop following immunization (Table 9–2). This result, and later *in vitro* experiments in which purified T and B cells were mixed and stimulated with antigens, showed that B cells would proliferate and differentiate in response to protein antigens only if helper T lymphocytes were also present. Subsequent studies have established that *most helper T cells are CD4$^+$, CD8$^-$, and class II MHC–restricted* in their recognition of foreign protein antigens (see Chapters 6 and 7). The availability of T cell help is often the limiting factor in antibody responses to protein antigens. Both helper T cells and B cells are stimulated by primary immunization, and both are responsible for enhanced antibody production in secondary responses.

There are two important questions about the functions of helper T cells in antibody responses:

1. How are these helper T cells stimulated by antigens in a way that enables them to interact with antigen-specific B lymphocytes?

2. What are the mechanisms by which helper T cells induce the growth and differentiation of B lymphocytes?

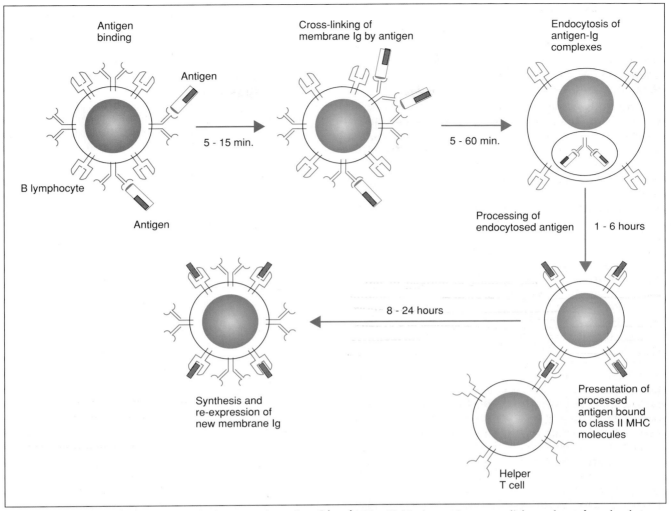

FIGURE 9-3. Fate of protein antigens after binding to membrane Ig on B lymphocytes. *Multivalent antigens cross-link membrane Ig molecules on a B cell, and the complexes are endocytosed. The antigen is processed inside the cell, and peptide fragments bound to class II MHC molecules are presented to helper T cells. Some of the membrane Ig may recycle back to the surface, but most of it is replaced by newly synthesized Ig molecules.*

TABLE 9-2. Identification of Helper T Cells in Antibody Responses to Protein Antigens

A. Adoptive Transfer

Cells Transferred into Irradiated Recipient			Anti-SRBC Antibody-Producing Cells in Spleen
SOURCE OF B CELLS	*SOURCE OF T CELLS*	Antigen	
Bone marrow cells	None	SRBC	−
None	Thoracic duct cells	SRBC	−
Bone marrow cells	Thoracic duct cells	SRBC	+
Bone marrow cells	Thoracic duct cells	—	−

B. Cell Culture

Cells Cultured	*Antigen*	Anti-SRBC Antibody-Producing Cells in Culture
Unfractionated spleen cells	SRBC	+
Splenic B cells	SRBC	−
Splenic T cells	SRBC	−
Splenic B cells and T cells	SRBC	+
Splenic B cells and T cells	–	−

Mouse B lymphocytes by themselves do not produce antibody against a T cell–dependent antigen, SRBC, *in vivo* (A) or *in vitro* (B). The addition of T cells allows the B cells to respond to SRBC. A response does not occur in the absence of antigen.

Abbreviation: SRBC, sheep red blood cells.

Mechanisms of Helper T Cell–B Cell Interactions

The sequence of events leading to helper T cell–dependent antibody responses to protein antigens is best understood by considering the immune response to hapten-protein conjugates. Haptens, such as dinitrophenol, are small chemicals that can be bound by B cell membrane Ig and by secreted antibodies but are not immunogenic by themselves. If, however, the haptens are coupled to proteins, which serve as carriers, the conjugates are able to induce antibody responses against the haptens.

There are three important characteristics of anti-hapten antibody responses stimulated by hapten-protein conjugates. First, such responses require cooperation between hapten-specific B cells and protein (carrier)-specific helper T cells. Second, in order to stimulate a response, the hapten and carrier portions have to be physically linked and cannot be administered separately. Third, the interaction is class II MHC–restricted; i.e., the helper T cells cooperate only with B lymphocytes that express class II MHC molecules recognized as self by the T cells. The same characteristics apply not only to hapten-protein conjugates but to all protein antigens in which one intrinsic determinant is recognized by B cells (and is, therefore, analogous to the hapten) and another determinant is recognized by helper T cells (and is analogous to the carrier).

The mechanism of T cell–B cell cooperation in the generation of antibody responses to protein antigens and hapten-protein conjugates became clear when it was appreciated that B lymphocytes are extremely efficient antigen-presenting cells. When an individual is exposed to an antigen, *specific B cells bind the native antigen to membrane Ig molecules (e.g., via the hapten determinant), internalize and process it, and present peptide fragments (carrier determinants) of the antigen associated with class II MHC molecules to specific helper T cells* (Fig. 9–4). The hapten is thus responsible for efficient carrier uptake, explaining why hapten and carrier must be physically linked. The helper T cells are then stimulated to perform their effector function, which is to promote B cell growth and differentiation. As we shall see later, this activation of B cells results from stimuli generated by physical contact with helper T cells and by cytokines secreted by the T cells.

The antigen-presenting function of B lymphocytes accounts for many features of antibody responses to protein antigens. It is responsible for the MHC restriction of T cell–B cell interactions. In any humoral immune response, B cells specific for the antigen that initiates the response are preferentially activated as compared with bystander cells that are not specific for the antigen. There are several reasons for this. First, only B cells expressing receptors (membrane Ig molecules) that bind the antigen receive the first signal for activation. Second, antigen-specific B cells are able to present the antigen at 10^4- to 10^6-fold lower concentrations than all other antigen-presenting cells (APCs).

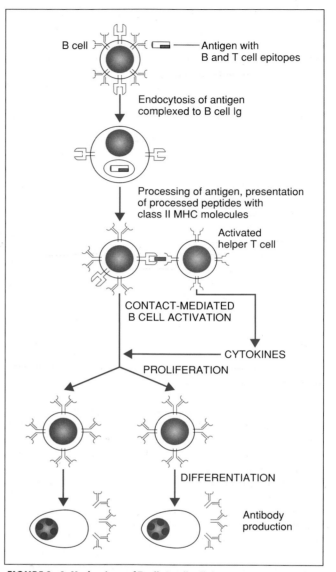

FIGURE 9–4. Mechanisms of T cell–B cell collaboration. *Antigen-specific B cells bind protein antigens via membrane Ig and internalize, process, and present MHC-associated peptide determinants to specific CD4⁺ helper T cells. The physical contact between activated helper T cells and B cells initiates B cell responses. Helper T cells secrete cytokines that stimulate the proliferation and differentiation of the B cells.*

This is because membrane Ig molecules specifically bind the antigen at low concentrations, and because antigens endocytosed with Ig are delivered to the intracellular protein processing pathway that is especially efficient at generating class II MHC–peptide complexes (see Chapter 6). Experimentally, this has been demonstrated with protein antigens conjugated to anti-Ig antibodies, and with bifunctional antibodies in which one arm of the antibody binds to membrane Ig and another to a foreign antigen. Antigens internalized in this way are more efficiently processed and presented to T cells than antigens internalized by pinocytosis or via B cell surface receptors other than Ig. As a result, whenever antigen concentrations are limiting, specific B cells are the preferential APCs. Third, the antigen-presenting B cells are the cells that form physical contacts with helper T cells and, because of proximity, are exposed to the highest concentrations of T cell–derived cytokines. Therefore, *antigen-specific B lymphocytes are the preferential recipients of T cell help, and are stimulated to proliferate and differentiate.* The antibodies that are subsequently secreted are specific for conformational determinants of the antigen, because membrane Ig on B cells is capable of binding conformational epitopes of native antigens. This feature determines the fine specificity of the antibody response, and is independent of the fact that helper T cells recognize only linear epitopes of processed peptides.

Although it is clear that B cells need to function as APCs for MHC-restricted T cell–B cell interactions to occur, it is likely that other APCs are required for initiating the activation of helper T cells in primary antibody responses. There are several reasons for this conclusion. Resting, or previously unstimulated, B lymphocytes are inefficient at stimulating resting T cells and may even induce T cell tolerance, mainly because resting B cells are deficient in costimulators (see Chapters 7 and 10). In unimmunized individuals, there may be so few B cells specific for a particular antigen that they cannot effectively initiate a T cell response. Furthermore, it is known that for generating optimal primary antibody responses to protein antigens the antigens have to be administered with adjuvants, and one function of adjuvants is to enhance the antigen-presenting functions of macrophages (see Chapter 10). Therefore, when an individual is exposed to a protein antigen for the first time, APCs such as macrophages and dendritic cells may process and present the antigen to resting helper T cells. These T cells are activated, then interact with B cells that also present the antigen, and a primary response ensues. In secondary responses, on the other hand, the expanded clones of antigen-specific memory B cells may be fully capable of functioning as APCs. This is supported by the observation that secondary antibody responses *in vitro* require only B cells, helper T cells, and antigen. Depletion of macrophages reduces or even abolishes primary antibody responses, but does not abrogate antibody production by previously stimulated lymphocytes. Accessory cells such as macrophages may also have functions other than antigen presentation in humoral immune responses; these functions are described later in the chapter.

The Role of T Cell–B Cell Contact in B Lymphocyte Activation

Activated helper T cells that recognize antigens presented by B lymphocytes deliver two types of stimuli that result in the proliferation and differentiation of B cells. As mentioned above, these stimuli are generated by the physical contact between T and B lymphocytes, and by the cytokines produced by helper T cells.

The importance of the physical, or cognate, interaction between antigen-presenting B cells and antigen-reactive helper T cells in the generation of humoral immune responses has been established by a variety of experiments (Fig. 9–5). For instance, supernatants of activated helper T cells, which contain multiple cytokines, are rarely, if ever, as effective in inducing antibody production by B cells as the helper T cells themselves, especially in cultures of B cells stimulated with low concentrations of soluble protein antigens. Furthermore, if helper T cells are first activated with antigen, chemically fixed, rendering them incapable of synthesizing or secreting cytokines, and then co-cultured with B cells, they are still capable of inducing RNA synthesis by and proliferation of the B cells. The same responses are seen if the B cells are cultured with purified plasma membranes of activated helper T lymphocytes. In the absence of cytokines, fixed T cells or membranes induce only modest B cell proliferation. The full proliferation of B cells, and their differentiation to antibody-secreting cells, require cytokines, as we shall discuss later.

Such results suggested that B cells express a membrane molecule(s) that binds to a complementary receptor on activated T lymphocytes, and this interaction provides the stimulus that initiates B cell responses. The principal molecules involved in T cell contact–mediated B cell stimulation are now known to be CD40 on B cells, and its complementary 39 kD ligand (called gp39) on activated helper T cells. CD40 is a ~50 kD glycoprotein that is expressed on most mature B lymphocytes but is lost after B cells differentiate to become antibody-secreting cells. CD40 is a member of a family of cell surface proteins that includes the receptors for tumor necrosis factor (TNF, see Chapter 12) and a protein called Fas (see Chapter 19). It is postulated that this family of proteins plays a role in regulating programmed cell death and cellular proliferation. Antibodies to CD40 can replace helper T cells in stimulating some B cell responses, and fibroblasts expressing the CD40 ligand (by gene transfection) stimulate B cells much like contact with helper T cells (Fig. 9–5). Mutations in the CD40 ligand result in an X-linked immunodeficiency disease called the hyper-IgM syndrome, which is characterized by defects in helper T cell–dependent antibody responses (see Chapter 21).

The interaction of gp39 on T cells with CD40 on B cells occurs independently of antigen and MHC molecules. Thus, the likely sequence of events in T cell–B cell interactions is as follows. B cells present MHC-associated antigenic peptides to helper T cells; the helper T cells are activated to express gp39; gp39 then binds to CD40 on the antigen-presenting B cell; this interaction initiates B cell growth; and subsequent responses of the B cells are stimulated by cytokines produced by the helper T cells. The biochemical nature of the signals generated by CD40 engagement, and the mechanisms by which these signals induce B cell growth, are not yet known.

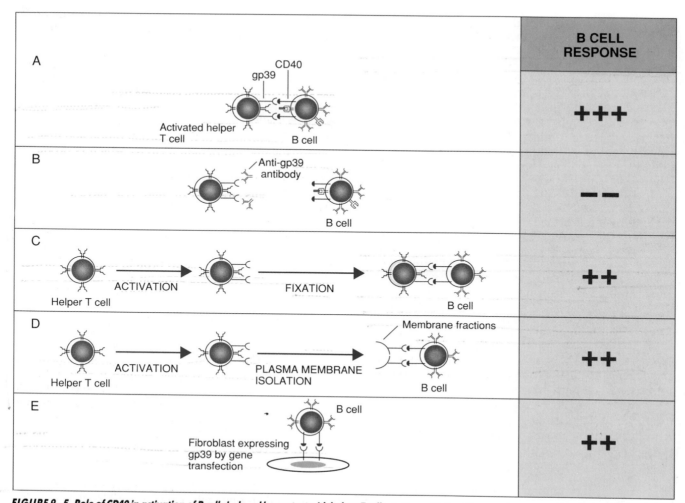

FIGURE 9–5. Role of CD40 in activation of B cells induced by contact with helper T cells. *Activated helper T cells recognize antigen presented by B cells and express gp39, which binds to CD40 on B cells and initiates B cell responses (A). Blocking antibodies against gp39 inhibit the T cell contact–mediated stimulation of B cells (B). Pre-activated and fixed helper T cells (C), gp39-containing plasma membrane fractions of activated T cells (D), and fibroblasts expressing gp39 (E) all can replace intact, viable T cells. Note that the full growth and differentiation of B cells require T cell–derived cytokines as well as T cell contact.*

Cytokines (Helper Factors) in Antibody Responses

Cytokines are soluble proteins secreted by T lymphocytes and by other cell types in response to activating stimuli. Cytokines mediate many of the effector functions of the cells that produce them, and are the principal mechanisms by which various immune and inflammatory cell populations communicate with one another. Although cytokines may be produced as a result of the stimulation of specific T cells by antigens, the cytokines themselves are not antigen-specific and do not bind to antigens. Their general properties, structural features, and functional effects are described in Chapter 12. The role of these secreted proteins in humoral immunity has been most clearly established by showing that various aspects of antibody responses can be inhibited by cytokine antagonists, or are deficient in mice in which particular cytokine genes are knocked out by homologous recombination.

Cytokines serve two principal functions in antibody responses: they determine the types of antibodies produced by selectively promoting switching to different heavy chain isotypes, and they provide amplification mechanisms by augmenting B cell proliferation and differentiation. The cytokines that function as helper factors in antibody responses have the following general properties:

1. *Different cytokines may stimulate B cell proliferation and differentiation to antibody-secreting cells.* Any one cytokine may function in different phases of the responses of B cells, and various cytokines may serve the same or overlapping functions in antibody production (an example of the "redundancy" of cytokine actions). Because of this realization, the old classification of helper factors into "B cell growth factors" and "B cell differentiation factors" is no longer considered valid.

2. *The most selective, and only known obligatory, roles of individual cytokines are in heavy chain class*

switching. Different cytokines may uniquely induce switching to different heavy chain classes, as described below. This is the reason why mice in which individual cytokine genes are knocked out, or animals treated with specific cytokine antagonists, often show complete deficits in selected isotypes.

3. *Combinations of particular cytokines may be synergistic or antagonistic in their effects on B cells.*

4. The most potent helper factors for B cells are cytokines produced by CD4+ helper T cells. However, some of the cytokines that stimulate B cell growth and differentiation may be secreted by macrophages and other non–T cells.

5. The production of cytokines contributes to the activation of "bystander" B cells that are not specific for the antigen initiating the response but are present in the vicinity of antigen-stimulated cells. Bystander B cell activation is readily observed *in vitro* and is presumably also responsible for the production of non-specific antibody following exposure to potent immunogens. For instance, infection with helminthic parasites stimulates 100-fold or greater increases in serum IgE, and only a small fraction of this IgE (probably less than 5 per cent) is specific for the particular helminth. Note, however, that even in such responses, the antigen-specific B cells are preferentially stimulated as compared with bystander cells.

The activation of B cells by cytokines is an evolving story, since new factors and new effects of previously described mediators continue to be discovered. Nevertheless, it is possible to construct a basic scheme of the stages of B cell activation and to identify the cytokines that act at each of these stages (Fig. 9–6).

1. *Proliferation.* Many different cytokines have been shown to stimulate the proliferation of B cells, especially in experimental systems using polyclonal activators. Three helper T cell–derived cytokines, interleukin-2 (IL-2), interleukin-4 (IL-4), and interleukin-5 (IL-5), all contribute to B cell proliferation and may act synergistically. Interleukin-6 (IL-6), which is produced by macrophages, T cells, and many other cell types, is a growth factor for already differentiated, antibody-secreting B cells. IL-1, IL-10, and TNF have also been shown to have B cell growth–promoting activity *in vitro.* The redundancy in the actions of these cytokines accounts for the observation that an antagonist that blocks the function of any one has virtually no effect on B cell growth in response to protein antigens. Furthermore, mice in which the gene for IL-2, IL-4, or IL-10 is knocked out have essentially normal numbers of B cells.

2. *Antibody secretion.* Antibody synthesis and secretion in response to protein antigens, like B cell proliferation, are also enhanced by cytokines. In the mouse, IL-4 and IL-5 are the most potent inducers of antibody secretion by B cells. Human B cells cultured with polyclonal activators secrete high levels of antibody if IL-2 or IL-6 is added. It is not clear whether these differences in the cytokine responses of human and mouse B cells are due to true species variations, or merely reflect differences in experimental conditions.

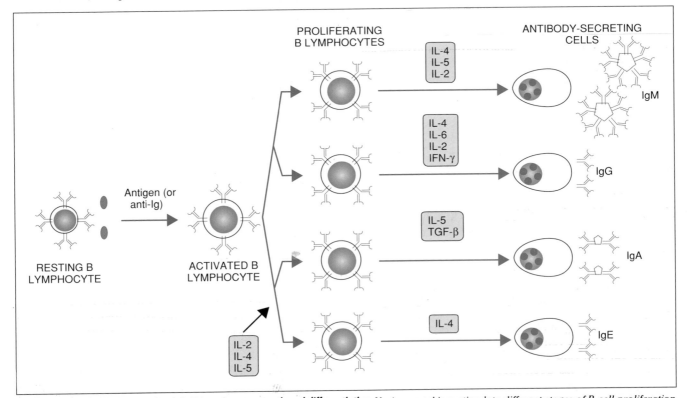

FIGURE 9–6. Functions of cytokines in B lymphocyte growth and differentiation. *Various cytokines stimulate different stages of B cell proliferation and differentiation in humans and mice. The same cytokines may have less striking effects at other stages that are not shown, and there may be differences among species.*

3. *Isotype switching.* We have mentioned previously that heavy chain isotype switching is typically seen with protein antigens and requires helper T cells. It is now known that different T cell–derived cytokines can selectively induce switching to particular Ig isotypes. For instance, *IL-4 is the principal switch factor for IgE in all species examined.* IgE production depends on IL-4, since IgE responses to antigen-specific or polyclonal stimulation *in vitro*, and to infection by helminthic parasites *in vivo*, are abrogated by antibodies that neutralize IL-4, and IL-4-deficient mice created by gene knockout have no serum IgE. These findings have many practical implications. IgE antibodies are important for host defense against parasitic infestations (see Chapter 16), and immediate hypersensitivity (allergic) reactions are due to IgE production (see Chapter 14). Therefore, therapeutic control of IL-4 secretion or function is potentially a powerful approach for the treatment of allergy. Similarly, the production of IgG2a in mice is dependent on interferon-γ (IFN-γ), which is also secreted by T cells. Therefore, addition of IL-4 or IFN-γ induces specific isotype switching in cultures of mature IgM and IgD–expressing B cells stimulated with antigens or polyclonal activators (Table 9–3). Interestingly, IFN-γ inhibits IL-4–induced B cell switching to IgE, and, conversely, IL-4 reduces IgG2a production. These are among the clearest examples of the antagonistic effects of different cytokines. Transforming growth factor-β (TGF-β), which is produced by many cell types, acts in concert with T cell–derived IL-5 to stimulate IgA production in mucosal lymphoid tissues (see Chapter 11). These two cytokines may, therefore, be especially important in mucosal immunity.

The mechanisms by which cytokines induce switching to different antibody isotypes are being actively studied. In mature B cells and cell lines that normally produce IgM, addition of IL-4 stimulates transcription through switch regions located 5' of the C_ϵ constant region genes in the heavy chain locus (Fig. 9–7). This leads first to the production of sterile or incomplete "germline" transcripts. Subsequently, the rearranged VDJ complex recombines with the C_ϵ gene

segment, producing a full-length functional ϵ heavy chain transcript. This process of switch recombination (see Chapter 4) leads to the synthesis of IgE antibodies.

4. *Affinity maturation and the generation of memory B cells.* Affinity maturation in secondary antibody responses and the generation of memory B cells are both helper T cell–dependent phenomena that occur only after immunization with protein antigens. However, it is not known if particular cytokines are involved in these aspects of humoral immune responses. Affinity maturation results from somatic mutations in the rearranged V genes of antigen and helper T cell–stimulated, rapidly proliferating B lymphocytes. Subsequently, B cells expressing receptors with the highest affinities for the antigen are selected to survive; the mechanism of this selection is described below. We do not know why some of the progeny of an antigen-stimulated B cell clone differentiate into antibody-secreting cells with brief life spans and others persist as long-lived memory cells.

Sequence of Events in Antibody Production in Response to Protein Antigens

Now that we have discussed the cellular interactions involved in humoral immune responses and the mechanisms of B cell stimulation, it is useful to summarize the sequence of events that occur in such responses *in vivo*. The process of antibody production is best defined in the spleen, but it is probably similar in lymph nodes and other lymphoid tissues.

The principal steps in antibody responses to protein antigens are the following (Fig. 9–8).

1. Within 1 or 2 days after administration of a protein antigen to a naive individual, the antigen is presented by macrophages and dendritic cells to naive, antigen-specific CD4$^+$ helper T lymphocytes in the T cell–rich zones of the spleen and lymph nodes. Clusters of activated T cells accumulate in these regions. Such T cells have been induced to express the CD40 ligand, gp39, and proceed to develop into cytokine-producing effector cells.

2. Specific B lymphocytes also encounter the antigen, may be stimulated to enter the cell cycle, and present peptide fragments of the antigen to activated helper T cells. As a result of cell-cell contact mediated by CD40 and gp39, as well as exposure to T cell cytokines, the antigen-presenting B cells begin to proliferate and differentiate into antibody-secreting cells. It is not known if the encounter between antigen-specific T and B cells is entirely random, or if it is regulated by stimuli that control cell migration and intercellular adhesion. These are the cognitive and activation phases of humoral immune responses. Small foci of antigen-producing B cells develop at the edges of T cell–rich zones, e.g., the periarteriolar lymphoid sheaths in the spleen, close to the sites of T cell stimulation (Fig. 9–9). Each focus of activated B cells is oligoclonal, being derived from one or a few lymphocytes.

TABLE 9–3. Heavy Chain Isotype Switching Induced by Cytokines

B Cells Cultured With		Ig Isotype Secreted (Per Cent of Total Ig)				
Polyclonal Activator	Cytokine	IgM	IgG1	IgG2a	IgE	IgA
LPS	None	85	2	<1	<1	<1
LPS	IL–4	70	20	<1	5	<1
LPS	IFN-γ	80	2	10	<1	<1
LPS	TGF-β and IL-5	75	2	<1	<1	15

Purified IgM$^+$ IgD$^+$ mouse B cells cultured with the polyclonal activator LPS, and various cytokines, show selective switching to different heavy chain isotypes. (The values of the isotypes shown are approximations, and do not add up to 100 per cent because not all were measured.)

Abbreviations: Ig, immunoglobulin; LPS, lipopolysaccharide; IL, interleukin; TGF, transforming growth factor; IFN, interferon.

Courtesy of Dr. Robert Coffman, DNAX Research Institute, Palo Alto, California.

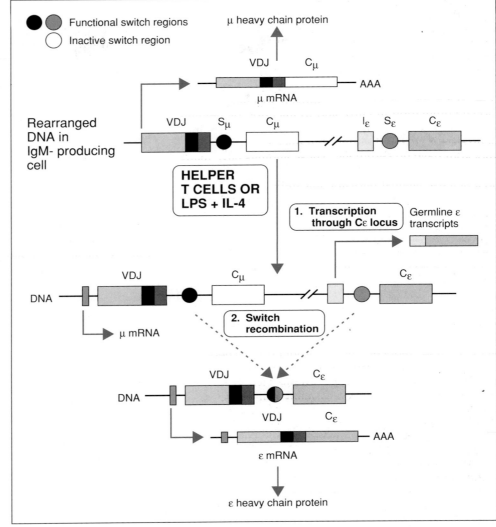

FIGURE 9–7. Mechanism of heavy chain class (isotype) switching induced by IL-4. *IL-4, acting in concert with helper T cells or a polyclonal activator such as LPS, initiates transcription through the ε switch region (S_ϵ), an adjacent gene segment called the initiator region (I_ϵ), and the downstream C region (C_ϵ). This is followed by switch recombination of the VDJ complex with the C_ϵ locus, and production of a full-length ε mRNA. (From Lederer, J. A., and Abbas, A. K. Cytokines in specific immune responses: regulators of lymphocyte growth and differentiation and activators of effector cells. In M. M. Frank, K. F. Austen, H. N. Claman, and E. R. Unanue (eds.). Samter's Immunological Diseases, 5th ed. Little, Brown & Co., Boston, 1994, with the permission of the publishers.)*

3. Heavy chain isotype switching is also seen in these foci of B cells, having been stimulated by helper T cell–derived cytokines.

4. Within 4 to 7 days after immunization, some of the foci of B cells develop into **germinal centers within lymphoid follicles,** and more activated B cells migrate into germinal centers. The development of germinal centers is a T cell–dependent process, perhaps triggered by gp39-CD40 interactions, and T cell–deficient individuals do not have germinal centers. Scattered CD4⁺ T cells are usually found within germinal centers, but no cytokine has been identified as being required for germinal center formation.

5. Three important changes occur in the B cells in germinal centers. First, the cells undergo rapid proliferation. It is estimated that the doubling time of germinal center B cells is 6 to 12 hours, so that within 5 days a single B cell may give rise to almost 5000 progeny. Second, the Ig V genes of these proliferating B cells are the targets of somatic hypermutation. It has been postulated that interactions with cells present in the germinal centers, such as helper T lymphocytes or follicular dendritic cells, may stimulate Ig mutations, but neither

the stimuli nor the mechanisms of hypermutation are known. The result of somatic hypermutation is that V gene mutations accumulate sequentially in the progeny of the proliferating B cell clones. As these processes are going on, antibodies that have been secreted into the circulation bind to residual antigen and may activate complement. These immune complexes are concentrated on the surfaces of **follicular dendritic cells** by binding to Fc and C3b receptors. (Follicular dendritic cells are found only in germinal centers, and are different from the dendritic cells that present peptides to CD4⁺ T cells.) Follicular dendritic cells constitutively express a cell surface ligand, vascular cell adhesion molecule-1, that binds activated B cells that express the counterreceptor, the VLA-4 integrin, in a high-affinity state. The third event in the lives of activated B cells is a consequence of the interaction of somatically hypermutated cells with the small amount of antigen being displayed on the follicular dendritic cells (Fig. 9–9). B lymphocytes whose membrane Ig molecules are able to recognize the displayed antigen with high affinity are selected to survive, and this is the basis for **affinity maturation** of the antibody response (see Chapter 4,

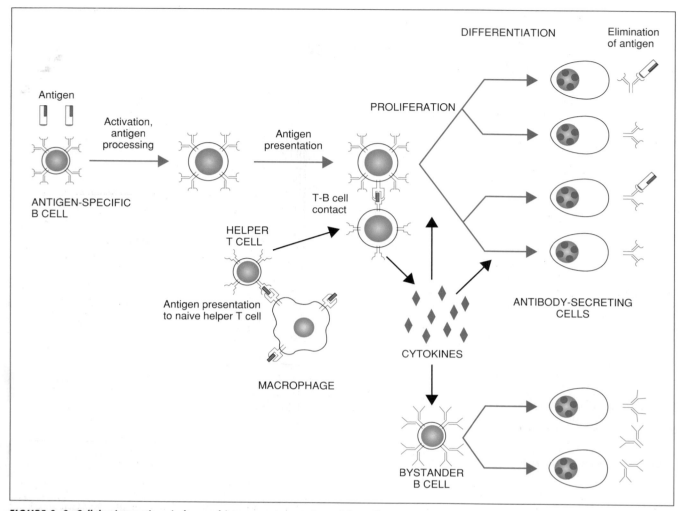

FIGURE 9–8. Cellular interactions in humoral immune responses to protein antigens. *Helper T cells, cytokines, and accessory cells, such as macrophages, act at different stages in humoral immune responses.*

Fig. 4–15). If, on the other hand, somatic mutations have generated B cell antigen receptors that no longer recognize the antigen, these cells die by a process of programmed cell death (apoptosis). Not surprisingly, germinal centers are sites of tremendous cell death, and macrophages present in germinal centers phagocytose and destroy these dead cells. Germinal centers gradually decrease in size and number by 1 to 2 weeks following immunization. After this time, affinity maturation also ceases unless the antigen is re-administered.

6. Some of the high-affinity B cells that exit germinal centers enter the areas adjacent to lymphoid follicles, where they develop into antibody-secreting cells. Plasma cells are found in the red pulp of the spleen and the deep cortex and medulla of lymph nodes. Antibody-secreting cells also migrate to and reside in the bone marrow, and at 2 or 3 weeks after immunization the marrow may be a major site of antibody production. Secreted antibodies enter the circulation, but most antibody-producing cells do not circulate actively and have finite life spans (probably a few weeks). Circulating antibodies bind antigens to initiate the effector phase of humoral immune responses. Other high-affin-

ity B cells that exit germinal centers develop into memory cells that circulate in the blood, and may live for months or years without overt antigenic stimulation. Memory cells typically bear high-affinity (mutated) antigen receptors and Ig molecules of switched isotypes more commonly than do naive B lymphocytes.

7. These processes are greatly accelerated in secondary antibody responses, because of the presence of memory cells that home to germinal centers and the rapid formation of immune complexes that can be concentrated by follicular dendritic cells.

Factors that Determine the Nature of Humoral Immune Responses to Protein Antigens

Different types of antigens and forms of antigen exposure stimulate antibody responses with distinct characteristics. The principal factors that determine the nature of antibody responses are the following:

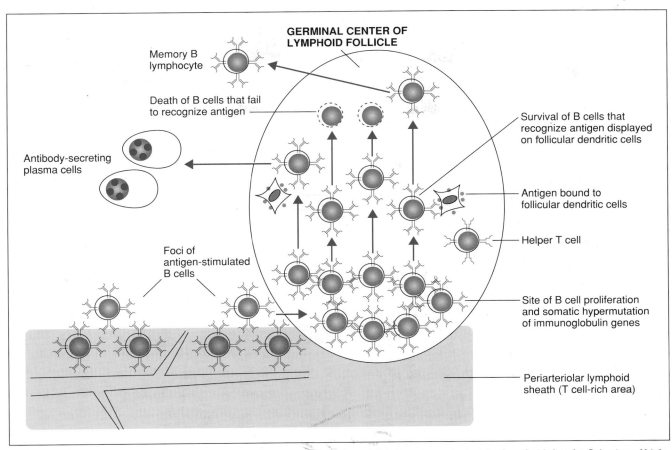

FIGURE 9–9. Antibody production in the spleen. *Foci of antigen-stimulated B cells develop near periarteriolar lymphoid sheaths. Selection of high-affinity antigen-specific B cell occurs in germinal centers, and antibody-secreting cells as well as memory cells exit germinal centers.*

1. *Types of cytokines produced:* An important general principle that has emerged from the study of cytokines is that the nature and magnitude of immune responses, such as antibody responses, are influenced by the relative amounts of different cytokines produced at sites of lymphocyte stimulation. This is because, as described above, various cytokines have selective effects on B cells, especially on heavy chain class switching, and because combinations of different cytokines may be synergistic or antagonistic.

Studies first done in mice, and subsequently in humans and other species, have shown that different antigens and immunization conditions preferentially activate subpopulations of CD4⁺ helper T cells that produce distinct sets of cytokines and, as a result, perform distinct effector functions. The two best-defined subsets of helper T cells are "T_H1" cells, which secrete IL-2 and IFN-γ, and "T_H2" cells, which produce IL-4, IL-5, IL-10, and IL-13. T_H1 cells are the principal inducers of cell-mediated immunity and delayed-type hypersensitivity reactions, which are often seen in infections by intracellular microbes (see Chapter 13). T_H2 cells, on the other hand, stimulate IgE production (because of IL-4) and eosinophilic inflammation (because IL-5 is a powerful eosinophil-activating cytokine). The development and properties of these T cell subsets will be discussed in more detail in Chapter 10. The important point here is that because T_H1 and T_H2 cells produce different cytokines that have different effects on B lymphocytes, preferential activation of one or the other subset by various antigens leads to qualitatively distinct humoral immune responses. This is of considerable importance for host defense mechanisms. For instance, the antibody response stimulated by T_H1 cells is dominated by IgG2a because of IFN-γ–mediated switching to this isotype. IgG2a opsonizes antigens for phagocytosis, since it activates complement and binds to FcγRI receptors on macrophages. Thus, this isotype participates in phagocyte-mediated host defense, complementing the macrophage activation induced by IFN-γ (see Chapter 13). Antibody isotypes triggered by T_H2 cells, such as IgE and IgG1 (in mice), or IgG4 (in humans), neither activate complement nor bind to macrophage Fc receptors. Rather, these antibodies are involved in host defense mediated by non-phagocytic effector cells, such as mast cells and eosinophils (see Chapter 14).

2. *Site of antigen exposure:* Antigens that enter the blood or lymph, and subsequently the peripheral lymphoid organs, such as the spleen and lymph nodes, induce the production of antibodies of multiple isotypes. Orally administered and inhaled antigens tend to stimulate high levels of IgA production, because B cells in mucosal lymphoid tissues readily switch to IgA. The

mechanisms of IgA production in mucosal tissues are discussed in Chapter 11.

3. *Nature of the antigenic stimulus:* Large doses of antigens, especially if they are administered systemically without adjuvants, often inhibit antibody production by inducing tolerance, or unresponsiveness, in helper T or B lymphocytes. The phenomenon of immunologic tolerance to foreign antigens is described in Chapter 10.

4. *Many of the features of secondary responses to protein antigens, and the differences from primary responses (see Table 9–1), are due to the increased activities of helper T cells that are stimulated by the first exposure to antigen.* Thus, heavy chain class switching, which is typical of secondary responses, is due to helper T cells and their cytokines. Affinity maturation, which increases with repeated antigenic stimulation, is also thought to be secondary to helper T cell–induced B cell activation. These features are usually seen in responses to protein antigens, because only proteins stimulate specific helper T cells. The more rapid and larger secondary response is because of the expansion of antigen-specific lymphocyte clones induced by prior antigenic stimulation.

THYMUS-INDEPENDENT ANTIGENS

The requirement for helper T cells explains why thymus-dependent protein antigens do not induce antibody responses in T cell–deficient animals, such as congenitally athymic (nude) or neonatally thymectomized mice. In contrast, many non-protein antigens stimulate antibody production in athymic mice, and these antigens are termed **thymus-independent** (TI). Their properties and the features of the antibody responses they induce are summarized in Table 9–4.

The most important TI antigens are polysaccharides, glycolipids, and nucleic acids, all of which induce specific antibody production in T cell–deficient animals. These antigens cannot be processed and presented in association with MHC molecules, and, therefore, they cannot be recognized by T cells. Most TI

antigens are polymeric, being composed of multiple identical antigenic epitopes; examples include dextrans, pneumococcal polysaccharide, and Ficoll. Such multivalent antigens may induce maximal cross-linking of membrane Ig on specific B cells, leading to activation without a requirement for cognate T cell help. B cell activation by TI antigens is the one situation in which membrane Ig-mediated signal transduction may be critical for subsequent responses of the cells. It is not clear if B cell responses to TI antigens are dependent on any second signals. Experiments with mice suggest that antibody responses to polysaccharides do require the presence of small numbers of macrophages and/or helper T cells. These cells may secrete cytokines that function as second signals for B cell responses to TI antigens, but neither the nature of these cytokines nor the mechanism(s) leading to their production are completely understood. Responses to most TI antigens consist largely of IgM antibodies of low affinity, and do not show significant heavy chain class switching, affinity maturation, or memory. However, some TI antigens do induce Ig isotypes other than IgM, probably because these antigens stimulate cytokine production. For instance, in humans the dominant antibody class induced by pneumococcal capsular polysaccharide is IgG2.

The practical significance of TI antigens is that many bacterial cell wall polysaccharides belong to this category, and humoral immunity is the major mechanism of host defense against such bacterial infections. For this reason, individuals with congenital or acquired deficiencies of humoral immunity are especially susceptible to life-threatening infections with encapsulated bacteria, such as pneumococcus, meningococcus, and *Haemophilus.* The circulation of normal individuals contains **"natural antibodies,"** which are apparently produced without overt antigen exposure. Most natural antibodies are low-affinity anti-carbohydrate antibodies, postulated to be specific for bacteria that colonize the gastrointestinal tract. Such antibodies may be physiologically important examples of responses to TI antigens. Antibody responses to TI antigens may occur at particular anatomic sites in lymphoid tissues. Macrophages located in the marginal zones of lymphoid follicles in the spleen are particularly efficient at trapping TI antigens, such as polysaccharides, when

TABLE 9–4. Properties of Thymus-Dependent and Thymus-Independent Antigens

Properties	Thymus-Dependent	Thymus-Independent (TI)
Chemical Nature	Proteins	Polymeric antigens, especially polysaccharides; also glycolipids, nucleic acids
Antibody Response in		
Athymic mice	No	Yes
T cell–depleted cultures	No	May be reduced
Features of Antibody Response		
Isotype switching	Yes	No (usually)
Affinity maturation	Yes	No
Secondary response (memory B cells)	Yes	No
Ability to Induce Delayed-Type Hypersensitivity	Yes	No

these are injected intravenously. Such antigens may either persist for prolonged periods on the surfaces of marginal zone macrophages, where they are recognized by specific B cells, or they may be transferred from the marginal zone to the adjacent follicle. Marginal zones are present only in the spleen. This may be the reason why splenectomized individuals have an increased susceptibility to infection by encapsulated bacteria like the pneumococcus, as a result of deficient antibody responses to capsular polysaccharides.

Based on experiments with mice, TI antigens have been classified into two groups. Polysaccharides and the other TI antigens mentioned above are called "TI-2" antigens; rigorous depletion of T cells (and macrophages) abolishes antibody responses to these. The prototypical "TI-1" antigen in mice is lipopolysaccharide (LPS), which stimulates B cells by itself, without a requirement for any other cells. LPS, also called endotoxin, is a major component of the cell walls of many gram-negative bacteria (see Chapter 12). At low concentrations, LPS stimulates specific antibody production. At high concentrations, it is a polyclonal B cell activator, stimulating the growth and differentiation of virtually all B cells without binding to the membrane Ig. It is postulated that a component of the LPS molecule binds to B cells and directly activates the cells, i.e., the antigen provides both the first and the second signals needed for B lymphocyte activation. However, neither the nature of the B cell receptor for LPS nor the biochemical mechanisms of LPS-induced B cell stimulation is clearly established. Also, LPS is a polyclonal B cell activator in mice but not in humans and most other species. In all species, LPS is one of the most potent activators of macrophages known (see Chapter 12).

ROLE OF ACCESSORY CELLS IN ANTIBODY RESPONSES

One of the first experiments suggesting the requirement for accessory cells in the responses of lymphocytes to antigens demonstrated that if spleen cells from unimmunized mice were depleted of adherent cells, they would not secrete antibody when stimulated by a model T cell–dependent antigen, sheep red blood cells. Responsiveness was restored by the addition of non-lymphoid cells such as macrophages, or, as shown later, by dendritic cells.

Macrophages and other accessory cells can perform various functions in the induction of humoral immunity.

1. *Macrophages and dendritic cells might be necessary for presenting antigens to helper T lymphocytes,* thereby inducing both cytokine secretion by and clonal proliferation of the T cells. As discussed above, this is probably most important for primary antibody responses, because in secondary responses B lymphocytes are available for antigen presentation to memory T cells. There is no evidence that B lymphocytes themselves need to recognize antigens presented by accessory cells, although this may occur *in vivo* with polysaccharides, which bind to marginal zone macrophages, and in secondary responses when follicular dendritic cells bind large amounts of opsonized antigens.

2. *Macrophages secrete cytokines,* which may augment the proliferation of both B and T lymphocytes. IL-1 and TNF may directly stimulate B cell proliferation, and IL-6 is a growth and differentiation factor for B cells.

Another accessory cell whose specialized function in humoral immune responses has been described above is the follicular dendritic cell. These cells can store and display antibody-complexed antigens for many years, and may be important for the periodic restimulation of memory B lymphocytes.

SUMMARY

Antibody responses are initiated by the interaction of antigen with specific membrane Ig molecules on B lymphocytes. This interaction stimulates resting B cells to enter the cell cycle, presumably via the production of a variety of intracellular second messengers. Thymus (or T cell)–dependent protein antigens are processed by the B cells and presented in association with class II MHC molecules to antigen-specific, class II MHC–restricted CD4$^+$ helper T lymphocytes. Activated helper T cells express a molecule called gp39 that specifically recognizes CD40 on B cells, and this interaction delivers activating signals to the B cells. In addition, helper T lymphocytes secrete cytokines that amplify antibody responses and regulate their nature. Different cytokines induce proliferation of B cells, secretion of antibody, and heavy chain isotype switching. Antigen-stimulated B cells undergo affinity maturation in the germinal centers of lymphoid follicles, and develop into antibody-secreting cells or long-lived memory cells. Accessory cells like macrophages may play a role, particularly in primary antibody responses, by presenting antigens to T cells to initiate T cell stimulation, and by secreting cytokines that promote the expansion and differentiation of both B and T lymphocytes.

Thymus-independent antigens induce antibody responses without the participation of antigen-specific helper T cells. Most TI antigens are polymeric polysaccharides, glycolipids, and nucleic acids that efficiently cross-link membrane Ig on B cells and may require small numbers of T cells (which are not antigen-specific and presumably provide cytokines) for inducing optimal antibody production by the B cells.

Elucidation of the mechanisms operative in humoral immunity is central to the understanding and potential treatment of disorders associated with excessive or deficient antibody production. In addition, the ability to specifically alter patterns of Ig gene expression by defined external stimuli provides valuable models for analyzing the mechanisms of signal transduction in B lymphocytes, and may lead to paradigms that are applicable to diverse biologic systems.

SELECTED READINGS

Banchereau, J., and F. Rousset. Human B lymphocytes: phenotype, proliferation, and differentiation. Advances in Immunology 52:125–262, 1992.

Clark, E. A., and P. J. L. Lane. Regulation of human B-cell activation and adhesion. Annual Review of Immunology 9:27–66, 1991.

Finkelman, F. D., J. Holmes, I. M. Katona, J. F. Urban, M. P. Beckmann, L. S. Park, K. A. Schooley, R. L. Coffman, T. R. Mosmann, and W. E. Paul. Lymphokine control of *in vivo* immunoglobulin isotype selection. Annual Review of Immunology 8:303–333, 1990.

Germinal centers in the immune response. Immunological Reviews volume 126, 1992 [entire volume devoted to this topic].

Gray, D. Immunological memory. Annual Review of Immunology 11:49–77, 1993.

Lanzavecchia, A. Receptor-mediated antigen uptake and its effect on antigen presentation to class II MHC–restricted T lymphocytes. Annual Review of Immunology 8:773–793, 1990.

Liu, Y.-J., G. D. Johnson, J. Gordon, and I. C. M. MacLennan. Germinal centers in T-cell–dependent antibody responses. Immunology Today 13:17–21, 1992.

MacLennan, I. C. M. The evolution of B-cell clones. Current Topics in Microbiology and Immunology 159:37–63, 1990.

Mosmann, T. R., and R. L. Coffman. Heterogeneity of cytokine secretion patterns and functions of helper T cells. Advances in Immunology 46:111–147, 1989.

Parker, D. C. T cell–dependent B cell activation. Annual Review of Immunology 11:331–360, 1993.

Reth, M. Antigen receptors on B lymphocytes. Annual Review of Immunology 10:97–121, 1992.

Szakal, A. K., H. M. Kosco, and J. G. Tew. Microanatomy of lymphoid tissues during humoral immune responses: structure function relationships. Annual Review of Immunology 7:91–109, 1989.

Vitetta, E. S., R. Fernandez-Botran, C. D. Myers, and V. M. Sanders. Cellular interactions in the humoral immune response. Advances in Immunology 45:1–105, 1989.

REGULATION OF

IMMUNE

RESPONSES

In previous chapters we have discussed how T and B lymphocytes recognize and respond to antigens, concentrating on the cellular and molecular mechanisms involved in antigen recognition and in the activation of antigen-specific clones of lymphocytes. Immune responses are qualitatively and quantitatively heterogeneous—different types of microbes and other antigens tend to stimulate responses with distinct features, and some forms of antigen exposure may be inhibitory rather than stimulatory. Moreover, immune responses are self-limited, and wane with time after antigen exposure. In this chapter, we will discuss the regulation of immune responses, and especially the mechanisms that inhibit and terminate lymphocyte activation.

The regulation of specific immune responses is a complex phenomenon, in which the antigen itself, accessory cells, and lymphocytes all contribute in multiple ways. Several mechanisms also function to prevent lymphocyte activation and to shut off responses that have been initiated. These mechanisms include the following:

1. **Elimination of the antigen** during the effector phase of immune responses

2. **Immunologic tolerance,** which is due to an antigen-induced block in the maturation and/or activation of specific lymphocytes, or death of antigen-specific lymphocytes under particular conditions of antigen exposure

3. Stimulation of populations of lymphocytes, called **suppressor T cells,** whose products inhibit the activation of specific T and B lymphocytes

4. Postulated responses to the idiotypic portions of antigen receptors, which result in **regulatory networks of idiotypes and anti-idiotypes**

5. **Feedback inhibition** of lymphocyte activation by the products of activated lymphocytes, namely antibodies and cytokines

We will first describe the factors that influence the magnitude and nature of immune responses, and then discuss the mechanisms that inhibit specific immunity.

FACTORS THAT DETERMINE THE NATURE AND MAGNITUDE OF IMMUNE RESPONSES

Exposure of the immune system to foreign antigens sets into motion the series of events that lead to lymphocyte activation and the generation of humoral and cell-mediated immunity. Different antigens and conditions of immunization lead to responses that vary both quantitatively and qualitatively. For instance, different antigens preferentially stimulate the production of antibodies of various heavy chain isotypes, activate T cells to produce distinct sets of cytokines, or generate cytolytic T lymphocytes (CTLs) or other effectors of cell-mediated immunity. Such diversity of immune effector mechanisms is important because it enables the immune system to protect an individual from the many distinct types of microbes present in the environment

that are most effectively eliminated by different mechanisms (see Chapter 16).

Three main factors influence the nature and magnitude of specific immune responses: (1) the type of antigen, as well as its dose and route of entry; (2) the numbers and types of accessory cells that initially interact with the antigen and induce lymphocyte activation; and (3) the nature of the responding lymphocytes. In the following section, we will discuss how each of these factors contributes to the development of specific immunity. Although these factors are considered individually, it should be kept in mind that antigens, accessory cells, and lymphocytes act in concert, influence one another in multiple ways, and are not separable in the induction or regulation of immune responses.

The Role of Antigen

Antigens are the obligatory first signals for lymphocyte activation. The nature of the antigen has a significant influence on the type and magnitude of the immune response that develops. These regulatory effects are of many different types:

1. *Chemically different antigens stimulate different types of immune responses.* Whereas protein antigens induce both humoral and cell-mediated immunity, polysaccharides and lipids are incapable of major histocompatibility complex (MHC)–associated presentation, so that they fail to stimulate MHC-restricted T cells and to induce cell-mediated immune responses. Antibody responses to polysaccharides and lipids are typically T cell–independent and consist largely of IgM antibodies (see Chapter 9). Proteins, on the other hand, stimulate isotype switching, affinity maturation, and the generation of memory B cells. Thus, encapsulated bacteria, whose principal immunogens are capsular polysaccharides, usually stimulate low-affinity IgM and some IgG antibodies, and immunity against these microbes is short-lived. In contrast, the protein antigens of some bacteria and most viruses induce strong humoral and cell-mediated immunity and long-lived immunologic memory. This is the reason why vaccination with bacterial capsular polysaccharides induces relatively short-lived protection, whereas individuals who are naturally infected with or actively vaccinated against many viruses remain resistant for many years, and often for life.

2. *The amount of antigen to which an individual is exposed influences the magnitude of the immune response generated.* Optimally immunogenic doses vary, depending on the antigen. In general, however, very large doses or repeated administration of protein antigens tends to induce specific T cell tolerance and inhibit immune responses. Large amounts of polysaccharide antigens may induce tolerance in specific B lymphocytes and thus inhibit antibody production.

3. *The immune response to an antigen varies according to the portal of entry of that antigen.* Antigens that are administered subcutaneously or intradermally are usually immunogenic, whereas large amounts of antigens administered intravenously or orally often in-

duce specific unresponsiveness. Such unresponsiveness has been attributed to tolerance induction in T and/or B lymphocytes or to the stimulation of specific suppressor T cells.

It has also been observed that individuals vary in their responsiveness to different foreign antigenic determinants. Unresponsiveness may be due to the absence of mature antigen-specific lymphocytes. Alternatively, individuals lacking MHC molecules capable of binding a foreign antigenic epitope cannot present this epitope to T cells, so that an immune response may not be induced against this epitope even if specific T cells are present.

The Role of Accessory Cells

As we discussed in Chapters 6 and 7, accessory cells such as macrophages, B lymphocytes, and dendritic cells are essential for the induction of T cell–dependent immune responses. Accessory cells present antigens to MHC-restricted T cells and produce membrane-associated and secreted costimulators that enhance the proliferation and differentiation of T lymphocytes. *Therefore, the presence of competent accessory cells stimulates T cell–dependent immune responses, and their absence leads to deficient responses.* Resting macrophages and naive, unstimulated B lymphocytes are deficient in costimulators. As a result, antigens presented by such antigen-presenting cells (APCs) may fail to stimulate naive CD4$^+$ T cells, and may even induce T cell tolerance (discussed later in the chapter). In contrast, dendritic cells and activated macrophages and B cells do express costimulators, as well as high levels of class II MHC molecules, and function as competent APCs. A postulated mechanism of action of **adjuvants** is to enhance the expression of costimulators on macrophages and other APCs. Because of this, the administration of protein antigens with adjuvants promotes cell-mediated immunity and T cell–dependent antibody production. Vaccines are most effective for generating systemic immunity when administered subcutaneously or intradermally together with adjuvants. Some microorganisms contain adjuvants in their cell walls that influence the type and strength of specific immune responses that these microbes induce. For instance, the cell walls of mycobacteria contain muramyl dipeptide, which is a potent adjuvant and is at least partly responsible for the propensity of mycobacteria to stimulate strong T cell–mediated immune responses.

Accessory cells may influence the development of immune responses by many other mechanisms. The role of MHC alleles expressed by APCs in the binding of antigenic peptides and the induction of T cell responses has been described in Chapter 6. It is also possible that even though an individual expresses MHC alleles capable of binding and presenting many different antigens, some of these antigens are processed and presented optimally by B cells and others by macrophages. In these cases, the magnitude of the immune response will depend on the relative numbers of B cells

and macrophages that are present at the site of antigen administration or in adjacent lymphoid organs. Different APCs may also process the same endocytosed antigen in distinct ways, leading to the expression of different MHC-associated peptide epitopes. As a result, the type of APCs involved in initiating T cell activation may influence the fine specificity of the response to a multideterminant protein antigen. Finally, different subpopulations of T cells may preferentially respond to antigens presented by different accessory cells. Examples of these are mentioned below.

The Types of Responding Lymphocytes

The nature of an immune response reflects the profile of antigen-specific lymphocytes that are stimulated by the immunization. *Lymphocytes, particularly T cells, consist of subpopulations that may be stimulated by different types of antigens and perform different effector functions.* For instance, as discussed in Chapter 6, in viral infections viral antigens are synthesized in infected cells and presented in association with class I MHC molecules, leading to the stimulation of CD8$^+$, class I MHC–restricted CTLs. In contrast, extracellular microbial antigens are endocytosed by APCs, processed, and presented preferentially in association with class II MHC molecules. This activates CD4$^+$, class II MHC–restricted helper T cells, leading to antibody production and macrophage activation but relatively inefficient development of CTLs.

Even within the population of CD4$^+$ helper T cells there are subsets that produce distinct cytokines in response to antigenic stimulation. Because most of the effector functions of helper T cells are mediated by cytokines, cells with distinct patterns of cytokine production perform different functions (discussed in Chapters 13 and 14). It is thought that naive CD4$^+$ T cells produce mainly the T cell growth factor, interleukin-2 (IL-2), upon initial encounter with antigen. Antigenic stimulation may lead to the differentiation of these cells, sometimes into a population called T$_H$0, which produces multiple cytokines, and subsequently into subsets called T$_H$1 and T$_H$2, which have relatively restricted profiles of cytokine production and effector functions (Fig. 10–1). T$_H$1 cells secrete IL-2 and interferon-γ (IFN-γ), which activates macrophages, and are the principal effectors of cell-mediated immunity against intracellular microbes and of delayed type hypersensitivity reactions (see Chapter 13). The antibody isotypes stimulated by T$_H$1 cells are effective at activating complement and opsonizing antigens for phagocytosis (see Chapter 9). Therefore, *T$_H$1 cells trigger phagocyte-mediated host defense.* Infections with intracellular microbes tend to induce the differentiation of naive T cells into the T$_H$1 subset, which promotes phagocytic elimination of these microbes. T$_H$2 cells, on the other hand, produce interleukin-4 (IL-4), which stimulates IgE antibody production, IL-5 (an eosinophil-activating factor), and IL-10 and IL-13 (which, to-

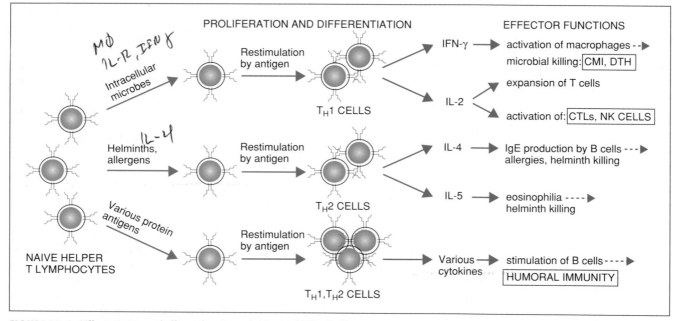

FIGURE 10-1. Differentiation and effector functions of subsets of CD4+ T cells. *(Redrawn from Lederer, J. A., and A. K. Abbas. Cytokines in specific immune responses: regulators of lymphocyte growth and differentiation and activators of effector cells. In M. M. Frank, K. F. Austen, H. N. Claman, and E. R. Unanue (eds.). Samter's Immunological Diseases, 5th ed. Little, Brown & Co., Boston, 1993, with the permission of the publishers.)*

gether with IL-4, suppress cell-mediated immunity). Therefore, *the T_H2 subset is mainly responsible for phagocyte-independent host defense*, e.g., against certain helminthic parasites, which is mediated by IgE and eosinophils (see Chapter 16), and for allergic reactions, which are due to IgE-dependent activation of mast cells and basophils (see Chapter 14). As one would expect, T_H2 cells develop after exposure to helminths and allergens. T_H0, T_H1, and T_H2 subsets were originally identified among cloned lines of mouse $CD4^+$ helper T cells. However, T cells that fit the cytokine patterns of these subsets have been found among uncloned populations of helper T cells in humans and experimental animals, especially in secondary or chronic immune responses to different types of antigens.

An important question that arises is why do different antigens stimulate the differentiation of naive helper T cells into a particular subset of effector cells. The preferential development of T_H1 and T_H2 subsets in response to different types of microbes or other antigens is not because these populations represent distinct lineages with distinct specificities. This is supported by the finding that naive $CD4^+$ cells from mice that express a single T cell receptor (TCR) as a transgene can be induced to develop into any of the subsets. Rather, *the conditions of antigen stimulation are the principal determinants of the pattern of differentiation of $CD4^+$ T cells*. The three factors that play major roles in driving naive $CD4^+$ cells toward T_H1- or T_H2-dominated populations are cytokines, the type of APCs, and the nature and amount of antigen. First, the cytokines that are produced early after antigen exposure, and which antigen-responsive T cells encounter during their differentiation, influence which subset is mainly induced (Table 10–1). IL-12 and IFN-γ promote the de-

velopment of T_H1 cells, and microbes that stimulate macrophages to produce IL-12 or natural killer (NK) cells to produce IFN-γ induce T_H1-dominated responses. In contrast, IL-4 stimulates differentiation toward T_H2 cells, and some parasites, such as helminths, may induce early IL-4 production. Second, the differentiation of $CD4^+$ T cells may be regulated by the type of APC that presents antigen. Activated macrophages are

TABLE 10–1. Factors That Control the Differentiation of $CD4^+$ T Cells

Naive $CD4^+$ T Cells Stimulated with	Cytokines Produced by Differentiated T Cells	
	IFN-γ	IL-4
Antigen + APCs	+ +	+ +
Antigen + APCs + IL-4	—	+ + +
Antigen + APCs + anti–IL-4 Ab	+ +	—
Antigen + APCs + IFN-γ	+ +	—
Antigen + APCs + IL-12	+ + +	—
Antigen + APCs (activated macrophages)	+ + +	—
Antigen + APCs (activated macrophages) + anti–IL-12 Ab	+	+

Naive $CD4^+$ T cells are isolated from TCR transgenic mice, which express a TCR specific for one antigen that they are not exposed to. The T cells are cultured with the specific antigen and APCs, with various cytokines or cytokine antagonists. Following 4 or 5 days, during which the T cells differentiate, the cells are restimulated with antigen + APCs, and cytokine production is assayed. IFN-γ secretion indicates differentiation to T_H1 cells, and IL-4 indicates T_H2 cells.

Abbreviation: AB, antibody.

especially potent at stimulating differentiation along the T_H1 pathway, in part because they are major sources of IL-12. This may provide a functionally useful bi-directional interaction, since macrophages induce the development of IFN-γ–producing T_H1 cells and are in turn activated by this cytokine. Third, the affinity with which naive T cells recognize antigen, or the concentration of MHC-associated peptide antigen to which the T cells are exposed, may also influence the relative development of T_H1 and T_H2 subsets. The mechanisms of these antigen-mediated effects are not understood. Considerable effort is currently being devoted to understanding the stimuli and mechanisms of differentiation of CD4$^+$ lymphocytes, because of the importance of these cells in controlling the nature of immune responses to infectious agents and other antigens.

Thus, many features of antigens, accessory cells, and lymphocytes determine the magnitude of specific immune responses (Table 10–2). In addition, different antigens and immunization conditions preferentially activate distinct subpopulations of lymphocytes, thus giving rise to responses with distinct characteristics.

TABLE 10–2. Factors That Determine the Nature and Magnitude of Immune Responses

	Factors That Favor	
	Stimulation of Immune Responses	*Inhibition or Lack of Immune Responses*
COGNITIVE PHASE		
Lymphocyte repertoire	Diversity of lymphocyte receptors for foreign antigens	Deletion of self-reactive lymphocytes
Antigen presentation	Presence of MHC molecules capable of binding processed antigens	Absence of MHC molecules capable of binding certain antigenic determinants
INDUCTION AND ACTIVATION PHASE		
Features of antigen		
Nature	Immunogenic forms	Tolerogenic forms
Amount	Optimal doses vary for different antigens	High doses favor tolerance
Portal of entry	Subcutaneous, intradermal	Intravenous, oral
Adjuvants	Recruitment and activation of accessory cells, induction of costimulators	Antigens without adjuvants are non-immunogenic or tolerogenic
Accessory cells	Presence of costimulators (for T cells)	Absence of costimulators
Antigen-specific T cells	Helper T cells	Suppressor T cells
Anti-idiotypic immune responses	Can be stimulating or inhibitory	Can be stimulating or inhibitory
Antibodies	Enhance antigen uptake and presentation by macrophages	Antibody feedback
Cytokines	Positive amplification loops	Antagonistic effects of different cytokines; immunosuppressive effects

MECHANISMS THAT INHIBIT IMMUNE RESPONSES

One of the cardinal features of specific immune responses is that normally such responses are self-limited. After exposure to an antigen, the immune response to that antigen develops following a brief lag period, reaches a peak, and gradually declines in intensity. *The principal reason why every normal immune response is self-limited is that the response eliminates the antigen that is the necessary first signal for lymphocyte activation.* In addition, the products of lymphocyte activation, such as cytokines and antibodies, are secreted for brief periods after antigen recognition and have short half-lives. The effector cells that develop as a result of antigen-stimulated lymphocyte differentiation, such as plasma cells and fully differentiated CTLs, are also short-lived and not self-renewing. Although memory cells survive for prolonged periods, they are functionally quiescent, and need antigenic stimulation to become effector cells. All these features contribute to the self-limitation of immune responses. In addition, as we shall discuss later in this chapter, stimulation of the immune system by antigens triggers mechanisms whose principal function is to inhibit lymphocyte activation. Such mechanisms lead to feedback inhibition of immune responses. Self-regulation is an important property of the immune system, because it ensures that immune responses persist only as long as they are needed, and it allows the system to respond to new antigens to which the individual is exposed.

IMMUNOLOGIC TOLERANCE TO FOREIGN ANTIGENS

The best defined mechanism of inhibition of immune responses is lymphocyte tolerance. Lymphocyte activation and tolerance are the two possible results of specific recognition of antigens by lymphocytes. Tolerance results from the interaction of antigens with antigen receptors on lymphocytes under conditions in which the lymphocytes are not activated but instead are killed or rendered unresponsive. Antigens that induce tolerance are called **tolerogens,** to be distinguished from **immunogens,** which generate immune responses. Tolerance to self antigens is a fundamental property of the immune system, and its loss leads to autoimmune diseases (see Chapter 19). Normally, all self antigens act as tolerogens. Many foreign antigens can be immunogens or tolerogens, depending on their physicochemical form, dose, and route of administration. Exposure of an individual to immunogenic antigens stimulates specific immunity, and for most immunogenic proteins subsequent exposures generate enhanced secondary responses. In contrast, exposure to a tolerogenic antigen not only fails to induce specific immunity but also inhibits lymphocyte activation by subsequent administration of immunogenic forms of the same antigen (Fig. 10–2). *This antigen-induced, im-*

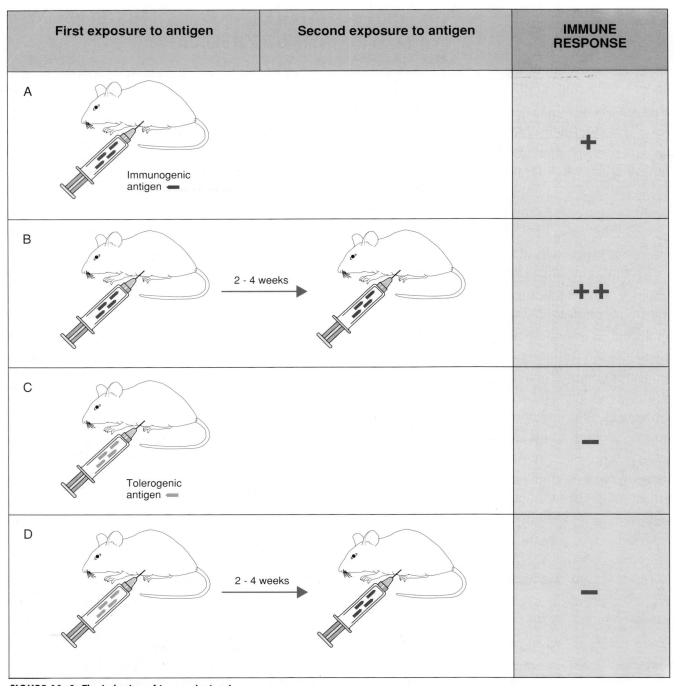

FIGURE 10–2. The induction of immunologic tolerance. *An immunogenic antigen stimulates a specific immune response (A) and a stronger secondary response upon subsequent immunization (B). A tolerogenic form of the same antigen does not induce an immune response (C) and prevents the response to subsequent immunization with the immunogenic antigen (D).*

munologically specific inactivation of lymphocytes is the hallmark of all forms of tolerance.

The mechanisms responsible for inducing and maintaining lymphocyte tolerance are important for several reasons:

1. Tolerance to self antigens protects the individual from harmful autoimmune reactions.

2. Exposure of an individual to foreign antigens in particular ways may lead to tolerance, and a subsequent failure to respond to the antigen.

3. A balance between lymphocyte activation and tolerance may influence the magnitude of specific immune responses.

4. Strategies for selectively inducing tolerance to defined antigens are now being tested for the treatment of autoimmune and allergic diseases, and for preventing the rejection of organ transplants.

In this section we will discuss tolerance to foreign antigens. Self-tolerance is described in Chapter 19, in the context of autoimmune diseases. Despite this divi-

sion, it is likely that the biochemical mechanisms of lymphocyte tolerance are essentially the same whether the tolerogen is a self antigen or a foreign antigen.

The classical studies of Peter Medawar and his colleagues in the 1950s demonstrated, for the first time, that tolerance was an immunologic phenomenon that could be analyzed experimentally. They showed that a mouse of one inbred strain could be made tolerant to the tissue histocompatibility antigens of a different strain by neonatal injection of lymphoid cells from the second strain. Once it became an adult, the recipient of the neonatal injection would accept a skin graft from the immunizing strain (Fig. 10–3). Moreover, lymphocytes from the recipient would not proliferate when cultured with cells from the donor strain in a mixed leukocyte reaction (see Chapter 17). This induced unresponsiveness to allogeneic molecules was highly specific, since the recipient mouse would reject skin allografts and would respond to stimulator cells from all strains that differed from the donor at the MHC locus.

Medawar's experiments were also the first to formally demonstrate that although adult animals rejected grafts of foreign cells, exposure of immature (neonatal) animals to foreign antigens, in this case allogeneic MHC molecules, induced long-lived and specific unresponsiveness to these antigens. This form of tolerance, although induced by a single injection of foreign cells, is long-lived probably because some of the injected allogeneic cells survive in the recipient, which becomes a chimera. Thus, immature lymphocytes specific for the donor MHC, which are generated throughout the life of the recipient animal, encounter the persisting donor cells, and this leads to tolerance induction.

Later studies showed that not only cell-associated MHC molecules but also soluble antigens could induce specific tolerance in immature lymphocytes, and that some forms of antigens were tolerogenic even for mature lymphocytes. Although the phenomenon of immunologic tolerance has been known for many years, the operative mechanisms are still not fully understood.

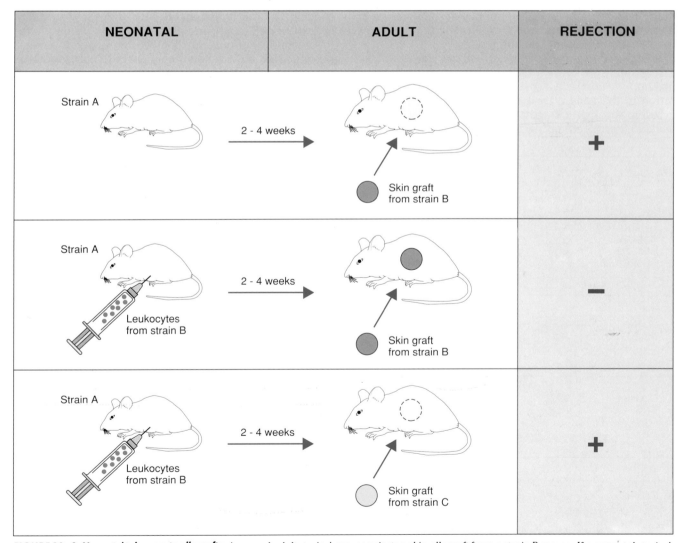

NEONATAL	ADULT	REJECTION
Strain A	2 - 4 weeks → Skin graft from strain B	+
Strain A — Leukocytes from strain B	2 - 4 weeks → Skin graft from strain B	−
Strain A — Leukocytes from strain B	2 - 4 weeks → Skin graft from strain C	+

FIGURE 10–3. Neonatal tolerance to allografts. *A normal adult strain A mouse rejects a skin allograft from a strain B mouse. If a neonatal strain A mouse is injected with strain B leukocytes, once the mouse becomes an adult, it fails to reject a skin graft from strain B. This form of tolerance is immunologically specific because the strain A mouse rejects a graft from a strain C donor. In this example, lymphocytes from the neonatally injected strain A mouse will not respond in vitro to strain B stimulators (in a mixed leukocyte reaction) but will respond normally to strain C stimulators.*

Moreover, much more is known about tolerance in CD4+ T cells than in other lymphocytes, as we shall discuss below.

General Properties of Immunologic Tolerance

Studies done in a variety of experimental systems have established the following general properties of immunologic tolerance.

1. *Tolerance is immunologically specific,* and, therefore, must be due to the deletion or inactivation of antigen-specific T and/or B lymphocytes. Both lymphocyte activation and tolerance are induced by interactions of antigens with the same types of clonally distributed receptors on antigen-specific cells, i.e., membrane immunoglobulin (Ig) on B cells or the T cell receptor on MHC-restricted T cells. Whether such interactions result in activation or tolerance depends on the maturational stage of the specific lymphocytes, the nature of the antigenic stimulus, and (for T cells) the nature of the APCs that present the antigen.

2. *Immature or developing lymphocytes are more susceptible to tolerance induction than are mature or functionally competent cells.* During their normal maturation in the generative lymphoid organs, all lymphocytes go through a stage at which antigen recognition leads to their death or inactivation. At this stage, poten-

tially self-reactive lymphocyte clones encounter self antigens and become tolerant to these antigens (see Chapter 19). This type of tolerance, which is induced in immature lymphocytes within the generative lymphoid organs, has been called "central tolerance."

3. *Tolerance to foreign antigens is induced even in mature lymphocytes when these cells are exposed to antigens under particular conditions.* We have emphasized, in previous chapters, the concept that lymphocyte activation requires two signals. The first signal is antigen, and the second may be costimulators for T cells, or T cell help for B lymphocytes and CTLs (see Chapters 7 and 9). Tolerance may be induced if the first signal, i.e., antigen binding to antigen receptors, directly inactivates specific lymphocytes, or if lymphocytes encounter antigen in the absence of second signals. Tolerance induced in mature lymphocytes that encounter antigens in peripheral tissues has been called "peripheral tolerance."

Immunologic tolerance results from two possible consequences of the encounter of clones of antigen-specific T and B lymphocytes with antigen: **clonal deletion,** or cell death, and **clonal anergy,** or functional inactivation without cell death (Fig. 10–4). It is also possible that an individual may develop unresponsiveness to a particular antigen despite the presence of mature, antigen-responsive lymphocytes. In these situations, the growth and differentiation of immunocompetent lymphocytes may be actively inhibited by other mechanisms, such as suppressor T cells. Thus,

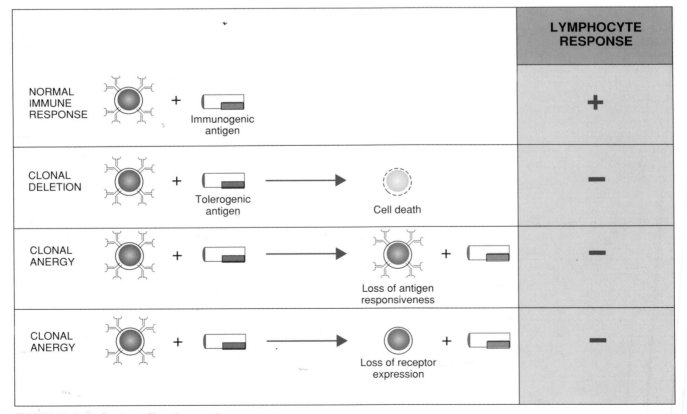

FIGURE 10–4. Mechanisms of lymphocyte tolerance. *A tolerogenic antigen may induce unresponsiveness in the antigen-specific clone of lymphocytes by causing cell death, blocking functional activation, or inhibiting antigen receptor expression.*

failure of an individual's immune system to respond to an antigen may be due to any combination of the absence or inactivation of T and/or B lymphocytes and the inhibitory effects of suppressor cells. We will first discuss how T and B lymphocytes are deleted or rendered unresponsive by interacting with tolerogenic antigens in peripheral tissues; regulation by suppressor cells is discussed later in this chapter.

Mechanisms of Peripheral T Lymphocyte Tolerance

Tolerogenic forms of protein antigens may inhibit specific immune responses by inducing tolerance in CD4$^+$ helper T cells. The best-documented mechanism of peripheral T cell tolerance is clonal anergy. *Several types of antigen exposure induce T cell tolerance*, including high doses of aqueous proteins administered systemically (e.g., intravenously) without adjuvants (called "high-dose tolerance"), protein antigens administered orally (called "oral tolerance"), and repeated administration of low doses of protein antigens without adjuvants (called "low-dose tolerance"). Tolerance in CD4$^+$ T cells may result in inhibition of both cell-mediated and humoral immune responses, because CD4$^+$ helper T cells are critical control elements in both types of responses to protein antigens. T cell tolerance is also induced at lower doses of antigens than is B cell tolerance, and T cell tolerance persists for longer periods.

Based largely on *in vitro* experiments with cloned lines of CD4$^+$ T cells, several mechanisms have been postulated to be responsible for peripheral T cell tolerance.

1. *If CD4$^+$ T cells recognize processed antigens presented by APCs that lack costimulators, the T cells survive but are rendered incapable of responding to the antigen even if it is later presented by competent APCs.* This is a form of clonal anergy. In Chapter 7, we introduced the concept that costimulators such as B7 were required for the development of full T cell responses. Experimentally, anergy can be induced in cloned lines of mouse CD4$^+$ T$_H$1 cells specific for known peptides and class II MHC molecules by exposing the T cells *in vitro* to peptide-MHC complexes on synthetic lipid membranes or on APCs that are treated with chemicals that presumably destroy costimulators (Fig. 10–5). Anergy may be prevented by adding accessory cells that do express costimulators, or by stimulating CD28, the T cell receptor for B7, with specific antibodies. Anergic T cells fail to secrete IL-2 and, therefore, to proliferate in response to antigen stimulation even with competent APCs. In some experimental models, anergy can be prevented if IL-2 is provided exogenously, allowing T cells exposed to the antigen to proliferate. The block of IL-2 transcription in anergic T cells may be due to a failure to activate nuclear factors that bind to the IL-2 promoter and stimulate transcription. The biochemical mechanisms that lead to the induction of anergy are incompletely understood. It is not due to a failure to express antigen receptors or accessory molecules required for T cell antigen recognition and stimulation. Anergy is also a long-lived process—*in vitro*, T cell clones that are rendered anergic may survive for 3 weeks or more in this "dormant" state.

The possibility that peripheral T cell tolerance is also induced *in vivo* if T cells recognize antigens without costimulation is suggested by a number of studies. If mice are given pancreas xenotransplants and treated with B7 antagonists, the grafts are accepted for long periods, even after the treatment is stopped. It is postulated that aqueous antigens administered in large amounts are presented by APCs lacking costimulators, and this is responsible for high-dose tolerance. Antigens can also be targeted for presentation by resting B lymphocytes, which express little or no B7, by administering the antigens conjugated to anti-Ig antibodies. This is another experimental method for inducing peripheral tolerance in CD4$^+$ T cells *in vivo*. The importance of deficient costimulation in oral tolerance and low-dose tolerance is not yet established.

2. Some *APCs may deliver negative or inhibitory signals to T cells* that result in tolerance rather than activation. For instance, human CD4$^+$ T cells become unresponsive when they recognize peptide antigens that are presented by other T cells (which express class II MHC molecules). This form of clonal anergy appears to be unrelated to an absence of costimulators. Whether or not T cell antigen presentation is of physiologic importance in inhibiting immune responses is not yet known. APCs that deliver negative signals to T lymphocytes have been called "veto cells."

3. The *affinity of antigen recognition by T cells* may determine whether the consequence will be activation or tolerance. In one experimental model, a mouse CD4$^+$ T cell clone specific for a particular peptide-class II MHC complex became anergic when cultured with competent (i.e., costimulator-expressing) APCs presenting a modified version of this peptide in which a single residue had been changed. It was postulated, but has not yet been proved, that the variant peptide binds to the T cells with a higher than normal affinity, and the result is tolerance rather than activation.

4. The *local microenvironment in which T cells recognize and respond to antigens* may also influence the balance between activation and tolerance. For instance, if CD4$^+$ T cells are exposed to high concentrations of IL-2 either just before or during antigenic stimulation, the T cells are killed by apoptosis. This may be a mechanism for preventing uncontrolled immune responses.

Although *in vitro* studies are providing valuable insights into the mechanisms of T cell tolerance, there remain important gaps in our knowledge. The biochemical mechanisms of antigen-induced tolerance (clonal anergy or deletion), and the relation of the *in vitro* models to peripheral tolerance *in vivo*, are incompletely understood. It is not known if anergy and deletion are induced by distinct types of antigen-receptor interactions, or if cell death may follow functional unresponsiveness in some situations. In addition, relatively

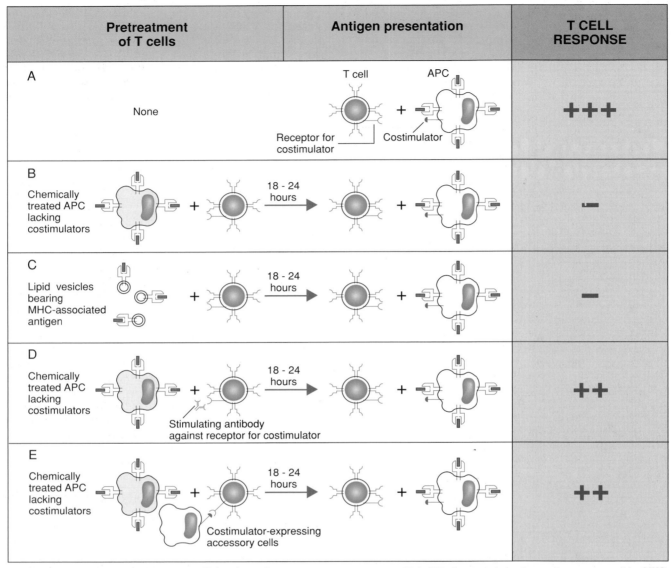

Pretreatment of T cells	Antigen presentation	T CELL RESPONSE
A None	T cell + APC — Receptor for costimulator / Costimulator	+++
B Chemically treated APC lacking costimulators	+ 18 - 24 hours → +	–
C Lipid vesicles bearing MHC-associated antigen	+ 18 - 24 hours → +	–
D Chemically treated APC lacking costimulators	+ Stimulating antibody against receptor for costimulator 18 - 24 hours → +	++
E Chemically treated APC lacking costimulators	+ Costimulator-expressing accessory cells 18 - 24 hours → +	++

FIGURE 10–5. Role of costimulators in T cell clonal anergy. *A peptide antigen-specific CD4+ T cell responds to that antigen presented by MHC-matched antigen-presenting cells (APCs) (A). Exposure of the T cell to the same peptide presented by chemically fixed APCs (B) or on class II MHC-bearing lipid vesicles (C) inhibits subsequent responses to the antigen presented by competent APCs. This form of clonal anergy is prevented by a stimulating antibody against a receptor for a costimulator (e.g., an anti-CD28 antibody) (D), or by costimulator (e.g., B7)-expressing accessory cells (E).*

little work has been done on tolerance in CD8+ T cells. It is thought that if CD8+ cells recognize class I MHC–associated antigens but do not receive T cell help, they are inactivated. This is similar to the postulated mechanism of tolerance induction in B lymphocytes. B7 is also a costimulator for CD8+ cells, but it is not known if antigen recognition by these cells in the absence of costimulation leads to anergy.

Mechanisms of B Lymphocyte Tolerance

Interactions of antigens with specific B lymphocytes (the first signal for B cell activation) in the absence of T cell help (the second signal) lead to toler-ance in the B cells and a failure to produce antibodies. In principle, this is analogous to tolerance in T lympho-cytes. Helper T cells and their secreted cytokines func-tion as "costimulators" for B cells (although by conven-tion the term "costimulator" is not used in this context). There are numerous examples of B cell anti-gen recognition without stimulation by helper cells leading to tolerance. For instance, systemic administra-tion of high doses of polysaccharide antigens or hap-ten-polysaccharide conjugates (which cannot be rec-ognized by T cells) induces tolerance in B lymphocytes, preventing subsequent antibody responses to immuno-genic doses or forms of the antigen. Presumably, the binding of protein antigens to B cells in the absence of T cell help can also lead to B cell tolerance. However, it is not clear to what extent B cell tolerance contributes to deficient antibody responses after administration of tolerogenic protein antigens, because tolerogenic proteins may rapidly inactivate helper T cells and this alone could account for inhibition of antibody responses.

Hypothetically, both clonal deletion and clonal anergy may lead to tolerance in antigen-specific B cell clones (Fig. 10–4). These mechanisms have been documented for B cell tolerance to self antigens, mainly using experimental models such as transgenic mice expressing various defined antigens throughout their development (see Chapter 19). It is not well known which of these mechanisms contributes to B cell tolerance to foreign antigens. The biochemical alterations that lead to B cell tolerance are also poorly understood. In general, tolerance induction in B lymphocytes requires higher concentrations of antigens than in T cells, and anergic B cells recover more rapidly than do anergic T cells after the tolerogen is removed.

It is clear that much remains to be learned about immunologic tolerance to foreign antigens, especially about the molecular mechanisms of tolerance and differences in the biochemical effects of immunogens and tolerogens on specific lymphocytes. The same problem will become apparent when we discuss self-tolerance and autoimmunity (see Chapter 19).

SUPPRESSOR T LYMPHOCYTES

Suppressor T cells are a class of lymphocytes thought to be distinct from helper and cytolytic T lymphocytes, whose function is to inhibit the activation phase of immune responses. The existence of suppressor cells was first demonstrated by experiments done in the late 1960s, using a complicated protocol that involved immunizing thymectomized and bone marrow–transplanted mice. A simpler demonstration of suppressor cell effects is shown in Table 10–3. Animals given an antigen in an immunogenic dose mount specific immune responses. If the antigen is injected under non-immunogenic conditions, e.g., high doses of aqueous antigen administered intravenously, the animals do not respond and may also be rendered unresponsive to subsequent administration of normally immunogenic antigen. This, of course, is often due to the induction of tolerance in specific lymphocytes. In other situations, however, if the lymphocytes from these unresponsive animals are adoptively transferred into syngeneic recipients, the recipients also fail to respond to the normally immunogenic antigen. This inhibition is immunologically specific because the recipients of the adoptive transfer respond normally to a different antigen. Subsequent studies showed that this form of unresponsiveness, which could be transferred from one individual to another, was mediated by T lymphocytes, which were termed **suppressor T cells.** From such studies evolved the hypothesis that the function of suppressor cells is to inhibit the activation of functionally competent antigen-specific T and/or B lymphocytes.

In the 1970s, many experimental systems were used to study suppressor cells, and their excessive or deficient function was invoked as the primary basis for a variety of immunologic abnormalities. However, for reasons that are discussed below, progress in our understanding of suppressor T cells has been slow, so that their significance and even their existence as a distinct class of T cells are doubted by many investigators.

Early studies with cultured human lymphocytes and experimental animals showed that *suppressor T cells have the following properties:*

1. Suppressor T cells are generally induced by the same immunization conditions that induce clonal anergy of lymphocytes, such as high concentrations of protein antigens or chemically reactive haptens administered without adjuvants or injected intravenously. It

TABLE 10–3. Identification of Antigen-Specific Suppressor T Cells

Mice Injected with		Antibody Response to	
T Lymphocytes from	Antigen	Antigen X	Antigen Y
None	Antigen X (immunogenic dose)	+	ND
None	Antigen X (suppressive dose)	—	ND
Mice previously given immunogenic dose of antigen X	Antigen X (immunogenic dose)	+	ND
Mice previously given suppressive dose of antigen X	Antigen X (immunogenic dose)	—	ND
Mice previously given suppressive dose of antigen X	Antigen Y (immunogenic dose)	ND	+

Normal mice respond to an immunogenic dose of antigen X but not to a suppressive dose (e.g., high dose of antigen without adjuvant). If T cells from mice given a suppressive dose of antigen X are adoptively transferred into normal syngeneic recipients, the response of the recipients to antigen X but not to antigen Y is inhibited. Thus, the immunosuppressive dose of antigen X induces specific suppressor T cells.

Abbreviation: ND, not done.

has been postulated that such conditions of immunization favor direct interactions of antigens with lymphocytes without the participation of APCs, and suppressor cells were thought to recognize antigens in the absence of MHC molecules.

2. In many experimental systems, the cells that inhibit immune responses are $CD8^+$. Their growth and differentiation may be dependent on $CD4^+$ cells.

3. In mice, different populations of suppressor T cells have been shown to be specific for antigens, such as proteins or haptens, or for the idiotypic determinants of lymphocyte receptors or secreted antibodies (see below). Most studies with human suppressor T lymphocytes have examined the inhibitory effects of $CD8^+$ cells on the responses of polyclonally stimulated B or T cells, and there are few documented examples of antigen-specific or idiotype-specific human suppressor cells. It is, therefore, difficult to draw general conclusions about the immunologic specificity of suppressor cells in humans.

4. The role of the MHC in the development and activation of suppressor T cells is also unclear. Some studies indicate that antigen recognition by suppressor cells, unlike that by most other mature T lymphocytes, is not MHC-restricted, because suppressor cells can bind to native antigens in the absence of APCs or MHC molecules. Other experiments done in mice indicated that the stimulation of suppressor T cells may be restricted by a region of the class II MHC that was called "I-J" and thought to be located between the I-A and I-E loci based on analyses of various inbred strains. However, sequencing of the entire mouse class II MHC has conclusively demonstrated that there is no DNA coding for a unique "I-J" molecule at this site, and attempts to demonstrate an "I-J"–encoded cell surface protein have generally failed. The explanation for this apparent artifact remains obscure.

5. The inhibitory effects of suppressor T cells are mediated by secreted proteins. Unlike the cytokines produced by other T lymphocytes, which are not antigen-specific, the suppressor factors secreted by murine suppressor T cells were found to have the same antigenic or idiotypic specificities as the T cells themselves. This led to the postulate that suppressor factors are functionally active secreted forms of T lymphocyte receptors, much as secreted and membrane Ig are two forms of the same antigen-specific B lymphocyte product. It is possible that soluble receptor molecules bind to MHC-associated antigens on APCs and competitively inhibit the activation of other T cells. However, it is not known whether this occurs *in vivo* or whether secreted T cell antigen receptors play a significant role in the physiologic down-regulation of specific immune responses.

A major problem in the study of suppressor T cells has been that attempts to purify these cells in numbers sufficient for biochemical analyses of receptors and secreted products or to establish stable cloned lines or hybridomas with specific suppressive activity have been largely unsuccessful. As a result, even basic questions, such as the nature of the receptors expressed by suppressor cells, are unresolved. The few suppressor clones and hybridomas that have been established show variable patterns of T cell receptor gene expression and often do not contain functionally rearranged $\alpha\beta$ or $\gamma\delta$ genes. Isolation, biochemical characterization, and molecular cloning of suppressor factors have also not been successful despite considerable effort. It is, therefore, not possible at present to construct a model for the specificity, mode of action, or function of suppressor T cells that fits all the available data.

Despite these concerns, it is likely that some antigens can stimulate lymphocyte populations whose major effect is the down-regulation of specific immune responses. *It may be that suppressor T cells are not a unique cell population but actually consist of lymphocytes that can inhibit immune responses in different ways.* Like other T lymphocytes, suppressor cells may recognize antigens in a specific manner and may function by various non-specific effector mechanisms. These inhibitory mechanisms could include the following:

1. Suppressor cells may produce an excess of cytokines with inhibitory function. Because cytokines have both stimulatory and inhibitory effects on lymphocytes, the nature and magnitude of the overall immune response are determined by the relative concentrations of different cytokines at the site of immune activation. For instance, transforming growth factor–β (TGF-β) is a powerful inhibitor of T and B cell proliferation. Therefore, an excess of TGF-β can inhibit immune responses, and cells that secrete large amounts of this cytokine may function as suppressor cells. In other situations, different cytokines may inhibit different types of immune responses. For instance, IFN-γ inhibits IL-4–mediated B cell switching to IgE, and conversely, IL-4, IL-10, and IL-13 inhibit IFN-γ–mediated macrophage activation. Therefore, IFN-γ–producing cells (e.g., T_H1 cells) may function as suppressors of IgE production, and cells that produce IL-4, IL-10 and IL-13 (i.e., T_H2 cells) may suppress cell-mediated immunity and delayed hypersensitivity. The important conclusion is that *various T cell populations are capable of suppressing different immune responses,* and there may not exist one unique population of "suppressor cells."

2. Suppressor cells can absorb necessary growth and differentiation factors. Mouse T cells stimulated with the lectin concanavalin A (ConA), a potent polyclonal activator, express large numbers of high-affinity receptors for IL-2, which is a lymphocyte growth and differentiation factor. ConA-activated T cells function as nonspecific suppressors of a variety of immune responses *in vitro*, presumably by absorbing IL-2 and inhibiting the stimulation of other lymphocytes in the culture. To date, however, there is no demonstrated example of such a phenomenon occurring *in vivo* or in cultures of lymphocytes stimulated with antigens. Some T cells may actively secrete cytokine receptors, which may suppress lymphocyte activation by competitively inhibiting the actions of the cytokines. Although soluble forms of receptors for several cytokines, including IL-2 and IL-4, have been detected in the circulation,

the physiologic importance or function of these soluble receptors is not established.

3. Suppressor cells may have cytolytic activity. Antigen-specific $CD8^+$ and some $CD4^+$ T lymphocytes can lyse target cells bearing the stimulating antigens in association with MHC molecules (class I and class II, respectively). This cytolysis results from direct cell-cell contact or the secretion of cytokines such as tumor necrosis factor (TNF) and lymphotoxin that lyse other cells (see Chapter 13). It is possible that CTLs can specifically lyse B and helper T cells that express foreign protein antigenic determinants in association with their MHC molecules and, therefore, serve as targets for the CTLs. This could result in an inhibition of specific immune responses.

4. In addition to the antigen-specific suppressors mentioned above, lymphocytes that inhibit various immune responses nonspecifically, called **natural suppressors,** have been demonstrated in neonatal animals and after total lymphoid irradiation or bone marrow transplantation. These natural suppressors may be related in lineage and function to NK cells (see Chapter 13). Their receptors, mode of induction, and mechanisms of action are incompletely understood. It has, however, been hypothesized that natural suppressors contribute to neonatal self-tolerance and to the immunodeficiency seen following irradiation and in graft-versus-host disease (see Chapter 17).

Such postulated mechanisms for the suppressive effects of certain T lymphocytes largely fit the paradigm wherein the cognitive functions of T cells are antigen-specific but their effector functions are non-specific. However, this does not explain the published reports of antigen-specific or idiotype-specific suppressor factors. It is clear that simple, quantitative experimental systems are needed to better analyze the role of suppressor T lymphocytes in the down-regulation of immune responses and the maintenance of tolerance to self and foreign antigens.

IDIOTYPIC REGULATION

The third mechanism for antigen-initiated immune regulation, in addition to tolerance and suppressor cells, is based on the observation that idiotypes, which are components of antigen receptors, are themselves potentially immunogenic, i.e., immune responses can be induced in an individual against antigen receptors expressed by the lymphocytes of that individual. The specificity of this type of regulation is not for the antigen but for the lymphocyte receptors that recognize the antigen. The idea that cells in an individual can respond to and discriminate between receptors on other similar cells is unique to the immune system, because only the immune system is endowed with sufficient diversity to allow such reciprocal recognition. This is a theoretical idea that continues to fascinate immunologists, although there is little formal proof that regulatory mechanisms based on recognition of idiotypes are important for the physiologic control of immune responses or as primary pathogenic mechanisms in immunologic diseases.

Idiotypes and Anti-idiotypic Immune Responses

The concept of idiotypic regulation evolved from the realization that antigen receptors on T and B lymphocytes are structurally diverse, containing variable regions that differ among different clones. These receptors are also capable of distinguishing between subtle variations in protein sequences, so that lymphocytes can recognize proteins that are only slightly different from self proteins. It is, therefore, conceivable that if one clone of lymphocytes is expanded during an immune response to a foreign antigen, other lymphocytes might specifically recognize and respond to the variable regions of the antigen receptors on the antigen-stimulated clone. Such receptor-specific lymphocytes may then interact with and alter the function of the receptor-bearing clone. The structures or determinants of antigen receptors that distinguish each clone of lymphocytes from all others are called **idiotopes,** and the collection of idiotopes on a given antigen receptor constitutes that receptor's **idiotype** (see Box 3-2, Chapter 3). Immune responses specific for idiotypes are called **anti-idiotypic.** Such responses can either augment or inhibit the activation of lymphocytes that produce the idiotypes. Thus, idiotypes and anti-idiotypes may constitute a system of self-regulation that is both stimulated by and acts on immunocompetent lymphocytes and consequently influences immune responses to foreign antigens.

The discovery of idiotypes came from studies showing that an antibody can be produced against one Ig molecule that would recognize that Ig but no others, even from the same species and inbred strain of animals. Most of these anti-idiotypic antibodies specifically recognize the antigen-combining sites of Ig molecules and, therefore, bind only to Ig molecules with a particular antigenic specificity. Combining site-specific anti-idiotypic antibodies can influence immune responses only against that antigen. In contrast, other anti-idiotypic antibodies have been produced that bind to hypervariable region determinants of Ig molecules that are close to but not within the antigen-combining site. Similar determinants may be present on Ig molecules of different specificities. Therefore, such anti-idiotypes may be induced by one antigen-specific Ig but may bind to immunoglobulins specific for other antigens and may, therefore, regulate immune responses against multiple antigens (Fig. 10–6). These principles, which were first established with secreted antibodies, may apply equally to the variable portions of membrane Ig molecules on B cells and to antigen receptors on T lymphocytes because all such receptors have unique idiotypes. Moreover, idiotypes may stimulate the production of antibodies and also of T cells specific for idiotypic determinants. Therefore, in theory, anti-idiotypic immune responses can be of both types, humoral and cell-mediated.

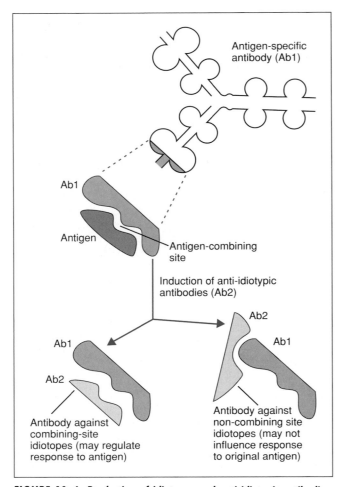

FIGURE 10–6. Production of idiotypes and anti-idiotypic antibodies.
The combining site of an antibody, Ab1, specific for an antigen has a shape complementary to that of the antigen. Anti-idiotypic antibodies (Ab2) against Ab1 may be specific for the combining site of Ab1, in which case they may influence responses to the antigen, or they may be specific for idiotypic determinants of Ab1 that are not part of the combining site.

(Labels in figure: Antigen-specific antibody (Ab1); Ab1; Antigen; Antigen-combining site; Induction of anti-idiotypic antibodies (Ab2); Ab1; Ab2; Antibody against combining-site idiotopes (may regulate response to antigen); Ab2; Ab1; Antibody against non-combining site idiotopes (may not influence response to original antigen))

Regulatory Functions of Idiotypic Networks

The potential regulatory role of anti-idiotypic immune responses was most clearly appreciated by Niels Jerne and enunciated in his **network hypothesis** in 1974. Jerne postulated that an antigen stimulates a specific T and/or B cell response, which in turn induces a wave of complementary anti-idiotypic responses (Fig. 10–6). Idiotype-specific antibodies can recognize the original antigen-specific responding lymphocytes and inhibit or augment their activation. Anti-idiotypic T cells may function in the same manner, perhaps by recognizing idiotypic determinants of the membrane Ig on B cells that is recycled, processed, and presented in association with MHC molecules by the idiotype-producing B cells themselves. According to Jerne's network hypothesis, a steady state in the immune system is maintained by this network of reciprocal idiotypes and anti-idiotypes. The introduction of antigen per-

turbs that balance and leads to detectable immune responses.

The analysis of idiotypic regulation has focused largely on two issues: (1) the production of anti-idiotypic antibodies following immunization with foreign antigens, and (2) the effects of anti-idiotypic antibodies on immune responses to foreign antigens. Much of the experimental evidence in support of the regulatory role of idiotypic interactions has come from experimental systems in which the immune response to an antigen is dominated by one or a few clones of responding lymphocytes. In such monoclonal or oligoclonal responses, one or a few antibodies with their unique idiotypes are dominant, so that their regulation can be manipulated and measured experimentally. A good example is the antibody response to the hapten phosphorylcholine (PC), which is a component of the cell walls of many bacteria. In BALB/c mice, almost 95 per cent of the antibodies produced in response to PC arise from B cells that express one particular V gene. Fortuitously, a chemically induced myeloma of BALB/c mice, called TEPC15 (abbreviated to T15), appears to have arisen by neoplastic transformation of a PC-specific B cell clone that expresses the same V gene. In other words, the antibody response of BALB/c mice to PC is dominated by the T15 idiotype. Since large amounts of this monoclonal Ig can be isolated from the myeloma, it is relatively simple to produce anti-idiotypic antibodies and to use these to measure levels of T15 idiotype following immunization with PC, as well as to alter the level of this idiotype following antigen administration. Similar **dominant idiotypes** are seen in immune responses to several other haptens in different inbred strains of mice. During the 1970s, interactions between idiotypes and anti-idiotypes were investigated in many such experimental systems. The potential importance of regulatory idiotypic interactions is supported by several studies, two illustrative examples of which are the following:

1. Injection of anti-T15 antibody into BALB/c mice inhibits the anti-PC antibody response to PC-coupled antigens, presumably by binding to and inhibiting PC-specific B cells, most of which express the T15 idiotype. In other experimental systems, different anti-idiotypic antibodies have been shown to either enhance or inhibit responses to antigens. Such results formally demonstrate the ability of anti-idiotypic immunity to regulate immune responses to foreign antigens.

2. Immunization of BALB/c mice with PC-containing antigens leads to production of anti-PC antibody expressing the T15 idiotype, followed some days later by the expansion of B cells specific for the T15 idiotype. As the number of anti-idiotypic B cells increases, the number of cells that secrete PC-specific antibody in the spleen decreases. Such findings demonstrate that lymphocytes producing the idiotype (i.e., antibody against the antigen) as well as cells producing the complementary anti-idiotype can be stimulated in the same animal in response to antigen alone, at least in situations in which only one or a few clones of lymphocytes are responding to the antigen.

Despite the demonstrated potential for regulation mediated by anti-idiotypic immune responses, the actual significance of this mechanism for controlling specific immunity is uncertain, for several reasons. Little is known about the role of idiotypic regulation in responses to multideterminant antigens, which presumably stimulate numerous clones of lymphocytes so that no single idiotype is dominant or even detectable. In such multiclonal responses, it is not possible to determine whether any anti-idiotypic antibodies or T cells are stimulated or whether they are at a level sufficient to mediate regulatory functions. Moreover, administration of some anti-idiotypic antibodies specific for a particular monoclonal Ig may induce or regulate immune responses that are unrelated in specificity to that Ig or to the antigen that initiated its production. This is probably because the anti-idiotypic antibody reacts with idiotypic determinants that are located outside antigen-combining sites and are, therefore, present on Ig molecules or antigen receptors of different specificities. In such situations, the effects of idiotypic regulation may be unrelated to the antigen-specific immune response, and their significance is unclear. In the final analysis, it has been difficult to establish the physiologic or pathologic role of idiotypes and anti-idiotypic immunity, and it will continue to be so until techniques are developed to measure and isolate antibodies and T cells with complementary idiotypes in conventional immune responses to a variety of antigens.

ANTIBODY FEEDBACK

Antibodies produced in response to an antigen are capable of inhibiting further immune responses to that antigen. For instance, if antigen-specific antibodies are administered to an animal either shortly before immunization with the target antigen or during an ongoing response, subsequent antibody production is reduced. This phenomenon, called **antibody feedback,** can down-regulate both humoral and cell-mediated immune responses. Feedback mediated by antibodies is important for ensuring that immune responses are self-limited and decrease in intensity with time after immunization.

This negative feedback function of antibodies is due to several mechanisms that may be operative at the same time:

1. *Antibodies eliminate and neutralize antigens and thereby remove the initiating stimulus for the immune response.* An injected antibody, or an antibody formed during an active response, complexes with the antigen. If the antigen-antibody complexes are formed by IgM or certain subclasses of IgG antibodies, they may subsequently activate the complement system (see Chapter 15). The complexes are avidly bound to and eliminated by Fcγ and/or complement receptor-bearing phagocytes and red blood cells. Clearance of antigens by enhancing their phagocytosis is one of the principal effector functions of antibodies. Antibodies also neutralize the stimulatory capacity of antigens by

binding to antigenic determinants and blocking their access to specific membrane Ig on B lymphocytes. This effectively limits B cell activation. For this reason, antibodies that mediate feedback inhibition are also called "blocking antibodies."

2. *Antibodies directly inhibit B lymphocyte activation by binding to Fc receptors on B cells.* Immune complexes composed of an antigen and specific IgG antibody have been shown to inhibit the activation of B lymphocytes specific for that antigen *in vitro* and *in vivo.* Such immune complexes can form in the circulation during a humoral immune response or can be artificially produced *in vitro.* It is thought that immune complex–mediated inhibition results from simultaneous interaction of the antigenic portion of the complex with membrane Ig molecules on specific B cells and of the antibody portion of the complex with Fcγ receptors (FcγRII) on the same cells (Fig. 10–7). This can occur only with multideterminant antigens, in which one epitope of the antigen will participate in the formation of the immune complex and another epitope will be available for binding to membrane Ig on specific B cells. This phenomenon can be mimicked by exposing B cells to intact anti-Ig antibodies whose combining sites bind to the B cell membrane Ig and whose Fc "tails" bind to Fc receptors (Fig. 10–7). It is, in fact, known that B cells are stimulated by F(ab')$_2$ fragments of anti-Ig antibodies or by intact anti-immunoglobulins that do not bind to Fc receptors. In contrast, intact anti-Ig antibodies that bind simultaneously to membrane Ig and to Fc receptors do not activate the B cells but, in fact, inhibit their responses even to polyclonal activators. The interaction of immune complexes or anti-Ig antibodies with Fc receptors on B cells may inhibit the generation of intracellular second messengers, such as increases

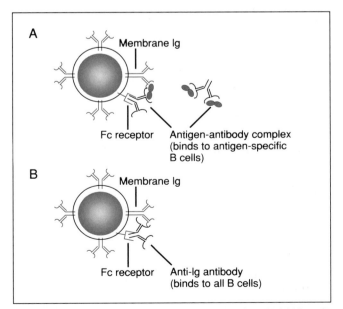

FIGURE 10–7. Antibody feedback: Fc receptor–mediated inhibition of B lymphocytes. *Simultaneous engagement of membrane Ig and Fcγ receptors inhibits B cell activation. This may occur when antigen-antibody complexes bind to antigen-specific B cells (A), or in an experimental situation when an anti-Ig antibody binds to the B cell (B).*

in phosphatidyl inositol metabolites and intracellular Ca^{++} (see Chapter 9). This leads to a block in the response of the B cells and, consequently, down-regulation of humoral immunity. Thus, the major physiologic function of Fcγ receptors on B lymphocytes may be their role in antibody-mediated feedback inhibition.

3. *Antigen-antibody complexes may regulate T cell responses*. It has been suggested that antigen-antibody complexes inhibit helper T cell activation and/or induce antigen-specific suppressor T lymphocytes, although there is little definitive evidence to support either mechanism. Some human peripheral blood T lymphocytes express Fc receptors specific for IgM or IgG antibody. Moreover, Fc receptors specific for different Ig isotypes can be induced on mouse and human T cells by exposing them to high concentrations of that isotype *in vivo* or *in vitro*. Therefore, the potential exists for antibodies or immune complexes to interact with T lymphocytes, although the functions of Fc receptor–bearing T cells in immune responses remain incompletely defined.

4. *Antibodies may induce or perturb regulatory idiotypic networks*. As discussed above, antibodies can trigger complementary anti-idiotypic responses, which may regulate both humoral and cell-mediated immunity.

5. *Antigen-antibody complexes may alter cytokine cascades*. For instance, macrophages exposed to immune complexes produce an IL-1 receptor antagonist that competitively inhibits binding of IL-1 to its receptor (see Chapter 12).

Antibody feedback is an excellent example of self-regulation because the effector molecules produced by the humoral immune response themselves serve to down-regulate the response. A practical application of antibody feedback is in the prevention of **Rh disease** (the main cause of erythroblastosis fetalis), which remains one of the most dramatic examples of successful immunologic intervention for a serious disorder. Rh disease affects infants born of mothers who do not express Rh blood group antigens and fathers who do. The erythrocytes of such a fetus are Rh-positive because of inheritance of the paternal Rh genes. Fetal blood enters the maternal circulation in small amounts during gestation and in substantial quantities during the delivery itself. The immune system of the Rh-negative mother recognizes the fetal Rh as a foreign antigen. Therefore, the mother makes increasing amounts of anti-Rh antibodies with each successive pregnancy. During pregnancy these maternal antibodies cross the placenta, enter the fetal circulation, bind to the fetal erythrocytes, and cause hemolysis, which increases in severity with each pregnancy and can lead to fetal death. In order to prevent this disease, when an Rh incompatibility between the mother and the father is detected, the mother is injected with a large dose of an anti-Rh antibody immediately after each delivery. This antibody presumably binds to fetal Rh$^+$ cells, inhibits the maternal immune response to fetal Rh antigens that are encountered at each delivery, and completely prevents the disease from developing.

REGULATORY EFFECTS OF CYTOKINES

In addition to immune regulation mediated by the products of B cells, cytokines produced by T lymphocytes and accessory cells exert both stimulatory and inhibitory effects on immune responses. These effects are generally not antigen-specific. The **stimulatory functions** of cytokines frequently generate amplification loops that enable the small number of lymphocytes specific for any one antigen to recruit the multiple effector mechanisms required to eliminate that antigen. Cytokine cascades, in which one cytokine enhances the production of or functional responses to others, are described in Chapter 12. Among the most striking examples of cytokine-mediated amplification of immune responses are the bidirectional interactions between T lymphocytes and macrophages. For instance, CD4$^+$T cells secrete IFN-γ, which enhances the expression of class II MHC molecules and costimulators such as B7 on mononuclear phagocytes. Since these T cells recognize foreign antigens in association with class II MHC products and need costimulators for activation, increased expression of class II MHC and costimulatory molecules makes the macrophages better APCs and promotes T cell activation (see Fig. 6–4, Chapter 6). Interleukin-4 (IL-4), secreted by CD4$^+$ T cells, increases class II MHC gene expression in B cells and may similarly enhance the avidity of antigen-specific, MHC-restricted T cell–B cell interactions. Some class I MHC–restricted CTLs secrete IFN-γ, lymphotoxin, and TNF, all of which stimulate class I MHC gene expression in target cells and enhance CTL-target interactions.

Cytokines also have profound **inhibitory effects** that might serve to regulate immune responses. The antagonistic effects of IL-4, IL-10, and IFN-γ on various immune responses, and the immunosuppressive effects of TGF-β, have been mentioned previously. Such phenomena are being appreciated more and more as immunologists begin to analyze the regulatory functions of cytokines.

SUMMARY

Immune responses to foreign antigens are regulated both quantitatively and qualitatively by numerous mechanisms. Factors that influence the induction of specific immunity include the type and amount of antigen, its portal of entry, and the participation of accessory cells in the immune response. These factors may determine which functionally distinct classes of lymphocytes are stimulated, and may influence the balance between lymphocyte activation and tolerance.

Immune responses decline as the antigenic stimulus is eliminated. In addition, several mechanisms serve mainly to inhibit lymphocyte activation. Antigen recognition by specific T lymphocytes in the absence of costimulators, or by B lymphocytes in the absence of T cell help, induces immunologic tolerance. This form of lymphocyte unresponsiveness is mainly due to anergy of antigen-specific clones. Ongoing responses may also be regulated by cells or molecules that are generated during the response itself. These include suppressor T lymphocytes, anti-idiotypic antibodies and T cells, secreted antibodies that mediate feedback inhibition, and cytokines that have inhibitory effects on lymphocyte activation and effector functions. Many of these regulatory interactions are incompletely understood, largely because regulation often has to be studied *in vivo* and involves multiple bidirectional interactions between the cells and molecules of the immune system. Despite this complexity, elucidating the mechanisms of immune regulation is one of the major challenges facing immunologists, because of its obvious importance in normal and abnormal immune responses.

SELECTED READINGS

Bloom, B. R., P. Salgame, and B. Diamond. Revisiting and revising suppressor T cells. Immunology Today 13:131–136, 1992.

Jerne, N. K. Towards a network theory of the immune system. Annals of Immunology (Institut Pasteur) 125C:373–389, 1974.

Miller, J. F. A. P., and G. Morahan. Peripheral T cell tolerance. Annual Review of Immunology 10:51–69, 1992.

Mosmann, T. R., and R. L. Coffman. Heterogeneity of cytokine secretion patterns and functions of helper T cells. Advances in Immunology 46:111–147, 1989.

Nossal, G. J. V. Cellular and molecular mechanisms of B lymphocyte tolerance. Advances in Immunology 52:283–331, 1992.

Rajewsky, K., and T. Takemori. Genetics, expression and functions of idiotypes. Annual Review of Immunology 1:569–607, 1983.

Romagnani, S. Human T_H1 and T_H2 subsets: doubt no more. Immunology Today 12:256–257, 1991.

Schwartz, R. H. A cell culture model for T lymphocyte clonal anergy. Science 248:1349–1356, 1990.

CHAPTER ELEVEN

FUNCTIONAL

ANATOMY OF

LOCAL AND

SYSTEMIC IMMUNE

RESPONSES

Much of our knowledge of specific immune responses is based on *in vitro* analyses of isolated cell populations exposed to antigens or to agents thought to be analogs of antigens, such as polyclonal activators specific for B and T lymphocytes. It is, however, obvious that in order to understand protective and pathologic immune responses, one needs to define how such responses occur *in vivo*, in intact organisms. This chapter will describe our current understanding of the initiation and development of immune responses *in vivo*, with an emphasis on the interactions between the different cells of the immune system and their microenvironments.

As we have seen in Chapter 10, the nature and magnitude of immune responses are determined in large part by the types of responding lymphocytes and accessory cells. In addition, there are several anatomic features of lymphoid cells and tissues that greatly influence the development of specific immune responses.

1. *The immune system has mechanisms for collecting antigens and concentrating them in tissues that are optimal sites of lymphocyte activation.* Most antigens enter the body through the skin and the mucosal epithelia of the gastrointestinal and respiratory tracts. From these sites, "samples" of the antigens are initially transported to and concentrated in regional lymphoid organs and may subsequently enter the systemic circulation. The cognitive and activation phases of primary immune responses are most efficiently initiated in the lymphoid organs that drain the sites of antigen entry. The remainder of the introduced antigens remains at the peripheral site of entry, and the effector phases of immune responses occur at these sites. In secondary T cell responses, the cognitive and activation phases may occur in the peripheral sites as well.

2. *The development of immune responses is greatly influenced by the recirculation, homing, and retention patterns of lymphocytes.* The ability of lymphocytes to exchange between the blood, lymph, lymphoid tissues, and peripheral (non-lymphoid) tissues is essential to enable the immune system to react to antigens virtually anywhere in the body. In addition, different classes of lymphocytes, or lymphocytes at different stages of activation or maturation, have quite distinct patterns of migration and recirculation. This property allows lymphocytes to be concentrated at sites where they most effectively respond to and eliminate foreign antigens.

3. *The special features of different tissues and their constituent cells may result in immune responses with distinct characteristics.* As a result, the nature of immune responses may vary depending on the portal of antigen entry and the anatomic location of lymphocyte activation. Examples illustrating this point will be mentioned throughout the chapter.

4. *Multiple amplification mechanisms enable the few lymphocytes that respond to any one antigen to perform the functions required for eliminating that antigen.* These amplification mechanisms include bidirectional interactions between accessory cells and lymphocytes (see Chapter 10); the ability of various

effector systems, such as complement (see Chapter 15) and cytokines (see Chapter 12), to perform multiple functions; and systems for antigen collection and lymphocyte homing that are described below.

We will begin this discussion of the functional anatomy of immune responses by describing lymphocyte recirculation. We will then discuss the sequence of events in lymphocyte activation *in vivo*, and the distinctive features of immune responses in lymphoid organs and in specialized tissues, such as the cutaneous and mucosal immune systems.

PATHWAYS AND MECHANISMS OF LYMPHOCYTE RECIRCULATION

As described in Chapters 4 and 8, antigen receptors on B and T cells are generated by somatic events that lead to the expression of different and unique receptor genes in each individual progenitor cell. All mature lymphocytes specific for one antigen are descended from a single progenitor, and thus constitute a single clone, bearing identical surface antigen receptors. The immune system contains a large number of lymphocyte clones (estimated to be $>10^9$), and any given foreign antigen, even a complex multideterminant antigen, can be recognized only by a very small percentage of the total lymphocyte pool, on the order of 1 in 100,000 or 1 in 1,000,000 T or B cells. This poses a major logistical problem for the immune system: *How can a small amount of a particular foreign antigen be efficiently recognized by the rare subpopulation of lymphocytes that are specific for that antigen so that a protective immune response can be initiated?* Two mechanisms maximize the efficiency of specific immune responses by bringing antigens and lymphocytes together in specialized tissues, namely the peripheral (secondary) lymphoid organs. First, antigens are collected from their portals of entry or sites of production and concentrated in the peripheral lymphoid organs. Second, lymphocytes pass through these lymphoid organs so that an antigen concentrated in any given organ can be seen by many more lymphocytes than those in residence in that tissue at any one time. This phenomenon of continuous, nonrandom migration of lymphocytes from the blood and lymphatic systems to lymphoid tissues and back to the blood stream is called **lymphocyte recirculation.**

Antigen Collection by the Lymphatic System

The function of collecting antigens from their portals of entry and delivering them to lymphoid organs is performed largely by the lymphatic system (Fig. 11–1). The skin, epithelia, and parenchymal organs contain numerous lymphatic capillaries that absorb and drain interstitial fluid (made of plasma filtrate) from these

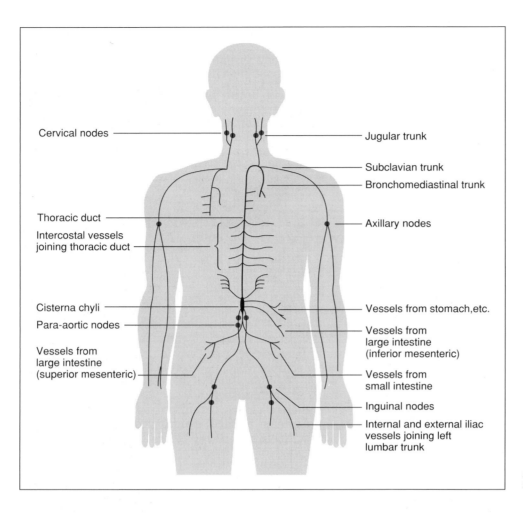

Cervical nodes

Jugular trunk

Subclavian trunk

Bronchomediastinal trunk

Thoracic duct

Intercostal vessels
joining thoracic duct

Axillary nodes

Cisterna chyli

Para-aortic nodes

Vessels from stomach,etc.

Vessels from
large intestine
(inferior mesenteric)

Vessels from
large intestine
(superior mesenteric)

Vessels from
small intestine

Inguinal nodes

Internal and external iliac
vessels joining left
lumbar trunk

FIGURE 11–1. Schematic illustration of the human lymphatic system.

sites. The absorbed interstitial fluid, called **lymph,** flows through the lymphatic capillaries into convergent, ever larger lymphatic vessels, eventually culminating in one large lymphatic vessel called the thoracic duct. Lymph from the thoracic duct is emptied into the superior vena cava, thus returning the fluid to the blood stream. Liters of lymph are normally returned to the circulation each day, and disruption of the lymphatic system may lead to rapid tissue swelling.

The lymph drained from the skin, mucosa, and other sites contains a sampling of all of the soluble and particulate self antigens and foreign antigens present in these tissues. (In some cases, antigen-presenting cells, displaying processed antigens, may also leave the tissue through these same lymphatics.) Lymph nodes are interposed along convergent networks of lymphatic vessels, and act as filters that "sample" the lymph at numerous points before it reaches the blood. Lymphatic vessels that carry lymph into a lymph node are referred to as **afferent;** those that drain the lymph from the node are called **efferent.** Since lymph nodes are connected in series along the lymphatics, an efferent lymphatic vessel exiting from one node may also serve as the afferent vessel for another.

When lymph enters a lymph node through an afferent lymphatic vessel, it percolates through the nodal stroma, where the lymph-borne antigens can be ex-

tracted from the fluid by resident antigen-presenting cells (APCs), such as macrophages and dendritic cells. Macrophages, through phagocytosis, are uniquely adept at extracting particulate and opsonized antigens. B cells in the node may also directly recognize soluble antigens, or they may recognize antigens that have been stored and concentrated, in the form of antigen-antibody complexes, on the surface of follicular dendritic cells. Macrophages, dendritic cells, and B cells that have taken up protein antigens can then process and present these antigens to T cells. The net result of antigen uptake by these various cell types is to accumulate and concentrate antigen in the lymph node, and display it in a form that can be recognized by specific T lymphocytes.

The collection and concentration of foreign antigens in lymph nodes are supplemented by two other anatomic adaptations that serve similar functions. First, the mucosal surfaces of the gastrointestinal and respiratory systems, in addition to being drained by lymphatic capillaries, also contain specialized mucosal collections of secondary lymphoid tissue that can directly sample the luminal contents of these organs for the presence of foreign antigens. The best characterized of these mucosal lymphoid organs are the Peyer's patches of the ileum, which are described in more detail later in this chapter. Second, the blood stream itself is monitored by APCs in the spleen for any antigens that reach the circulation. Such antigens may reach the blood either directly from the tissues or by way of the lymph from the thoracic duct.

Lymphocyte Recirculation

The pathways of migration of lymphocytes among lymphoid organs and peripheral tissues are best described for T cells (Fig. 11–2). When mature T cells first leave the thymus, they enter the blood stream. At this point in their development they are "naive" or "virgin" cells because they have not yet encountered and responded to their specific antigen. As we discussed in Chapter 2, such T cells characteristically express a high molecular weight isoform of the transmembrane molecule CD45, called CD45RA. CD45RA$^+$ T cells preferentially and efficiently leave the blood stream within the lymph nodes. As we shall discuss later, a lymphocyte surface molecule called L-selectin is expressed at high levels on naive T cells, binds to specialized endothelium in lymph nodes, and mediates homing of naive T cells to lymph nodes. If the T cells that have entered a lymph node fail to see their specific antigen within that node, they exit through an efferent lymphatic vessel and eventually return to the blood via the thoracic duct. One cycle of recirculation may take about an hour. Overall, the net flux of lymphocytes through lymph nodes is quite high, and it has been estimated that approximately 25×10^9 cells pass through lymph nodes each day. It is likely that a similar sequence of events occurs during lymphocyte migration through other peripheral lymphoid organs, such as the spleen.

If a naive T cell encounters its specific antigen in a lymph node, it becomes activated and enters into cell cycle. During the activation process, T cells increase their expression of several cell surface proteins that mediate adhesion to other cells and to extracellular matrix molecules. These surface proteins include LFA-1 (CD11aCD18), VLA-4 (CD49dCD29), VLA-5 (CD49eCD29), VLA-6 (CD49fCD29), and CD44, which have been discussed earlier as T cell accessory molecules (see Chapter 7). Activation also increases the affinities of integrins, especially LFA-1, for their ligands. As a consequence of these changes in surface receptor expression and affinity, activated T cells are more adherent to accessory cells and extracellular matrices and remain resident in the lymph node. The progeny of each activated T cell may differentiate into effector cells or into memory cells. As the T cells differentiate, they maintain high levels of adhesion molecules, but the affinity of these molecules (especially of the integrins) for their ligands rapidly declines after antigenic stimulation. Consequently, differentiated effector and memory T cells are less adhesive for lymph node cells and matrix molecules than recently activated cells and, like unstimulated naive T cells, return to the blood stream via the efferent lymphatics and the thoracic duct.

Previously activated T cells can be distinguished from naive cells because they express a different, lower molecular weight isoform of CD45, called CD45RO. Most previously activated and memory T cells no longer efficiently home to lymph nodes, because they express lower levels of L-selectin than naive cells, as will be described below. Instead, CD45RO$^+$ T cells preferentially home to sites of inflammation, which are often the sites of antigen entry, because the adhesion molecules expressed on previously activated T cells preferentially bind to peripheral endothelium at sites of inflammation. It is controversial whether T cells in the memory state are permanently altered or whether they revert to a "naive" state unless periodically restimu-

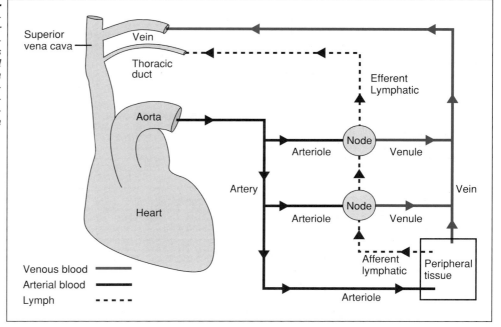

FIGURE 11–2. Pathways of lymphocyte recirculation. *Naive T cells preferentially leave the blood and enter lymph nodes across the high endothelial venules (HEVs). Memory T cells leave the blood and enter peripheral tissues through flat venules and reach the lymph nodes through afferent lymphatics. Lymphocytes return to the circulation through the efferent lymphatics and the thoracic duct, which empties into the superior vena cava.*

lated by antigen. The important point here is that *effector and memory T cells show a pattern of recirculation that is different from that of naive T cells,* and this difference is largely due to the expression of different endothelium-binding molecules on previously activated versus naive lymphocytes. The selective migration of naive T cells to lymphoid organs or of memory T cells to sites of inflammation is referred to as **homing.** The physiologic importance of these distinct homing pathways is that naive T cells preferentially home to the lymphoid organs, where they recognize and respond to foreign antigens (the cognitive and activation phases of primary immune responses), whereas memory T cells preferentially home to inflamed peripheral tissues, where they are needed to eliminate antigens (the effector phase of immune responses). Furthermore, the entry of memory T cells into the recirculating pool ensures that immunologic memory is systemic, i.e., that effector responses can be elicited at any site in the body, even if the memory cells were generated in the lymphoid tissues draining a single site of initial antigen entry. Finally, it should be noted that *the recirculation and tissue-specific homing of lymphocytes are largely independent of antigen recognition,* although the patterns of homing and extravascular retention of antigen are influenced by the presence of antigen and by the inflammation that often accompanies the entry of foreign antigens.

The efficient homing of naive T cells to the lymph nodes was initially described in the late 1950s and early 1960s by James Gowans and his colleagues. These investigators showed that lymphocyte extravasation into a peripheral lymph node occurred selectively at modified post-capillary venules within the stroma of the node. These specialized venules are lined by plump endothelial cells that, on cross section, protrude into the vessel lumen. Because of this morphologic appearance of the endothelial cells, such vessels are called **high endothelial venules** (HEVs). HEVs are also present in mucosal lymphoid tissues, such as Peyer's patches in the gut, but not in the spleen. Intravital videomicroscopy has shown that the *key characteristic of the HEV that leads to lymphocyte extravasation is increased adhesiveness of the high endothelium for circulating lymphocytes* (Fig. 11–3). Normally, lymphocytes coursing through the microcirculation randomly collide with vessel walls and either immediately rebound or adhere to the lining endothelial cells for only a fraction of a second before they are dislodged by the shear force of flowing blood. In contrast, when T cells collide with the endothelium lining an HEV, they remain loosely attached for several seconds. During this crucial window of time, a proportion of T cells are able to further increase their strength of attachment, to spread out into motile forms, and to crawl between (or through) the endothelial cells into the stroma of the secondary lymphoid organ. Within the mucosa of the gut, the prolonged time of attachment of lymphocytes to the endothelial lining of HEVs provides such an advantage for extravasation that 50 per cent of the T cells entering the mucosa do so through the HEVs despite the fact that the surface area of flat venules exceeds that of HEVs by over fifty to one!

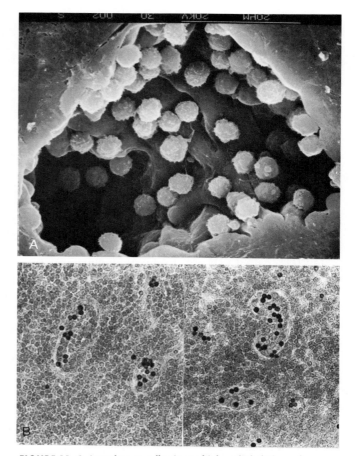

FIGURE 11–3. Lymphocyte adhesion to high endothelial venules.
A. *Scanning electron micrograph of a high endothelial venule with lymphocytes attached to the luminal surface of the endothelial cells. (Courtesy of J. Emerson and T. Yednock, University of California San Francisco School of Medicine, San Francisco. From Rosen, S. D., and L. M. Stoolman. Potential role of cell surface lectin in lymphocyte recirculation. In K. Olden, and J. Parent [eds.]. Vertebrate Lectins. Van Nostrand Reinhold, New York, 1987.)*
B. *A frozen section binding assay showing preferential attachment of added lymphocytes (stained darkly) to high endothelial venules, which are seen in cross section. (Reproduced with permission from Rosen, S. D. Lymphocyte homing: progress and prospects. Current Opinion in Cell Biology 1:913–919, 1989.)*

Because of their important place in the recirculation of lymphocytes, much study has been devoted to the characterization of HEVs. HEVs develop after birth from flat endothelial venules present in the secondary lymphoid organs. Several lines of evidence indicate that HEV formation is a consequence of local T cell activation and cytokine production triggered by antigen.

1. HEVs develop only when animals are exposed to environmental antigens, and HEVs fail to develop in animals that are raised in germ-free environments.
2. HEVs revert to flat endothelial venules when delivery of antigen to a lymph node is prevented, for instance, by surgically disrupting the afferent lymphatics. HEVs are always found in the peripheral lymph nodes and mucosal lymphoid tissues of normal adults. It is likely that they are maintained by continuous, low-level stimulation of the immune system by environmental antigens.

3. HEVs are not found in animals that do not have functional T lymphocytes.

4. The endothelial cells of HEVs express proteins that can also be induced in cultured endothelial cells by adding cytokines, such as interferon-γ (IFN-γ), that are secreted by activated T cells during immune response.

5. High endothelial morphologic patterns can similarly be induced in cell culture and *in situ* in the skin by adding T cell–derived cytokines.

Analysis of neonatal mice has revealed that lymphocytes preferentially home to lymph nodes even prior to the development of HEVs, suggesting that the venular endothelium of peripheral lymphoid organs may possess an intrinsically high adhesiveness for circulating naive lymphocytes. HEVs, which develop under the influence of cytokines, may serve to increase the efficiency of extravasation at these sites, but are not solely responsible for the tissue preference of naive T cells.

Molecular Basis of Lymphocyte Homing

The attachment of lymphocytes to the endothelium of various tissues is mediated by several homing receptors and other cell adhesion molecules on the lymphocytes and their corresponding ligands on endothelial cells (Table 11–1). The key tool in the analysis of homing receptors was the development of an *in vitro* assay for lymphocyte binding to endothelium by Judith Woodruff and colleagues. In brief, an isolated peripheral lymphoid organ (lymph node, spleen, or Peyer's patch) is rapidly frozen, and a 5 to 10 μm thick section is cut with a cryomicrotome. The frozen section of the organ is attached to a glass slide and gently fixed. A slurry of lymphocytes is placed on the slide over the section, and incubated with the section by gentle shaking at 8° C. Under these conditions, lymphocytes preferentially bind to the endothelium of the HEVs rather than to other elements of lymph nodes (Fig. 11–3). This frozen section binding assay has been used to establish two key points:

1. *Lymphocytes display tissue-specific discrimination between HEVs in different organs.* Different populations of normal lymphocytes preferentially bind to HEVs in peripheral lymph nodes or in mucosal lym-

phoid organs, such as Peyer's patch, depending on the anatomic site from which the cells were isolated. Thus, lymphocytes isolated from lymph nodes bind best to lymph node HEVs, cells from Peyer's patches bind to Peyer's patch HEVs, and blood lymphocytes contain populations of both types. Moreover, different lymphoid tumor cell lines, which are derived from individual clones of lymphocytes, preferentially bind to lymph node HEVs or to Peyer's patch HEVs, but not to both. In contrast to the tissue-specific attachment of lymphocytes to various HEVs, the binding of memory T cells to activated endothelium at sites of inflammation shows little specificity for different tissues.

2. *There are specific surface proteins that mediate the attachment of lymphocytes to HEVs of different tissues.* Monoclonal antibodies raised against lymphoid tumor cell lines have been identified as inhibitors of binding in this assay, and have been used to characterize lymphocyte surface proteins, called **homing receptors,** that can mediate tissue-specific attachment. The presence of distinct lymphocyte homing receptors that confer binding specificity for lymph node HEVs versus Peyer's patch HEVs implies that there are also distinct tissue-specific HEV ligands for these homing receptors. Some of these endothelial cell ligands, called **addressins,** have also been identified by monoclonal antibodies using the same frozen section binding assay.

The best characterized lymphocyte homing receptor is the molecule that mediates the binding of naive lymphocytes to the HEVs of peripheral lymph nodes. This molecule is a 90 kD glycoprotein, originally identified by a monoclonal antibody called MEL-14, and is called **L-selectin.** It is a carbohydrate-binding protein that shares a high degree of homology with two other proteins involved in leukocyte–endothelial cell adhesion. These three molecules are collectively called **selectins** (i.e., lectins, or carbohydrate-binding proteins, that mediate selective leukocyte adhesion). The lymph node homing receptor is called L-selectin because it was first identified on lymphocytes (Box 11–1). L-selectin is expressed at high levels by CD45RA+ (naive) T cells and is down-regulated upon T cell activation, so that it is less abundantly expressed on most CD45RO+ (memory) T cells. The endothelial ligand, or addressin, for L-selectin is a complex sialylated carbohydrate bound to one or more surface proteins preferentially expressed by lymph node HEVs. One of these proteins is a lymph node–specific sulfated proteoglycan that may also be secreted by HEVs. It has been called "GlyCAM-1" (for glycan-bearing cell adhesion molecule–1). Since the glycan moiety is recognized by L-selectin, tissue specificity of lymphocyte binding may be determined more by the enzymes that synthesize the distinct carbohydrate moieties in endothelial cells from lymph node than by unique structural proteins of the lymph node endothelial cells. L-selectin is also expressed by other leukocytes, such as neutrophils and monocytes, and may play a role in the homing of these non-lymphoid cells to sites of inflammation. Although naive T cells express relatively low levels of LFA-1, *in vivo* experiments have implicated this cell adhesion molecule in T cell homing to lymph nodes as well.

TABLE 11–1. Lymphocyte Homing Receptors

	T Cell Homing Receptor	Endothelial Ligand
A. Homing of naive T cells to peripheral lymph nodes	L-selectin LFA-1	GlyCAM-1 ?
B. Homing of T cells to mucosal tissues (e.g., Peyer's patches)	α4β7 integrin CD44	MadCAM-1 ?
C. Homing of memory and effector T cells to peripheral tissues	VLA-4 LFA-1 CD44	VCAM-1 ICAM-1, 2 Hyaluronate

BOX 11–1. SELECTINS

The selectins, sometimes called lectin adhesion molecules (LECAMs), are a family of three separate but closely related proteins that mediate adhesion of leukocytes to endothelial cells (see table). One member of this family of adhesion molecules is expressed on leukocytes, and two other members on endothelial cells, but all three participate in the process of leukocyte-endothelium attachment. Each of the selectin molecules is a single chain transmembrane glycoprotein with a similar modular structure. The amino terminus, expressed extracellularly, is related to the family of mammalian carbohydrate-binding proteins known as C-type lectins. Like other C-type lectins, ligand binding by selectins is calcium dependent. The lectin domain is followed by a domain homologous to part of the epidermal growth factor, which, in turn, is followed by a number of tandemly repeated domains related to structures previously identified in complement regulatory proteins as "short consensus repeats" (see Chapter 15). These short consensus repeats, which have six cysteine residues per domain in the selectins instead of the four found in complement regulatory proteins, are followed by a hydrophobic transmembrane region and a short cytoplasmic carboxy terminal region.

L-selectin, or CD62L, the family member that serves as a homing receptor for lymphocytes to lymph node HEVs, is also expressed on other leukocytes. On neutrophils, it serves to bind these cells to cytokine (TNFα, IL-1, and IFN-γ)-activated endothelial cells found at sites of inflammation. L-selectin recognition of its ligand is thought to happen quickly but is of low affinity; this property allows L-selectin to mediate rolling of neutrophils on endothelium. The rolling is followed by more stable LFA-1–mediated attachment of the neutrophils to endothelial cell ICAM-1, spreading, and LFA-1–mediated transmigration. The HEV ligand for L-selectin is a complex sialylated carbohydrate, which is, in part, carried by a sulfated proteoglycan called GlyCAM-1.

E-selectin, also known as endothelial leukocyte adhesion molecule 1 (ELAM-1) or CD62E, is exclusively expressed by cytokine-activated endothelial cells, hence the designation "E." E-selectin recognizes complex sialylated carbohydrate groups related to the Lewis X or Lewis A family found on various surface proteins of granulocytes, monocytes, and certain memory T cells. On a subset of T cells these carbohydrate groups have been called cutaneous lymphocyte antigen–1 (CLA-1), and have been implicated in homing of certain T cells to the epidermis. Endothelial cell expression of E-selectin is a hallmark of acute cytokine-mediated inflammation, and antibodies to E-selectin can block neutrophil accumulation *in vivo*. The role of E-selectin in lymphocyte homing is less clear; it may be involved in the homing of memory T cells to peripheral sites of inflammation.

P-selectin (CD62P) was first identified in the secretory granules of platelets, hence the designation "P." It has since been found in secretory granules of endothelial cells, which are called Weibel-Palade bodies. When endothelial cells or platelets are stimulated to secrete stored proteins, P-selectin is translocated within minutes to the cell surface as part of the exocytic secretory process. Upon reaching the cell surface, P-selectin mediates binding of neutrophils and monocytes. The ligands recognized by P-selectin appear similar to those recognized by E-selectin.

The structural relationship of the selectins to each other has been reinforced by the finding that the three selectin genes are located in tandem on chromosome 1 in both mice and humans. The selectin structural motif clearly arose from duplication of an ancestral selectin gene. The differences among the three selectins serve to confer both differences in binding specificity and differences in tissue expression. However, it is thought that all three selectins mediate rapid low-affinity attachment of leukocytes to endothelium, an early and important step in leukocyte homing, although E-selectin may mediate high-affinity attachment as well.

The Selectin Family

Selectin	Size	Distribution	Ligand	Principal Function
L-selectin (CD62L)	90–110 kD (variation due to glycosylation)	Leukocytes (expression on T cells is high on naive cells, generally low on memory cells)	1. GlyCAM-1 (lymph node HEV) 2. ? (Cytokine-activated endothelium)	1. Naive T cell homing 2. Inflammatory leukocyte homing
E-selectin (CD62E)	110 kD	Cytokine-activated endothelium (TNF, LT, IL-1)	Sialylated Lewis X and related glycans	Binding of leukocytes at sites of cytokine-induced inflammation
P-selectin (CD62P)	140 kD	1. Storage granules of endothelium 2. Storage granules of platelets	Sialylated Lewis X and related glycans	1. Binding of leukocytes early in cytokine-independent inflammation 2. Binding of activated platelets to monocytes at sites of inflammation

The homing receptor(s) that mediate lymphocyte migration to mucosal sites are less well defined. Most circulating lymphocytes that home to Peyer's patches appear to be B cells; in fact, this may be a major recirculation pathway for B lymphocytes. One monoclonal antibody directed against an epitope of CD44 on T cells can block the binding of human lymphocytes to Peyer's patch HEVs in the frozen section binding assay. CD44 is also a cell receptor for hyaluronic acid, a glycosaminoglycan. HEVs from both Peyer's patches and lymph nodes show increased synthesis of glycosaminoglycans, a change that is also inducible in cultured endothelial cells by cytokines; but no role for glycosaminoglycans has yet been established in lymphocytes homing to Peyer's patches. A second group of antibodies that inhibit binding of lymphocytes to Peyer's patches has been found to react with the α chain of the VLA-4 integrin (see Box 7–3, Chapter 7). In lymphocytes that home to Peyer's patches, the VLA-4 α chain (CD49d) may pair with an unusual integrin light chain (called β7). Vascular cell adhesion molecule–1 (VCAM-1), the normal cellular ligand for VLA-4, is not expressed on Peyer's patch HEVs. A murine Peyer's patch addressin, called MadCAM-1 (for mucosal addressin cell adhesion molecule–1), that binds the α4β7 integrin has been identified recently; it contains three Ig domains and a polypeptide backbone that could be modified by attachment of glycosaminoglycans to also interact with CD44. It is also possible that homing to mucosa could involve memory T cell homing to sites of chronic, low-level inflammation as well as tissue-specific homing. Such inflammation could well result from the presence of bacteria in the lumen of the gut. Consistent with this idea is the observation that both CD44 and VLA-4, the two molecules thought to be involved in homing to Peyer's patches, are also increased in expression on CD45RO$^+$ memory T cells that home to sites of inflammation (see Chapter 13).

There is little current information about the nature of homing receptors or addressins involved in lymphocyte homing to respiratory mucosa or to the spleen. This is a major gap in our knowledge since the rate of lymphocyte passage through the spleen is about 250 × 10^9 cells each day, or about half of the total lymphocyte population every 24 hours. The spleen does not contain morphologically identifiable HEVs, and the role of selectins or other adhesion molecules in homing to the spleen is largely unknown. It is possible that homing of lymphocytes to the spleen does not show the same degree of selectivity for naive cells as do lymph nodes.

The homing of effector and memory T cells to sites of inflammation, and the retention of these cells in extravascular peripheral tissues, will be described more fully in Chapter 13. As we have mentioned earlier, such T cells do not recirculate efficiently through lymph nodes because they express low levels of L-selectin. Instead, memory and effector T cells express high levels of adhesion molecules (e.g., LFA-1, VLA-4, and CD44), the ligands for which are present or induced on endothelium in peripheral tissues, especially after exposure to inflammatory cytokines. Therefore, effector and memory T cells preferentially home to sites of inflammation. Note that lymph nodes draining sites of inflammation may themselves be exposed to inflammatory cytokines, so that memory T cells may home to such inflamed nodes as they do to peripheral tissues.

Lymphocytes not only home to particular sites but are retained at these sites. We have mentioned above the mechanisms that may mediate the transient retention of naive T cells that encounter antigen in peripheral lymphoid organs. Activated and memory T cells tend to be retained in peripheral tissues because these cells express adhesion molecules for extracellular matrix proteins. For instance, VLA-4 and VLA-5 bind to fibronectin, and CD44 to hyaluronate. Interestingly, the adhesiveness of several integrins for their ligands is enhanced by antigen recognition as well as by other stimuli, such as cytokines. Thus, activated and memory T cells may home to sites of inflammation irrespective of antigen specificity. The cells that recognize antigen rapidly up-regulate their adhesiveness for other cells and for extracellular matrices (via LFA-1, VLA-4, and VLA-5). As a result, antigen-stimulated cells are preferentially retained at the site of specific antigen recognition. We will return to a discussion of this process in Chapter 13.

Finally, relatively little is known about the recirculation and tissue-specific homing of B lymphocytes. Some memory B cells bind to germinal centers, and VLA-4 on the B cells and VCAM-1 on follicular dendritic cells may be involved in this interaction. Previously activated, IgA-producing B cells have a propensity to home to Peyer's patches (see below).

IMMUNE RESPONSES IN SPLEEN AND LYMPH NODES

The morphology of the spleen and lymph nodes, and the anatomic compartmentalization of different cell populations in these organs, were described in Chapter 2. These organs are the principal sites for the initiation of most primary immune responses, and for the activation of B lymphocytes and the production of antibodies. Recent studies using combinations of morphologic and molecular techniques, as well as analyses of homogeneous lymphocyte populations (e.g., in antigen receptor transgenic mice), are providing fascinating insights into the anatomy of immune responses in lymphoid organs.

The Fate of Antigens *In Vivo*

The localization of antigens in lymphoid tissues has been studied mainly in experimental animals. The *in vivo* fate of administered antigens is determined by several factors.

1. The nature of the antigen. Particulate substances, soluble proteins, and polysaccharides tend to be concentrated in different areas of lymphoid tissues, as described below.

2. The route of antigen entry. Intravenously administered antigens are trapped mainly in the spleen, which is the principal site of immune responses to blood-borne antigens. In contrast, antigens that enter via the skin and mucosa, or from parenchymal organs and connective tissues, are carried by the lymphatic drainage to regional lymph nodes. Some immune responses may also be initiated locally at the site of antigen entry, particularly in mucosal and cutaneous lymphoid tissues.

3. The immunization status of the animal. The fates of antigens vary in naive and previously immunized individuals.

Most of our current knowledge about what happens to antigens *in vivo* is based on analyses of the spleens in animals given antigens intravenously. Antigens enter the spleen via the central arterioles, which divide into progressively smaller branches that end in the marginal zones and from where the blood enters the vascular sinusoids of the red pulp. Intravenously injected particulate and soluble antigens are trapped largely by macrophages in the marginal zones and red pulp of the spleen. In previously unimmunized individuals, a fraction of injected soluble antigen can be found in the periarteriolar lymphoid sheaths, which are rich in interdigitating dendritic cells and T lymphocytes. Polysaccharide antigens injected intravenously are first trapped by marginal zone macrophages and then rapidly transported to lymphoid follicles, where they stimulate B cell responses. In previously immunized individuals, injected antigens are rapidly complexed with antibodies, and most of the complexes are phagocytosed and destroyed. A small fraction is displayed on the surfaces of follicular dendritic cells in lymphoid follicles, and this depot of antigen may persist for many weeks, providing a long-lasting stimulus for memory lymphocytes.

Antigens are transported to lymph nodes either in soluble form or attached to surfaces of APCs. For instance, some cutaneously administered antigens are picked up by epidermal Langerhans cells and carried to draining lymph nodes, where they initiate T cell responses. The fate of antigens once they enter lymph nodes is not as well understood, although the general features are probably similar to those of the spleen.

Antigen Presentation in Lymphoid Tissues

In Chapter 6, we introduced the concept that several cell types, notably dendritic cells, macrophages, and B lymphocytes, have the ability to present protein antigens to CD4$^+$ T cells. The relative contributions of

these APCs to the induction of T cell responses *in vivo* are not yet established. There is considerable experimental evidence supporting the ability of dendritic cells to present antigens to naive T cells both *in vitro* and *in vivo*. The anatomic co-localization of dendritic cells and T cells in the periarteriolar lymphoid sheaths of the spleen and the parafollicular cortex of lymph nodes also supports the importance of this APC type in initiating T cell responses. Macrophages, which are abundant in the red pulp of the spleen and the medulla of lymph nodes, are efficient at picking up particulate antigens. These macrophages may migrate within lymphoid tissues to T cell–rich zones, where they may stimulate the development of CD4$^+$ cells to effector cells. B cells present antigens to activated helper T cells to initiate antibody responses. As discussed in Chapters 9 and 10, B cells may be inefficient at activating naive T cells, and their role as APCs may be most important in secondary antibody responses.

Activation of T and B Lymphocytes in the Spleen and Lymph Nodes

Following intravenous administration of antigen to naive animals, T cell activation is probably initiated near the periarteriolar lymphoid sheaths of the spleen. This is the zone of greatest mitotic activity. Activated T cells may then migrate from the lymphoid sheaths into the marginal zone. As they do so, they encounter B cells migrating in the opposite direction, and this presumably maximizes the chances of cell-cell interactions. Clusters of cytokine-producing T cells, often in close proximity to antibody-producing B cells, are most numerous in the marginal zones, adjacent to the terminal branches of the central arterioles. Such clusters may persist for many days after antigen exposure, suggesting that T cell activation continues in the marginal

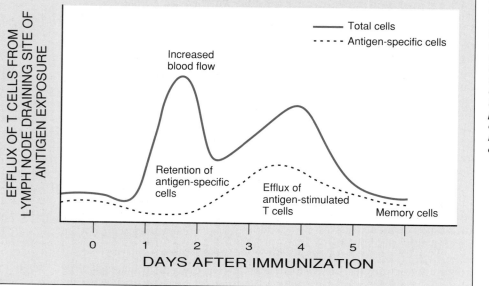

FIGURE 11–4. Trafficking of T cells through a lymph node draining a site of antigen entry. *Cells leaving the node shut down shortly after antigen exposure. Blood flow and efflux of cells then increase, but antigen-specific cells are retained in the node. Antigen-stimulated cells later appear in the efferent lymph. These results are from experiments with sheep in which the efferent lymphatics of selected nodes (e.g., the popliteal node) can be cannulated.*

Legend (within figure):
Total cells
Antigen-specific cells

Increased blood flow

Retention of antigen-specific cells

Efflux of antigen-stimulated T cells

Memory cells

EFFLUX OF T CELLS FROM LYMPH NODE DRAINING SITE OF ANTIGEN EXPOSURE

DAYS AFTER IMMUNIZATION
0   1   2   3   4   5

zones. The activation of B lymphocytes in the spleen was described in Chapter 9.

In lymph nodes draining sites of antigen administration, the first change is seen within a few hours after antigen exposure. Blood flow through the node increases by more than 20-fold, allowing an increased number of naive lymphocytes access to the site where antigen is concentrated (Fig. 11–4). Efflux of cells from the node may decrease at the same time. These changes are probably due to an inflammatory reaction to adjuvants associated with the antigen or due to inflammatory cytokines produced as a result of antigen entry. During the next day or so, antigen-specific cells are preferentially retained in the node, presumably because they recognize the antigen and up-regulate their expression of adhesion molecules. The first wave of mitotic activity is seen within 1 or 2 days in the T cell–rich parafollicular areas of the cortex. Cytokine-producing T cells are also found in the parafollicular regions of the cortex. Shortly thereafter, there is a rapid efflux of activated cells out of the node; the mechanisms responsible for this emigration of activated cells are not fully understood. The activated cells then enter the peripheral circulation and home to different sites. For instance, activated T cells home to peripheral tissues where the antigen entered and has persisted (see Chapter 13). Some B cells may remain in the lymph nodes, where they differentiate into antibody-secreting cells and undergo affinity maturation (see Chapter 9). IgA-producing B cells migrate to mucosal lymphoid tissues. The output of antigen-stimulated cells decreases by about a week after antigen exposure. After this time, memory T and B cells that have developed in the lymph node exit and enter the circulating pool.

With this background of the general features of immune responses *in vivo*, we will proceed to a description of responses in specialized tissues.

THE CUTANEOUS IMMUNE SYSTEM

The skin is the largest organ in the body and the principal physical barrier between the organism and the external environment. In addition, the skin is an active participant in host defense, with the ability to generate and support local immune and inflammatory reactions. Many foreign antigens gain entry into the body via the skin, so that many immune responses are initiated in this tissue.

Cellular Components of the Cutaneous Immune System

The skin consists of an epidermis separated from the underlying dermis by a basement membrane. Each of these tissues contains cell populations that may play active roles in immune reactions (Fig. 11–5).

KERATINOCYTES. The epithelial cells of the epidermis, or keratinocytes, produce a number of cytokines, including interleukin-1 (IL-1), GM-CSF, IL-3, TNF, and IL-6; and after activation by T cell–derived cytokines such as IFN-γ, keratinocytes secrete chemokines that stimulate the chemotaxis and activation of leukocytes. (The properties and actions of these cytokines are discussed in more detail in Chapter 12.) Although these findings suggest that keratinocytes may augment local inflammation and lymphocyte activation, it is not known if the cytokines produced by keratinocytes can reach the dermis, where most of the lymphocytes and other leukocytes are located.

In addition to serving as sources of cytokines, keratinocytes can be induced to express class II MHC molecules by exposure to IFN-γ. This is similar to the induction of class II expression on macrophages and other cell populations (see Chapters 5 and 6). Keratinocytes also express costimulators that may be distinct from costimulators on dendritic cells, macrophages, and B lymphocytes. It is, however, unclear if keratinocytes function as APCs for initiating T cell reactions.

EPIDERMAL LANGERHANS CELLS. Langerhans cells are bone marrow–derived cells with long dendritic processes located in the suprabasilar portion of the epidermis. It is thought that a bone marrow precursor gives rise to cells that reside in the skin as epidermal Langerhans cells, some of which then migrate to lymphoid organs

FIGURE 11–5. *Cellular components of the cutaneous immune system.*

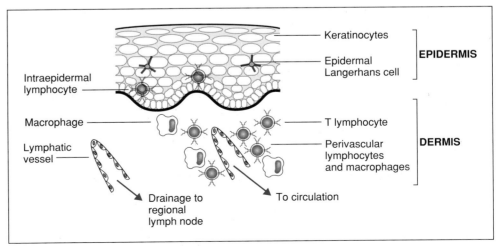

Keratinocytes
Epidermal Langerhans cell
EPIDERMIS

Intraepidermal lymphocyte

Macrophage

Lymphatic vessel

T lymphocyte
Perivascular lymphocytes and macrophages
DERMIS

Drainage to regional lymph node

To circulation

where they are identified as interdigitating dendritic cells (see Chapter 2). The function of Langerhans cells in the presentation of protein antigens to CD4+ T cells is described below.

INTRAEPIDERMAL LYMPHOCYTES. Within the epidermis there is a small population of lymphocytes. In humans, these constitute only about 2 per cent of skin-associated lymphocytes (the rest residing in the dermis), and the majority are CD8+ T cells. Intraepidermal T cells may express a more restricted set of antigen receptors than T lymphocytes in most extracutaneous tissues. In mice, many intraepidermal lymphocytes are T cells that express the γδ form of the antigen receptor (see Chapter 7). As we shall see later, this is also true of intraepithelial lymphocytes in the intestine, raising the possibility that γδ T cells, at least in some species, may be uniquely committed to recognizing antigens encountered at epithelial surfaces. However, neither the specificity nor the function of this T cell subpopulation is clearly defined.

The homing of some T cells to the epidermis may be controlled by specific adhesion molecules. Intraepidermal T cells as well as some T cells in the dermis express a sialylated carbohydrate, called cutaneous lymphocyte antigen-1 (CLA-1), which is recognized by E-selectin, originally identified as an endothelial molecule induced early in inflammatory responses (see Chapter 13 and Box 11–1). Most of the CLA-1 determinant is synthesized when T cells become activated in the skin microenvironment, perhaps in response to cytokines. A small number of circulating T cells express CLA-1, and these cells may adhere to endothelial cells expressing E-selectin. Whether E-selectin is expressed on epidermal cells, and plays a role in the epidermotropism of some T lymphocytes, is not known.

DERMAL LYMPHOCYTES AND MACROPHAGES. The connective tissues of the dermis contain T lymphocytes (both CD4+ and CD8+), predominantly in a perivascular location, and scattered macrophages. This is essentially similar to connective tissues in other organs. The T cells usually express phenotypic markers typical of activated or memory cells, such as CD45RO and high levels of the IL-2 receptor α chain (CD25).

Initiation of Immune Responses in the Skin

When protein antigens are introduced into the skin, either by topical application or by injection, three cell types function as APCs. *Langerhans cells provide the major pathway of presentation of cutaneously encountered antigens to naive T cells.* Langerhans cells bind the antigen to their surfaces and process it, and bearing processed antigen, they migrate from the epidermis into lymphatic vessels and thence into regional lymph nodes, where they come to reside in the parafollicular regions of the cortex. Here the Langerhans cells, which are now called interdigitating dendritic cells, present the antigen to naive CD4+ T cells that have entered the node through HEVs. In their resting state,

i.e., without extrinsic stimulation, dendritic cells are the most potent APCs in the body. (In contrast, as we discussed in Chapters 6 and 10, other APCs such as macrophages and B lymphocytes may need to be activated in order to develop the capacity to present antigens to and stimulate T cells.) The main reason for this is that dendritic cells constitutively express high levels of class II MHC molecules as well as costimulators, such as the B7 glycoprotein. Interestingly, freshly isolated Langerhans cells do not activate T lymphocytes, but acquire the ability to do so after brief (1 to 2 days) culture. It is postulated that this culture period is the *in vitro* analog of the migration of antigen-bearing Langerhans cells from the epidermis to draining lymph nodes. Langerhans cells differentiate into potent APCs during this migration, ensuring that naive T lymphocytes are activated in the lymph nodes and not in the skin where antigen initially entered. Dermal macrophages and venular endothelial cells may present antigens to T lymphocytes in the dermis. Most of these dermal T cells are previously activated or memory cells. Therefore, T cell reactions to macrophage or endothelium-associated antigens in the dermis may be more important for generating effector responses to antigen challenge in previously immunized individuals than for initiating primary responses to antigens encountered for the first time.

Effector Phases of Immune Responses in the Skin

The major type of T cell–mediated immune response in the skin is **delayed-type hypersensitivity (DTH).** This is a reaction to soluble protein antigens or to chemicals that can bind to and modify self proteins, creating new antigenic determinants. DTH is a cell-mediated immune response that results from the activation of T cells and the secretion of cytokines. It is described in more detail in Chapter 13.

Much less is known about humoral immunity in the skin. Secretory IgA is present in secretions in the skin, such as sweat, and its importance is suggested by the clinical observation that patients with IgA deficiency are susceptible to pyogenic skin infections. Since B lymphocytes are rarely encountered in cutaneous tissues, it is likely that IgA is produced by B cells activated in draining lymph nodes and is transported back to the skin via the circulation. The skin is also an important site of IgE-mediated immediate hypersensitivity reactions, which are caused by the release of chemical mediators from dermal mast cells (see Chapter 14).

THE MUCOSAL IMMUNE SYSTEM

Although lymphocytes have been recognized in the mucosa and submucosa of the gastrointestinal and respiratory tracts for many decades, the idea of a specialized mucosa-associated immune system is relatively new. Like the skin, these mucosal epithelia are barriers between the internal and external environments, and are, therefore, an important first line of defense. Moreover, *immune responses to oral antigens differ in some fundamental respects from responses to antigens encountered at other sites.* The two most striking differences are the high levels of IgA production associated with mucosal tissues, and the tendency of oral immunization with protein antigens to induce T cell tolerance rather than activation. Such observations have convincingly established both the physiologic importance and the functional uniqueness of the mucosal immune system. Much of our knowledge of mucosal immunity is based on studies of the gastrointestinal tract, and this is emphasized in the discussion that follows. In comparison, little is known about immune responses in the respiratory mucosa, even though the airways are a major portal of antigen entry. It is likely, however, that the features of immune responses are basically similar in all mucosa-associated lymphoid tissues.

Cellular Components of the Mucosal Immune System

In the mucosa of the gastrointestinal tract, lymphocytes are found in large numbers in three main regions—scattered throughout the lamina propria, in Peyer's patches, and within the epithelial layer (Fig. 11–6). Cells at each site have distinct phenotypic and functional characteristics.

INTRAEPITHELIAL LYMPHOCYTES. The majority of intraepithelial lymphocytes are T cells. In humans, most of these are CD8+ cells. Strikingly, in mice about 50 per cent of intraepithelial lymphocytes express the $\gamma\delta$ form of the TCR, similar to intraepidermal lymphocytes in the skin. In most other species, including humans, only about 10 per cent of intraepithelial lymphocytes are $\gamma\delta$ cells. Although this proportion is not impressive, it is still higher than the proportions of $\gamma\delta$ cells found among T cells in other tissues. Both the $\gamma\delta$ and the $\alpha\beta$ TCR-expressing intraepithelial lymphocytes show limited diversity of antigen receptors, with a few V genes being

dominant. All these findings support the idea mentioned previously that intraepithelial lymphocytes have a limited range of specificities that is distinct from that of most T cells, and may have evolved to recognize commonly encountered intraluminal antigens.

Intraepithelial lymphocytes express a novel integrin called HML-1 (human mucosal lymphocyte antigen-1), which is composed of a unique α chain in association with a $\beta 7$ chain. It is postulated that this adhesion molecule mediates the homing of particular T cells to or retention within intestinal epithelia.

LAMINA PROPRIA LYMPHOCYTES. The intestinal lamina propria contains a mixed population of cells. These include T lymphocytes, most of which are CD4+ and have the phenotype of activated cells. It is likely that T cells initially recognize and respond to antigens in regional mesenteric lymph nodes, and migrate back to the intestine to populate the lamina propria. This is similar to the postulated origin of T cells in the dermis of the skin. In addition, the lamina propria contains large numbers of activated B lymphocytes and plasma cells, as well as macrophages, eosinophils, and mast cells.

MUCOSAL LYMPHOID FOLLICLES. **Peyer's patches** are organized mucosal lymphoid follicles in the small intestine. Morphologically and functionally similar follicles are abundant in the appendix, and are found in smaller numbers in much of the gastrointestinal and respiratory tracts. **Pharyngeal tonsils** are also mucosal lymphoid follicles analogous to Peyer's patches. Like lymphoid follicles in the spleen and lymph nodes, the central regions of the mucosal follicles are B cell–rich areas that often contain germinal centers. Peyer's patches also contain small numbers of CD4+ T cells, mainly in the interfollicular regions. In adult mice, 50 to 70 per cent of Peyer's patch lymphocytes are B cells, and 10 to 30 per cent are T cells. Some of the epithelial cells overlying Peyer's patches are specialized "M (membranous) cells." M cells lack microvilli, are actively pinocytic, and transport macromolecules from the intestinal lumen into subepithelial tissues. They are thought to play an important role in delivering antigens to Peyer's patches. (Note, however, that M cells do not themselves function as antigen-presenting cells.)

FIGURE 11–6. Cellular components of the mucosal immune system.

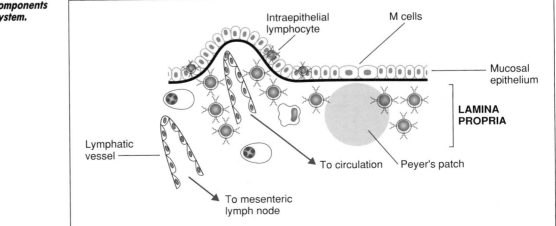

Induction of Immune Responses in Mucosal Tissues

The bulk of orally administered antigen enters from the intestinal lumen into lymphatics and is carried to draining mesenteric lymph nodes, where immune responses are initiated. Some ingested protein antigens may be transported through M cells into Peyer's patches, where they are capable of stimulating both T and B lymphocytes. Although intestinal epithelial cells can be induced to express class II MHC molecules, e.g., by exposure to IFN-γ, there is no evidence that these cells are capable of presenting antigens to and stimulating T lymphocytes. Lymphocytes that are activated in mesenteric lymph nodes may return to populate the lamina propria. Lymphocytes stimulated in Peyer's patches may also migrate to the lamina propria, or into mesenteric lymph nodes and ultimately the systemic circulation. Thus, the compartments of the mucosal immune system are connected with one another and with the rest of the immune system.

Production of IgA

IgA is the major class of antibody that can be actively and efficiently secreted through epithelia. Therefore, it plays a critical role in defense against intestinal and respiratory pathogens, and in the passive transfer of immunity in milk and colostrum from mothers to infants. The size of the intestinal surface accounts for the enormous quantity of IgA that is produced. It is estimated that a normal 70 kg adult secretes about 3 gm of IgA per day, accounting for 60 to 70 per cent of the total output of antibodies.

In the gastrointestinal tract, the process of IgA production is initiated by the entry of protein antigens into the Peyer's patches. Here the antigens stimulate specific T lymphocytes in the inter-follicular regions as well as B lymphocytes in the follicles. Some of the B lymphocytes differentiate into IgA-producing cells and migrate to the lamina propria. The two cytokines that are mainly responsible for switching to the IgA isotype

are TGF-β (which may be produced by T cells as well as non-lymphoid stromal cells) and IL-5 (see Chapter 9). Some activated B cells migrate into the germinal centers of the Peyer's patches, where they undergo proliferation and somatic mutations of Ig genes, leading to affinity maturation of antibodies. This is probably similar to the sequence of events in lymphoid follicles in the spleen and lymph nodes. After they are generated, IgA-producing B cells may reside in the lamina propria, or may migrate to other mucosal tissues or lymphoid organs.

There are several reasons why the amounts of IgA produced in the mucosal immune system are higher than in other tissues. First, IgA-expressing B cells tend to home to Peyer's patches and lamina propria. This has been demonstrated by injecting antigen-stimulated, IgA-expressing B cells into the systemic circulation of normal, unimmunized animals. The homing receptors and addressins responsible for this homing are unknown. Second, IL-5–producing helper T cells are more numerous in Peyer's patches than in other lymphoid tissues. Although the mucosal immune system is the site of greatest IgA production and the source of secretory IgA, this isotype may also be produced by B cells in other lymphoid tissues and in the bone marrow, giving rise to serum IgA.

Secretory IgA forms a dimer that is held together by the coordinately synthesized and secreted J chain (see Chapter 3). (In contrast, serum IgA is usually a monomer lacking the J chain.) Once this dimer is secreted into the lamina propria, it is transported through epithelial cells into the intestinal lumen by a protein called the **secretory component** (or poly-Ig receptor). Secretory component is synthesized by mucosal epithelial cells and expressed on their basal and lateral surfaces. The membrane-associated form is a ~100 kD glycoprotein with five extracellular domains homologous to Ig domains, and is thus a member of the Ig superfamily. The secreted, dimeric IgA containing the J chain binds to and forms covalent complexes with the membrane-associated secretory component on mucosal epithelial cells (Fig. 11–7). This complex is endocytosed into the epithelial cell and transported in vesicles to the luminal surface. Here the extracellular domain of

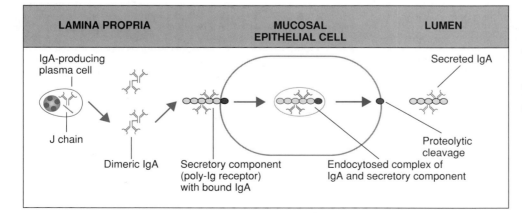

LAMINA PROPRIA   MUCOSAL EPITHELIAL CELL   LUMEN

IgA-producing plasma cell

Secreted IgA

J chain

Dimeric IgA

Secretory component (poly-Ig receptor) with bound IgA

Endocytosed complex of IgA and secretory component

Proteolytic cleavage

FIGURE 11–7. Mechanisms of IgA transport and secretion in mucosal epithelia. *IgA is produced by plasma cells in the lamina propria and binds to secretory component. The complex is actively transported through the epithelial cell, and the bound IgA is released by proteolytic cleavage.*

the secretory component, carrying the IgA molecule, is proteolytically cleaved, leaving the transmembrane and cytoplasmic domains attached to the epithelial cell and releasing the bound IgA into the intestinal lumen. Secretory component is also responsible for the secretion of IgA into bile, milk, sputum, and saliva. Although its ability to transport IgA has been studied most extensively, secretory component is capable of transporting IgM into intestinal secretions as well. (Note that secreted IgM is also a polymer associated with the J chain.) In secretions, IgA serves to neutralize microbes and toxins.

Oral Tolerance

The oral administration of a protein antigen often leads to a marked suppression of systemic humoral and cell-mediated immune responses to immunization with the same antigen. The inhibition is antigen-specific and fulfills the criteria for immunologic tolerance (see Chapter 10). The physiologic importance of oral tolerance may be as a means of preventing immune responses to bacteria that normally reside as commensals in the intestinal lumen and are needed for digestion and absorption. Despite extensive analysis, there is no consensus on the mechanisms responsible for oral tolerance. Some studies have shown that orally administered proteins induce T cell clonal anergy, which resembles anergy induced by antigen presentation by costimulator-deficient APCs (see Chapter 10). However, it is not known which APCs present antigens administered via the enteric route to induce T cell tolerance, or how anergy induced by oral antigen is manifested as systemic unresponsiveness. An alternative possibility is that oral antigens may stimulate the production of cytokines, such as TGF-β, that inhibit lymphocyte proliferation, resulting in the suppression of immune responses. In fact, TGF-β may participate in both the distinctive responses to oral immunization, because it is known to induce B cell switching to IgA and to inhibit lymphocyte proliferation. TGF-β–producing cells may migrate to distant sites and even inhibit immune responses in the periphery. Anergy and suppression are not mutually exclusive mechanisms, and both may contribute to oral tolerance. Whatever its precise mechanism, the phenomenon of oral tolerance has obvious practical relevance. It is a potential treatment for autoimmune diseases in which the autoantigen is known, and for other clinical situations in which it may be desirable to inhibit specific immune responses to defined protein antigens.

SUMMARY

The immune system copes with the problem of efficient recognition of foreign antigens by collecting and concentrating antigens in the secondary lymphoid organs and by rapidly circulating lymphocytes among these organs to sample the collected antigens. The migration of lymphocytes into the secondary lymphoid organs occurs through specialized high endothelial venules (HEVs), where tissue-specific lymphocyte homing receptors recognize endothelial ligands, called addressins. The receptor responsible for homing of lymphocytes to peripheral lymph nodes is called L-selectin, and is expressed at high levels on naive T cells, accounting for the preferential migration of these cells into lymph node. Most memory T cells have little if any L-selectin and do not home to lymph nodes. Instead, memory T cells express increased levels of adhesion molecules that promote their preferential migration through vessels at sites of antigen exposure or inflammation.

Immune responses in different tissues have distinctive characteristics. Priming of T lymphocytes occurs mainly in lymph nodes and spleen. These organs are also the principal sites of antibody production. Immune responses in the skin are initiated largely by antigen presentation by epidermal Langerhans cells. The typical response in the skin is the T lymphocyte–mediated delayed-type hypersensitivity reaction. The mucosal immune system is specialized to produce large quantities of IgA, which is the only class of antibody that is efficiently secreted through epithelial cells into the lumen of the gastrointestinal and respiratory tracts. In addition, protein antigens that are administered orally tend to induce T cell tolerance.

SELECTED READINGS

Bevilacqua, M. P. Endothelial-leukocyte adhesion molecules. Annual Review of Immunology 11:767–804, 1993.

Kupper, T. S. Immune and inflammatory processes in cutaneous tissues: mechanisms and speculations. Journal of Clinical Investigation 86:1783–1789, 1990.

Picker, L. J., and E. C. Butcher. Physiological and molecular mechanisms of lymphocyte homing. Annual Review of Immunology 10:561–591, 1992.

Pober, J. S., and R. S. Cotran. Immunologic interactions of T lymphocytes with vascular endothelium. Advances in Immunology 50:261–302, 1991.

Van den Ertwegh, A. J. M., W. J. A. Boersma, and E. Claasen. Immunological functions and in vivo cell-cell interactions of T cells in the spleen. Critical Reviews in Immunology. 11:337–380, 1992.

Van Rooijen, N. Antigen processing and presentation in vivo: the microenvironment as a critical factor. Immunology Today 11:436–439, 1990.

EFFECTOR MECHANISMS OF IMMUNE RESPONSES

The physiologic function of all specific immune responses is to eliminate the initiating antigen. The mechanisms by which specific lymphocytes recognize and respond to foreign antigens, i.e., the cognitive and activation phases of immune responses, were discussed in Section II. Section III describes the effector mechanisms that are recruited and stimulated by antigen-activated lymphocytes. In Chapter 12 we describe cytokines that are produced by T lymphocytes and by some non-lymphoid cells. These molecules are the soluble mediators of cell-mediated immunity as well as non-immune inflammatory reactions. Chapter 13 presents the effector cells of cell-mediated immunity, including T lymphocytes, macrophages, and natural killer cells, which participate in immune-mediated inflammatory reactions and function as the primary defense mechanisms against intracellular microbes. Chapter 14 discusses immediate hypersensitivity, an inflammatory reaction caused by the activation of a specialized subset of CD4$^+$ T cells, which leads to the production of IgE antibody, activation of mast cells and basophils, and recruitment of eosinophils. Chapter 15 deals with the complement system, one of the major effector mechanisms of the humoral immune response.

CYTOKINES

In Chapter 1, we introduced the concept that defense against foreign organisms, such as viruses or bacteria, is mediated by natural (or innate) and by specific (or acquired) immunity. The effector phases of both natural and specific immunity are in large part mediated by protein hormones called **cytokines.** In natural immunity, the effector cytokines are mostly produced by mononuclear phagocytes and are therefore often called **monokines.** Although monokines can be elicited directly by microbes, they also can be secreted by mononuclear phagocytes in response to antigen-stimulated T cells, i.e., as part of specific immunity. Most cytokines in specific immunity are produced by activated T lymphocytes, and such molecules are commonly called **lymphokines.** T cells produce several cytokines that serve primarily to regulate the growth and differentiation of various lymphocyte populations and thus play important roles in the (**activation phase**) of T cell–dependent immune responses. Other T-cell–derived cytokines function principally to activate and regulate inflammatory cells, such as mononuclear phagocytes, neutrophils, and eosinophils. These T cell–derived cytokines are the effector molecules of cell-mediated immunity and are also responsible for communication between the cells of the immune and inflammatory systems. Finally, both lymphocytes and mononuclear phagocytes produce other cytokines, such as **colony-stimulating factors** (CSFs), which stimulate the growth and differentiation of immature leukocytes in the bone marrow, providing a source of additional leukocytes to replace the cells that are consumed during inflammatory reactions.

In this chapter, we discuss the structure, production, and biologic actions of cytokines. Before describing the specific molecules, we will begin with a brief historical overview of cytokine research and a review of the general properties shared by cytokines that allow us to consider them as a group.

DISCOVERY AND CHARACTERIZATION OF CYTOKINES

The discovery of particular cytokines can often be traced to investigation of infectious disease or of antigen-induced immune responses. Early studies of cytokines, extending from about 1950 to 1970, largely involved the description of numerous protein factors produced by different cells that mediated particular functions in particular bioassays. It was in this era, for example, that antiviral interferons, fever-producing pyrogens, and macrophage-activating factor were discovered. The second phase of cytokine research, encompassing roughly the 1970s, involved the partial purification and characterization of many individual cytokines as well as production of specific neutralizing antisera. In this period, it was first appreciated that diverse cytokine-mediated effects being studied by different investigators were often mediated by the same molecules. For example, interferon-γ (IFN-γ) was discovered by virologists as a T cell–derived antiviral protein and independently discovered by immunologists as a T cell–derived activator of macrophage functions. Similarly, interleukin-1 (IL-1) was discovered as an endogenous mediator of fever (a pyrogen) produced in response to bacterial infections and was discovered by immunologists as a costimulator of thymocyte proliferation. An important hypothesis generated at this time was that cytokines were principally synthesized by leukocytes and primarily acted on (other) leukocytes, and thus could be called **interleukins** (ILs). For example, a macrophage-derived costimulator activity for thymocytes was designated interleukin-1, and a T cell–derived T cell growth factor was called interleukin-2. However, preparations of cytokines available in the 1970s were often impure, and many of the available anticytokine antibodies were not absolutely specific for one cytokine. These methodological limitations prevented firm identification of the active factors as the same or distinct molecules.

The golden age of cytokine research occupied the 1980s. It was characterized by the molecular cloning and expression of individual cytokine molecules and by the production of completely specific, often monoclonal, neutralizing antibodies. These reagents allowed definitive identification of the structure and properties of individual cytokine molecules. The 1980s were more than a culmination of the early work because, in addition, many new cytokines were discovered and many previously unexpected properties of known cytokines were revealed. As a result of these studies, there is now a wealth of information about the sources and biologic activities of particular cytokines.

There are two continuing challenges in cytokine research. First, although much has been learned about the effects of cytokines *in vitro*, it is still largely unknown which biologic actions of a particular cytokine are important *in vivo* and which effects are necessary for a particular biologic response to occur. Experiments designed to answer these questions are in progress using recombinant cytokine molecules, specific cytokine antagonists, transgenic animals expressing cytokine genes, and animals that lack specific cytokines through gene knockout technology. Second, the availability of recombinant cytokines and specific antagonists has opened the possibility for clinicians to modify immune and inflammatory responses in a predictable fashion to influence the course of a disease. The task is to discover the most efficacious ways to use these **biological response modifiers** to achieve a desired outcome. Some of these clinical uses of cytokines and their antagonists will be discussed in subsequent chapters on immunologic diseases, transplantation, and tumor immunity.

GENERAL PROPERTIES OF CYTOKINES

Although cytokines are a diverse group of proteins, there are a number of properties shared by these molecules:

1. *Cytokines are produced during the effector phases of natural and specific immunity and serve to mediate and regulate immune and inflammatory responses.* In natural immunity, microbial products, such as lipopolysaccharide (LPS), directly stimulate mononuclear phagocytes to secrete their cytokines. In contrast, T cell–derived cytokines are elicited primarily in response to specific recognition of foreign antigens. However, these distinctions are not absolute because cytokines produced by one cell type often regulate the synthesis of cytokines by other cells.

2. *Cytokine secretion is a brief, self-limited event.* In general, cytokines are not stored as pre-formed molecules, and their synthesis is initiated by new gene transcription. Such transcriptional activation is usually transient, and the mRNAs encoding cytokines are unstable. The combination of a short period of transcription and a short-lived mRNA transcript ensures that cytokine synthesis is transient. Some cytokines may be additionally controlled by post-transcriptional mechanisms, such as proteolytic release of an active product from an inactive precursor. Once synthesized, cytokines are usually rapidly secreted, resulting in a burst of cytokine release as needed.

3. *Many individual cytokines are produced by multiple diverse cell types.* To emphasize that the cellular source of these molecules is usually not a distinguishing characteristic, investigators are increasingly adopting the convention followed in this book, namely to refer to these molecules collectively as cytokines rather than as lymphokines or monokines, regardless of their cellular source in a particular experiment.

4. *Cytokines act upon many different cell types.* This property is called **pleiotropism.** The earlier view that cytokines are primarily molecules produced by leukocytes that act particularly on leukocytes ("interleukins") is now considered too restricted a concept.

5. *Cytokines often have multiple different effects on the same target cell.* Some effects may occur simultaneously, whereas others may occur over different time frames (i.e., minutes, hours, or days).

6. *Cytokine actions are often redundant.* Many functions originally attributed to one cytokine have proved to be shared properties of several different cytokines. This observation has been reinforced by the study of knockout mice that lack particular cytokine genes yet display only subtle abnormalities in their immune responses.

7. *Cytokines often influence the synthesis of other cytokines,* leading to cascades in which a second or third cytokine may mediate the biologic effects of the first cytokine. The ability of one cytokine to enhance or suppress the production of others may provide important positive and negative regulatory mechanisms for immune and inflammatory responses.

8. *Cytokines often influence the action of other cytokines.* Two cytokines may interact to antagonize each other's action, to produce additive effects, or, in some cases, to produce greater than anticipated or even unique effects, a kind of interaction commonly referred to as synergy.

9. *Cytokines, like other polypeptide hormones, initiate their action by binding to specific receptors on the surface of target cell* (Box 12–1). The relevant target cell may be the same cell that secretes the cytokine (**autocrine** action), a nearby cell (**paracrine** action), or, like true hormones, a distant cell that is stimulated via cytokines that have been secreted into the circulation (**endocrine** action). Receptors for cytokines often show very high affinities for their ligands, with dissociation constants (K_d) in the range of 10^{-10} to 10^{-12} M. (For comparison, recall that antibodies typically bind antigens with a K_d of 10^{-7} M to 10^{-11} M, and major histocompatibility complex [MHC] molecules bind peptides with a K_d of only about 10^{-6} M.) As a consequence, only very small quantities of a cytokine need be produced to elicit a biologic effect.

10. *The expression of many cytokine receptors is regulated by specific signals.* This signal may be another cytokine or even the same cytokine that binds to the receptor, permitting positive amplification or negative feedback.

11. *Most cellular responses to cytokines require new mRNA and protein synthesis.* The mechanism by which cytokine binding to cell surface receptors stimulates transcription is still not completely known (Box 12–2). Some recent studies have identified nucleotide sequences in the 5′ flanking regions of genes whose transcription is activated by cytokine action. It is presumed that cytokines stimulate the production or binding of specific nuclear regulatory factors to these target sequences, and such binding, in turn, causes transcription.

12. *For many target cells, cytokines act as regulators of cell division, i.e., as growth factors.* Some immunologists now feel that cytokines should be categorized with epithelial and mesenchymal cell growth factors into a larger functional group of polypeptide regulatory molecules. However, we will continue to distinguish those molecules whose primary actions are as mediators of host defense (i.e., cytokines) from those molecules whose primary role resides in tissue repair (i.e., the epithelial and mesenchymal cell polypeptide growth factors).

FUNCTIONS OF CYTOKINES

We have organized our discussion of specific cytokines into four broad categories of function: (1) *mediators of natural immunity,* which are elicited by infectious agents from mononuclear phagocytes; (2) *regulators of lymphocyte activation, growth, and differentiation,* which are elicited in response to specific antigen recognition by T lymphocytes; (3) *regulators of immune-mediated inflammation,* which activate nonspecific inflammatory cells elicited in response to specific antigen recognition by T lymphocytes; and (4) *stimulators of immature leukocyte growth and differentiation,* which are produced by both stimulated lymphocytes and other cells. This classification is based on what appear to be the principal biologic actions of a

BOX 12–1. CYTOKINE RECEPTORS

The principal function of cytokine receptors is to convert an extracellular signal, namely the presence of a specific cytokine, into an intracellular signal, such as activation of an enzyme, that can trigger a target cell response. All known cytokine receptors are transmembrane proteins, and it is thought that the extracellular domains bind cytokine, thereby providing the means of detection of the extracellular signal. Signal transduction may involve the extracellular, transmembrane, or (most likely) intracellular portions of the cytokine receptor.

Cytokine receptors have been grouped into five large families based upon the presence of conserved folding motifs or sequence homologies (see figure, part A). The first motif to be noted in cytokine receptors was the Ig domain, and certain cytokine receptors (e.g., the type I and type II IL-1 receptors) contain several extracellular domains that belong to the Ig superfamily. This motif is also common in mesenchymal cell growth factor receptors, e.g., for platelet-derived growth factor or fibroblast growth factor receptors and in receptors for certain colony-stimulating factors such as c-kit ligand and M-CSF.

The second motif to be characterized in cytokine receptors involves a conserved extracellular sequence of five amino acid residues, tryptophan-serine-X-tryptophan-serine (written as WSXWS in the single letter amino acid code), where amino acid residue X is variable. This sequence motif is found in a large number of cytokine receptors, and is typically located just proximal to the transmembrane region. All cytokine receptors bearing this motif bind cytokines that share a four α-helical strand structure, including IL-2, IL-3, IL-4, IL-5, IL-6, IL-7, GM-CSF, and G-CSF. Interestingly, the IL-6 receptor contains both an Ig domain and the WSXWS motif in its extracellular portions. Receptors bearing the WSXWS motif are sometimes called members of the "type I family of cytokine receptors."

A third group of receptors, to date defined only at sequence level, includes the type I and type II interferon receptors. This group may also include the initiating protein of the coagulation cascade, tissue factor, but this is less certain. This sequence pattern is said to define the "type II family of cytokine receptors." The fourth structure identified in cytokine receptors is that found in the two TNF receptors (called p55 and p75). These sequences are homologous to the Fas protein, the B cell surface molecule CD40, and receptors for nerve growth factor. These molecules have been called type III cytokine receptors. The final motif described in cytokine receptors is a seven transmembrane α-helical structure displayed by the receptors for the chemokines. This

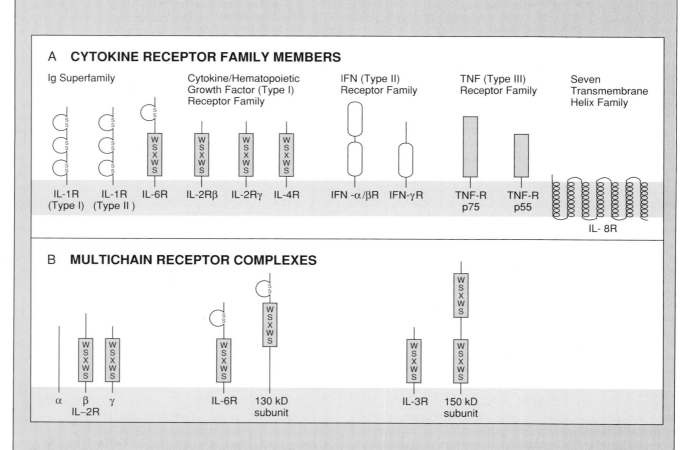

Cytokine receptors share various structural motifs, allowing them to be categorized into families (A). Several of these receptor proteins are known to function as parts of multichain complexes (B). The 130 kD subunit that transduces IL-6 signals also interacts with other polypeptide receptors, whereas the 150 KD subunit that transduces IL-3 signals is shared by the IL-5 and GM-CSF receptors.

Continued

motif was originally found in β-adrenergic receptors and retinal rhodopsin and is widely shared by receptors that are coupled to heterotrimeric GTP-binding proteins.

Several cytokine receptors actually consist of two or more separate transmembrane polypeptide chains that function as a complex (see figure, part B). For example, the high affinity IL-2 receptor contains three separate chains (α, β, and γ). Both β and γ, but not α, contain the WSXWS motif. IL-2R$\beta\gamma$ heterodimers bind IL-2 and mediate signal transduction. IL-2Rα serves to increase the affinity of the receptor for the cytokine, but does not contribute to signaling. The γ subunit may also associate with the IL-4 and IL-7 receptors. The IL-6 receptor interacts with a separate transmembrane signal-transducing 130 kD glycoprotein

that, like the IL-6 receptor itself, also contains an Ig domain and a WSXWS motif. At least three other protein hormones (ciliary neurotropic factor, oncostatin M, and leukemia inhibitory factor) also have receptors that interact with the same 130 kD signal-transducing molecule. Several other cytokine receptors (for IL-3, IL-5, and GM-CSF) are believed to share a 150 kD signal-transducing subunit in humans; in mice, the IL-3 receptor has a unique but homologous signal-transducing subunit.

Except for the M-CSF receptor and c-kit, which are tyrosine kinases, the molecular features of cytokine receptors that are involved in signal transduction are not well defined. This may change in the near future as many laboratories are currently working on this question.

particular cytokine, although, as we shall see, many cytokines may function in more than one of these categories.

Cytokines That Mediate Natural Immunity

The cytokines that mediate natural immunity include those that protect against viral infection and those that initiate inflammatory reactions that protect against bacteria. The cytokines discussed here are summarized in Table 12–1.

TYPE I INTERFERON

Type I interferons (IFNs) comprise two serologically distinct groups of proteins. The first group, collectively called IFN-α, is a family of about 20 structurally related polypeptides of approximately 18 kD, each encoded by a separate gene. (Some investigators now subdivide the IFN-α family into two groups, IFN-α1 and IFN-α2/IFN-ω, on the basis of the relatedness of amino acid sequences within the family.) Natural IFN-α preparations are usually a mixture of these molecules, and neutralizing sera react with all members of the IFN-α family. The major cell source for production of IFN-α is

TABLE 12–1. Mediators of Natural Immunity

Cytokine	Number of Genes	Polypeptide Size	Cell Source	Cell Target	Primary Effects on Each Target
Type I IFN	~20 IFN-α; 1 IFN-β	18 kD (monomer)	Mononuclear phagocyte, other (α); fibroblast, other (β)	All NK cell	Antiviral, antiproliferative, increased class I MHC expression Activation
Tumor necrosis factor	1	17 kD (homotrimer)	Mononuclear phagocyte, T cell	Neutrophil Endothelial cell Hypothalamus Liver Muscle, fat Thymocyte	Activation (inflammation) Activation (inflammation, coagulation) Fever Acute phase reactants (serum amyloid A protein) Catabolism (cachexia) Costimulator
Interleukin-1	2 (IL-1α, IL-1β)	17 kD (monomer)	Mononuclear phagocyte, other	Thymocyte Endothelial cell Hypothalamus Liver Muscle, fat	Costimulator Activation (inflammation, coagulation) Fever Acute phase reactants (serum amyloid A protein) Catabolism (cachexia)
Interleukin-6	1	26 kD (homodimer)	Mononuclear phagocyte, endothelial cell, T cell	Thymocyte Mature B cell Liver	Costimulator Growth Acute phase reactants (fibrinogen)
Chemokines	20+ related genes	8–10 kD (monomer)	Mononuclear phagocyte, endothelial cell; fibroblast; T cell; platelet	Leukocytes	Leukocyte chemotaxis and activation

Abbreviations: MHC, major histocompatibility complex; NK, natural killer; kD, kilodalton; IFN, interferon; IL, interleukin.

BOX 12-2. CYTOKINE SIGNAL TRANSDUCTION

Most cytokine actions depend upon new gene transcription and are thought to be mediated by cytokine-induced activation of specific DNA-binding proteins (transcription factors). The intracellular pathways by which cytokines activate transcription factors are diverse and not yet completely defined, but several clues have recently emerged about how some of these signals are transduced. Four current models are listed below.

INTERFERONS. IFNs are thought to cause activation of receptor-associated tyrosine kinases. The best evidence for this model is the observation that IFN-α signaling is lost in cells deficient in a particular tyrosine kinase, Tyk-2. IFN-γ signaling is maintained in Tyk-2–negative cells, but is lost in cells deficient in a different tyrosine kinase, JAK-2. Neither type of IFN functions in cells deficient in JAK-1. One substrate for the IFN-α–activated tyrosine kinase is a multi-subunit transcription factor called ISGF-3; upon tyrosine phosphorylation of several subunits, this factor assembles and moves from the cell cytoplasm to the nucleus, where it binds to specific sequences (called interferon sequence response elements, or ISREs) in the promoters of various IFN-α–inducible genes. IFN-γ activates a different tyrosine kinase that selectively phosphorylates only one subunit of ISGF-3. Upon tyrosine phosphorylation, this subunit can act as an independent transcription factor (called the gamma-activated factor, or GAF) that recognizes different sequences (called gamma-activated sequences, or GAS) from those seen by the entire ISGF-3 complex. Consequently, IFN-γ induces a different set of genes from those activated by IFN-α.

TNF/IL-1. These two cytokines share an ability to cause rapid translocation of a pre-existing NF-κB complex (p50-p65) from cell cytoplasm to nucleus, where it binds to specific regulatory DNA sequences in the promoters of several cytokine-inducible genes. (See Box 4–4 in Chapter 4 for discussion of NF-κB and related transcription factors.) One pathway thought to be involved in translocation of NF-κB begins with receptor-mediated activation of a phosphatidylcholine-specific phospholipase C (PC-PLC). This PC-PLC enzyme releases diacylglycerol from membrane-bound phosphatidylcholine. Free diacylglycerol activates a sphingomyelinase enzyme that liberates ceramide from membrane-bound sphingomyelin. Ceramide binds to and activates a specific ceramide-activated protein kinase, which, in turn, is thought to release NF-κB from its interaction with a cytoplasmic binding subunit, called I-κB. Once dissociated from I-κB, NF-κB moves to the nucleus and activates transcription of genes containing κB-binding sequences.

CHEMOKINES. Chemokines bind to seven transmembrane α-helical receptors. Upon ligand binding, these receptors are thought to catalyze the exchange of GTP for GDP bound to the α subunit (G$_\alpha$) of a heterotrimeric GTP-binding protein. When GTP is bound, G$_\alpha$ dissociates from the heterodimeric complex of G$_\beta$G$_\gamma$. Different G$_\alpha$-GTP isoforms, activated by different receptors, are capable of activating different cellular enzymes (such as adenylyl cyclase), and free G$_\beta$G$_\gamma$ may activate yet other enzymes. Eventually, G$_\alpha$-GTP hydrolyzes its bound GTP back to GDP. G$_\alpha$-GDP rapidly rebinds to G$_\beta$G$_\gamma$, terminating the signal. Among the enzymes activated by chemokines through heterotrimeric GTP-binding proteins are two isoforms of phosphatidylinositol-specific phospholipase C (PI-PLC-β1 and -β2). As we discussed in Chapter 7, PI-PLCs cleave membrane-bound phosphatidylinositol to yield inositol triphosphate, which elevates the levels of cytoplasmic free calcium, and diacylglycerol, which, in the presence of elevated calcium, activates isoforms of protein kinase C (PKC). Calcium, binding to calmodulin, activates yet other enzymes. Both calcium-activated kinases and PKC are thought to contribute to leukocyte motility by their interactions with cytoskeletal proteins such as myosin light chain.

HEMATOPOIETIC GROWTH FACTORS (CSFs). Homodimeric hematopoietic growth factors, such as IL-3, cause clustering of their WSXWS-containing receptors and associated signal-transducing subunits. This clustering is thought to activate receptor-associated tyrosine kinases analogous to the events initiated by cross-linking of the TCR complex (see Chapter 7), although the precise kinases that are activated by cytokine receptors are not yet known. As discussed in Chapter 7, receptor-associated tyrosine kinases typically act in two steps. First, they phosphorylate specific tyrosine residues in the cytoplasmic domains of the receptors themselves or in receptor-associated signal-transducing subunits. These phosphorylated tyrosine residues in the receptor are recognized by cytoplasmic proteins that contain SH2 domains, so that various SH2-containing proteins bind to the receptor and are clustered at the membrane. Second, the receptor-associated tyrosine kinases then phosphorylate additional tyrosine residues in the newly bound SH2-containing proteins, causing these proteins to become activated. In the T cell, some of these SH2-containing proteins are enzymes, such as PI-PLC-γ1, which (like PI-PLC-β1 and -β2) initiates a cascade that elevates cytoplasmic calcium and activates PKC (see Chapter 7). Recently, a pathway has been described that connects tyrosine kinase activation to mitogenesis. Specifically, tyrosine phosphorylation of a growth factor receptor leads to binding of a nonenzymatic SH2-containing protein called GRB-2. GRB-2 contains an SH-3 domain that binds another protein called SOS. Upon tyrosine phosphorylation, SOS catalyzes the exchange of GTP for bound GDP in a monomeric GTP-binding protein called ras. Ras-GTP (but not ras-GDP) activates a cascade of serine/threonine kinases that eventually leads to phosphorylation and activation of several transcription factors, including AP-1 and c-myc, that trigger cell division.

---

the mononuclear phagocyte, and IFN-α is sometimes called **leukocyte interferon.** The second serological group of type I IFN consists of a single gene product, a 20 kD glycoprotein called IFN-β. The usual cell source for isolation of IFN-β is the cultured fibroblast, and IFN-β is sometimes called **fibroblast interferon.** However, many cells make both IFN-α and IFN-β. The most potent natural signal that elicits type I IFN synthesis is viral infection. Experimentally, production of type I IFN is commonly elicited by synthetic double-stranded RNA

molecules, which may mimic a signal produced during viral replication. Both IFN-α and IFN-β are also secreted during immune responses to antigens. In this case, antigen-activated T cells stimulate mononuclear phagocytes to synthesize IFN. IFN-α and IFN-β show little structural similarity to each other. Nevertheless, all type I IFN molecules bind to the same cell surface receptor and appear to induce a similar series of cellular responses. The type I IFN receptor is a single chain polypeptide, homologous to the type II (immune or gamma) IFN receptor. It may also share folding motifs with other proteins, such as tissue factor (see Box 12–1).

There are four principal biologic actions of type I IFN:

1. *Type I IFN inhibits viral replication.* IFN causes cells to synthesize a number of enzymes, such as 2'-5' oligoadenylate synthetase, that collectively interfere with replication of viral RNA or DNA. The antiviral action of type I IFN is primarily paracrine, in that a virally infected cell secretes IFN to protect neighboring cells not yet infected. A cell that has responded to IFN and is resistant to viral infection is said to be in an **antiviral state.**

2. *Type I IFN inhibits cell proliferation.* This may be due to induction of the same enzymes that inhibit viral replication but also may involve other enzymes that prevent amino acid synthesis, especially of essential amino acids such as tryptophan. Although the mechanisms may be partly different, the antiviral effects and the antiproliferative effects of IFN cannot be uncoupled. It has been proposed that IFN-β is a physiologic inhibitor of normal cell growth. IFN-α is used as an antiproliferative agent for certain tumors (e.g., hairy cell leukemia and childhood hemangiomas).

3. *Type I IFN increases the lytic potential of natural killer (NK) cells.* As will be discussed in Chapter 13, a major function of NK cells is to kill virally infected cells.

4. *Type I IFN modulates MHC molecule expression.* In general, type I IFN increases expression of class I MHC molecules and profoundly inhibits class II MHC molecule expression. Because most cytolytic T lymphocytes (CTLs) recognize foreign antigens bound to class I MHC molecules, type I IFN boosts the effector phase of cell-mediated immune responses by enhancing the efficiency of CTL-mediated killing. At the same time, type I IFN may inhibit the cognitive phase of immune responses by preventing the activation of class II MHC–restricted helper T lymphocytes.

Thus, three of the principal activities of type I IFN, namely the induction of the antiviral state, the activation of NK cell lytic functions, and the increase in class I MHC molecule expression on virally infected cells, all act in concert to eradicate viral infections.

TUMOR NECROSIS FACTOR

Tumor necrosis factor (TNF) *is the principal mediator of the host response to gram-negative bacteria* and may also play a role in the response to other infectious organisms. (Some investigators refer to TNF as TNF-α and refer to lymphotoxin [LT] as TNF-β; this practice is controversial and increasingly confusing since the introduction of the term "LT-β" to refer to yet another member of this cytokine family. We shall use the simpler nomenclature of TNF and LT throughout this book.) The active components of gram-negative bacteria are **lipopolysaccharide** (LPS) molecules (also called **endotoxin**) derived from the bacterial cell wall (Fig. 12–1). TNF was originally identified (and was so named) as a mediator of tumor necrosis present in the

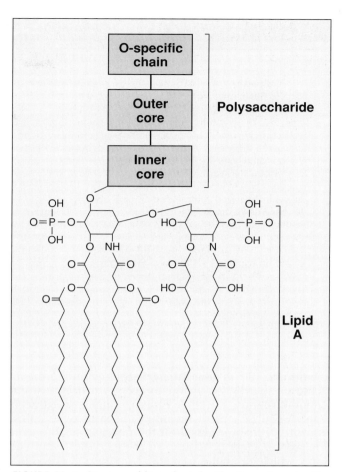

FIGURE 12–1. Structure of lipopolysaccharide. *Lipopolysaccharides are released when the cell walls of gram-negative bacteria, such as E. coli, are degraded. The lipid A moiety, which contains most of the biologic activity, is hydrophobic. The polysaccharide, which can contain 50 or more hexose moieties, can be divided into more conserved core regions and bacterial stain-specific ("O-specific") regions.*

serum of animals treated with LPS. At low concentrations, LPS stimulates the functions of mononuclear phagocytes and (in mice) acts as a polyclonal activator of B cells (see Chapters 9 and 13), host responses that contribute to elimination of the invading bacteria. However, high concentrations of LPS cause tissue injury, disseminated (widespread) intravascular coagulation (DIC), and shock, often resulting in death. The Shwartzman reaction is an experimental model for studying the pathologic effects of LPS (Box 12–3). It is now clear that TNF is one of the principal mediators of these effects of LPS.

The major cellular source of TNF is the LPS-activated mononuclear phagocyte, although antigen-stimulated T cells, activated NK cells, and activated mast cells can also secrete this protein. IFN-γ, produced by T cells, augments TNF synthesis by LPS-stimulated mononuclear phagocytes. Thus, TNF is a mediator of both natural and acquired immunity and an important link between specific immune responses and acute inflammation. In the mononuclear phagocyte, TNF is initially synthesized as a nonglycosylated transmembrane protein of approximately 25 kD. The orientation of

BOX 12-3. THE SHWARTZMAN REACTION

The mechanism of LPS-mediated tissue injury was investigated by Shwartzman, who found that two intravenous injections of a sublethal quantity of LPS, administered 24 hours apart, would cause DIC in the rabbit. This is called the **systemic Shwartzman reaction** and is due to widespread intravascular thrombus formation on the surfaces of endothelial cells. If the first LPS injection is given intradermally, the second intravenous injection causes hemorrhagic necrosis of skin exclusively at the intradermal injection site. In this **localized Shwartzman reaction**, tissue injury is caused by activated neutrophils and by inadequate perfusion of the tissue. The inadequate tissue perfusion results from local intravascular coagulation (fibrin formation) and from cellular plugging of the microcirculation by neutrophils and platelets. Recent studies have shown that TNF can in large part substitute for LPS in eliciting both the local Shwartzman reaction and the systemic toxicity of LPS. Moreover, neutralizing antibody to TNF affords protection against both the injurious and the lethal effects of LPS. Thus, TNF is thought to be an obligatory mediator of LPS-induced tissue injury.

The Shwartzman reaction is an exaggerated form of a host response to microbes, which, under less extreme physiologic conditions, functions primarily to eliminate microbes and limit their spread. Although TNF is now known to be one of the principal cytokines involved in such host responses, TNF was first identified as a factor present in the plasma of LPS-treated animals that could cause hemorrhagic necrosis of tumors. Some of the anti-tumor action of TNF is mediated by direct tumor cell lysis, a process not well understood but believed to involve TNF binding to surface receptors on tumor cells, thereby initiating phospholipase activation and perhaps free radical–mediated cell injury. Mostly, however, TNF induces tumor necrosis by causing a local Shwartz-man-like reaction to occur in the tumor vascular bed. The basis for the selective effect on tumor blood vessels is not known, but tumor cells appear to release factors that increase the sensitivity of local endothelial cells to TNF. These tumor factors act like the first injection of LPS.

---

membrane TNF is unusual, in that the amino terminus is intracellular, the transmembrane segment is near the amino terminus, and the carboxy terminus is extracellular. A 17 kD fragment, including the carboxy terminus, is proteolytically cleaved off the plasma membrane of the mononuclear phagocyte to produce the "secreted" form, which circulates as a stable homotrimer of 51 kD. Native TNF assumes a triangular pyramidal shape such that each side of the pyramid is formed by a different monomeric subunit. The receptor binding sites are at the base of the pyramid, allowing simultaneous binding to more than one receptor.

TNF actions are initiated by binding of the soluble trimer to cell surface receptors. There are two distinct TNF receptors, of 55 and 75 kD, respectively, each encoded by a separate gene. The affinity of TNF for its receptors is unusually low for a cytokine, the K_d being only approximately 5×10^{-10} M for binding to the 75 kD receptor and 1×10^{-9} M for binding to the 55 kD receptor. However, TNF is synthesized in very large quantities and can easily saturate its receptors. TNF receptors are present on almost all cell types examined. Activated cells shed their TNF receptors; such soluble receptors may act as competitive inhibitors of the cell surface receptor.

Many TNF responses involve increased rates of transcription of particular target genes, often through activation of NF-κB or AP-1 transcription factors. A model for the activation of NF-κB by TNF is described in Box 12–2.

The biologic actions of TNF, like those of LPS, are best understood as a function of quantity (Fig. 12–2). *At low concentrations, i.e., at approximately 10^{-9} M, TNF acts locally as a paracrine and autocrine regulator of leukocytes and endothelial cells.* The principal biologic actions of TNF at low concentrations are the following:

1. TNF causes vascular endothelial cells to express new surface receptors (**adhesion molecules**) that make the endothelial cell surface become adhesive for leukocytes, initially for neutrophils and subsequently for monocytes and lymphocytes. TNF also acts on neutrophils to increase their adhesiveness for endothelial cells. These actions contribute to accumulation of leukocytes at local sites of inflammation and are probably the physiologically most important local effects of TNF (see Chapter 13).

2. TNF activates inflammatory leukocytes to kill microbes. TNF is especially potent at activating neutrophils but also affects eosinophils and mononuclear phagocytes.

3. TNF stimulates mononuclear phagocytes and other cell types to produce cytokines, including IL-1, IL-6, TNF itself, and chemokines.

4. TNF exerts an interferon-like protective effect against viruses and augments expression of class I MHC molecules, potentiating CTL-mediated lysis of virally infected cells.

These effects of TNF are critical for inflammatory responses to microbes. If inadequate quantities of TNF are present, e.g., in animals treated with neutralizing anti-TNF antibodies, a consequence may be a failure to contain infections.

If the stimulus for TNF production is sufficiently strong, greater quantities of the cytokine are produced. In this setting, TNF enters the blood stream, where it can act as an endocrine hormone. *The principal systemic actions of TNF in physiologic host responses to infections are the following:*

1. TNF is an *endogenous pyrogen* that acts on cells in hypothalamic regulatory regions of the brain to induce fever. It shares this property with IL-1, and both cytokines are found in the serum of animals or people

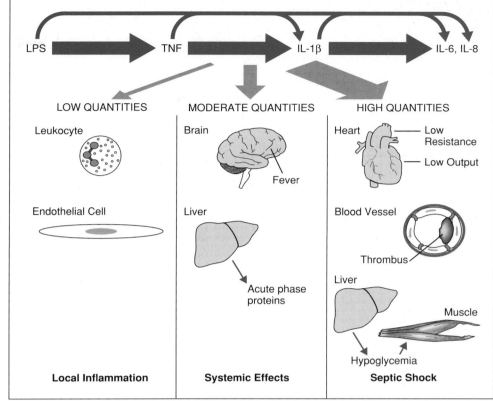

FIGURE 12–2. The LPS-induced cytokine cascade. *Bacterial LPS acts on macrophages to release TNF. TNF induces macrophages to release IL-1β. IL-1β acts on macrophages and vascular endothelial cells to release IL-6 and IL-8. (The thinner arrows indicate that LPS directly induces IL-1β, IL-6, and IL-8 and that TNF directly induces IL-6 and IL-8, but these actions are amplified through the cascade.) When low quantities of cytokine are released, the effects are local. With moderate quantities, systemic effects can be detected. At high levels, these cytokines produce the syndrome of septic shock.*

exposed to LPS, which functions as an exogenous pyrogen. Fever production in response to TNF or IL-1 is mediated by increased synthesis of prostaglandins by cytokine-stimulated hypothalamic cells. Prostaglandin synthesis inhibitors, such as aspirin, reduce fever by blocking this action of TNF or IL-1.

2. TNF acts on mononuclear phagocytes and perhaps vascular endothelial cells to stimulate secretion of

IL-1 and IL-6 into the circulation (Fig. 12–3). This is one example of a cascade of cytokines that share many biologic activities.

3. TNF acts on hepatocytes to increase synthesis of certain serum proteins, such as serum amyloid A protein. The spectrum of hepatocyte proteins induced by TNF is identical to that induced by IL-1 but differs from that induced by IL-6 (described below). The com-

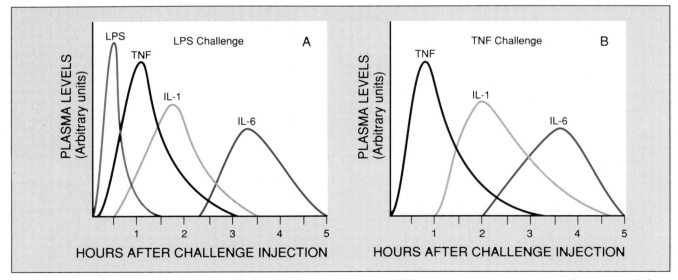

FIGURE 12–3. Cytokine cascades in sepsis. *Following injection of lipopolysaccharide (LPS) (A), there are successive waves of tumor necrosis factor (TNF), IL-1, and IL-6 detectable in plasma. Injection of TNF (B) produces successive waves of IL-1 and IL-6. In the presence of antibody to TNF, LPS-induced plasma elevations of IL-1 and IL-6 are inhibited; and in the presence of antibody to IL-1, plasma elevations of IL-6 are inhibited. These data suggest that there are ordered cascades of cytokine production: LPS induces TNF, which induces IL-1, which induces IL-6 synthesis.*

bination of hepatocyte-derived plasma proteins induced by TNF or IL-1 plus those induced by IL-6 constitutes the **acute phase response** to inflammatory stimuli (Box 12–4).

4. TNF activates the coagulation system, primarily by altering the balance of the procoagulant and anticoagulant activities of vascular endothelium.

5. TNF suppresses bone marrow stem cell division. Chronic administration of TNF may lead to lymphopenia and immunodeficiency.

6. Long-term systemic administration of TNF to experimental animals causes the metabolic alterations of **cachexia,** a state characterized by wasting of muscle and fat cells. The cachexia is produced largely by TNF-induced appetite suppression. TNF also suppresses synthesis of lipoprotein lipase, an enzyme needed to release fatty acids from circulating lipoproteins so that they can be utilized by the tissues. Although TNF by itself can produce cachexia in experimental animals, other cytokines, such as IL-1, may also contribute to the cachectic state accompanying certain chronic diseases such as tuberculosis and cancer.

The combination of fever, elevated IL-6 levels, elevated acute phase reactants, bone marrow suppression, and activation of coagulation has been noted in patients treated with intravenous TNF for cancer chemotherapy.

In the setting of gram-negative bacterial sepsis, massive quantities of TNF are produced, and serum concentrations of TNF can transiently exceed 10^{-7} M.

Animals producing this much TNF die of circulatory collapse and disseminated intravascular coagulation. Neutralizing antibodies to TNF can prevent mortality, implicating this cytokine as a critical mediator of septic or endotoxin shock (Fig. 12–4). Moreover, infusion of high levels of TNF is by itself lethal, producing a shock-like syndrome. *Several specific actions of TNF may contribute to its lethal effects at extremely high concentrations.*

1. TNF reduces tissue perfusion by depressing myocardial contractility. The mechanism of this action appears to involve induction of an enzyme in cardiac myocytes, nitric oxide synthase (NOS), that converts arginine to citrulline and NO. NO made by this enzyme inhibits myocardial contractility.

2. TNF further reduces blood pressure and tissue perfusion by relaxing vascular smooth muscle tone. TNF may act directly on smooth muscle cells and also can act indirectly by stimulating production of vasodilators, such as prostacyclin and NO by vascular endothelial cells.

3. TNF causes intravascular thrombosis, leading to reduced tissue perfusion. This is due to a combination of endothelial and mononuclear phagocyte alterations, which promote coagulation, and activation of neutrophils leading to vascular plugging by these cells. These TNF-mediated actions account for many of the effects of LPS seen in the Shwartzman reaction of rabbits and disseminated intravascular coagulation in humans.

4. TNF causes severe metabolic disturbances,

BOX 12–4. THE ACUTE PHASE RESPONSE

The acute phase response consists of a rapid adjustment of plasma protein composition in response to injurious stimuli, including infection, burns, trauma, and neoplasia. Several different plasma proteins rise in concentration, whereas others fall. Among the proteins whose levels increase are C-reactive protein, which functions as a nonspecific opsonin to augment phagocytosis of bacteria; α_2 macroglobulin and other anti-proteinases; the clotting protein fibrinogen; and serum amyloid A protein, a molecule of uncertain function. Albumin and transferrin, the iron transport protein, decline. Most of these changes in plasma concentrations can be directly attributed to alterations in the levels of synthesis of these plasma proteins by hepatocytes. Experiments using whole animals, liver slices, cultured hepatocytes, or hepatocyte-derived tumor cell lines have revealed that these changes in biosynthesis are caused by alterations in gene transcription regulated primarily by IL-6 (on fibrinogen) and IL-1/TNF (on serum amyloid protein).

The precise function of the acute phase response is largely unknown. The increases in opsonizing proteins and anti-proteinases are believed to aid natural immunity and protect against tissue injury, respectively. Elevation in fibrinogen, caused by IL-6, is of uncertain benefit but has had major impact on clinical medicine. Specifically, elevated levels of fibrinogen can cause red blood cells to form stacks (rouleaux). When blood is collected and allowed to stand at unit gravity, rouleaux sediment more rapidly than individual red blood cells. Rouleaux in venous blood may sediment before the red blood cells are fully oxygenated, leading

to a dark mass at the bottom of the container. In ancient times, this mass of dark, deoxygenated red blood cells was called "black bile," and ancient and medieval physicians would perform bleeding of patients to remove this "sickly humor." In modern times, the realization that the more rapid red blood cell sedimentation reflected the presence of illness, rather than representing its cause, allowed measure of the **erythrocyte sedimentation rate** to become a useful diagnostic test for the presence of the acute phase response. In the past few years, more specific measures of the acute phase response, for example, of C-reactive protein or of IL-6, have now largely supplanted this useful tool.

Although the acute phase response is characterized by rapid onset, it can persist in the setting of chronic inflammation. In some patients with chronic inflammatory disease (e.g., rheumatoid arthritis; see Chapter 20), persistent elevations of serum amyloid A protein may lead to deposition of this protein in the interstitium of tissues. Such deposited protein, in the form of fibrils rich in β-pleated sheet structure, can interfere with normal organ function (e.g., myocardial contraction, glomerular filtration). Such patients are said to have developed **amyloidosis** because such protein deposits stain with acidic iodine, a reaction originally developed for amylose or animal starch. Similar fibrils can develop in other settings (e.g., multiple myeloma, Alzheimer's disease, or endocrine cell tumors); however, in these cases, the protein fibrils are not of serum amyloid A protein origin and are unrelated to the acute phase response.

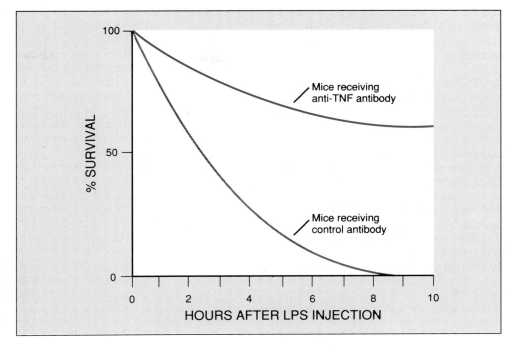

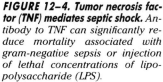

FIGURE 12–4. Tumor necrosis factor (TNF) mediates septic shock. Antibody to TNF can significantly reduce mortality associated with gram-negative sepsis or injection of lethal concentrations of lipopolysaccharide (LPS).

such as a fall in blood glucose concentrations to levels that are incompatible with life. This is due to overutilization of glucose by muscle and failure to replace glucose by the liver.

Many of the biologic actions of TNF are augmented by IFN-γ. In some cells that are targets of TNF effects, this interaction may be explained by IFN-γ–stimulated increases in TNF receptor numbers. However, in many cases, IFN-γ enhancement of TNF activity is noted without any effect on TNF binding. The full significance of this interaction is not clear, but activated T cells often secrete TNF and IFN-γ coordinately. Coordinate secretion of these two cytokines may provide a means of locally enhancing the actions of TNF without requiring concentrations that produce systemic toxicity.

INTERLEUKIN-1

Interleukin-1 was first defined as a polypeptide derived from mononuclear phagocytes that enhanced the responses of thymocytes to polyclonal activators, i.e., as a costimulator of T cell activation. A convenient bioassay for this activity is the costimulation (with concanavalin A or phytohemagglutinin) of murine thymocyte proliferation. It is now appreciated that this assay is not specific for IL-1 and may also detect other cytokines such as IL-6. Although IL-1 was discovered as a costimulator of T cells, *it is now clear that the principal function of IL-1, similar to TNF, is as a mediator of the host inflammatory response in natural immunity.* Indeed, there is little evidence to support a role of IL-1 as a physiologically important costimulator of mature T cell activation.

The major cellular source of IL-1, like that of TNF, is the activated mononuclear phagocyte. IL-1 production by mononuclear phagocytes can be triggered by

bacterial products such as LPS, by macrophage-derived cytokines such as TNF or IL-1 itself, and by contact with CD4+ T cells. Like TNF, IL-1 can be found in the circulation following gram-negative bacterial sepsis, where it can act as an endocrine hormone. In this case, it is produced mainly in response to TNF (see Fig. 12–3). IL-1 synthesis differs from that of TNF in two important regards. First, T cells are more effective than LPS at eliciting synthesis of IL-1 by mononuclear phagocytes. Second, IL-1 is made by many diverse cell types, such as epithelial and endothelial cells, providing potential local sources of IL-1 in the absence of macrophage-rich infiltrates.

Biochemical purification of IL-1 secreted by mononuclear phagocytes revealed that the biologic activity of this cytokine actually resided in two major polypeptide species, each approximately 17 kD but with distinct isoelectric points of 5.0 and 7.0. It is now known that these two forms, called IL-1α and IL-1β, respectively, are products of two different genes. The two forms of IL-1 show less than 30 per cent structural homology to each other, but both species bind to the same cell surface receptors and their biologic activities are essentially identical. A third member of the IL-1 family, called IL-1 receptor antagonist, will be discussed below. The IL-1 molecules are also related structurally to the various forms of fibroblast growth factor.

Both IL-1 polypeptides are synthesized as approximately 33 kD precursors that are proteolytically cleaved to generate the mature 17 kD proteins. The 17 kD forms fold in a barrel-like structure, rich in strands of β-pleated sheet. The 33 kD IL-1α precursor is biologically active, but IL-1β must be processed to the 17 kD form before it can exert biologic effects. An IL-1–specific protease has been identified in mononuclear phagocytes that is responsible for most of the conversion of IL-1β to its active form. The complete amino acid sequence of both IL-1 species presents a theoretical problem: unlike conventionally secreted proteins, neither IL-1 polypeptide has a hydrophobic signal sequence to target the nascent polypeptide to the endoplasmic reticulum, and both proteins appear to be synthesized as cytoplasmic proteins. It is therefore unknown how these molecules are secreted. The N terminal region of IL-1α contains a nuclear targeting sequence that may transport IL-1α into the nucleus of the cell that synthesizes it. Most of the IL-1 activity found in the circulation is IL-1β.

Two different membrane receptors for IL-1 have been characterized, both of which are members of the Ig superfamily. The type I receptor was initially characterized from a T cell line where it mediates IL-1 stimulation; it has slightly higher affinity for IL-1β than for IL-1α. The type II receptor was initially characterized from a B cell; it has greater affinity for IL-1α than for IL-1β. It is not clear, at present, whether the type II receptor mediates IL-1 actions or merely serves to competitively inhibit IL-1 binding to the type I receptor. The K_d for IL-1 binding to its receptors may be as high as 1×10^{-12} M; however, IL-1 may be active on some target cells at concentrations as low as 1×10^{-15} M, suggesting that additional IL-1 binding proteins may exist. Many IL-1–induced transcriptional effects, like those of TNF, involve NF-κB (see Box 12–2).

The biologic effects of IL-1, similar to those of TNF, depend on the quantity of cytokine released (see Fig. 12–2). At low IL-1 concentrations, the principal biologic effects are as a mediator of local inflammation. Specifically, IL-1 acts on mononuclear phagocytes and vascular endothelium to increase further synthesis of IL-1 and induce synthesis of IL-6. It also shares many of the inflammatory properties of TNF. For example, IL-1 acts on endothelial cells to promote coagulation and to increase expression of surface molecules that mediate leukocyte adhesion. IL-1 does not directly activate inflammatory leukocytes, such as neutrophils, but it causes mononuclear phagocytes and endothelial cells to synthesize chemokines that do activate leukocytes (see below).

When secreted in larger quantities, IL-1 enters the blood stream and exerts endocrine effects. *Systemic IL-1 shares with TNF the ability to cause fever, to induce synthesis of acute phase plasma proteins* (such as serum amyloid A protein) *by the liver, and to initiate metabolic wasting (cachexia).*

It was initially very surprising to note the extensive similarities of IL-1 actions with those of TNF, a striking example of the redundancy of cytokine effects. However, there are several important differences between these cytokines. First, IL-1 does not produce tissue injury by itself, although it is secreted in response to LPS and can potentiate tissue injury caused by TNF. Moreover, even at very high systemic concentrations, IL-1 is not lethal. Second, although IL-1 mimics many of the inflammatory and procoagulant properties of TNF, IL-1 cannot replace TNF as a mediator of the Shwartzman reaction and does not cause hemorrhagic necrosis of tumors. Third, most tumor cell lines are not directly lysed by IL-1 *in vitro*. Fourth, IL-1 does not share with

TNF an ability to increase expression of MHC molecules. Finally, IL-1 potentiates rather than suppresses the actions of CSFs on bone marrow cells.

IL-1 is the only cytokine to date for which **naturally occurring inhibitors** have been described. The best defined of these is produced by human mononuclear phagocytes. It is structurally homologous to IL-1 and binds to IL-1 receptors but is biologically inactive, so that it functions as a competitive inhibitor of IL-1. It is therefore commonly called IL-1 receptor antagonist (IL-1ra). In monocytes, IL-1ra is synthesized with a signal sequence and is efficiently secreted, thereby inhibiting the actions of IL-1. In other cell types, IL-1ra mRNA may be spliced to remove the signal sequence so it is not secreted; the functions of intracellular IL-1ra are unknown. Type I and type II IL-1 receptors are also shed by activated cells. Both IL-1ra and soluble receptors may be endogenous regulators of IL-1 action. It may also be possible to use cytokine inhibitors as biologic response modifiers in disease states that are caused by excessive or unregulated cytokine production, such as septic shock.

INTERLEUKIN-6

Interleukin-6 (IL-6) is a cytokine of approximately 26 kD that is synthesized by mononuclear phagocytes, vascular endothelial cells, fibroblasts, and other cells in response to IL-1 and, to a lesser extent, TNF. It is also made by some activated T cells. IL-6 can be detected in the circulation following gram-negative bacterial infection or TNF infusion and appears to be secreted in response to TNF or IL-1 rather than LPS itself (see Fig. 12–3). IL-6 does not cause vascular thrombosis or the tissue injury that is seen in response to LPS or TNF. The functional form of IL-6 is probably a homodimer.

The receptor for IL-6 consists of a 60 kD binding protein and 130 kD signal-transducing subunit. The binding protein contains both an Ig domain and a tryptophan-serine-X-tryptophan-serine (WSXWS, where X stands for a variable amino acid residue) motif characteristic of receptors that interact with cytokines sharing a four α-helical folding pattern (see Box 12–1). The signal transducing subunit also contains both an Ig domain and the WSXWS motif, but it is not specific for IL-6 and can interact with other polypeptides as well. Clustering of the 130 kD subunit by interactions with cytokine and specific binding protein is thought to trigger signaling. Shed IL-6 receptors can also bind IL-6 and signal through the 130 kD subunit.

The two best described actions of IL-6 are on hepatocytes and B cells:

1. *Interleukin-6 causes hepatocytes to synthesize several plasma proteins, such as fibrinogen, that contribute to the acute phase response* (Box 12–4).

2. *Interleukin-6 serves as a growth factor for activated B cells late in the sequence of B cell differentiation.* IL-6 similarly acts as a growth factor for many malignant plasma cells (plasmacytomas or myelomas), and many plasmacytoma cells that grow autonomously actually secrete IL-6 as an autocrine growth factor. Moreover, IL-6 can promote the growth of somatic cell

hybrids produced by fusing normal B cells with plasma-cytoma cells, i.e., the "hybridomas" that produce monoclonal antibodies (Box 3–1, Chapter 3). Transgenic mice that over-express the IL-6 gene develop massive polyclonal proliferation of plasma cells.

In addition to these well described actions, *in vitro* experiments suggest that IL-6 may serve as a costimulator of T cells and of thymocytes. IL-6 also acts as a cofactor with other cytokines for the growth of early bone marrow hematopoietic stem cells. Finally, it should be noted that one of the first activities ascribed to IL-6, that of an interferon, has not been confirmed using recombinant preparations of IL-6, and the alternative name of IFN-β_2 for this cytokine has now been abandoned.

CHEMOKINES

A recent discovery in the cytokine field is the existence of a large family of structurally homologous cytokines, approximately 8 to 10 kD in size. These molecules share the ability to stimulate leukocyte movement (**chemokinesis**) and directed movement (**chemotaxis**) and have been collectively called "chemokines," a contraction of **chemo**tactic cyto**kines.** All of these molecules contain two internal disulfide loops. Some investigators separate these factors into two subfamilies, based on whether the two amino terminal cysteine residues are immediately adjacent (cys-cys) or separated by one amino acid (cys-X-cys). These differences correlate with organization of the two subfamilies into separate gene clusters.

The chemokines of the cys-X-cys subfamily are produced largely by activated mononuclear phagocytes as well as by tissue cells (endothelium, fibroblasts) and megakaryocytes (which give rise to platelets containing stored chemokine). These molecules act predominantly on neutrophils as mediators of acute inflammation. The best characterized member of this subfamily is interleukin-8. The cys-cys subfamily is produced largely by activated T cells. These molecules act predominantly on subsets of mononuclear inflammatory cells. For example, a chemokine called RANTES acts on memory CD4$^+$ T cells and monocytes. An exception to this generalization is monocyte chemotactic protein–1 (MCP-1), a cys-cys chemokine that acts only on monocytes but is made by activated mononuclear phagocytes and tissue cells as well as by T cells. Chemokines of both subfamilies bind to heparan sulfate proteoglycans on the endothelial cell surface, and may function principally to stimulate chemokinesis of leukocytes that attach to cytokine-activated endothelium through induced adhesion molecules.

Several chemokine receptors have recently been characterized, and all of these belong to the seven transmembrane α-helical family (see Box 12–1). Interestingly, some chemokine receptors appear to interact with several different chemokines; the significance of this molecular promiscuity is not yet known.

Cytokines That Regulate Lymphocyte Activation, Growth, and Differentiation

Some cytokines function principally to regulate the growth and differentiation of lymphocytes and mediate the activation phase of specific immune responses. Most of these cytokines are produced by T cells, especially antigen-specific CD4$^+$ T lymphocytes. Such T cells provide help for both cell-mediated and humoral immune response, in large part through the secretion of cytokines. The cytokines that act primarily to regulate lymphocytes themselves are interleukin-2, interleukin-4, and transforming growth factor–β (TGF-β). The properties of the cytokines discussed in this section are listed in Table 12–2.

INTERLEUKIN-2

*Interleukin-2 (IL-2), originally called **T cell growth factor** (TCGF), is the principal cytokine responsible for progression of T lymphocytes from the G_1 to S phase of the cell cycle.* IL-2 is produced by CD4$^+$ T cells, and in lesser quantities by CD8$^+$ T cells. IL-2 acts on the same cells that produce it; i.e., it functions as an **autocrine**

TABLE 12–2. Mediators of Lymphocyte Activation, Growth, and Differentiation

Cytokine	Number of Genes	Polypeptide Size	Cell Source	Cell Target	Primary Effects on Each Target
Interleukin-2	1	14–17 kD (monomer)	T cells	T cell	Growth; cytokine production
				NK cell	Growth, activation
				B cell	Growth, antibody synthesis
Interleukin-4	1	20 kD (monomer)	CD4$^+$ T cell, mast cell	B cell	Isotype switching to IgE
				Mononuclear phagocyte	Inhibit activation
				T cell	Growth
Transforming growth factor–β	Several	14 kD (homodimer)	T cells, mononuclear phagocyte, other	T cell	Inhibit activation and proliferation
				Mononuclear phagocyte	Inhibit activation
				Other cell types	Growth regulation

Abbreviations: NK, natural killer; kD, kilodalton; Ig, immunoglobulin.

growth factor. IL-2 also acts on nearby T lymphocytes, including both CD4$^+$ and CD8$^+$ cells, and is also therefore a **paracrine growth factor.** During physiologic immune responses, IL-2 does not circulate in the blood to act at a distance, and thus it is not considered to be an endocrine growth factor.

Secreted IL-2 is a 14 to 17 kD glycoprotein encoded by a single gene on chromosome 4 in humans. The size heterogeneity of the mature protein is due to variable extents of glycosylation of an approximately 130 amino acid residue polypeptide. Native IL-2 is folded into a globular protein containing two sets of paired parallel α-helices, each sheet oriented at a slight angle to the other. This α-helical folding motif is common to all cytokines that interact with receptors with the WSXWS sequence, including IL-3, IL-4, IL-5, IL-6, GM-CSF, and G-CSF. Normally, IL-2 is transcribed, synthesized, and secreted by T cells only upon activation by antigens. IL-2 synthesis is usually transient, with an early peak of secretion occurring about 4 hours after activation. The mechanisms of transcriptional regulation of IL-2 synthesis have been described in Chapter 7 (Box 7–5).

The principal actions of IL-2 are on lymphocytes:

1. *Interleukin-2 is the major autocrine growth factor for T lymphocytes, and the quantity of IL-2 synthesized by activated CD4$^+$ T cells is an important determinant of the magnitude of T cell-dependent immune responses.* IL-2 also stimulates synthesis of other T cell–derived cytokines such as IFN-γ and lymphotoxin (LT). Failure to synthesize adequate quantities of IL-2 has been described as a cause of antigen-specific T cell anergy (see Chapter 10).

The action of IL-2 on T cells is mediated by binding to IL-2 receptor proteins. This system is perhaps the best understood of all cytokine receptors. Two distinct cell surface proteins on T cells bind IL-2. The first to be identified, called IL-2Rα, is a 55 kD polypeptide (p55) that appears upon T cell activation and was originally called Tac (for T activation) antigen. IL-2Rα binds IL-2 with a K$_d$ of approximately 10^{-8} M. Binding of IL-2 to cells expressing only IL-2Rα does not lead to any detectable biologic response. The second IL-2–binding protein, called IL-2Rβ, is about 70 to 75 kD (called variously p70 or p75) and is a member of the receptor family characterized by the WSXWS motif (see Box 12–1). The affinity of binding of IL-2 to this receptor is higher than to IL-2Rα, with a K$_d$ of approximately 10^{-9} M. IL-2Rβ is expressed coordinately with a 64 kD polypeptide, called IL-2Rγ, which is also a member of the WSXWS family, forming a complex designated as IL-2Rβγ. IL-2 causes growth of cells expressing only IL-2Rβγ, with half maximal growth stimulation occurring at the same concentration of IL-2 that produces half maximal binding. Cells that express IL-2Rα as well as IL-2Rβγ can bind IL-2 much more tightly, with a K$_d$ of approximately 10^{-11} M. Growth stimulation of such cells occurs at a similarly low IL-2 concentration. Both IL-2 binding and growth stimulation can be blocked by antibodies to either IL-2Rα or IL-2Rβ and most efficiently by a combination of antibodies to both receptor subunits. These observations have been interpreted to mean that *IL-2Rα forms a complex with IL-2Rβγ, increasing the affinity of the IL-2Rβγ receptor for IL-2 and thereby allowing a growth signal to be delivered at significantly lower IL-2 concentrations.* It is believed that IL-2 first binds rapidly to IL-2Rα, and this facilitates association with IL-2Rβγ. As depicted in Figure 12–5, resting T cells express IL-2Rβγ but not IL-2Rα and can be stimulated only by high levels of IL-2. Upon antigen receptor-mediated T cell activation, IL-2Rα is rapidly expressed, thereby reducing the concentration of IL-2 needed for growth stimulation. In fact, IL-2 itself can further increase IL-2Rα synthesis. Although much is known about the interaction of IL-2 with its receptor, the intracellular signals produced by cytokine binding have not been identified. There is some evidence that a tyrosine kinase may be involved in IL-2-mediated T cell growth stimulation, but its identity is not yet known.

2. *IL-2 stimulates the growth of NK cells and enhances their cytolytic function,* producing so-called lymphokine-activated killer (LAK) cells (see Chapter 13). NK cells, like resting T cells, express IL-2Rβγ and can be stimulated by high levels of IL-2. NK cells, however, do not express IL-2Rα and therefore do not reduce their requirement for IL-2, even after activation. Thus, only high concentrations of IL-2 will lead to LAK cell formation. IL-2 synergizes with other cytokines, notably IL-12, to induce IFN-γ secretion by NK cells.

3. *IL-2 acts on human B cells both as a growth factor and as a stimulus for antibody synthesis.* It does not appear to cause isotype switching. These activities of IL-2 are discussed more fully in Chapter 9.

Actions of IL-2 on other cell populations are less well established. IL-2 receptor proteins have been detected on mononuclear phagocytes. However, a specific IL-2 function in this cell type has not been described. Mice in which the IL-2 gene is disrupted by knockout technology appear to have a relatively normal immune system. These observations suggest that many IL-2 actions may be redundant or, more likely, that IL-2–independent T cells can arise and be selected for in the thymus.

Chronic T cell stimulation leads to shedding of IL-2Rα. Shed receptor proteins may bind free IL-2, preventing its interaction with cells. However, the much greater affinity of IL-2Rαβγ for IL-2 compared with IL-2Rα alone suggests that serum IL-2Rα is not likely to contribute significantly to immunosuppression. Clinically, an increased level of shed IL-2Rα in the serum is a marker of strong antigenic stimulation, e.g., acute rejection of a transplanted organ. Infection of T cells by human T lymphotrophic virus–1 (HTLV-1) activates IL-2Rα synthesis and also leads to shed IL-2Rα in the serum.

INTERLEUKIN-4

Interleukin-4 (IL-4) was initially identified as a helper T cell–derived cytokine of approximately 20 kD that stimulated the proliferation of mouse B cells in the presence of anti-Ig antibody (an analog of antigen) and

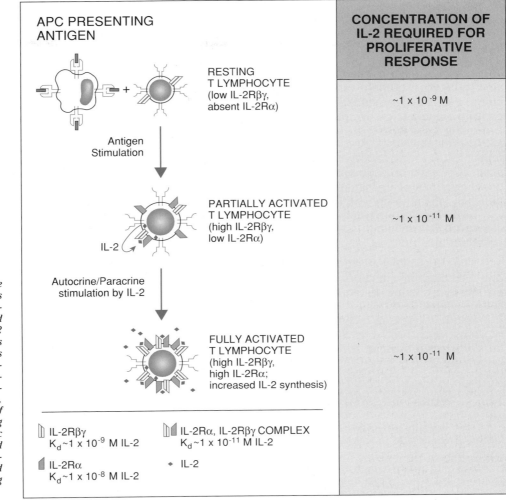

APC PRESENTING ANTIGEN	CONCENTRATION OF IL-2 REQUIRED FOR PROLIFERATIVE RESPONSE
RESTING T LYMPHOCYTE (low IL-2Rβγ, absent IL-2Rα)	~1 x 10^{-9} M
PARTIALLY ACTIVATED T LYMPHOCYTE (high IL-2Rβγ, low IL-2Rα)	~1 x 10^{-11} M
FULLY ACTIVATED T LYMPHOCYTE (high IL-2Rβγ, high IL-2Rα; increased IL-2 synthesis)	~1 x 10^{-11} M

Antigen Stimulation

Autocrine/Paracrine stimulation by IL-2

IL-2Rβγ K$_d$~1 x 10^{-9} M IL-2

IL-2Rα K$_d$~1 x 10^{-8} M IL-2

IL-2Rα, IL-2Rβγ COMPLEX K$_d$~1 x 10^{-11} M IL-2

IL-2

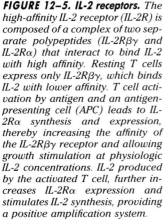

FIGURE 12–5. IL-2 receptors. The high-affinity IL-2 receptor (IL-2R) is composed of a complex of two separate polypeptides (IL-2Rβγ and IL-2Rα) that interact to bind IL-2 with high affinity. Resting T cells express only IL-2Rβγ, which binds IL-2 with lower affinity. T cell activation by antigen and an antigen-presenting cell (APC) leads to IL-2Rα synthesis and expression, thereby increasing the affinity of the IL-2Rβγ receptor and allowing growth stimulation at physiologic IL-2 concentrations. IL-2 produced by the activated T cell, further increases IL-2Rα expression and stimulates IL-2 synthesis, providing a positive amplification system.

caused enlargement of resting B cells as well as increased expression of class II MHC molecules. It is now known that the main physiologic function of IL-4 is as a regulator of allergic reactions (see Chapter 14). IL-4 is a member of the four α-helical cytokine family, and its receptor is a 130 kD protein that contains the conserved WSXWS motif (see Box 12–1). It is thought that IL-4 signaling involves clustering of the receptor by IL-4 homodimers, activating a receptor-associated tyrosine kinase. The principal cellular sources of IL-4 are CD4+ T lymphocytes, specifically of the T$_H$2 subset (see Chapter 10). In fact, IL-4 production is used as the criterion for classifying CD4+ T cells into this subset, with IFN-γ being the hallmark of the T$_H$1 cells. Activated mast cells and basophils, as well as some CD8+ T cells, are also capable of producing IL-4.

IL-4 has important actions on several cell types.

1. *IL-4 is required for the production of IgE and is the principal cytokine that stimulates switching of B cells to this heavy chain isotype.* The mechanisms of this effect were described in Chapter 9. IgE is the principal mediator of immediate hypersensitivity (allergic) reactions, and enhanced production of IL-4 is believed to be central to the development of allergies (see Chapter

14). IgE antibodies also play a role in defense against helminthic infections, this being the principal known physiologic function of the T$_H$2 subset of helper T cells (see Chapter 16). Mice in which the IL-4 gene is disrupted fail to produce IgE. IL-4 also inhibits switching to IgG2a and IgG3 in mice, all of which are augmented by IFN-γ. This is one of several reciprocal antagonistic actions of IL-4 and IFN-γ.

2. IL-4 inhibits macrophage activation and blocks most of the macrophage activating effects of IFN-γ, including increased production of cytokines such as IL-1, nitric oxide, and prostaglandins. These effects are shared with those of IL-10, which is also produced by T$_H$2 cells. This is one of the main reasons why activation of T$_H$2 cells is often associated with a suppression of macrophage-mediated immune reactions (see Chapter 10).

3. IL-4 is a growth and differentiation factor for T cells, in particular for cells of the T$_H$2 subset. IL-4 promotes the development of IL-4 + IL-5–secreting T$_H$2 cells from naive T cells stimulated with antigen. Thus, stimuli that favor IL-4 production early after antigen exposure favor the development of T$_H$2 cells. This early source of IL-4 is not yet known. IL-4 also functions as the autocrine growth factor for differentiated T$_H$2 cells,

further promoting expansion of this subset. Mice lacking the IL-4 gene show a deficiency in the development and maintenance of T_H2 cells, even after stimuli (such as helminthic infections) that are normally potent inducers of this subset.

4. IL-4 stimulates the expression of certain adhesion molecules, notably vascular cell adhesion molecule–1 (VCAM-1), on endothelial cells, resulting in increased binding of lymphocytes, monocytes, and especially eosinophils. IL-4–treated endothelial cells also secrete the chemokine monocyte chemotactic protein–1 (MCP-1) and an as yet undefined chemokine that acts specifically on eosinophils. As a result, high local concentrations of IL-4 induce monocyte- and eosinophil-rich inflammatory reactions.

5. IL-4 is a growth factor for mast cells, and synergizes with interleukin-3 (IL-3) in stimulating mast cell proliferation.

Thus, IL-4 plays a critical role in IgE- and eosinophil-mediated inflammatory reactions. IL-4 antagonists are currently being tested in patients for controlling severe allergic reactions.

Another cytokine recently identified as a product of mouse T_H2 T cells is IL-13. Its biologic activities largely overlap those of IL-4 and will not be discussed separately.

TRANSFORMING GROWTH FACTOR-β

The original description of transforming growth factor–β was made in the field of tumor biology. It was noted that certain tumors produced activities, called transforming growth factor, that would allow normal cell types to grow in soft agar, a characteristic of malignant ("transformed") cells. Subsequently, it was found that growth stimulation was caused by one polypeptide, called TGF-α, but that survival in soft agar required a second factor, called TGF-β. TGF-α is a polypeptide growth factor for epithelial and mesenchymal cells and will not be discussed further. TGF-β is a family of closely related molecules, encoded by distinct genes, commonly designated TGF-β1, TGF-β2, and TGF-β3. (The TGF-β family also includes other members thought to be involved in normal development rather than immunity; these will not be discussed here.) Cells of the immune system (e.g., T cells and monocytes) synthesize mainly TGF-β1, but certain anatomic sites (e.g., within the central nervous system) may contain high levels of TGF-β3. Native TGF-β1 is a homodimeric protein of approximately 28 kD. TGF-β1 is synthesized in a latent form that must be activated by proteases. Both antigen-activated T cells and LPS-activated mononuclear phagocytes secrete biologically active TGF-β1. TGF-β receptors are not yet well defined, although one TGF-β–binding protein may be a serine/threonine kinase.

The actions of TGF-β are highly pleiotropic. TGF-β inhibits the growth of many cell types and stimulates the growth of others. Often, TGF-β can either inhibit or stimulate growth of the same cell type, depending upon culture conditions such as degree of confluence. TGF-β causes synthesis of extracellular matrix proteins, such as collagens, and of cellular receptors for matrix proteins. (The ability of TGF-β to induce extracellular matrix probably underlies its ability to promote cell growth in soft agar.) *In vivo*, TGF-β causes the growth of new blood vessels, a process called angiogenesis.

As a cytokine, TGF-β is potentially important because it antagonizes many responses of lymphocytes. For example, TGF-β inhibits T cell proliferation to polyclonal mitogens or in mixed leukocyte reactions (see Chapter 17) and inhibits maturation of CTLs. It can also inhibit macrophage activation. TGF-β also acts on other cells, such as polymorphonuclear leukocytes and endothelial cells, again largely to counteract the effects of pro-inflammatory cytokines. In this sense, TGF-β is an "anti-cytokine" and may be a signal for shutting off immune responses. Mice in which the TGF-β1 gene has been disrupted by knockout technology develop uncontrolled inflammatory reactions. Signals that cause T cells to synthesize TGF-β may cause them to behave as suppressor cells (see Chapter 10). *In vivo*, certain tumors may escape an immune response by secreting large quantities of TGF-β.

Although TGF-β is largely a negative regulator of immune responses, it may have some positive effects as well. For example, in mice, TGF-β has been shown to switch B cells to the IgA isotype, and it may therefore be important in the generation of mucosal immune responses that are mediated by IgA (discussed in Chapter 11).

Cytokines That Regulate Immune-Mediated Inflammation

We will now discuss a group of cytokines derived principally from antigen-activated CD4$^+$ and CD8$^+$ T lymphocytes that serve primarily to activate the functions of nonspecific effector cells. Thus, these cytokines play key roles in the effector phase of cell-mediated immune responses. The molecules described in this section are summarized in Table 12–3.

INTERFERON-γ

Interferon-γ (IFN-γ), also called immune or type II interferon, is a homodimeric glycoprotein containing approximately 21 to 24 kD subunits. The size variation of the subunit is caused by variable degrees of glycosylation, but each subunit contains an identical 18 kD polypeptide encoded by the same gene. IFN-γ is produced both by naive (T_H0) and T_H1 CD4$^+$ helper T cells and by nearly all CD8$^+$ T cells. Transcription is directly initiated as a consequence of antigen activation and is enhanced by IL-2 and IL-12. IFN-γ is also produced by natural killer (NK) cells, which are the principal source of this cytokine in T cell–deficient mice. (In this setting, IFN-γ may function as a mediator of natural immunity.)

As its name implies, IFN-γ shares many activities with type I IFN. Specifically, IFN-γ induces an antiviral state and is antiproliferative. However, IFN-γ binds to a unique cell surface receptor, different from but structurally related to that utilized by type I IFN. More importantly, IFN-γ has several properties related to im-

TABLE 12–3. Mediators of Immune-Mediated Inflammation

Cytokine	Number of Genes	Polypeptide Size	Cell Source	Cell Target	Primary Effects on Each Target
Gamma interferon	1	21–24 kD (homodimer)	T cell, NK cell	Mononuclear phagocyte Endothelial cell NK cell All	Activation Activation Activation Increased class I and class II MHC molecules
Lymphotoxin	1	24 kD (homotrimer)	T cell	Neutrophil Endothelial cell NK cell	Activation Activation Activation
Interleukin-10	1	20 kD (homodimer)	T cell	Mononuclear phagocyte B cell	Inhibition Activation
Interleukin-5	1	20 kD (homodimer)	T cell	Eosinophil B cell	Activation Growth and activation
Interleukin-12	2	35–40 kD (heterodimer)	Macrophages	NK cells T cells	Activation Activation (growth and differentiation)
Migration inhibition factor	?	?	T cell	Mononuclear phagocyte	Conversion from motile to immotile state

Abbreviations: NK, natural killer; kD, kilodalton; MHC, major histocompatibility complex.

munoregulation that separate it functionally from type I IFN.

1. *IFN-γ is a potent activator of mononuclear phagocytes.* It directly induces synthesis of the enzymes that mediate the respiratory burst, allowing macrophages to kill phagocytosed microbes. Along with second signals, such as LPS and perhaps TNF, it allows macrophages to kill tumor cells. Cytokines that cause such functional changes in mononuclear phagocytes have been called **macrophage-activating factors** (MAFs). *IFN-γ is the principal MAF and provides the means by which T cells activate macrophages.* Other MAFs include GM-CSF, and, to a lesser extent, IL-1 and TNF. Macrophage activation is described in more detail in Chapter 13. It is worth noting here that macrophage activation actually involves several different responses, and macrophages are said to be activated when they perform a particular function being assayed. For example, IFN-γ fully activates macrophages to kill phagocytosed microbes but only partly activates macrophages to kill tumor cells.

2. *IFN-γ increases class I MHC molecule expression and, in contrast to type I IFN, also causes a wide variety of cell types to express class II MHC molecules.* Thus, IFN-γ amplifies the cognitive phase of the immune response by promoting the activation of class II–restricted CD4$^+$ helper T cells (see Chapter 6, Fig. 6–5). *In vivo,* IFN-γ can enhance both cellular and humoral immune responses through these actions at the cognitive phase.

3. *IFN-γ acts directly on T and B lymphocytes to promote their differentiation.* IFN-γ promotes the differentiation of naive CD4$^+$ T cells to the T$_H$1 subset and inhibits the proliferation of T$_H$2 cells. IFN-γ is one of the cytokines required for the maturation of CD8$^+$ CTLs (see Chapter 13). It also acts on B cells to promote switching to the IgG2a and IgG3 subclasses in mice and to inhibit switching to IgG1 and IgE.

4. *IFN-γ activates neutrophils,* upregulating their respiratory burst. It is a less potent activator of neutrophils than TNF or lymphotoxin.

5. *IFN-γ stimulates the cytolytic activity of NK cells,* more so than type I IFN.

6. *IFN-γ is an activator of vascular endothelial cells,* promoting CD4$^+$ T lymphocyte adhesion and morphologic alterations that facilitate lymphocyte extravasation. As mentioned earlier, IFN-γ also potentiates many of the actions of TNF on endothelial cells.

The net effect of these varied activities of IFN-γ is to promote T$_H$1 and macrophage-rich inflammatory reactions, while suppressing T$_H$2 and eosinophil-rich reactions. Mice in which the IFN-γ or IFN-γ receptor genes have been disrupted show several immunologic defects, including increased susceptibility to infections with intracellular microbes (which cannot be cleared because of defective macrophage activation), reduced production of nitric oxide by macrophages from mice infected with mycobacteria, reduced serum levels of IgG2a and IgG3 antibodies, reduced expression of class II MHC molecules on macrophages from mycobacteria-infected mice, and defective NK cell function.

LYMPHOTOXIN

Lymphotoxin is a 21 to 24 kD glycoprotein that is approximately 30 per cent homologous to TNF and competes with TNF for binding to the same cell surface receptors. (As noted earlier, LT is sometimes called TNF-β.) In humans, LT and TNF genes are located in tandem within the MHC on chromosome 6 (see Chapter 5). LT is produced exclusively by activated T lymphocytes and is often produced coordinately with IFN-γ by such cells. Human LT, unlike TNF, contains one or two N-linked oligosaccharides (accounting for the variability in molecular sizes). In further contrast to TNF, LT is synthesized as a true secretory protein without a membrane-spanning region. A third member of the TNF/LT family has recently been described. The gene product, tentatively named LT-β, is a cell surface protein that binds LT to form a cell surface complex that mediates the effects of LT on other cells.

Most studies have found little difference between the biologic effects of TNF and LT, consistent with their binding to the same receptor. The most important distinction between these cytokines appears to be that LT is synthesized exclusively by T cells, whereas TNF, although made by T cells, is predominantly derived from mononuclear phagocytes. In general, the quantities of LT synthesized by T cells are much less than the amounts of TNF made by LPS-stimulated mononuclear phagocytes, and LT is not readily detected in the circulation. Therefore, LT is usually a locally acting paracrine factor and not a mediator of systemic injury. Although neither TNF nor LT is toxic for normal (nonneoplastic) cells, both cytokines may contribute to CTL-mediated lysis of target cells (see Chapter 13). Like TNF, LT is a potent activator of neutrophils and thus provides lymphocytes with a means of regulating acute inflammatory reactions. It is more potent than IFN-γ as an activator of neutrophils, and the actions of LT are enhanced by IFN-γ. LT is also an activator of vascular endothelial cells, causing increased leukocyte adhesion, cytokine production, and morphologic changes that facilitate leukocyte extravasation. These effects, like those of TNF, are also enhanced by IFN-γ.

INTERLEUKIN-10

Interleukin-10 (IL-10) is an 18 kD cytokine produced by the T_H2 subset of CD4$^+$ helper cells. It is also produced by some activated B cells, by some T_H1 cells (in humans), by activated macrophages, and by some non-lymphocytic cell types (e.g., keratinocytes). IL-10 is a member of the four α-helical cytokine family and probably functions as a homodimer. The two major activities of IL-10 are to inhibit cytokine (i.e., TNF, IL-1, chemokine, and IL-12) production by macrophages, and to inhibit the accessory functions of macrophages in T cell activation. The latter effect is due to reduced expression of class II MHC molecules and reduced expression of certain costimulators (e.g., B7). The net effect of these actions is to inhibit T cell–mediated immune inflammation. In addition to its inhibitory effects on macrophages, IL-10 has stimulatory actions on B cells. It may be a switching factor for the production of IgG4 in humans (homologous to IgG1 in mice).

Studies of mice in which the IL-10 gene has been disrupted by knock-out technology reveal few immunologic abnormalities. Such mice develop intestinal inflammatory lesions, the basis of which is unexplained.

Interestingly, the genome of the Epstein-Barr virus contains a gene homologous to IL-10, and viral IL-10 shares *in vitro* activity with the T cell–derived cytokine. This raises the intriguing possibility that the virus has acquired the human gene as a means of inhibiting antiviral immunity.

INTERLEUKIN-5

Interleukin-5 (IL-5) is an approximately 40 kD homodimeric cytokine produced by the T_H2 subset of

CD4$^+$ T cells and by activated mast cells. It belongs to the four α-helical cytokine family, although each bundle of four helices consists of three strands from one monomer and one strand from the other. The receptor contains the WSXWS motif and interacts with a 150 kD signal-transducing subunit shared with IL-3 and GM-CSF (see Box 12–1).

The major action of IL-5 is to stimulate the growth and differentiation of eosinophils and to activate mature eosinophils in such a way that they can kill helminths. In mice, neutralizing antibodies to IL-5 inhibit the eosinophilia seen in response to helminthic infection. This activity of IL-5 is complemented by the activities of IL-4 (e.g., IgE switching and eosinophil recruitment) and of IL-10 (e.g., IgG4 switching), contributing to T_H2-mediated allergic reactions (see Chapter 14). IL-5 also acts as a costimulator for the growth of antigen-activated mouse B cells and was previously called either B cell growth factor 2 or T cell replacing factor. IL-5 may function synergistically with other cytokines, such as IL-2 and IL-4, to stimulate the growth and differentiation of B cells. IL-5 has also been found to act on more mature B cells to cause increased synthesis of immunoglobulin, especially of IgA. These actions are discussed in greater detail in Chapter 9.

INTERLEUKIN-12

Interleukin-12 is a 70 kD heterodimer consisting of two covalently linked polypeptide chains, one of 35 kD (p35) and the other of 40 kD (p40). The p35 subunit is produced by many cell types, including T and B lymphocytes, NK cells, and monocytes. The p40 chain is produced mainly by activated monocytes and B cells, so that these are the principal sources of the complete cytokine. (In this functional category of cytokines, IL-12 is the only one that is not produced by T cells, and because of its action on NK cells, can also be considered a mediator of natural immunity.) The p35 protein has a four α-helix structure, similar to that of many other cytokines. Interestingly, the p40 component of IL-12 is homologous to the IL-6 receptor, containing an Ig domain and a WSXWS motif. Thus, the intact heterodimer appears to be composed of one cytokine-like protein and one cytokine receptor–like protein. Binding studies indicate that the true receptor for IL-12 is expressed on activated T and NK cells, but this receptor has not yet been fully characterized.

IL-12 is an important regulator of cell-mediated immune responses because of its effects on NK cells and T lymphocytes.

1. *IL-12 is the most potent NK cell stimulator known.* It induces transcription of IFN-γ by NK cells, and shows a strong synergy with IL-2. In addition to stimulating IFN-γ production, IL-12 enhances the cytolytic activity of NK cells and is a growth factor for these cells.

2. *IL-12 stimulates the differentiation of naive CD4$^+$ T cells to the T_H1 subset.* The development of a T_H1 versus T_H2 dominant T cell response may be controlled by the relative production of IL-12 and IFN-γ, which

favor T$_H$1 differentiation, and IL-4 and IL-10, which promote T$_H$2 differentiation (see Chapter 10).

3. *IL-12 stimulates the differentiation of CD8$^+$ T cells into mature, functionally active CTLs.* Because of this effect, IL-12 has some potential in the treatment of disseminated cancers.

Thus, IL-12 is an important regulator of the effector phase of cell-mediated immune reactions. It serves this function by directly activating some effector cells, and by regulating the development of other effector cells.

MIGRATION INHIBITION FACTOR

We conclude our discussion of cytokines that regulate effector cells by considering the issue of migration inhibition factor (MIF). One early view of cell-mediated immune reactions proposed that mononuclear phagocyte accumulation in tissues depended on the retention of such cells in response to locally produced cytokines that inhibit motility. It now seems more likely that retention of leukocytes in the tissues is controlled primarily by expression of specific receptors for extracellular matrix molecules, such as integrins (see Box 7–3, Chapter 7), and CD44. Nevertheless, one of the first cytokine activities identified was one that inhibited macrophage motility *in vitro*, called migration inhibition factor. MIF has still not been identified as a unique cytokine. At present, both the biochemical identity and biologic significance of MIF remain unclear.

Cytokines That Stimulate Hematopoiesis

Several of the cytokines generated during both natural immunity and antigen-induced specific immune responses have potent stimulatory effects on the growth and differentiation of bone marrow progenitor cells. Thus, immune and inflammatory reactions, which consume leukocytes, also elicit production of new leukocytes to replace inflammatory cells. All of the various mature leukocyte cell populations arise as a consequence of progressive expansion and irreversible differentiation of the progeny of self-renewing pluripotent stem cells. Maturation of hematopoietic cells involves commitment to a particular lineage and occurs concomitantly with loss of ability to develop into other mature cell types. This process has been depicted as a simple tree. The cytokines that stimulate expansion and differentiation of bone marrow progenitor cells are collectively called **colony-stimulating factors** (CSFs) because they are often assayed by their ability to stimulate the formation of cell colonies in bone marrow cultures. These colonies of cells mature during the *in vitro* assay, acquiring characteristics of specific cell lineages (e.g., granulocytes, mononuclear phagocytes). Different CSFs act on bone marrow cells at different stages of maturation and preferentially promote development of colonies of different lineages (Fig. 12–6). The names assigned to CSFs reflect the types of colonies that arise

in these assays. Interestingly, many of the CSFs are located in a gene cluster on human chromosome 5, including IL-3 and GM-CSF. IL-4 and IL-5 have been mapped to this same complex.

Some of the actions of CSFs are influenced by other cytokines. For example, TNF, LT, IFN-γ, and TGF-β all inhibit growth of bone marrow progenitor cells. In contrast, IL-1 and IL-6 enhance responses to CSFs. In general, cytokines are thought both to be necessary for normal marrow function and to provide a means of fine tuning function in response to stimulation. Some of the specific CSFs are listed in Table 12–4.

c-KIT LIGAND

The pluripotent stem cell expresses a tyrosine-kinase membrane receptor that has been identified as the protein product of the cellular oncogene, *c-kit*. The extracellular portion of this receptor contains five Ig domains. The cytokine that interacts with the receptor has been called **c-kit ligand,** and is also referred to as "stem cell factor." c-Kit ligand is synthesized by stromal cells of the bone marrow (including adipocytes, fibroblasts, and endothelial cells) in two forms: a transmembrane protein of about 27 kD and a secreted form of about 24 kD. These different products result from alternative splicing of the same gene. The soluble form of this ligand is absent in a mutant mouse strain called steel, and the soluble form of the c-kit ligand is thus sometimes called *steel factor*. The steel mouse has only selective gaps in its bone marrow–derived cell populations (e.g., inadequate mast cell and eosinophil production), which has led to the conclusion that the cell surface form of c-kit ligand is more important than the soluble form for stimulating stem cells to mature into various hematopoietic lineages. Elimination of both forms of c-kit ligand, by complete knockout of the gene, is lethal.

It is not yet possible to purify large numbers of stem cells for direct analysis. Many of the conclusions about c-kit ligand and other early acting CSFs are derived from experiments in which populations enriched from stem cells are exposed to the cytokines in culture, and the types of colonies that develop are analyzed. From this kind of experiment, it is believed that c-kit ligand is needed to make stem cells responsive to other CSFs, but that it does not cause colony formation by itself. Bone marrow cell cultures that contain stromal cells do not have a requirement for exogenous c-kit ligand since the stromal cells express this gene product.

INTERLEUKIN-3

Interleukin-3 (IL-3), also known as **multilineage colony-stimulating factor** (multi-CSF), is a 20 to 26 kD product of CD4$^+$ T cells that acts on the most immature marrow progenitors and promotes the expansion of cells that differentiate into all known mature cell types. IL-3 is a member of the four α-helix family of cytokines. In humans, the receptor consists of a unique WSXWS-containing subunit and a 150 kD signal-transducing

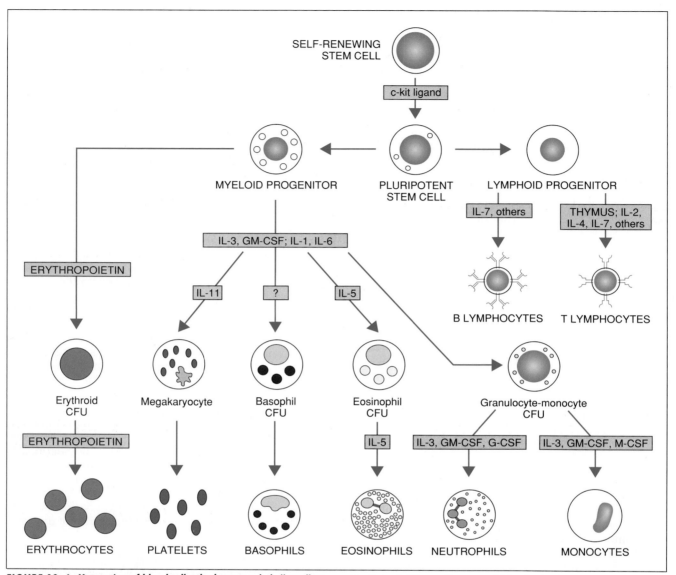

FIGURE 12–6. Maturation of blood cells: the hematopoietic "tree." The maturation of different lineages of blood cells is regulated by various cytokines. CFU, colony-forming unit; IL, interleukin; GM-CSF, granulocyte-macrophage colony-stimulating factor.

subunit shared with IL-5 and GM-CSF. In the mouse, the signal-transducing subunit is unique. Most functional analyses of IL-3 have been performed in mice. It has been found that IL-3 also promotes the growth and development of mast cells from bone marrow–derived progenitors, an action enhanced by IL-4. IL-3 is produced by CD4$^+$ helper T cells of both the T$_H$1 and T$_H$2 subsets. Human IL-3 has been identified by the complementary DNA (cDNA) cloning of a molecule homologous to mouse IL-3. Although IL-3 is made by some human T cell clones, it has been harder to establish a role for this cytokine in experimental systems of hematopoiesis in humans. In fact, many actions attributed to murine IL-3 appear to be performed by human granulocyte-macrophage CSF (see below). It is not known whether these experimental results reflect differences in species or in experimental conditions. If these are a

species difference, they may be related to the differences in IL-3 receptor structure described above.

Granulocyte-Macrophage Colony-Stimulating Factor

Granulocyte-macrophage colony-stimulating factor (GM-CSF) is a 22 kD glycoprotein made by activated T cells and by activated mononuclear phagocytes, vascular endothelial cells, and fibroblasts. GM-CSF is a member of the four α-helix family of cytokines. Its receptor consists of a unique WSXWS-containing subunit and a 150 kD signal-transducing subunit. As noted above, this latter subunit is shared with the IL-5 receptor and, in humans but not mice, with the IL-3 receptor. GM-CSF in the mouse acts primarily on bone marrow progenitors already committed to develop into leuko-

TABLE 12–4. Mediators of Immature Leukocyte Growth and Differentiation

Cytokine	Number of Genes	Polypeptide Size	Cell Source	Cell Target	Primary Effects on Each Target
c-Kit ligand	1	24 kD (monomer)	Bone marrow stromal cell	Pluripotent stem cell	Activation
Interleukin-3	1	20–26 kD (dimer)	T cell	Immature progenitor	Growth and differentiation to all cell lines
Granulocyte-macrophage CSF	1	22 kD (dimer)	T cell, mononuclear phagocyte, endothelial cell, fibroblast	Immature progenitor Committed progenitor Mononuclear phagocyte	Growth and differentiation to all cell lines Differentiation to granulocytes and mononuclear phagocytes Activation
Macrophage CSF	1	40 kD (dimer)	Mononuclear phagocyte, endothelial cell, fibroblast	Committed progenitor	Differentiation to mononuclear phagocytes
Granulocyte CSF	1	19 kD (dimer)	Mononuclear phagocyte, endothelial cell, fibroblast	Committed progenitor	Differentiation to granulocytes
Interleukin-7	1	25 kD (monomer)	Fibroblast, bone marrow stromal cells	Immature progenitor	Growth and differentiation to B lymphocytes

Abbreviations: CSF, colony-stimulating factor; kD, kilodalton.

cytes and thus presumably acts on a more differentiated population than IL-3. In human systems, however, GM-CSF also promotes growth of cells not yet committed to form leukocytes (e.g., platelets and progenitors of red blood cells), replacing IL-3. GM-CSF also activates mature leukocytes. For example, it mimics some of the actions of IFN-γ as an activator of macrophages, although it is less potent.

GM-CSF is not detected in the circulation and presumably acts locally at sites of production. Thus, in peripheral tissues T cell– and macrophage-derived GM-CSF may function mainly to activate mature leukocytes at sites of immune inflammatory responses, whereas hematopoietic effects may be mediated by GM-CSF produced by T cells, endothelial cells, or stromal fibroblasts in the bone marrow. Recombinant GM-CSF has been used to stimulate the bone marrow of patients with defects in hematopoiesis and to stimulate bone marrow recovery after cytotoxic chemotherapy or bone marrow transplantation.

MONOCYTE-MACROPHAGE COLONY-STIMULATING FACTOR

Monocyte-macrophage colony-stimulating factor (M-CSF), also called CSF-1, is made by macrophages and by endothelial cells and fibroblasts. The secreted polypeptide is approximately 40 kD and forms a stable dimer. The M-CSF receptor is structurally related to c-kit. It contains five extracellular Ig domains and an intracellular tyrosine kinase. The M-CSF receptor gene was initially identified as the normal cellular counterpart of a viral oncogene, *v-fms*.

M-CSF acts primarily on those progenitors that are already committed to develop into monocytes and are presumably more mature than the targets for GM-CSF. Like GM-CSF, M-CSF does not circulate, and the major colony-stimulating effect may be derived from local production within the marrow cavity.

GRANULOCYTE COLONY-STIMULATING FACTOR

Granulocyte colony-stimulating factor (G-CSF) is made by the same cells that make GM-CSF. The secreted polypeptide is approximately 19 kD and probably forms a dimer. G-CSF is a member of the four α-helical cytokine family, and its receptor contains the WSXWS motif. In contrast to other CSFs, G-CSF does normally circulate. It acts primarily on marrow progenitors already committed to develop into granulocytes, again a more mature population than that responsive to GM-CSF. Because G-CSF can act at a distance, neutrophil maturation and release from bone marrow are highly influenced by inflammatory reactions occuring in the periphery, outside the marrow.

INTERLEUKIN-7

Interleukin 7 (IL-7) is a cytokine secreted by marrow stromal cells that acts on hematopoietic progenitors committed to the B lymphocyte lineage. Most models of hematopoiesis suggest that lymphocyte progenitors differentiate from common stem cells very early in maturation, so that IL-7 is probably acting on cells at the same level of development as IL-3 or GM-

CSF. Recent studies suggest that IL-7 may also stimulate the growth and maturation of immature CD4⁻CD8⁻ T cell precursors in the thymus. However, this is based on *in vitro* experiments, and the cellular source of IL-7 in the thymus is not known. Transgenic mice that overexpress IL-7 show markedly increased numbers of pre–B cells in the bone marrow and peripheral lymphoid tissues.

OTHER COLONY-STIMULATING CYTOKINES

IL-9 is a 30 to 40 kD protein that supports the growth of some T cell lines and of bone marrow–derived mast cell progenitors. It may also stimulate development of other lineages from marrow-derived precursors. However, it is not known whether IL-9 has an effect on normal lymphocytes (other than cell lines) or if it plays a role in the regulation of immune responses or hematopoiesis *in vivo*.

IL-11 is a ~20 kD cytokine produced by bone marrow stromal cells, especially after activation (which may be achieved experimentally by pharmacologic agents such as phorbol esters). IL-11 stimulates megakaryopoiesis and may prove to be of therapeutic benefit in patients with platelet deficiencies. It also enhances the development of macrophages and perhaps other cell lineages from marrow precursors.

SUMMARY

Cytokines are a family of protein mediators of both natural and acquired immunity. The same cytokines are often made by many cell types, and individual cytokines often act on many cell types. The actions of different cytokines are often redundant and influence the action of other cytokines. In general, cytokines are synthesized in response to inflammatory or antigenic stimuli and act locally, in an autocrine or paracrine fashion, by binding to high affinity receptors on target cells. Certain cytokines may be produced in sufficient quantity to circulate and exert endocrine actions. For many cell types, cytokines serve as growth factors.

We have classified cytokines into four groups, according to their principal actions:

The first group consists of those cytokines that mediate natural immunity and includes the antiviral type I interferons and the pro-inflammatory cytokines—tumor necrosis factor, interleukin-1, interleukin-6, and members of the newly described family of chemokines. The predominant cellular source of these molecules is mononuclear phagocytes.

The second group of cytokines is derived largely from antigen-stimulated CD4⁺ T lymphocytes and serves to regulate the activation, growth, and differentiation of B and T cells. This group includes interleukin-2, the principal T cell growth factor; interleukin-4, the major regulator of IgE synthesis; and transforming factor–β, which inhibits lymphocyte responses.

The third group of cytokines, produced by antigen-activated CD4⁺ and CD8⁺ T lymphocytes, serves to activate inflammatory leukocytes and places these effector cells under T cell regulation. This group includes interferon-γ, the principal activator of mononuclear phagocytes; lymphotoxin, an activator of neutrophils; interleukin-10, a negative regulator of mononuclear phagocyte function; interleukin-5, an activator of eosinophils; and interleukin-12 (produced by mononuclear phagocytes), a stimulator of NK cells and T cells.

The fourth group, collectively called colony-stimulating factors, consists of cytokines derived from marrow stromal cells and T cells, which stimulate the growth of bone marrow progenitors, thereby providing a source of additional inflammatory leukocytes.

Thus, cytokines serve many functions that are critical to host defense against pathogens and provide links between specific and natural immunity. Cytokines also regulate the magnitude and nature of immune responses by influencing the growth and differentiation of lymphocytes. Finally, cytokines provide important amplification mechanisms that enable small numbers of lymphocytes specific for any one antigen to activate a variety of effector mechanisms to eliminate the antigen. Excessive production or actions of cytokines can lead to tissue injury and even death. The administration of cytokines or their inhibitors is a potential approach for modifying biologic responses associated with disease.

SELECTED READINGS

Arai, K., F. Lee, A. Miyajima, S. Miyatake, N. Arai, and T. Yokota. Cytokines: coordinators of immune and inflammatory responses. Annual Review of Biochemistry 59:783–836, 1990.

Dinarello, C. A. Role of interleukin-1 in infectious diseases. Immunological Reviews 127:119–146, 1992.

Farrar, M. A., and R. D. Schreiber. The molecular cell biology of interferon-gamma and its receptor. Annual Review of Immunology 11:571–611, 1993.

Minami, Y., T. Kono, T. Miyazaki, and T. Taniguchi. The IL-2 receptor complex: its structure, function and target genes. Annual Review of Immunology 11:245–268, 1993.

Moore, K. W., A. O'Garra, R. de W. Malefyt, P. Vieira, and T. R. Mosmann. Interleukin-10. Annual Review of Immunology 11:165–190, 1993.

Nicola, N. A. Hematopoietic cell growth factors and their receptors. Annual Review of Biochemistry 58:45–77, 1989.

Oppenheim, J. J., C. O. C. Zachariae, N. Mukaida, and K. Matsushima. Properties of the novel proinflammatory supergene "intercrine" cytokine family. Annual Review of Immunology 9:817–848, 1991.

Palladino, M. A., R. E. Morris, H. F. Starnes, and A. D. Levinson. The transforming growth factor-betas. A new family of immunoregulatory molecules. Annals of The New York Academy of Sciences 593:181–187, 1990.

Sen, G. C., and P. Lengyel. The interferon system. A bird's eye view of its biochemistry. Journal of Biological Chemistry 267:5017–5020, 1992.

Smith, K. A. Interleukin-2: inception, impact and implications. Science 240:1169–1176, 1988.

Stadnyk, A. W., and J. Gauldie. The acute phase response during parasitic infection. Immunology Today 12:A7–A11, 1992.

Taga, T., and T. Kishimoto. Cytokine receptors and signal transduction. FASEB Journal 7:3387–3396, 1993.

Trinchieri, G., M. Wysocka, A. D'Andrea, M. Rengaraju, M. Aste, M. Kubin, N. M. Valiante, and J. Chehimi. Natural killer cell stimulatory factor (NKSF) or interleukin-12 is a key regulator of immune response and inflammation. Progress in Growth Factor Research 4:355–368, 1993.

Vassalli, P. The pathophysiology of tumor necrosis factors. Annual Review of Immunology 10:411–452, 1992.

CHAPTER THIRTEEN

EFFECTOR MECHANISMS OF T CELL–MEDIATED IMMUNE REACTIONS

Historically, specific immunity has been divided into *humoral immunity*, which can be adoptively transferred from an immunized donor to a naive host by antibodies in the absence of cells, and *cell-mediated immunity*, which can be adoptively transferred only by viable T lymphocytes. This classification, first evident through adoptive transfer experiments, is actually quite general, because it is based on fundamental differences among various effector mechanisms in the immune system. The effector phase of the immune response is initiated and targeted by specific antigen recognition. *In humoral immunity, specific recognition of antigen in the effector phase is mediated by the binding of secreted antibody molecules to antigen.* Antibody is thus sufficient to adoptively transfer humoral immunity. *In cell-mediated immunity, in contrast, the effector phase, as well as the cognitive phase, is initiated through specific antigen recognition by T cells.* In this chapter, we will discuss the various effector mechanisms of cell-mediated immune reactions.

In some forms of cell-mediated immunity, antigen-specific T cells directly perform the effector function, as when cytolytic T lymphocytes (CTLs) lyse specific target cells; in others, antigen-activated T cells secrete cytokines that recruit and activate effector cells that are not specific for the antigen, such as macrophages and natural killer (NK) cells. When the effector cells are nonspecific, antigen specificity is conferred by proximity to the antigen-stimulated T cells. T cells can recognize and respond to foreign antigen only when it is presented in a complex with a self major histocompatibility complex (MHC) molecule on the surface of an appropriate antigen-presenting cell (APC) or target cell. *Therefore, cell-mediated immunity is directed at or near cells that bear foreign antigens on their surface, and cell-mediated immune reactions are physiologically most important for eradicating microbes or viruses that live intracellularly, i.e., within APCs.* Indeed, the original description of cell-mediated immunity was the adoptive transfer of protection against *Listeria monocytogenes,* an intracellular bacterium (see Chapter 16). Cell-mediated immune reactions may also be important for elimination of cells that express foreign MHC molecules, as in an allograft (see Chapter 17), or express tumor-specific antigens, as in a malignant tumor (see Chapter 18).

Different types of cell-mediated immune reactions may result from T cell recognition of antigen.

1. In **delayed type hypersensitivity** (DTH), antigen-activated T cells secrete cytokines, which have several effects. Some cytokines activate venular endothelial cells to recruit monocytes from the blood at the site of antigen challenge. Other cytokines convert the monocytes into activated macrophages that serve to eliminate the antigen. The T cells that mediate DTH are usually CD4$^+$ T$_H$1 cells, but cytokines produced by CD8$^+$ T cells can initiate the same reaction.

2. In **CTL responses** to viral infections or organ transplants, antigen-activated CD8$^+$ T cells differentiate into functional CTLs, which lyse target cells expressing specific antigen-MHC complexes. This process of differentiation often requires "help" in the form of cytokines secreted by antigen-activated CD4$^+$ T cells.

3. In the initial response to viral infections, **natural killer (NK) cells** serve to eradicate infected cells prior to the appearance of specific CTLs (see Chapter 16). In graft-versus-host reactions, NK cells, stimulated by cytokines from antigen-activated CD4$^+$ T cells, differentiate into **lymphokine-activated killer (LAK) cells,** which nonspecifically lyse target cells.

4. In helminthic infections and in allergic inflammation, antigen-activated CD4$^+$ T$_H$2 cells secrete cytokines that activate mast cells and recruit and activate basophils and eosinophils. This kind of immune reaction and its effector mechanisms will be discussed in Chapter 14.

This chapter begins with a discussion of the T cells that regulate cell-mediated immune reactions and then considers the various effector cell populations that are involved in each of these distinct reaction patterns.

T Lymphocytes and the Initiation of Cell-Mediated Immune Reactions

T cells initiate specific immunity, both cell-mediated and humoral, by recognizing portions of protein antigens (peptides) bound to self class II MHC molecules on the surface of APCs. Upon activation by specific antigen, these T cells secrete cytokines, many of which act on other cell populations involved in host defense. For example, tumor necrosis factor (TNF) and lymphotoxin (LT) activate neutrophils and vascular endothelial cells; interleukin-5 (IL-5) activates eosinophils; interferon-γ (IFN-γ) activates mononuclear phagocytes; and interleukin-2 (IL-2) activates NK cells as well as both T and B lymphocytes. *By means of cytokine secretion, T cells stimulate the function and focus the activity of nonspecific effector cells of natural immunity, thereby converting these cells into agents of specific immunity.* Indeed, the first function of T cells in the evolutionary development of specific immunity may well have been to augment and direct the effector mechanisms of natural immunity. As antigen-specific effector cells such as CTLs and B lymphocytes evolved, the general pattern of T cell function remained the same: through the secretion of cytokines, such as IL-2 and IL-4, T cells provide "help" necessary for the activation of other lymphocytes.

The multitude of cytokines produced by antigen-activated T cells, each with distinct but overlapping sets of cellular targets, raised the question of how particular antigens elicit particular types of immune reactions. As we discussed in Chapter 10, there is now considerable evidence that T cells differentiate into subsets that produce distinct patterns of cytokines and perform distinct functions. In this chapter, we will focus on reactions induced by CD4$^+$ T$_H$1 and CD8$^+$ T cells, i.e., those that produce IFN-γ, TNF, LT, and IL-2. In Chapter 14, we will discuss reactions triggered by CD4$^+$ T$_H$2 cells, i.e., those that produce IL-4, IL-5, and IL-10. We do not yet fully understand how different antigens activate and expand different T cell subsets (see Chapter 10).

DELAYED TYPE HYPERSENSITIVITY AND ITS EFFECTOR CELLS

*Delayed type hypersensitivity is a form of cell-mediated immune reaction in which the ultimate effector cell is the activated **mononuclear phagocyte (macrophage)**.* This type of cell-mediated immunity is part of the primary defense mechanism against intracellular bacteria, such as *Listeria monocytogenes* and mycobacteria. Such microbes cannot be killed by normal unactivated phagocytes and, indeed, may even preferentially survive within the phagolysosomes or cytoplasm of monocytes. Eradication of these organisms requires enhancement of the microbicidal function of phagocytes by T cell–derived cytokines. The same sequence of T cell and macrophage activation can be elicited by soluble protein antigens or chemically reactive haptens. In this situation, as in host defense, macrophage activation can cause tissue injury. If the antigen is not a microbe, DTH reactions produce tissue injury without providing a "protective" function, hence the term "hypersensitivity."

The classical animal model of DTH is the response of an immunized guinea pig to antigen applied by "skin painting" or introduced by intradermal injection. Such reactions may be induced in humans by contact sensitization with chemicals and environmental antigens, or by intradermal injection of microbial antigens in individuals immunized by prior infection (Fig. 13–1). For example, purified protein derivative (PPD), a protein prepared from *Mycobacterium tuberculosis,* will elicit a DTH response when injected into individuals who have recovered from primary tuberculosis or who have been vaccinated against tuberculosis. The characteristic response of DTH evolves over 24 to 48 hours. About 4 hours after injection of antigen, neutrophils accumulate around the post-capillary venules at the injection site. The neutrophil infiltrate rapidly subsides, and by about 12 hours the injection site becomes infiltrated by T cells and blood monocytes, also organized in a perivenular distribution (Fig. 13–2). The endothelial cells lining these venules become plump, show increased biosynthetic organelles, and become leaky to plasma macromolecules. Fibrinogen escapes from the blood vessels into the surrounding tissues, where it is converted into fibrin. The deposition of fibrin and, to a lesser extent, accumulation of T cells and monocytes within the extravascular tissue space around the injec-

tion site cause the tissue to swell and become hard ("indurated"). Induration, the hallmark of DTH, is detectable by about 18 hours after injection of antigen and is maximal by 24 to 48 hours. The lag in the onset of palpable induration is the reason for calling the response "delayed type."

Although experimental DTH was first described in guinea pigs, DTH-like reactions may be elicited in other animals such as mice or rats. Histologically, these murine reactions differ from DTH responses in guinea pig or man in that the inflammatory infiltrate at 18 to 24 hours shows a paucity of T cells and activated macrophages, but rather consists largely of neutrophils. The basis of this difference is not known, but may reside in the inflammatory functions of vascular endothelium or species differences in the production or effects of cytokines. Nevertheless, in all species examined, DTH reactions to most protein antigens may be adoptively transferred by antigen-sensitized CD4$^+$ T cells. CD8$^+$ T cells are also capable of adoptively transferring DTH-like reactions. *In vivo,* it is likely that DTH reactions elicited by viruses are predominantly mediated by CD8$^+$ T cells, whereas those that are elicited by phagocytosed bacteria are predominantly mediated by CD4$^+$ T$_H$1 T cells. Presumably, this is because cytoplasmic viral proteins are largely presented to T cells in association with class I MHC molecules, whereas protein antigens in phagolysosomes are largely presented to T cells in association with class II MHC molecules (see Chapter 6). As we shall discuss later, both kinds of DTH responses may be complemented by CTL responses, predominantly involving CD8$^+$ T cells.

In clinical practice, loss of DTH responses to universally encountered antigens (e.g., candidal antigens) is an indication of deficient T cell function, a condition known as **anergy.** (This general loss of immune responsiveness should be distinguished from "clonal anergy," a mechanism for providing tolerance to specific antigens, discussed in Chapter 10.) Anergic individuals are extremely susceptible to infection by microorganisms that are normally resisted by cell-mediated immunity, such as mycobacteria and fungi.

DTH reactions, like other types of specific immunity, consist of three sequential processes (Fig. 13–3).

1. The *cognitive phase,* in which CD4$^+$ and sometimes CD8$^+$ T cells recognize foreign protein antigens presented on the surface of APCs.

2. The *activation phase,* in which the T cells secrete cytokines and proliferate.

3. The *effector phase.* In DTH, the effector phase can be further subdivided into two steps: (a) **inflammation,** in which vascular endothelial cells, activated by cytokines, recruit circulating leukocytes into the tissues at the local site of antigen challenge; and (b) **resolution,** in which macrophages, activated by cytokines, act to eliminate the foreign antigen. This process may be accompanied by tissue injury.

These stages will be discussed in the context of the cell type central to each step of the process.

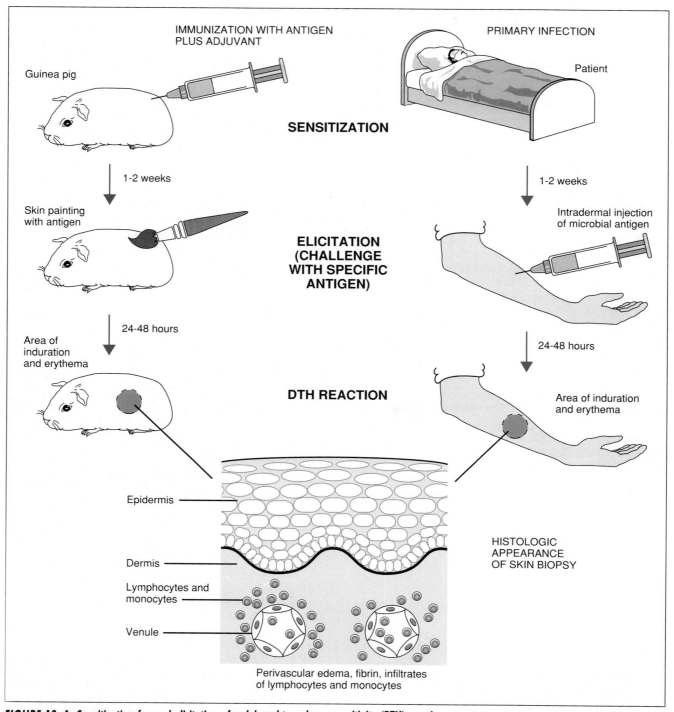

FIGURE 13–1. Sensitization for and elicitation of a delayed type hypersensitivity (DTH) reaction. *A guinea pig is sensitized experimentally by injection of antigen or by skin painting with antigen (not shown); in humans, sensitization occurs through infection or by vaccination (not shown). In these two species, subsequent challenge of sensitized individuals with specific antigens then elicits histologically similar DTH reactions.*

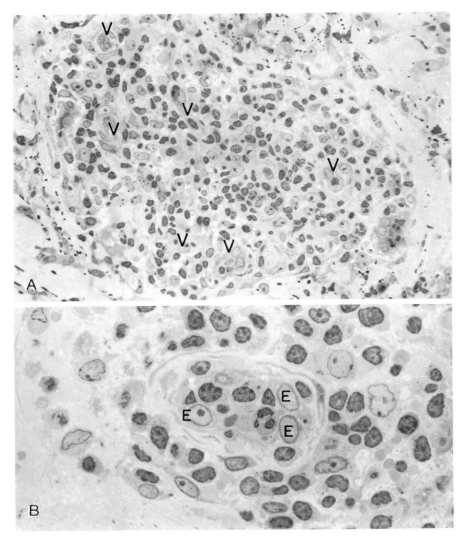

FIGURE 13-2. Morphology of a DTH reaction.
A. *Low-power photomicrograph depicting mononuclear cell infiltrates surrounding venules (V) in human skin in a reaction to foreign antigen. (Reproduced with permission from Dvorak, H. F., and M. C. Mihm, Jr. Basophilic leukocytes in allergic contact dermatitis. Journal of Experimental Medicine 135:235–254, 1972. Copyright permission of the Rockefeller University Press, New York.)*
B. *High-power photomicrograph showing morphologically altered venular endothelium (E) in the midst of the inflammatory infiltrates. (Reproduced with permission from Dvorak, H. F., S. J. Galli, and A. M. Dvorak. Expression of cell mediated hypersensitivity in vivo: recent advances. International Review of Experimental Pathology 21:119–194, 1980.)*

Antigen-Presenting Cells and the Cognitive and Activation Phases of Delayed Type Hypersensitivity

Experimentally, DTH reactions are produced in two separate steps (see Fig. 13–1). In the first or "sensitization" step, foreign antigen is presented to naive T cells, resulting in antigen-specific CD4$^+$ T cell activation, expansion, and differentiation. In the second or "elicitation" step, the same antigen is presented to an expanded population of memory CD4$^+$ T cells at the peripheral site where the antigen is introduced. Different APCs are believed to participate in these two stages (Fig. 13–4). In the first step, *specialized resident APCs, such as Langerhans cells in the epidermis,* carry antigen from the portal of entry (e.g., the skin) to the draining lymph nodes, where contact with antigen-specific naive T cells is more likely to occur. Activated T cells both expand in number and increase their ability to cross

endothelial barriers. Both changes serve to enhance the likelihood of encounter with antigen at the peripheral site. Although Langerhans cells present antigen for initial immunization, this process is probably too slow to account for elicitation of DTH reactions in sensitized individuals.

The elicitation step is also initiated by antigen presentation, in this case to memory CD4$^+$ T cells found in the circulation. It seems likely that an important APC for this situation is the **vascular endothelial cell,** particularly endothelial cells lining the post-capillary venules. These cells express both MHC molecules and costimulators, and are capable of activating T cells *in vitro.*

Antigen presentation by endothelium is not responsible for the generalized homing of memory T cells once the response is under way. As we discussed in Chapter 11, the vast majority of T cells are recruited to the inflammatory site by mechanisms that are independent of antigen. Once T cells extravasate into the tissue, they may be restimulated by antigen presented on **resident macrophages.** Antigen presentation by macro-

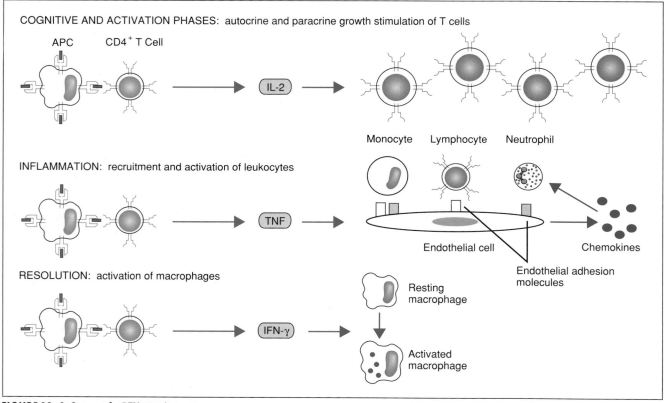

FIGURE 13–3. Stages of a DTH reaction. *DTH reactions are initiated by T cell recognition of an MHC-associated antigen on an antigen-presenting cell (APC); in the example shown, this is a class II–associated antigen recognized by a CD4+ T cell, but a CD8+ T cell is capable of inducing a similar reaction. Different cytokines secreted by the T cell in response to antigen recognition play predominant roles in different phases of the reaction, as shown. Other cytokines that are not shown may play auxiliary roles.*

phages probably serves to amplify and sustain the response until the foreign antigen has been eliminated. Consequently, antigen-specific T cells are preferentially expanded and retained. Furthermore, presentation of antigen by macrophages may initiate the elicitation step, bypassing the endothelium, if nonspecific inflammatory irritants that cause antigen-independent homing of T cells (e.g., adjuvants) are included with the antigen.

Once activated by antigen in the peripheral tissue, the T cells that mediate DTH do so by secretion of cytokines. Four cytokine-mediated effects appear most important for development of the characteristic inflammatory reaction.

1. IL-2 causes autocrine and paracrine proliferation of antigen-activated T cells. Higher concentrations of IL-2 can also stimulate bystander T cells not specific for the antigen. Indeed, by the time lymphocytic infiltrate becomes pronounced, more than 90 per cent of the activated T cells present at the site of antigen challenge are not specific for the eliciting antigen. In addition to its effects on proliferation, IL-2 augments the synthesis of cytokines by CD4+ T cells, especially IFN-γ, TNF, and (at later times) LT.

2. IFN-γ acts on APCs, such as endothelium or macrophages, to increase class II MHC molecule expression, increasing the efficiency of antigen presentation to CD4+ T cells at the local site. This is another

important amplification mechanism for the induction of DTH.

3. TNF and LT act on venular endothelial cells to augment their capacities to bind and activate leukocytes, leading to inflammation. IFN-γ and IL-4 may have similar actions on endothelial cells, resulting in specific recruitment of mononuclear cells.

4. IFN-γ acts on monocytes infiltrating the inflammatory site to enhance their ability to eliminate antigen. *Because IFN-γ is the most potent macrophage-activating cytokine in all species examined, it is the most important mediator of DTH.* IFN-γ also acts on B cells to promote switching to the IgG2a isotype (in mice), an isotype of antibody that is particularly effective in binding to macrophage Fcγ receptors and augmenting the efficiency of phagocytosis.

Venular Endothelial Cells and Inflammation

Venular endothelial cells at sites of antigen administration may play two roles in the DTH reaction. First, as discussed above, venular endothelial cells may act as APCs to initiate T cell activation. Second, *venular endothelial cells regulate the infiltration of leukocytes into the inflammatory reaction.*

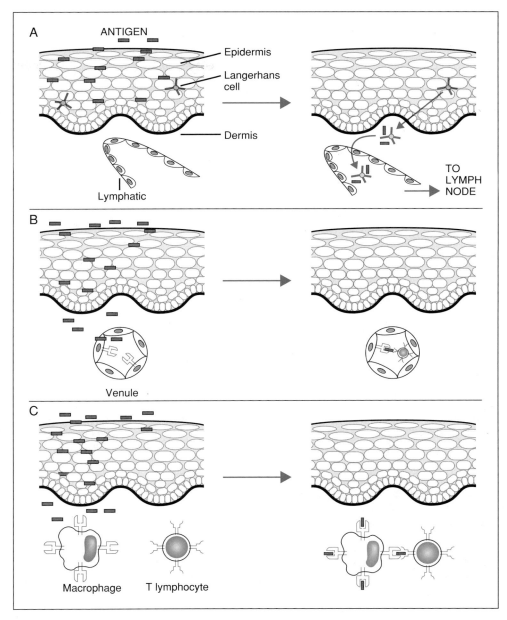

FIGURE 13–4. Antigen-presenting cells (APCs) in DTH reactions. *Three different cell types present antigen to T cells in various phases of DTH reactions. Specialized APC, such as Langerhans cells (A), endocytose and process foreign protein antigens during the sensitization phase. Langerhans cells transport these antigens to the lymph nodes and then present them to antigen-specific naive T cells, triggering a primary immune response. During the elicitation phase, venular endothelial cells (B) present antigen to circulating memory T cells to initiate a local secondary immune response. Resident macrophages (C) in the tissues present antigen to recruited T cells to amplify and sustain the reaction until the source of foreign antigen is eliminated.*

Under the influence of TNF and other cytokines produced by T cells and macrophages responding to antigen challenge, endothelial cells perform four functions that contribute to inflammation (Fig. 13–5):

1. By production of vasodilator substances such as prostacyclin (PGI_2) and nitric oxide (NO), endothelial cells cause increased blood flow and optimize delivery of leukocytes at the site of inflammation. TNF increases the expression of enzymes in endothelial cells that synthesize prostacyclin, and, in combination with IFN-γ, increases production of NO.

2. By expression of new or increased levels of certain surface proteins, endothelial cells become adhesive for leukocytes. In this adhesive state, a random encounter of a circulating leukocyte with a venular endothelial cell will result in an increase in the residence time of leukocytes on the venular surface. As has been shown for lymphocyte diapedesis across high endothelial venules in organized lymphoid tissues (see Chapter 11), such increased residence time can serve to increase the likelihood of extravasation. Several leukocyte adhesion molecules on vascular endothelium are induced in peripheral tissues in response to cytokines. Three cytokine-induced endothelial molecules are well characterized, and have been demonstrated to be important in the development of antigen-induced inflammation (Figs. 13–6 and 13–7). **E-selectin** (also called endothelial-leukocyte adhesion molecule–1 or ELAM-1) is the first molecule to be induced by TNF (onset 1 to 2 hours). E-selectin is structurally related to the peripheral lymph node homing receptor on T cells, L-selectin (see Chapter 11). On venules of peripheral tissues, E-selectin mediates the initial attachment of neutrophils.

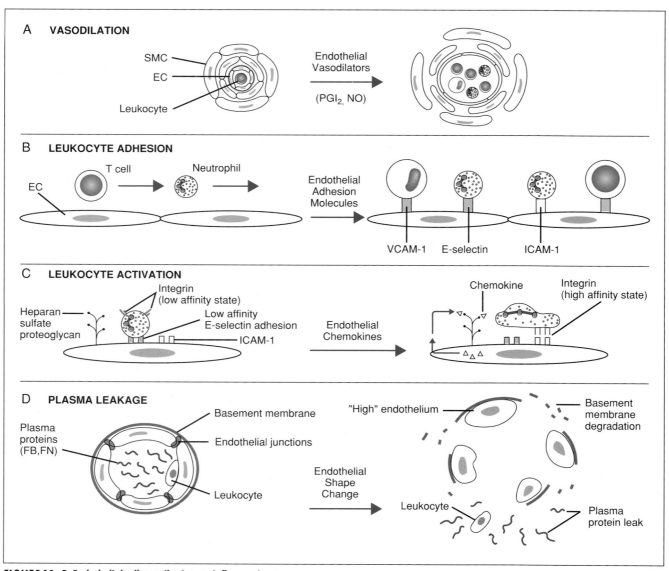

FIGURE 13–5. Endothelial cell contributions to inflammation. *Vascular endothelial cells, in response to TNF and other cytokines, produce vasodilators (PGI₂ and NO) that increase leukocyte delivery to tissues (A); express adhesion molecules (E-selectin, VCAM-1, ICAM-1) that bind leukocytes (B); synthesize and express chemokines (IL-8, MCP-1, etc.) that activate leukocytes, increasing integrin affinity and cell motility (C); and allow plasma proteins (fibrinogen fibronectin) to leak into the tissues, forming a scaffolding for leukocytes (D). EC, endothelial cell, FB, fibrinogen; FN, fibronectin; SMC, smooth muscle cell.*

In areas of flowing blood, E-selectin–mediated interactions with neutrophils may result in rolling. E-selectin may also contribute to the initial binding of other inflammatory cell types, but this is less clear. **Vascular cell adhesion molecule–1** (VCAM-1) is induced somewhat more slowly (onset 4 to 6 hours) and mediates the initial attachment of memory T cells and other leukocytes expressing the VLA-4 integrin molecule. **Intercellular adhesion molecule–1** (ICAM-1 or CD54) is induced with a time course similar to that of VCAM-1. ICAM-1 is most critical for transmigration of leukocytes. T cells interact with ICAM-1 through LFA-1, whereas neutrophils engage ICAM-1 predominantly through Mac-1. Leukocyte L-selectin may also contribute to leukocyte recruitment, but its ligand on endothelial cells of peripheral tissues is not known. *These sequential changes in the endothelial cell surface are caused by cytokines and lead to sequential adhesion, first of neutrophils and then of lymphocytes and monocytes.*

3. TNF causes endothelial cells to secrete chemokines such as IL-8 and monocyte chemotactic protein–1 (MCP-1). The secreted chemokines bind to endothelial cell surface heparan sulfate glycosaminoglycans, where they preferentially interact with leukocytes that are bound to endothelial cell adhesion molecules. The chemokines have three separate actions on the leukocytes. First, they increase the affinity of Mac-1 and LFA-1 for ICAM-1 (and perhaps of VLA-4 for VCAM-1). Second, they cause leukocyte spreading from a round immotile form to a flat migrating form. And third, they stimulate cell locomotion. Collectively, these changes trigger leukocyte extravasation.

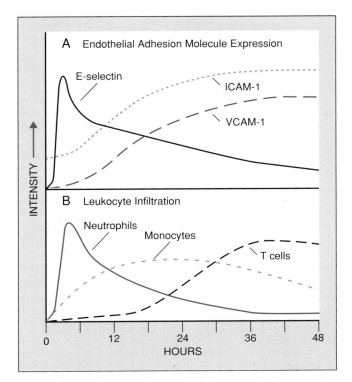

FIGURE 13–6. Time course of endothelial adhesion molecule expression and leukocyte infiltration following antigen rechallenge in the skin. *Similar responses can be elicited with intradermal injection of TNF.*

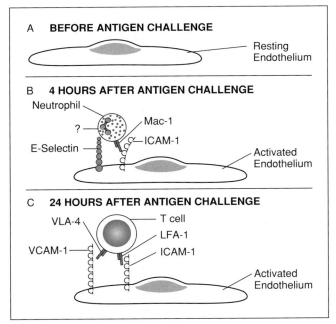

FIGURE 13–7. Adhesion molecules in DTH. *As the inflammatory reaction develops, different endothelial ligands are expressed that interact with different leukocytes. At 4 hours, E-selectin interacts with its neutrophil ligand and ICAM-1 interacts principally with Mac-1 (CD11bCD18). Neutrophil LFA-1 may also interact with ICAM-1 or (not shown) ICAM-2. By 24 hours, T cells interact with VCAM-1 (via VLA-4) and ICAM-1 (via LFA-1). E-selectin may play a lesser role. L-selectin, expressed on both neutrophils and T cells, may also mediate adhesion (not shown).*

4. TNF, acting in concert with IFN-γ, causes endothelial cells to undergo shape changes and basement membrane remodeling that favor leakage of macromolecules and extravasation of cells. The shape changes are indistinguishable from those of endothelial cells lining high endothelial venules (see Chapter 11). Leakage of plasma macromolecules, especially fibrinogen, is the basis of induration. The deposition of fibrinogen (and its insoluble cleavage product, fibrin) as well as plasma fibronectin in the tissues forms a scaffolding that facilitates leukocyte migration and subsequent retention in extravascular tissues. Plasma leakage also serves to reduce the shear force imparted by flowing blood, thereby favoring leukocyte attachment to endothelium.

Activated T cells and macrophages within the tissue also produce chemokines. The principal role of these molecules may be to stimulate chemotaxis within the tissue, rather than the initial recruitment of leukocytes from the circulation.

Once leukocytes enter the tissues, they may die in a few days (especially characteristic of neutrophils), may become activated (especially characteristic of T cells and monocytes), or may leave, probably through lymphatic vessels. The molecules controlling these processes are not yet defined. T cells that are stimulated by antigen in the extravascular tissue remain at the site of inflammation because cell activation increases the expression of receptors for extracellular matrix molecules. The members of the β1 integrin family (see Chapter 7, Box 7–3) are particularly important. VLA-4 and VLA-5 allow leukocytes to bind to fibronectin, and VLA-6 mediates attachment to laminin. Chronically activated T cells express additional integrin receptors (e.g., VLA-2) that mediate attachment to collagen.

The Role of Activated Macrophages in Delayed Type Hypersensitivity

Once blood monocytes leave the circulation and enter the extravascular tissues at sites of DTH reactions, they differentiate into macrophages, which are the ultimate effector cells of these reactions. The macrophages function to eliminate microorganisms and other sources of antigen. The differentiation of monocytes into effector cells is called **macrophage activation.**

The activation of macrophages is not a single process. A macrophage is considered to be activated if it performs a function measured in a specific assay, e.g., killing a microbe. In other assays, e.g., initiating blood coagulation or killing a tumor cell, the same macrophage may appear to be unactivated. Because such functional assays are biologically complex, it is preferable to divide the process of activation into more simple components. The unstimulated blood monocyte is usually considered to be at rest. *Activation consists of quantitative alterations in the expression of various gene products (proteins) that endow the activated macrophage with the capacity to perform some function that cannot be performed by the resting monocyte.* In general, macrophage activation thus results from new or increased gene transcription. For example, activation may consist of increasing expression of a cytochrome enzyme that catalyzes the generation of reactive oxygen species. As a consequence of increased enzyme expression, the activated macrophage may be able to perform a function, e.g., killing of phagocytosed bacteria, that cannot be performed by the resting monocyte. The agents that cause gene transcription and thus macrophage activation are soluble cytokines, bacterial products (e.g., lipopolysaccharide [LPS]), and extracellular matrix molecules. The best-described macrophage-activating cytokine is IFN-γ. However, IFN-γ is not the only cytokine that can activate macrophages, and IFN-γ does not activate all possible capacities of the macrophage. Macrophages may also be activated by T cell contact perhaps through CD40, similar to the activation of B cells (see Chapter 9). Some specific examples of the functions of activated macrophages follow:

1. *Activated macrophages kill microorganisms.* Killing of bacteria by macrophages involves phagocytosis and generation of reactive oxygen species. Cytokines such as IFN-γ augment both endocytosis and phagocytosis by monocytes. Phagocytosis of specific particles can be further enhanced by opsonizing bacteria, that is, coating the bacteria with specific IgG molecules or complement components (see Chapters 3 and 15). IFN-γ causes macrophages to increase expression of high affinity receptors for the Fc portion of IgG, promoting uptake of opsonized bacteria. Once in the cell, macrophages kill bacteria by generating reactive oxygen species, and, as noted above, IFN-γ induces transcription of the gene encoding the enzyme that generates active oxygen. *IFN-γ is thus sufficient to fully activate macrophages for killing of microorganisms.*

Mouse macrophages, but probably not human macrophages, have a second important inducible microbicidal mechanism. Upon treatment of mouse macrophages with IFN-γ in combination with LPS, TNF, or IL-1, these cells express a high-output nitric oxide synthase that, unlike the endothelial cell enzyme, is constitutively active (i.e., independent of calcium). Nitric oxide made in large quantities by this enzyme can contribute to bacterial killing. NO also inhibits viral replication.

2. *Activated macrophages stimulate acute inflammation, often through secretion of short-lived inflammatory mediators.* Many of these mediators, such as platelet-activating factor (PAF), prostaglandins, and leukotrienes, are lipids. Some are synthesized by macrophages themselves, and others are generated from plasma molecules in response to enzymes and related molecules secreted by the macrophages. For example, macrophages produce a protein called tissue factor, which can initiate the extrinsic clotting cascade; thrombin, a blood protease activated during the clotting cascade, causes neutrophils and endothelial cells to synthesize PAF. Treatment with cytokines, such as IFN-γ, enhances the biosynthetic capacities of the macrophage to generate mediators such as tissue factor. The collective action of these macrophage-derived mediators is to produce local inflammation. The inflammatory reaction that results is rich in neutrophils and serves to contain and destroy infectious organisms and to get rid of injured tissue. Thus, the activated macrophage acts as an endogenous surgeon to cauterize the wound, leading to elimination of antigen and resolution of the DTH reaction.

3. *Activated macrophages become more efficient APCs.* A significant part of the enhanced antigen-presenting capacity may be attributed to increased surface expression of class II MHC molecules. IFN-γ is the best known activator of the transcription of class II MHC genes, but in macrophages, granulocyte-macrophage colony-stimulating factor (GM-CSF) may also have some effect. It is also likely that costimulatory functions are enhanced in activated macrophages. Specifically, activated macrophages express the B7 molecule. Activated macrophages also express increased levels of ICAM-1 and LFA-3 (see Chapter 7).

4. *Activated macrophage products, such as cytokines and growth factors, progressively modify the local tissue environment, initially leading to destruction of tissue and later, i.e., in chronic DTH reactions, causing replacement by connective tissue.* IFN-γ facilitates synthesis of cytokines by macrophages but is not sufficient to completely activate these functions. Often, a microorganism can supply a necessary second signal for cytokine synthesis, such as LPS from a bacterial cell wall. Other T cell–derived cytokines can substitute for LPS and work with IFN-γ to stimulate macrophages to secrete cytokines. The effects of macrophage-derived cytokines and growth factors occur in two phases. Acutely, TNF, IL-1, and macrophage-derived chemokines augment inflammatory reactions initiated by T cells. Cytokines act in concert with the inflammatory mediators described above to recruit and activate neutrophils and monocytes, causing local tissue destruction. Chronically, these same cytokines also stimulate fibroblast proliferation and collagen production. These slow actions of cytokines are augmented by the actions of macrophage-derived polypeptide growth factors. Platelet-derived growth factor, produced by activated macrophages, is a potent stimulator of fibroblast proliferation, whereas macrophage-derived transforming growth factor–β (TGF-β) augments collagen synthesis. Macrophage secretion of fibroblast growth factor causes endothelial cell migration and proliferation, leading to new blood vessel formation (**angiogenesis**). The consequence of these slow actions of cytokines and growth factors is that prolonged activation of macrophages in a tissue, e.g., in the setting of chronic antigenic stimulation, leads to replacement of differentiated tissues by fibrous tissue, a process called **fibrosis** (or scarring). *Fibrosis is the outcome of chronic DTH, when elimination of antigen and rapid resolution are unsuccessful.*

5. *Activated macrophages kill tumor cells.* Although the activated macrophage is usually thought of

as an effector of host defense against infectious organisms, tumor biologists have observed that activated macrophages also selectively kill malignant cells. This phenomenon is discussed in greater detail in Chapter 18. Suffice it to say here that much of the antitumor effect of activated macrophages may be attributed to the ability of TNF, produced by these cells, to cause tumor cell death. A second anti-tumor mechanism of murine (but probably not human) macrophages is the production of NO; this response was discussed earlier as an antimicrobial mechanism.

In chronic DTH reactions, activated macrophages themselves undergo changes. Such macrophages develop increased cytoplasm and cytoplasmic organelles. In standard histologic sections stained with hematoxylin and eosin, activated macrophages may resemble skin epithelial cells and have therefore been called "epithelioid." Sometimes, these macrophages can fuse to form multinucleate giant cells. Individual clusters of activated macrophages, often focused about particulate sources of antigen such as *Mycobacterium*, produce palpable nodules of inflammatory tissue called **granulomas** (i.e., granular masses) (Fig. 13–8). Granuloma-

tous inflammation is a characteristic response to some persistent microbes, such as *Mycobacterium tuberculosis*, and simply represents a form of chronic DTH. Experimentally, granulomas can be elicited by attaching soluble protein antigens to undigestible latex beads so they are particulate and persistent in tissues. Granulomatous inflammation is frequently associated with tissue fibrosis. Although fibrosis is a "healing reaction" to injury, it can also interfere with normal tissue function. Much of the respiratory difficulty associated with tuberculosis or fungal infections of the lung is caused by replacement of normal lung with scar tissue.

The pathologic consequences of DTH raise a more general point that was alluded to earlier in the chapter. All of the various effector mechanisms of the immune system have evolved as mechanisms of host defense, yet all can cause "hypersensitivity," i.e., injurious reactions. Activated macrophages contribute to cell-mediated immunity by containing and eradicating infectious organisms, such as mycobacteria or fungi, that can survive within phagocytes. Although DTH reactions are targeted by T cells to be selective for the invading microorganisms, they are still somewhat injurious to normal host tissues. When DTH is elicited experimentally with a non-injurious agent, such as a protein or heat-killed bacteria, one sees only the destructive aspects and not the protective functions. Similarly, when the protective functions are ineffective or incompletely effective, the reaction persists and the destructive consequences can accumulate, as in granulomatous diseases.

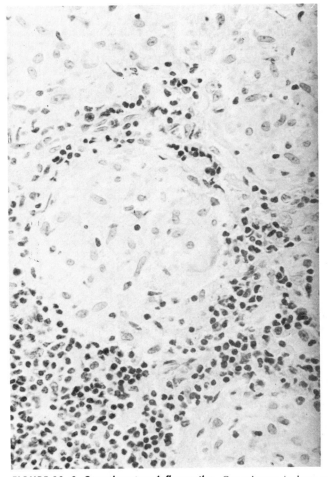

FIGURE 13–8. Granulomatous inflammation. *Granulomas in human lung, showing T cells surrounding nodular collections of activated macrophages. (Courtesy of Dr. Carol Farver, Department of Pathology, Brigham and Women's Hospital, Boston.)*

CYTOLYTIC T LYMPHOCYTES

Cytolytic T lymphocytes are a subset of T cells that kill target cells expressing specific antigen. CTLs appear to be important effector cells in three settings: intracellular infections of non-phagocytic cells or infections that are not completely contained by phagocytosis, such as viral infections or infection by bacteria such as *Listeria monocytogenes*; acute allograft rejection; and rejection of tumors. Each of these processes is discussed in more detail in Section IV. In this chapter, we focus upon the characteristics of CTLs and their mechanisms of action.

The majority of CTLs express the CD8 molecule and specifically recognize foreign peptides derived from intracellularly synthesized antigens associated with self class I MHC molecules. Rare CTLs express the CD4 molecule and recognize peptides associated with class II molecules. As discussed in Chapters 7 and 8, the T cell antigen receptor genes utilized by CD8+ CTLs are indistinguishable from those utilized by CD4+ helper T cells. The preference of CD8+ T cells for class I MHC molecules is instead related to the direct binding of CD8 to nonpolymorphic regions of the class I MHC molecule. Like helper T cells, CTLs undergo maturation and selection in the thymus.

Development and Differentiation of Functional CTLs

CTLs are not fully differentiated when they exit the thymus. Although they express functional $\alpha\beta$ T cell receptor molecules and recognize antigen, they cannot lyse target cells. Indeed, very few, if any, functional CTLs specific for an allograft can be detected in the blood of a potential allograft recipient prior to transplantation (see Chapter 17). However, if T lymphocytes are cultured with leukocytes from the donor of an allograft, i.e., in a mixed leukocyte reaction (see Chapter 17), graft-specific CD8$^+$ CTLs can be detected in the culture after 7 to 10 days. Similarly, if T cells from a virus-infected individual are stimulated with virus-infected syngeneic cells *in vitro*, virus-specific self MHC–restricted CD8$^+$ CTLs are detected within 5 to 10 days. The appearance of functional CTLs depends upon a process of differentiation.

The principal features of CTL differentiation are the following:

1. *CTLs develop or differentiate from "pre-CTLs."* Pre-CTLs are T cells that are committed to the CTL lineage, have undergone thymic maturation, and are already specific for a particular foreign antigen. These cells express CD3-associated $\alpha\beta$ T cell receptors (TCRs) and CD8, but they lack cytolytic function.

2. *Pre-CTLs do not require a special microenvironment for differentiation and can develop within the infected or foreign tissue.* Pre-CTLs are normally present at low frequency in the blood and peripheral lymphoid tissues and can be detected by stimulating differentiation *in vitro* before assessing cytolytic function.

3. *Differentiation of pre-CTLs to functional CTLs requires at least two separate kinds of signals: the first is specific recognition of antigen on a target cell, and the second depends on T cell–derived cytokines* (Fig. 13–9). There are two currently unresolved issues about the cytokine requirement for CTL differentiation. First, the precise cytokines required are not known. It is likely that IL-2 and IFN-γ are important, but several other cytokines, including IL-4, IL-6, IL-7, and IL-12 have been found to play a role in some *in vitro* experiments. Second, the identity of the T cells responsible for providing these cytokines is not well established. In most experiments, there appears to be a requirement for CD4$^+$ T cells (presumably of the T$_H$1 subset) that respond to antigens presented by class II+ APCs; in other models, CD8$^+$ T cells stimulated by antigens presented by professional APCs are sufficient to provide the requisite cytokines. Indeed, it is possible that such cytokines may be produced by CD8$^+$ cells and act in an autocrine manner, giving rise to "helper-independent" CTLs.

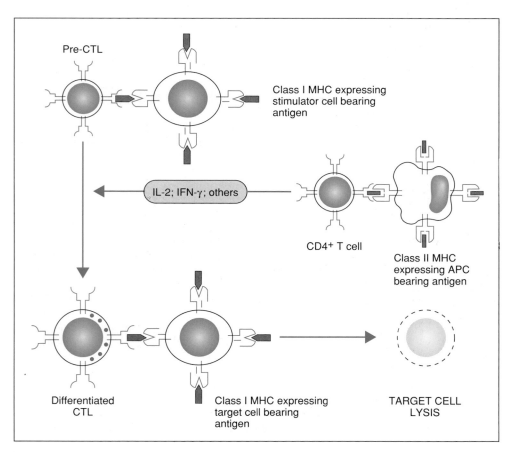

Pre-CTL

Class I MHC expressing stimulator cell bearing antigen

IL-2; IFN-γ; others

CD4$^+$ T cell

Class II MHC expressing APC bearing antigen

Differentiated CTL

Class I MHC expressing target cell bearing antigen

TARGET CELL LYSIS

FIGURE 13–9. Stimuli for the differentiation of cytolytic T lymphocytes (CTLs). *In order to differentiate into fully functional CTLs, CD8$^+$ pre-CTLs require two signals: recognition of class I MHC–associated antigen on a stimulator cell, and cytokines provided by helper T cells. These cytokines may be provided by CD4$^+$ T$_H$1 T cells, as shown here, or by CD8$^+$ T cells.*

Functions of CTLs

The function of differentiated CTLs is to lyse (i.e., kill) target cells. Differentiation from pre-CTLs involves the acquisition of the machinery to perform cell lysis. Two parallel sets of changes occur during this process. First, CTLs develop specific membrane-bound cytoplasmic granules. These granules contain several macromolecules, including a membrane pore-forming protein called **perforin** or **cytolysin;** enzymes that contain reactive serines in their active site (commonly called "serine esterases"); protein toxins, which are either identical or structurally related to LT; and proteoglycans. Second, CTLs develop the capacity to transcribe and secrete cytokines and other proteins upon activation, most specifically IFN-γ, LT, TNF, and, to a lesser degree, IL-2. As discussed below, both granule contents and secreted cytokines may be directly involved in CTL-mediated lysis.

Mechanisms of CTL-Mediated Lysis

There are several key features of CTL-mediated lysis.

1. *CTL killing is antigen-specific.* Only target cells that bear the same class I MHC–associated antigen that triggered pre-CTL differentiation can be killed by an individual CTL.

2. *CTL killing requires cell contact.* This requirement arises from the need of CTLs to be triggered by recognition of a target antigen associated with a cell surface MHC molecule. CTLs kill only those cells to which they attach, and bystander cells are not injured. This is because the lytic mechanisms of CTLs are directed toward the point of contact of the T cell receptor (TCR) molecule with antigen.

3. *CTLs themselves are not injured during lysis of target cells.* Moreover, each individual CTL is capable of sequentially killing multiple target cells. The mechanisms that protect CTLs from lysis are, as will be discussed below, not fully understood.

The process of CTL-mediated lysis consists of five steps (Fig. 13–10):

1. *Recognition of antigen and conjugate formation.* The CTL binds to the target cell using its specific antigen receptor and other accessory molecules, such as CD8, CD2, and LFA-1. Target cell recognition, therefore, involves class I MHC molecules (the ligand for CD8), complexed to specific peptide (the complex serving as the ligand for the TCR), LFA-3 (the ligand for CD2), and ICAM-1 or ICAM-2 (the ligands for LFA-1). It may be that transient conjugate formation can occur via CD2 and LFA-1–mediated adhesion in the absence of or prior to specific antigen recognition, or that antigen recognition may enhance the ability to form conjugates by augmenting the binding function of the adhesion mole-

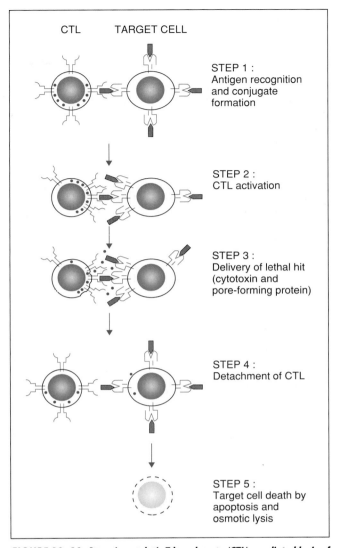

FIGURE 13–10. Steps in cytolytic T lymphocyte (CTL)–mediated lysis of target cells. Note that conjugate formation (step 1) also requires interactions between CTL accessory molecules (LFA-1, CD8) on the CTLs and their specific ligands on the target cell; these are not shown (see Fig. 7–8, Chapter 7).

cules. CTL-mediated killing of target cells that do not express ICAM-1 or (in humans) LFA-3 is very inefficient.

2. *Activation of the CTL.* The CTL is activated by cross-linking of its antigen receptor. Cross-linking or clustering of TCR:CD3 complexes on CTLs may be a simple consequence of multivalent recognition of MHC-peptide complexes on the target cell. The intracellular signals generated by the TCR may be augmented by signals delivered through the various accessory molecules. The process of CTL activation is thus entirely analogous to the activation of helper T cells described in Chapter 7.

3. *Delivery of a "lethal hit" by the activated CTL to its conjugated target* (see below).

4. *Release of the CTL.* The CTL is released from its target cell, a process that may be facilitated by de-

creases in the affinity of accessory molecules for their ligands.

5. *Programmed death of the target cell as a consequence of receiving a lethal hit.*

Delivery of the lethal hit appears to occur by two parallel mechanisms, either one of which is adequate for target cell lysis. *In the first mechanism, CTLs focus and then secrete (exocytose) the contents of some of their cytoplasmic granules in the areas of contact with their target cells.* Focusing of the granules is initiated by clustering of TCR:CD3 molecules and involves the cytoskeleton. The microtubule organizing center of the CTL is moved to the area of the cytoplasm near the contact with the target cell, and granules are clustered in this same region. As a consequence of granule content exocytosis, the pore-forming protein, present as a monomer in the granule, comes in contact with extracellular concentrations of calcium (typically 1 to 2 mM) and undergoes polymerization. Polymerization of the pore-forming protein preferentially occurs in a lipid bilayer such as the plasma membrane of the target cell. The polymerized form of the protein acts as an ion-permeable channel in the target cell plasma membrane. If a sufficient number of these channels are present, the target cell will be unable to exclude ions and water, leading to osmotic swelling and lysis. This method of cell killing is analogous to that produced by the membrane attack complex of complement, and the CTL pore-forming protein is structurally homologous to the ninth component of complement, the principal constituent of the membrane attack complex (see Chapter 15). Purified pore-forming protein can be used experimentally to lyse cells. The additional components of the granule, i.e., the serine esterases, the cell toxins, and the proteoglycans, may also injure cells, but the mechanisms by which they do so are less well understood.

The second mechanism of lysis involves activating enzymes within the target cell to digest its own DNA. The signal(s) that induce DNA degradation have not been unequivocally identified. Two major candidates are LT, possibly conjugated on the CTL surface to the LT-β subunit (see Chapter 12), and adenosine triphosphate (ATP). It is also possible that a CTL surface protein, perhaps LT, recognizes the Fas antigen on target cells, and this leads to target cell apoptosis. It is clear, however, that delivery of this signal does not depend upon granule exocytosis. Once the nuclear DNA is fragmented, target cell nuclei also undergo fragmentation, a process called **apoptosis.** Killing of target cells by osmotic swelling and killing by apoptosis are mechanistically independent and are complementary.

As noted above, CTLs themselves are not killed during the lytic process. However, CTLs can be killed by other CTLs and by high concentrations of the pore-forming proteins or the CTL-derived cell toxin. This raises the question of why CTLs are not injured during target cell lysis. The answer is probably quantitative: *CTLs are relatively resistant to CTL-mediated lysis.* The mechanism of this relative resistance is not known; one possibility is that CTLs express high levels of membrane proteins that disassemble the pore-forming complex.

Much of our understanding of CTL development and function is based on studies of these cells in the experimental setting of allograft rejection. Indeed, CTLs are readily isolated from rejecting allografts, and adoptive transfer of mature CTLs can cause allograft rejection (see Chapter 17). Although suitable experimental systems for *in vivo* study are less well developed, *it is believed that the physiologic function of CTLs is the eradication of viral infection.* CTLs inhibit viral replication in two ways:

1. *CTLs act to destroy infected host cells that are the source of replicating virus particles.* An important additional effect of CTL-induced apoptosis may be to activate cellular enzymes that degrade viral genomes.

2. *CTLs produce IFN-γ,* which stimulates the microbicidal activities of macrophages that have phagocytosed viruses. IFN-γ also promotes production of IgG2a antibody (in mice), which neutralizes virus, activates complement (see Chapter 15) and opsonizes viral particles for phagocytosis. Finally, IFN-γ shares antiviral activities with the type I IFNs.

CTL function *in vivo* is likely to occur in conjunction with other cell-mediated immune defense mechanisms, such as activated macrophages. Indeed, these two mechanisms may complement each other. A good example of the cooperative action of CD4$^+$ and CD8$^+$ T cells is in immunity to *Listeria monocytogenes*, which is described in Chapter 16 (see Fig. 16–4).

NATURAL KILLER CELLS

Natural killer (NK) cells are a subset of lymphocytes found in blood and lymphoid tissues, especially spleen. NK cells are derived from the bone marrow and appear as large lymphocytes with numerous cytoplasmic granules, because of which they are sometimes called **large granular lymphocytes** (LGLs). NK cells are best thought of as phylogenetically primitive CTLs that lack the specific T cell receptor (TCR) for antigen recognition. NK cells possess the ability to kill certain tumor cells and normal cells infected by virus. Killing by NK cells is not specific for particular viral antigenic determinants and is not restricted by MHC molecules. Such killing is "natural," in that it is not induced by specific antigen and is thus part of natural rather than specific immunity. Although the target specificity of NK cells is broader than that of CTLs, it is nevertheless not random. NK cells can lyse normal cells infected by some viruses, but not others, and will not lyse uninfected cells. NK activity can cause lysis of certain tumor cell lines, particularly of hematopoietic origin, but not of others. The existence of NK specificity is most clearly demonstrated by the phenomenon of "cold target inhibition"; i.e., one NK target cell type can inhibit lysis of a different NK target type by competing for effector cells, whereas cells that are not NK targets do not compete (Fig. 13–11).

EXPERIMENTAL CONDITIONS	LYSIS (RELEASE OF LABEL)

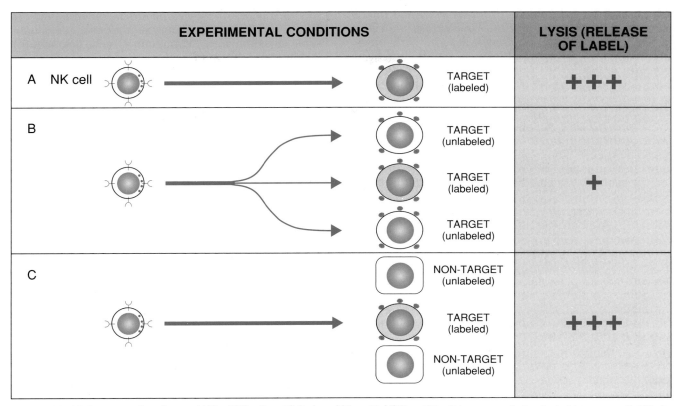

FIGURE 13–11. Demonstration of natural killer (NK) cell specificity by cold target inhibition. *NK cells can cause lysis of suitable target cells (A). An excess of unlabeled target cells inhibits NK cell–mediated lysis of labeled targets (B), whereas cells that are not NK targets do not function as competitive inhibitors (C). By this approach, it has been shown that NK cells recognize a variety of virus-infected cells and hematopoietic tumors (all of which serve as cold target inhibitors for one another), but MHC molecules are not involved in this recognition. (In contrast, cold target inhibition of virus-specific CD8⁺ cytolytic T lymphocyte (CTL) killing requires that the cold target express the same viral antigen and class I MHC molecules as the labeled target.)*

By surface phenotype and lineage, NK cells are neither T nor B cells. NK cells do not undergo thymic maturation and may be increased in animals that lack a thymus. Moreover, NK cells do not undergo Ig or TCR gene rearrangements and do not express CD3 molecules. However, NK cells do express the CD2 molecule and a low-affinity receptor for the Fc portion of IgG, called FcγRIII or CD16 (see Chapter 3). NK cells can be induced to proliferate and secrete cytokines by cross-linking either CD2 or CD16. In this regard, it is worth noting that despite lacking CD3, NK cells do express homodimers of the ζ chain, identical to those which associate with TCR complexes in MHC-restricted T cells. In NK cells, the ζ chain or a homodimeric protein called γ, which is structurally homologous to ζ, is associated with CD16. Both ζ and γ homodimers are thought to be involved in signal transduction initiated by IgG binding to CD16.

NK cells express the signal-transducing β and γ subunits of the IL-2 receptor, but not the affinity-enhancing α subunit, and can be induced to proliferate only by high concentrations of IL-2. In addition, NK cells may share with CTLs certain other surface markers. For example, in mice, both CTLs and NK cells express a surface ganglioside called asialo GM-1. Although markers such as asialo GM-1 are useful for

identifying NK cells, their relationship to NK function is unclear. There are several recently described non-polymorphic genes that are uniquely expressed in NK cells; it has been speculated that one or more of these genes encodes the as yet unidentified NK cell antigen receptor.

The molecular structure recognized by NK cells on the surface of susceptible target cells is not yet defined. Such a structure would presumably be shared by primitive cells, tumor cells, and virally infected cells, since all are recognized by NK cells. Part of the difficulty in identifying an NK target structure may arise from the possibility that NK cells are heterogeneous, so that different NK populations may recognize different classes of molecules (and different types of target cells). Two competing ideas about the molecular basis of NK cell recognition are currently under active consideration. In the first model, NK cells recognize a target molecule, perhaps encoded within the MHC, that is constitutively expressed on embryonic cells and on certain tumor cells and may be induced on virally infected cells. This structure could be a protein or a carbohydrate. In the second model, NK cells lyse target cells that lack expression of a normal molecule on the target cell. It has been proposed that this missing molecule is a class I molecule, particularly (in humans) HLA-C, associated with a specific self peptide. Primitive cells and tumor cells are targets because class I molecules are often expressed at low levels on these cell types. Viral infection renders a cell susceptible because virally derived peptides are thought to displace the critical self peptide. This second model does not address the question of how the NK cell can detect the absence of a target cell molecule.

Unlike CTLs, NK cells do not appear to require prior contact with target antigens to develop cytolytic capacities. They share with CTLs a responsiveness to cytokines, although NK cells do not need antigen contact to acquire cytokine responsiveness. NK cells can be activated to increase their ability to lyse target cells by treatment with type I IFN, IFN-γ, IL-12, TNF, or IL-2. NK cells can acquire additional specificities by virtue of CD16-mediated recognition of targets coated with IgG antibodies. This form of cytolysis is called **antibody-dependent cell-mediated cytotoxicity** (ADCC), and NK cells are its principal mediator (see Chapter 3).

Killing of targets by NK cells involves similar mechanisms as killing by CTLs, namely granule exocytosis and induction of target cell DNA fragmentation and apoptosis. NK granules, like CTL granules, contain pore-forming protein, cytotoxins, serine esterases, and proteoglycans. It is not known whether the apoptosis-inducing signal produced by NK cells is the same as or different from that of CTLs. NK cells synthesize TNF but not LT. NK cells also secrete IFN-γ, especially in response to IL-2 and IL-12 (see Chapter 12). In mice lacking functional T cells, NK cell–derived IFN-γ can activate macrophages to kill infectious organisms such as *Listeria monocytogenes*.

The role of NK cells in normal immunity is not clearly established. Since these cells were originally detected, in part, by their ability to kill virally infected cells, it has been hypothesized that they serve to lyse infected cells until antigen-specific CTLs can differentiate from pre-CTLs (see Chapter 16). Rare individuals lacking NK cells are more susceptible to severe viral infections. Because NK cells can lyse certain tumor cells, it has also been proposed that NK cells serve to kill malignant clones *in vivo*. However, neither viral infection–associated nor tumor-associated inflammatory infiltrates show significant numbers of NK cells. The one setting in which large numbers of NK cells predominate in the lesions is in graft-versus-host disease (GVHD) in recipients of bone marrow transplants. We will discuss GVHD in greater detail in Chapter 17; suffice it to say here that NK cells infiltrate into epithelium such as skin and can be found adjacent to necrotic epithelial cells, the hallmark of GVHD. The mechanism by which NK cells lyse normal epithelial cells is not fully known. It has been observed that when NK cells are treated with sufficient concentration of IL-2 to be stimulated through IL-2Rβγ, they differentiate into lymphokine-activated killer (LAK) cells. LAK cells demonstrate enhanced cytolytic capacity and a very broad target specificity, killing a wide variety of tumor cells and normal cell types, including epithelial cells. Thus, in GVHD, transplanted CD4+ T cells may recognize and respond to the alloantigens of the host. These T cells produce IL-2, which may stimulate the differentiation of NK cells into LAK cells. This is another example of how, in specific cell-mediated immunity, T cells augment the functions and focus the actions of the effector cells of natural immunity.

SUMMARY

Cell-mediated immunity consists of immune responses that are initiated by antigen recognition by specific T lymphocytes and in which T lymphocytes participate in the effector stage as well. There are several forms of cell-mediated immune reactions, which are initiated by activation of T cells in response to specific antigen. Activated T cells secrete cytokines, which, in turn, activate various effector cell populations. In delayed type hypersensitivity reactions, T cells secrete tumor necrosis factor, which causes endothelial cells to recruit inflammatory leukocytes, and interferon-γ, which activates macrophages to kill microorganisms, initiate acute inflammatory responses, and produce tissue remodeling.

Cytolytic T lymphocytes, which usually bear CD8, are important effector cells in settings of intracellular microbial infection and allograft rejection. CTLs differentiate from pre-CTLs in response to two signals: (1) a target cell bearing endogenously synthesized peptide antigens presented in association with self class I MHC molecules or a target expressing specific foreign class I MHC molecules, and (2) a combination of several T cell–derived cytokines. Upon differentiation, CTLs acquire the ability to kill target cells expressing the appropriate MHC-associated antigen. CTL-mediated killing involves two complementary mechanisms: (1) granule exocytosis of a membrane pore-forming protein that causes osmotic lysis of target cells, and (2) provision of a signal that activates DNA degrading enzymes in target cells.

Natural killer cells are a population of large granular lymphocytes that normally serve to kill target cells bearing undefined target molecules (or those lacking in a protective molecule) or cells coated with specific IgG molecules. NK cell–mediated killing uses the same mechanisms employed in CTL-mediated killing. NK cells are activated by cytokines produced by CD4+ T cells. In response to high levels of IL-2, NK cells differentiate into lymphokine-activated killer cells that kill target cells in relatively indiscriminate fashion. By recruiting and activating NK cells, CD4+ T cells can cause lysis of normal cell types in response to antigen stimulation, characteristic of the reaction found in acute graft-versus-host disease.

SELECTED READINGS

Adams, D. O., and T. A. Hamilton. The cell biology of macrophage activation. Annual Review of Immunology 2:283–318, 1984.

Bevilacqua, M. P. Endothelial-leukocyte adhesion molecules. Annual Review of Immunology 11:767–804, 1993.

Cerottini, J. C., and H. R. MacDonald (organizers). 17th Forum in Immunology: Molecular mechanism of T-cell–mediated cytotoxicity. Annales de L'Institut Pasteur Immunology 138:287–342, 1987.

Dannenberg, A. M., Jr. Delayed-type hypersensitivity and cell-mediated immunity in the pathogenesis of tuberculosis. Immunology Today 12:229–233, 1991.

Doherty, P. C., J. E. Allan, F. Lynch, and R. Ceredig. Dissection of an inflammatory process induced by CD8+ T cells. Immunology Today 11:55–59, 1990.

Herberman, R. B., C. W. Reynolds, and J. Ortaldo. Mechanisms of cytotoxicity by natural killer (NK) cells. Annual Review of Immunology 4:651–680, 1986.

Kovacs, E. J. Fibrogenic cytokines: the role of immune mediators in the development of scar tissue. Immunology Today 12:17–23, 1991.

Kupfer, A., and S. J. Singer. Cell biology of cytotoxic and helper T-cell functions. Annual Review of Immunology 7:309–337, 1989.

Mosmann, T. R., and R. L. Coffman. Heterogeneity of cytokine secretion patterns and functions of helper T cells. Advances in Immunology 46:111–147, 1989.

Pober, J. S., and R. S. Cotran. Immunologic interactions of T lymphocytes with vascular endothelium. Advances in Immunology 50:261–302, 1991.

Podack, E. R., H. Hengartner, and M. G. Lichtenheld. A central role of perforin in cytolysis? Annual Review of Immunology 9:129–157, 1991.

Trinchieri, G. Biology of natural killer cells. Advances in Immunology 47:187–376, 1989.

Versteeg, R. NK cells and T cells: mirror images? Immunology Today 13:244–247, 1992.

Young, J. D., C. C. Liu, P. M. Persechini, and Z. A. Cohn. Perforin-dependent and -independent pathways of cytotoxicity mediated by lymphocytes. Immunological Reviews 103:161–202, 1988.

CHAPTER FOURTEEN

EFFECTOR MECHANISMS OF IMMUNOGLOBULIN E– INITIATED IMMUNE REACTIONS

One of the most powerful effector mechanisms of the immune system is the reaction initiated by IgE-dependent stimulation of tissue mast cells and their circulating counterparts, the basophils. When antigen binds to IgE molecules preattached to the surface of these cells, there is a rapid release of a variety of mediators that collectively cause increased vascular permeability, vasodilation, bronchial and visceral smooth muscle contraction, and local inflammation. This reaction is called **immediate hypersensitivity** because it begins rapidly, within minutes of antigen challenge. In its most extreme systemic form, called **anaphylaxis,** mast cell–derived or basophil-derived mediators can restrict airways to the point of asphyxiation and produce cardiovascular collapse leading to death. (The term anaphylaxis was coined to indicate that antibodies, especially IgE antibodies, could confer the opposite of protection [prophylaxis] on an unfortunate individual.) Individuals prone to develop strong immediate hypersensitivity responses are called **atopic** and are said to suffer from **allergies.** Atopy meant "unusual," but we now realize that allergy is in fact quite common. Indeed, allergy is the most common disorder of immunity, affecting 20 per cent of all individuals in the United States. In different individuals, atopy may take different forms such as hay fever, asthma, urticaria (hives), or chronic eczema (skin irritation). All of these conditions are forms of immediate hypersensitivity induced by mast cell or basophil activation.

Mast cell and basophil activation is most characteristically initiated when specific antigen binds to and cross-links preattached surface IgE molecules. Thus, *the typical sequence of events in immediate hypersensitivity* is as follows: (1) production of IgE by B cells in response to the first exposure to an antigen, called "sensitization," (2) binding of the IgE to specific Fc receptors on the surfaces of mast cells and basophils, and (3) interaction of re-introduced antigen with the bound IgE, leading to (4) activation of the cells and release of mediators, some of which are stored in the cytoplasmic granules of the mast cells and basophils (Fig. 14–1). The clinical and pathologic manifestations of immediate hypersensitivity are due to the actions of the released mediators.

Until recently, the existence of immediate hypersensitivity posed a conundrum: for what purpose has the organism developed this potentially lethal, disease-causing arm of the immune system? The answer may be that immediate hypersensitivity is part of a larger response that leads to inflammatory infiltrates rich in eosinophils called the **late phase reaction.** The late phase reaction is a host defense mechanism against some helminthic infections and insect larval infestations. Although we now better appreciate that eosinophilic inflammation plays a protective function, it is also more apparent that eosinophil-mediated tissue injury is a major component of allergic diseases such as asthma. Thus, IgE-initiated protective immunity and immediate hypersensitivity are mediated by the same effector mechanisms. Recall that we made the same point when discussing cell-mediated immunity and delayed type hypersensitivity in Chapter 13.

This chapter focuses on IgE-initiated reactions. We begin by describing experimental models of immediate hypersensitivity and eosinophilic inflammation. We then turn to the biology of IgE and to the Fc receptors that bind IgE on the surface of mast cells or basophils. Next, we discuss the biology of mast cells and related cell types, including a description of how these cells are activated in response to antigen. We then describe the structure of the mediators produced by activated mast cells, basophils, and eosinophils, and the biologic effects of these mediators. Finally, we conclude with a more detailed description of different allergic diseases, integrating features of IgE-initiated reactions and the responses of various target tissues to explain specific clinical syndromes associated with immediate hypersensitivity.

FEATURES OF IMMEDIATE HYPERSENSITIVITY

The classic example of immediate hypersensitivity in humans is the "wheal and flare reaction" (Fig. 14–2). When a sensitized individual is challenged by intradermal injection of an appropriate antigen, the injection site becomes red from locally dilated blood vessels engorged with red blood cells. In the second phase, the site rapidly swells as a result of leakage of plasma from the venules. This soft swelling is called a **wheal** and can involve an area of skin as large as several centimeters in diameter. In the third phase, blood vessels at the margins of the wheal dilate and become engorged with red blood cells, producing a characteristic red rim called a **flare.** The full wheal and flare reaction can appear within 5 to 10 minutes after administration of antigen and usually subsides in less than an hour. By electron microscopy, the venules in the area of the wheal show slight separation of the endothelial cells, which accounts for the escape of macromolecules and fluid, but not cells, from the vascular lumen.

The first clue to the mechanism of this reaction also came from histologic examination. Mast cells in the area of the wheal and flare show evidence of release of pre-formed mediators, i.e., their cytoplasmic granules have been discharged. A causal association of IgE and mast cells with immediate hypersensitivity has been deduced from three kinds of experiments:

1. Immediate hypersensitivity reactions can be elicited in nonresponsive individuals if the local skin site is first injected with IgE from a responsive individual. *Thus, IgE is responsible for specific recognition of antigen and can be used to adoptively transfer immediate hypersensitivity.* Such adoptive transfer experiments were first performed with serum from immunized individuals in the 1920s. Some 40 years later, it was shown that the serum protein responsible for transferring this reaction was a class of antibody, which was named IgE. This serum factor was originally called "reagin," and for this reason IgE molecules are still sometimes called "reaginic antibodies."

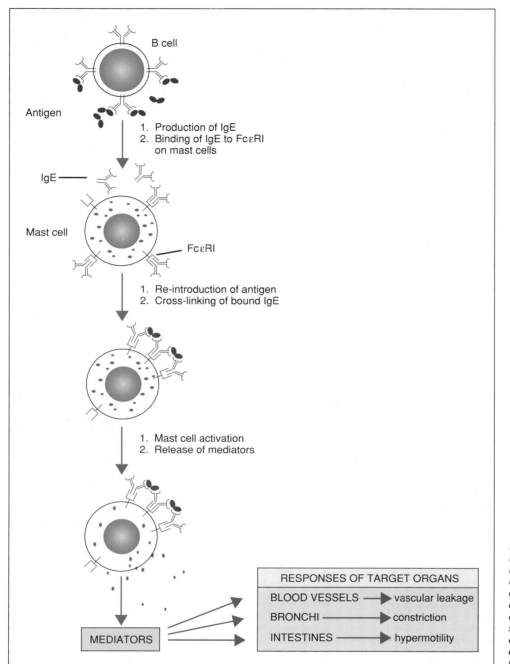

1. Production of IgE
2. Binding of IgE to FcεRI on mast cells

1. Re-introduction of antigen
2. Cross-linking of bound IgE

1. Mast cell activation
2. Release of mediators

RESPONSES OF TARGET ORGANS	
BLOOD VESSELS	➝ vascular leakage
BRONCHI	➝ constriction
INTESTINES	➝ hypermotility

MEDIATORS

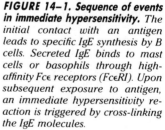

FIGURE 14–1. Sequence of events in immediate hypersensitivity. *The initial contact with an antigen leads to specific IgE synthesis by B cells. Secreted IgE binds to mast cells or basophils through high-affinity Fcε receptors (FcεRI). Upon subsequent exposure to antigen, an immediate hypersensitivity re-action is triggered by cross-linking the IgE molecules.*

2. *Immediate hypersensitivity reactions can be mimicked by injecting anti-IgE antibody instead of antigen.* Anti-IgE elicits a reaction both in atopic individuals who have high levels of antigen-specific IgE antibodies and in non-atopic individuals who have low but measurable levels of IgE. Anti-IgE antibodies act as an analog of antigen and directly activate mast cells and basophils that have bound IgE on their surface. This use of anti-IgE to activate mast cells is similar to the use of anti-IgM or anti-IgD antibodies as analogs of antigen to activate B cells (see Chapter 9), except that in the case of mast cells or basophils, secretory IgE, made by B

cells, is bound to high-affinity Fc receptors on the cell surface rather than being synthesized as membrane IgE.

3. *Immediate hypersensitivity reactions can be mimicked by injection of other agents that directly cause mast cell activation, such as C5a, or by local trauma, which causes mechanical disruption of mast cells; and can be inhibited by agents that prevent mast cell activation.* Mast cells can also be activated by locally released neurotransmitters, such as substance P.

Although these classic experiments in immediate hypersensitivity were originally performed in humans,

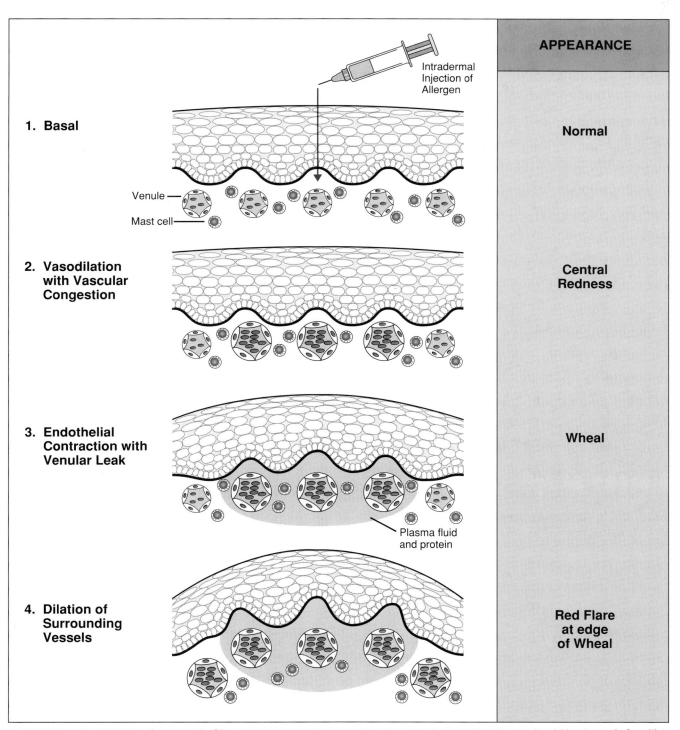

FIGURE 14–2. The IgE-initiated response in skin. *In response to antigen-stimulated release of mast cell mediators, local blood vessels first dilate and then become leaky to fluid and macromolecules, producing redness and local swelling (a wheal). Subsequent dilation of vessels on the edge of the swelling produces the appearance of a red rim (the flare).*

immunologists often use animal models to permit greater ease of experimental manipulation. The guinea pig consistently mounts strong immediate hypersensitivity reactions and has proved to be the most useful animal model.

A **late phase reaction** begins between 2 and 4 hours after elicitation of many immediate hypersensi-

tivity reactions. At this time, the wheal and flare of the immediate hypersensitivity reaction have subsided. This late phase reaction consists of accumulation of inflammatory leukocytes, including neutrophils, eosinophils, basophils, and CD4$^+$ T cells. These T cells are enriched for cells that produce IL-4 but not IFN-γ, the hallmark of the T$_H$2 subset. The inflammation is maximal by about 24 hours and then gradually subsides. Late phase reactions in atopic individuals are rich in eosinophils. Atopic individuals have elevated numbers of activated eosinophils in their peripheral blood, and the composition of the infiltrate may partly reflect the blood count. However, it is also clear that IL-4 produced by mast cells or T_H2 T cells can selectively recruit eosinophils into the tissue. The late phase reaction is part of immediate hypersensitivity, since, like the wheal and flare reaction, it can be adoptively transferred with IgE and can be mimicked by anti-IgE antibodies or mast cell activating agents. The principal protective function of IgE-initiated immune reactions is the eradication of parasites. Eosinophil-mediated killing of IgE-coated helminths is an effective defense against these organisms (see Chapter 16). It has also been speculated that IgE-dependent mast cell activation in the gastrointestinal tract promotes expulsion of parasites by increasing peristalsis and by an outpouring of mucus. A genetically mast cell-deficient mouse strain shows increased susceptibility to infection by tick larvae, and immunity can be provided to these mice by adoptive transfer of specific IgE and mast cells (but not by either component alone). The larvae are eradicated by the specific late phase reaction. The importance of this defense mechanism has been further underscored by studies of mice treated with anti–IL-4 antibody, and of IL-4 knockout mice. As discussed in Chapter 12, such mice do not make IgE, and appear to be less resistant than normal animals to some helminthic infections.

BIOLOGY OF IgE

As we have noted, IgE antibody provides recognition of antigen for immediate hypersensitivity reactions. IgE is the isotype of immunoglobulin that contains the ϵ heavy chain (see Chapter 3). It circulates as a bivalent antibody and is normally present in plasma at a concentration of less than 1 μg/ml. In pathologic conditions, such as helminthic infections and severe atopy, this level can rise to over 1000 μg/ml. The IgE heavy chain V regions and IgE light chains are products of the same genes as other Ig molecules. The heavy chain C regions are encoded by the ϵ gene located in the Ig heavy chain gene cluster. Thus, IgE is produced as a result of heavy chain isotype switching (see Chapter 4).

Regulation of IgE Synthesis

There is a critical difference in IgE production between atopic and normal individuals: The former produce high levels of IgE in response to particular antigens, whereas the latter generally synthesize other Ig isotypes, such as IgM and IgG, and only small amounts of IgE. Four interacting factors contribute to regulation of IgE synthesis: (1) heredity, (2) the natural history of antigen exposure, (3) the nature of the antigen, and (4) helper T cells and their cytokines.

HEREDITY

Abnormally high levels of IgE synthesis and associated atopy often run in families. Although the full inheritance pattern is probably multigenic, family studies have shown that there is clear autosomal transmission of atopy. However, the target organ of atopic disease is variable. Thus, hay fever, asthma, and eczema can be present to various degrees in different members of the same kindred. All of these individuals, however, will show higher than average plasma IgE levels. In addition to this general proclivity to synthesize IgE, the ability to make specific IgE antibodies to certain antigens, e.g., ragweed pollen, is also inherited and may be linked to particular class II major histocompatibility complex (MHC) alleles. This may be an example of an "immune response gene" (Ir gene) effect (see Chapter 6). In the case of a complex antigen such as ragweed pollen, different class II alleles may serve to present different peptides to specific T cells.

NATURAL HISTORY OF ANTIGEN EXPOSURE

The natural history of antigen exposure is an important determinant of the level of specific IgE antibodies. In general, repeated exposure to a particular antigen is necessary to develop an atopic reaction to that antigen. Individuals with allergic rhinitis or asthma often benefit from a geographic change of residence with a change in indigenous plant pollens, although local antigens in the new residence may trigger an eventual return of the symptoms. The most dramatic examples of the influence of the natural history of exposure to antigen are seen in cases of insect, e.g., bee stings. The protein toxins in the insect venoms are usually not of concern on the first encounter because the atopic individual has no pre-existing specific IgE antibodies. However, an IgE response may occur after a single encounter with antigen, and a second sting by an insect of the same species may induce fatal anaphylaxis!

NATURE OF THE ANTIGEN

Antigens that elicit strong immediate hypersensitivity reactions are called **allergens** and are proteins or chemicals bound to proteins. It is not known why some antigens cause strong allergic responses whereas other antigens, which may be encountered by the same route of administration, are simply not allergenic and instead result in non-IgE humoral or cell-mediated immune responses. The property of being allergenic may reside in the antigen itself, perhaps in epitopes seen by certain T cells. Some drugs, such as penicillin, characteristically elicit strong IgE responses. It is thought that these drugs bind to self proteins, forming hapten-carrier conjugates that function as "neoantigens."

Some protein antigens are naturally encountered with adjuvant substances that favor IgE synthesis. For example, an antigen and an adjuvant may be present in the same parasite. If the adjuvant triggers IL-4 release (perhaps from mast cells), T cells activated in this environment are more likely to differentiate into T_H2 cells that promote isotype switching to IgE.

HELPER T CELLS AND CYTOKINES

IgE- and eosinophil-mediated immune reactions are dependent on the activation of CD4+ helper T cells of the T_H2 subset. These T cells secrete IL-4, which is required for isotype switching to IgE (see Chapter 9) and promotes eosinophil recruitment, and IL-5, which activates eosinophils. Accumulations of T_H2 cells have been demonstrated at sites of immediate hypersensitivity reactions in the skin and bronchial mucosa. Atopic individuals contain larger numbers of allergen-specific IL-4–secreting T cells in their circulation than do nonatopic persons. In addition, in atopic patients, the allergen-specific T cells produce more IL-4 per cell than in normal individuals. All these factors contribute to the increased IgE production associated with atopy. Because immediate hypersensitivity reactions are dependent on T cells, T cell–independent antigens such as polysaccharides cannot elicit such reactions unless they become attached to proteins.

As we discussed in Chapter 10, the activation of T_H1 or T_H2 cells in response to protein antigens leads to quite distinct classes of immune reactions. The cytokines produced by T_H1 cells are responsible for delayed type hypersensitivity (see Chapter 13). In contrast, T_H2 cells not only elicit IgE production and eosinophilic inflammation but also limit macrophage activation, because they do not produce IFN-γ and because two T_H2-derived cytokines, IL-4 and IL-10, antagonize the macrophage-activating actions of IFN-γ. The effects of these helper T cell subsets on antibody production are also distinct, and cooperate with their effects on inflammatory cells. Thus, the IFN-γ produced by the T_H1 subset promotes the secretion of antibodies, such as IgG2a in mice, that bind to Fcγ receptors on macrophages, enhancing phagocytosis of opsonized particles. At the same time, IFN-γ inhibits switching to IgE. In contrast, IL-4 produced by T_H2 cells induces IgE production, and IgE is the isotype preferentially utilized in antibody-dependent cell-mediated cytotoxicity (ADCC) mediated by eosinophils.

Fc Receptors for IgE

IgE, like all other antibody molecules, is exclusively made by B cells, yet IgE functions as an antigen receptor on the surface of mast cells and basophils. On these cells, IgE is bound by Fc receptors specific for ε heavy chains, called FcεR. Two classes of FcεR have been identified on different cell types. Mast cells and basophils express high-affinity receptors, called FcεRI. The dissociation constant (K_d) of these receptors for IgE is about 1×10^{-10} M. The serum concentration of IgE, although quite low compared with other Ig isotypes in normal individuals (i.e., less than 1 μg/ml or ~5 × 10^{-10} M), is still sufficiently high to bind to the FcεRI receptors. FcεRI has recently been detected on epidermal Langerhans cells and some dermal macrophages; its function on these cells is not known.

Each FcεRI molecule contains four separate polypeptides, one α, one β, and two identical γ chains (Fig.

14–3). As deduced from transfection experiments, all three subunits must be present to have cell surface expression. The α chain mediates binding of IgE. The predicted amino acid sequence of the α chain of the rat FcεRI contains 222 amino acid residues, yielding a predicted size of 25 kilodaltons (kD). The 180 amino terminal residues form two extracellular 90 amino acid residue repetitive sequences that are members of the Ig superfamily. The IgE binding site, formed by these Ig domains, is highly homologous to the IgG binding sites of the FcγRII and FcγRIII receptors described in Chapter 3. Each FcεRI α chain has an approximately 20 amino acid residue hydrophobic sequence that is believed to cross the cell membrane once and approximately 20 carboxy terminal amino acids that form a cytoplasmic domain. The β chain of FcεRI is a 243 amino acid residue hydrophobic polypeptide whose predicted structure crosses the membrane four times. The two identical γ chain polypeptides are only 62 amino acid residues long and are highly homologous to the ζ chains of the T cell antigen receptor complex (see Chapter 7). From its predicted structure, only five amino terminal amino acid residues of the γ chain are extracellular. Each γ chain crosses the membrane once, and the remaining residues are intracellular. In NK cells, the FcεRI γ chain associates with FcγRIII.

The cytoplasmic portions of the FcεRI β and γ chains contain the "antigen recognition activation motif" found in the cytoplasmic domains of the CD3 γ, δ, and ε chains in T cells as well as in the Igα and Igβ chains associated with membrane IgM and IgD in B cells (see Chapters 7 and 9). These features suggest that both the β and γ chains of FcεRI are involved in signal transduction.

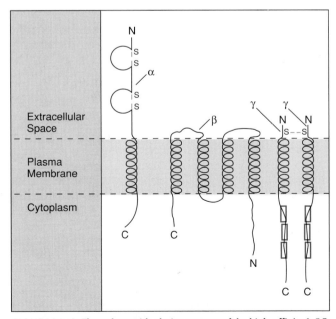

FIGURE 14–3. The polypeptide chain structure of the high-affinity IgE Fc receptor (FcεRI). *IgE binds to the Ig-like domains of the α chain. The β chain and the γ chains are thought to mediate signal transduction. The boxes in the cytoplasmic region of the γ chain are antigen receptor activation motifs similar to those found in the TCR complex (see Fig. 7–6).*

A second receptor for IgE, FcεRII, is an approximately 30 kD protein related to C-type mammalian lectins, a family which includes the selectins (see Chapter 11, Box 11–1). The affinity of FcεRII for IgE is much lower than that of FcεRI and appears to vary considerably among different cell types. In addition, several monoclonal antibodies appear to distinguish FcεRII expressed on eosinophil cell lines from those on B cells. Recent molecular cloning studies of the IgE binding chain of FcεRII suggest that two polypeptides may be generated by alternative translational start sites and alternative splicing of messenger RNA (mRNA) from the same gene. One product is B cell–specific and is expressed constitutively (FcεRIIa); the other product (FcεRIIb, also called CD23) is induced on B cells, monocytes, and eosinophils by IL-4. The eosinophil receptor is used in IgE-dependent killing of parasites by eosinophils. The role of FcεRII on B cells and monocytes is less well defined.

BIOLOGY OF MAST CELLS, BASOPHILS, AND EOSINOPHILS
Properties of Mast Cells and Basophils

All mast cells are derived from progenitors present in the bone marrow. Normally, mast cells are not found in the circulation. Progenitors are believed to migrate to the peripheral tissues as immature cells and undergo differentiation *in situ*. Mature mast cells are found throughout the body, predominantly located near blood vessels and nerves, and beneath epithelia. By light microscopy, human mast cells may be round, oval, or even spindle-shaped. The nuclei are typically round. The cytoplasm contains populations of membrane-bound granules and often lipid bodies (Fig. 14–4). The granules contain acidic proteoglycans, which bind basic dyes. Some of these dyes assume a different color when bound by the granules than they do when staining nuclear DNA, so that the granules are sometimes called "metachromatic."

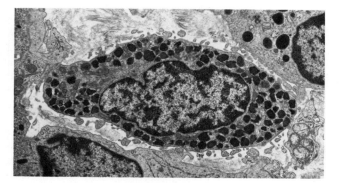

FIGURE 14–4. Electron micrograph of a human mast cell. *Note the characteristic numerous cytoplasmic granules, known to contain histamine, heparin, and various enzymes. (Courtesy of Dr. Noel Weidner, Department of Pathology, Brigham and Women's Hospital, Boston.)*

A recent advance in the understanding of mast cell biology is the appreciation that in rodents mature mast cells may assume one of two phenotypes (Table 14–1). Mast cells found in the mucosa of the gastrointestinal tract have chondroitin sulfate as their major granule proteoglycan. Such "mucosal" mast cells contain little histamine. The second phenotype has been found in the lung and in the serosa of body cavities. These "connective tissue" mast cells contain heparin as their major granule proteoglycan and produce large quantities of histamine. Mast cells may also be cultured from rodent bone marrow in the presence of IL-3. Such cultured mast cells resemble mucosal mast cells based on granule content of chondroitin sulfate and low histamine. Moreover, the presence of mucosal mast cells *in vivo* appears to depend upon T cells, the presumed source of IL-3, since they are absent in athymic mice. Bone marrow–derived mucosal mast cells can be changed to a connective tissue mast cell phenotype by co-culture with fibroblasts. Repopulation experiments in mast cell–deficient mice further suggest that the mucosal and connective tissue phenotypes are not fixed and that bidirectional changes may be possible in suitable microenvironments. However, it is likely that in normal development there is a maturational sequence of bone marrow precursor to mucosal type mast cell to connective tissue mast cell. The key point is that *the precise nature of the mast cell and the mediators it can produce vary with its anatomic location.*

In humans, the factors that regulate mast cell growth and development are less well defined. There appears to be a similar pattern of T cell–independent connective tissue mast cells and T cell–dependent mucosal mast cells. However, human mast cell phenotypes are not as clearly differentiated as those of the mouse. Major differences between types of human mast cells reside in the composition of serine proteases found in the granules (trypsin-like or chymotrypsin-like in substrate specificity) and in the ultrastructural morphology of the granules. Nevertheless, it does appear that in humans as well as in mice the pattern of mediators produced by mast cells may vary with anatomic location.

Basophils share a number of similarities with mast cells. Like mast cells, basophils are derived from bone marrow progenitors and contain granules that bind basic dyes. Basophils are capable of synthesizing many of the same mediators as mast cells. Most significantly, both basophils and mast cells express the same high-affinity Fcε receptor (FcεRI) and can be triggered by antigen binding to IgE. Therefore, basophils, like mast cells, may mediate immediate hypersensitivity reactions to antigen. Despite these similarities, basophils appear to be a distinct cell type from mast cells. Basophils mature in the bone marrow and circulate in their differentiated form. Like other granulocytes, basophils enter tissues only when they are recruited into inflammatory sites. Basophils, like neutrophils, express a number of adhesion molecules important for homing, such as LFA-1 (CD11aCD18), Mac-1 (CD11bCD18), and CD44. Thus, basophils are best thought of as an inflammatory granulocyte, with structural and functional sim-

TABLE 14–1. Mast Cell Heterogeneity

	Connective Tissue	Mucosal	Bone Marrow–Cultured
T cell dependence	No	Yes	Yes
Histamine content	High	Low	Low
Major proteoglycan	Heparin	Chondroitin sulfate	Chondroitin sulfate
Major arachidonate metabolite	PGD_2	$LTC_4 > PGD_2$	$LTC_4 = PGD_2$

In rodents, mast cells isolated from connective tissue or gastrointestinal mucosa, or cultured from bone marrow in the presence of IL-3, differ in several properties, the most important of which are listed here.

Abbreviations: PGD_2, prostaglandin D_2; LT, leukotrienes.

ilarities to mast cells but derived from a different cell lineage.

Activation of Mast Cells and Basophils

The event that initiates immediate hypersensitivity is the binding of antigen to IgE on the mast cell or basophil surface. Mast cells and basophils are activated by cross-linking of FcεRI molecules, which is thought to occur by binding of multivalent antigens to the attached IgE molecules (Fig. 14–5). Experimentally, antigen binding can be mimicked by polyvalent anti-IgE or by anti-FcεRI antibodies. In fact, such antibodies can activate mast cells from atopic as well as non-atopic individuals, whereas allergens activate mast cells only in atopic persons. The reason for this is that in an individual allergic to a particular antigen, a significant proportion of the IgE bound to mast cells is specific for that antigen. Administration of the antigen will cross-link sufficient IgE molecules to trigger mast cell activation. In contrast, in non-atopic individuals, the mast cell–associated IgE is specific for many different antigens (all of which may have induced low levels of IgE production). Therefore, no single antigen will cross-link enough of the IgE molecules to cause mast cell activation. Anti-IgE antibodies, on the other hand, can cross-link these IgE molecules and lead to comparable triggering of mast cells from both atopic and non-atopic individuals.

Activation of mast cells (and basophils) results in three types of biologic responses:

1. Mast cells undergo regulated secretion in which the *pre-formed contents of their granules are released by exocytosis.*

2. Mast cells enzymatically synthesize *lipid mediators* derived from precursors stored in cell membranes and, in some cases, in the lipid bodies.

3. Mast cells initiate transcription, translation, and *secretion of cytokines.*

The mechanisms of granule exocytosis are partly understood, largely from studies of rat mast cell and basophil leukemia cell lines. The cross-linking of FcεRI results in activation of a phosphatidylinositol-specific phospholipase C (PI-PLC) that catalyzes phosphatidylinositol bisphosphate breakdown to inositol triphos-

phate (IP_3) and diacylglycerol (DAG). The coupling of FcεRI to the activation of PI-PLC may involve tyrosine kinases, as is established for other antigen receptors (see Chapters 7 and 9), or a heterotrimeric GTP-binding protein, as is established for chemokine receptors (see Chapter 12, Box 12–2), or both. IP_3 causes elevation of cytoplasmic calcium, and DAG activates protein kinase C. In the basophil, the activated protein kinase C phosphorylates myosin light chains. This event is thought to lead to disassembly of actin-myosin complexes beneath the plasma membrane, thus allowing granules to come in contact with the plasma membrane, resulting in membrane fusion and exocytosis of the granule contents. The role of elevated calcium is less clear, but calcium binding to calmodulin leads to activation of myosin light chain kinase, which phosphorylates myosin light chain at distinct amino acid residues from protein kinase C. Calcium-calmodulin complexes may activate other proteins involved in the fusion of granules with the plasma membrane. Free calcium also may activate phospholipase A_2, the rate limiting enzyme involved in the generation of lipid mediators (see below).

Cross-linking of FcεRI also activates the enzyme adenylyl cyclase through a heterotrimeric GTP-binding protein. This, in turn, elevates cyclic adenosine monophosphate (cAMP) levels and cAMP activates protein kinase A. Protein kinase A inhibits degranulation, suggesting that this pathway is a negative feedback loop.

Mast cells may be activated by mechanisms other than cross-linking FcεRI. For example, mast cells or basophils may respond to mononuclear phagocyte–derived chemokines produced as part of natural immunity, to as yet undefined T cell–derived cytokines produced as part of cell-mediated immunity (Chapter 13), and to complement-derived anaphylatoxins, such as C5a, produced during humoral immune responses (see Chapter 15). Mast cells may also be recruited into inflammatory reactions and activated by neutrophil granule contents or by neurotransmitters such as norepinephrine and substance P. These latter agents are potentially important as links between the nervous system and the immune system. The nervous system is known to affect the expression of immediate hypersensitivity reactions. The "flare," produced at the edge of the wheal in elicited immediate hypersensitivity reactions, is in part mediated by the nervous system, as shown by the observation that the flare is markedly diminished in skin sites lacking innervation.

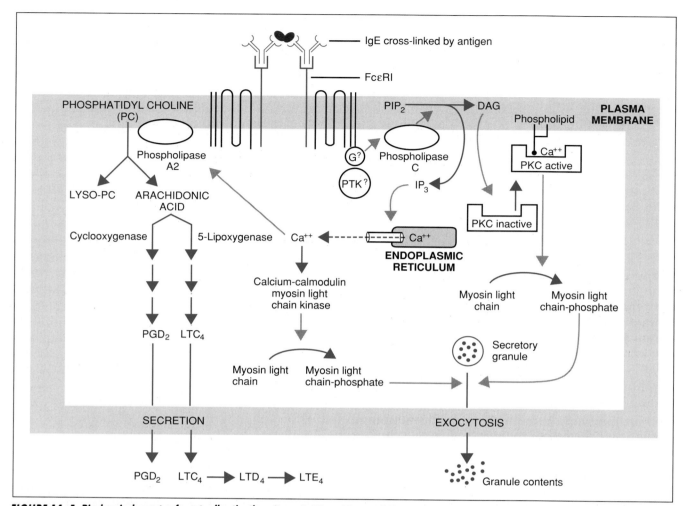

FIGURE 14–5. Biochemical events of mast cell activation. *Cross-linking of bound IgE by antigen is thought to activate a protein tyrosine kinase (PTK) and/or a heterotrimeric guanosine triphosphate (GTP)–binding (G) protein that in turn causes activation of a phosphatidylinositol-specific phospholipase C. This enzyme catalyzes release of inositol triphosphate (IP₃) and diacylglycerol (DAG) from membrane PIP₂. IP₃ causes release of intracellular calcium (Ca⁺⁺) from the endoplasmic reticulum. Ca⁺⁺ in the cytoplasm directly activates certain enzymes, such as phospholipase A₂, and, in complex with calmodulin, activates other enzymes such as myosin light chain kinase. Ca⁺⁺ and DAG combine with membrane phospholipids to activate protein kinase C (PKC), which also phosphorylates myosin light chain protein substrates. These intracellular events are similar to those that occur in T and B cells in response to cross-linking their antigen receptors (see Fig. 7–11). In mast cells, the result of activation is the generation of lipid mediators, such as prostaglandin D₂ (PGD₂) or leukotriene C₄, and the exocytosis of secretory granules.*

Eosinophils

The inflammatory infiltrates of late phase reactions are typically rich in eosinophils. Eosinophils are bone marrow–derived granulocytes whose granules contain basic proteins that bind acidic dyes such as eosin. Indeed, the two major proteins of the eosinophil granule are called major basic protein and eosinophil cationic protein. Major basic protein is toxic for helminths, and eosinophils are the principal effector cells of antibody-dependent cell-mediated cytotoxicity (ADCC) against helminthic infections. Major basic protein also causes damage to normal tissues.

The production and activation of eosinophils are under the control of the same T cells (of the T_H2 subset) that regulate IgE synthesis. Interleukin-5 (IL-5) acts as an eosinophil-activating factor, converting resting eosinophils to a larger "hypodense" state that is more potent at mediating ADCC. IL-5 also augments eosinophil production, and this is supported by the ability of anti–IL-5 antibody to inhibit the eosinophilia that occurs in mice infected with helminthic parasites.

There is increasing evidence that hypodense eosinophils are selectively recruited into late phase inflammatory reactions. Eosinophils, like neutrophils, bind to endothelial cells expressing E-selectin. However, unlike neutrophils, eosinophils express VLA-4 (CD49dCD29) and also adhere to endothelial cells that express vascular cell adhesion molecule–1 (VCAM-1). IL-4 can induce endothelial cells to express VCAM-1 without inducing expression of E-selectin. IL-4 may also induce endothelial cells to express an eosinophil-selective chemokine. Consequently, inflammatory sites enriched for IL-4–producing T_H2 T cells or basophils will efficiently attract eosinophils.

Once recruited into an inflammatory site, eosinophils act as effector cells. We have already discussed the fact that these cells release toxic granule proteins that can kill helminths by ADCC or cause tissue damage in allergic reactions. ADCC may be mediated through the FcεRII receptor for IgE or through an as yet uncharacterized F_c receptor for IgA. Little is known about the mechanisms involved in eosinophil degranulation. Stimulated eosinophils also produce vasoactive lipid mediators, which may augment the effects of mediators produced by mast cells and basophils.

MAST CELL–DERIVED AND BASOPHIL–DERIVED MEDIATORS

This section of the chapter describes the various mediators of immediate hypersensitivity released by mast cells or basophils upon activation. It should be remembered that mast cells are heterogeneous and that not all mast cells will release the same mediators or the same combinations of mediators. Nevertheless, the same general classes of mediators appear to be made by most mast cells as well as by basophils. These may be divided into **pre-formed mediators,** which include biogenic amines and granule macromolecules, and **newly synthesized mediators**, which include lipid-derived mediators and cytokines. Some cytokines, such as tumor necrosis factor (TNF) in human dermal mast cells, may also exist as pre-formed stores that are released during degranulation.

Biogenic Amines

The granules of mast cells contain non-lipid, low molecular weight vasoactive mediators. In humans, the prototypic mediator of this class is **histamine,** but in certain rodents serotonin may be of equal or greater import. Because these substances have in common the structural features of an amine group and share common functional effects on blood vessels, they have been collectively called "biogenic" or "vasoactive" amines. Histamine acts by binding to target cell receptors, and different cell types express distinct classes of receptors (e.g., H_1, H_2, H_3) that can be distinguished by pharmacologic inhibitors. Upon binding to cellular receptors, histamine initiates intracellular events, such as phosphatidylinositol breakdown to IP_3 and DAG, which cause different changes in different cell types. In vascular endothelial cells, binding of histamine leads to endothelial cell contraction and leakage of plasma into the tissues. Histamine also causes endothelial cells to synthesize vascular smooth muscle cell relaxants, such as prostacyclin and nitric oxide, which cause vasodilation. These actions of histamine produce the wheal and flare response of immediate hypersensitivity. Moreover, H1 histamine receptor antagonists (commonly called

antihistamines) can inhibit the wheal and flare response to intradermal allergen or anti-IgE antibody.

Histamine also causes constriction of intestinal and bronchial smooth muscle. Thus, histamine may contribute to the increased peristalsis or bronchospasm associated with food allergies or asthma, respectively. However, in these instances, especially in asthma, antihistamines are not effective at blocking the reaction. Moreover, bronchoconstriction in asthma is more prolonged than the effects of histamine, which is rapidly removed from the extracellular milieu by amine-specific transport systems. Thus, other mast cell–derived mediators are clearly important in some forms of immediate hypersensitivity.

Granule Proteins and Proteoglycans

In addition to vasoactive amines, mast cell granules contain several enzymes, such as serine proteases and aryl sulfatase, as well as proteoglycans such as heparin or chondroitin sulfate. The enzymes may cause tissue injury when released upon mast cell degranulation. One function of the negatively charged proteoglycans may be to bind and store the positively charged biogenic amines. However, it is not clear how important these substances are as mediators of immediate hypersensitivity reactions.

Lipid Mediators

Three classes of lipid mediators are synthesized by activated mast cells (Fig. 14–6). In general, these reactions are all initiated by the actions of phospholipase A_2, which releases substrates from precursor phospholipids stored in membranes or in the lipid bodies. The substrates are then converted by enzyme cascades into the ultimate mediators.

1. The first mast cell lipid mediator to be described was **prostaglandin D_2** (PGD_2). Released PGD_2 binds to receptors on smooth muscle cells and acts as a vasodilator and as a bronchoconstrictor. Moreover, PGD_2 is released from lung mast cells during asthmatic bronchoconstriction. PGD_2 is synthesized from arachidonic acid derived from phospholipid by the sequential actions of enzymes. The synthesis of PGD_2, like that of other prostaglandins, depends upon the enzyme cyclooxygenase, and PGD_2 synthesis can be prevented by inhibitors of cyclooxygenase, such as aspirin and nonsteroidal anti-inflammatory agents. Surprisingly, doses of these drugs that completely prevent PGD_2 synthesis paradoxically exacerbate asthmatic bronchoconstriction. Thus, PGD_2 is unlikely to be a key mediator of this form of immediate hypersensitivity.

2. The second class of mast cell arachidonic acid–derived mediators is the **leukotrienes.** Mast cells convert arachidonic acid, by the action of 5-lipoxygenase and other enzymes, into three main leukotrienes (LT), LTC_4, LTD_4, and LTE_4. (Lesser amounts of LTB_4 may be

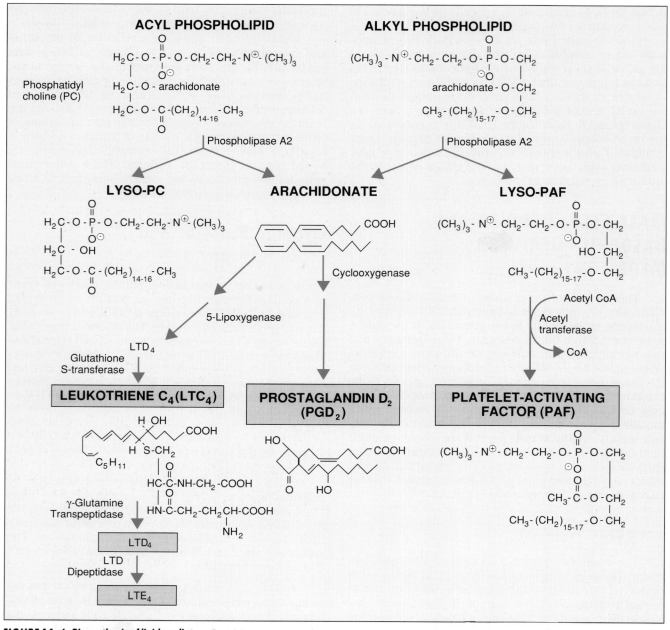

FIGURE 14–6. Biosynthesis of lipid mediators. *Breakdown of membrane phospholipids by phospholipase A_2 leads to generation of leukotriene C_4, prostaglandin D_2, and platelet-activating factor (PAF).*

made as well, but this leukotriene is more characteristically a product of blood phagocytes.) Mast cell–derived leukotrienes bind to specific receptors on smooth muscle cells, different from the receptors for PGD_2, and cause prolonged bronchoconstriction. When injected into skin, these leukotrienes produce a characteristic long-lived wheal and flare reaction. Collectively, LTC_4, LTD_4, and LTE_4 constitute what was once called "slow-reacting substance of anaphylaxis" (SRS-A) and are now thought to be major mediators of asthmatic bronchoconstriction. Pharmacologic inhibitors of 5-lipoxygenase also block anaphylactic reactions in experimental systems; such agents are in clinical trials. The probable reason why aspirin exacerbates asthma is that

PGD_2 and leukotriene synthesis are the two major competitive fates for arachidonic acid in mast cells, and inhibition of cyclooxygenase shunts arachidonic acid into the 5-lipoxygenase pathway, leading to increased leukotriene production.

3. The third lipid mediator produced by mast cells is called **platelet-activating factor** (PAF) for its original bioassay as an inducer of rabbit platelet aggregation. PAF is synthesized by acylation of lysoglyceryl ether phosphorylcholine, which is derived from a membrane phospholipid by phospholipase A_2 release of a fatty acid. (If the fatty acid is arachidonic acid, then phospholipase A_2 can generate the precursors of all three lipid mediators in one reaction.) PAF has direct

bronchoconstricting actions. It also causes retraction of endothelial cells and can relax vascular smooth muscle. However, PAF is very hydrophobic and is rapidly destroyed by enzymes in plasma. It is uncertain whether mast cell–released PAF can reach its target cells. Nevertheless, pharmacologic inhibitors of PAF receptors do ameliorate some aspects of immediate hypersensitivity in rabbit lung. PAF may be of particular importance in late phase reactions, where it can activate inflammatory leukocytes. In this situation, the major source of PAF may be the surface of vascular endothelial cells (stimulated by histamine or leukotrienes) rather than mast cells.

Cytokines

Within the last few years, it has been appreciated that cultured mast cells are significant sources of cytokines, including TNF, IL-1, IL-4, IL-5, IL-6, and various colony-stimulating factors (CSFs) such as IL-3 and granulocyte-monocyte colony-stimulating factor (GM-CSF). Many of these cytokines, especially IL-3 and IL-4, were once thought to be exclusively produced by T cells. The relative contributions of mast cells versus T cells to the production of these molecules *in vivo* are not yet clear. Nevertheless, it now appears likely that cytokines, released upon IgE-mediated mast cell activation or upon T_H2 cell recruitment, are predominantly responsible for the late phase reaction. TNF in particular may account for sequential polymorphonuclear and mononuclear cell infiltrates by the same mechanisms described in Chapter 13 for DTH reactions. The key differences between the inflammatory infiltrates of the late phase reaction and those of DTH are the abundance of eosinophils and T_H2 cells in the former compared with activated macrophages and T_H1 cells in DTH. As mentioned earlier, IL-4, through its selective induction of endothelial VCAM-1 and an eosinophil-selective chemotactic substance, is responsible for selective recruitment of eosinophils. It is not yet known how T_H2 cells may be selectively recruited in the late phase reaction.

CLINICAL ALLERGY IN HUMANS

Now that we have described the cells and mediators of immediate hypersensitivity, we can return to consideration of various allergic diseases. As we noted earlier, severely atopic individuals are characterized by elevated levels of serum IgE. In addition, these individuals have more high-affinity Fcε receptors on each mast cell, and a larger proportion of these receptors are occupied by IgE compared with non-atopic individuals.

Atopic individuals characteristically present with one or more manifestations of atopic disease. The most common forms of atopic disease are allergic rhinitis (hay fever), bronchial asthma, and atopic dermatitis (eczema). The clinical and pathologic features of allergic reactions vary with the anatomic site because of several factors: (1) the point of contact with and the

nature of the allergen, (2) the concentrations of mast cells in various target organs, (3) the local mast cell phenotype, and (4) the sensitivity of target organs to mast cell–derived mediators. Furthermore, only certain kinds of antigens, including plant pollens, dust mites, and some drugs and foods, typically produce immediate hypersensitivity reactions.

Immediate Hypersensitivity Reactions in the Skin

When an allergen is introduced into the skin of a sensitized, atopic individual, the reaction that ensues is mediated largely by histamine. Histamine binds to venular endothelial cells, which express numerous histamine receptors. Most immediately, the endothelial cells synthesize and release prostacyclin, nitric oxide, and PAF. These mediators cause vascular smooth muscle cell relaxation, and the injection site becomes red from local accumulation of red blood cells. The endothelial cells also retract, allowing plasma to extravasate. The initial redness (erythema) is then replaced by soft swelling, the wheal. Finally, the blood vessels on the edge of the wheal dilate in a reaction augmented by the nervous system, producing the flare. Antihistamines (H_1 receptor antagonists) can block this response almost completely. Skin mast cells appear to produce little in the way of long-acting mediators, such as leukotrienes, and the wheal and flare response typically subsides after about 15 to 20 minutes. Clinically, this reaction can occur after contact of the skin with an allergen, or after an allergen enters the circulation via the intestinal tract or by injection. The cutaneous reaction to systemic allergens, called urticaria, may persist for several hours, probably because antigen persists in the plasma.

In many atopic patients, a late phase reaction begins after about 2 to 4 hours. Tumor necrosis factor, IL-4, and other cytokines, probably derived from mast cells, act on the venular endothelial cells to promote inflammation, involving the production of vasodilators, adhesion molecules, and chemokines that facilitate leukocyte diapedesis (see Chapter 13). As may be expected for a cytokine-mediated response, the late phase inflammatory reaction is not inhibited by antihistamines. It can be blocked by pretreatment with corticosteroids, which inhibit cytokine synthesis. Chronic eczema is probably a clinical manifestation of the late phase reaction in the skin. Eczema is often treated with topical corticosteroids.

Immediate Hypersensitivity Reactions in the Lung

Immediate hypersensitivity (asthmatic) reactions in the lung resemble skin reactions in some ways, but differ in others. In the lung, mast cell mediators act not only on the blood vessels but also on bronchial smooth

BOX 14—1. BRONCHIAL ASTHMA

Asthma is best considered as a clinical-pathologic triad of intermittent (and reversible) airway obstruction, chronic bronchial inflammation with eosinophils, and bronchial smooth muscle cell hyper-reactivity to bronchoconstrictors. Asthma affects about 10 million people in the United States. The prevalence rate is similar in other industrialized countries, but may be lower in less developed areas of the world. Affected individuals may suffer considerable morbidity, and there is an increasing awareness that asthma causes death in some patients.

Several lines of evidence have established that most asthma is a form of immediate hypersensitivity. About 75 per cent of patients show positive skin test responses (i.e., wheal and flare reactions) to injection of one or more common allergens. Furthermore, airway obstruction can be triggered in many asthmatic patients by inhalation of specific allergen. Finally, many asthmatics and their family members have other manifestations of atopy, such as rhinitis (hay fever) or eczema. Even among non-atopic

asthmatics, the pathophysiology of airway constriction is similar, suggesting that alternative mechanisms of mast cell degranulation (e.g., by locally produced neurotransmitters) may underlie the disease.

Most investigators now believe that asthma should be considered primarily as an inflammatory disease. In this view, the primary lesion of asthma is the accumulation of T_H2 T cells and eosinophils in the airway mucosa, an example of a late phase reaction. Smooth muscle cell hypertrophy and hyper-reactivity are thought to result from leukocyte-derived mediators and cytokines. The pathophysiologic sequence may be initiated by mast cell activation in response to allergen binding to IgE. Mast cell–derived cytokines lead to recruitment of eosinophils, basophils, and T_H2 cells. Mast cells, basophils, and eosinophils all produce mediators that constrict airway smooth muscle. The most important of the bronchoconstricting mediators are LTC_4 and its breakdown products, LTD_4 and LTE_4. In clinical experiments, antagonists of

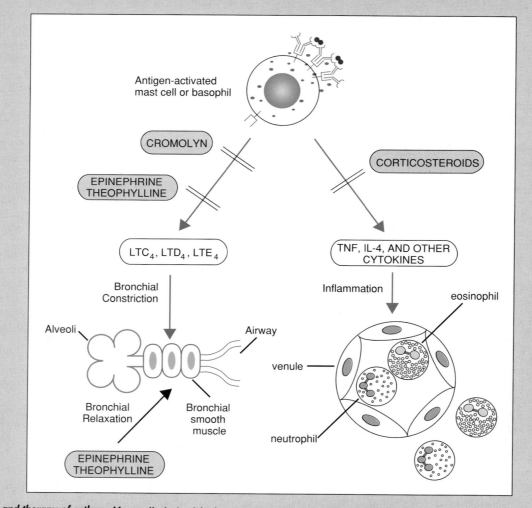

Mediators and therapy of asthma. *Mast cell–derived leukotrienes are thought to be the major mediators of acute airway constriction. Therapy is targeted both at reducing mast cell activation with inhibitors such as cromolyn and at countering leukotriene actions on bronchial smooth muscle by bronchodilators such as epinephrine and theophylline. These drugs also inhibit mast cell activation. Mast cell–derived cytokines are thought to be the major mediators of sustained airway inflammation, an example of a late phase reaction, and corticosteroid therapy is used to inhibit cytokine synthesis.*

Continued

LTC_4 synthesis or leukotriene receptor antagonists prevent allergen-induced airway constriction. Aspirin, which blocks cyclooxygenase and shunts more arachidonic acid into leukotriene biosynthesis, can exacerbate or even trigger asthmatic attacks. Histamine plays little role in airway constriction, and antihistamines (H_1 receptor antagonists) have no role in treatment of asthma. Indeed, since many antihistamines are also anticholinergics, these drugs may worsen airway obstruction by causing thickening of mucous secretions, an action opposed by acetylcholine.

Current therapy has two major targets: prevention and reversal of inflammation, and relaxation of airway smooth muscle. In recent years, the balance of therapy has shifted towards anti-inflammatory agents as the primary mode of treatment. Two major classes of drugs are in current use: corticosteroids, which block cytokine production, and sodium cromolyn. The mechanism of action of sodium cromolyn is not clear, but it appears to antagonize IgE-induced release of mediators. Both agents can be used prophylactically as inhalants. Corticosteroids may also be given systemically, especially once an attack is under way, to reverse inflammation. Newer anti-inflammatory therapies are in pre-clinical and clinical trials, including inhibitors of leukocyte adhesion to endothelial cells (e.g., antibodies to VCAM-1, ICAM-1, or E-selectin) and inhibitors of platelet-activating factor, a pro-inflammatory lipid derived from IgE-activated mast cells. It remains to be seen if these agents are effective in treating asthma.

Bronchial smooth muscle cell relaxation has principally been achieved by elevating intracellular cAMP in the smooth muscle cells, which inhibits contraction. The major drugs used are activators of adenylyl cyclase, such as epinephrine and related β_2-adrenergic agents, and inhibitors of the phosphodiesterase enzymes that degrade cAMP, such as theophylline. These drugs also raise cAMP in mast cells, acting to inhibit mast cell degranulation. Inhalants of epinephrine-like drugs have been widely used as prophylactic therapy, but long-term cardiovascular side effects are limiting use of these agents. Inhibitors of leukotriene synthesis and leukotriene receptor antagonists are in current clinical trial as newer approaches to prevent bronchoconstriction.

muscle. Bronchial asthma (Box 14–1) is characterized by paroxysms of bronchial constriction and increased production of thick mucus, which leads to bronchial obstruction and exacerbates respiratory difficulties. The smooth muscle cells in the airways of asthmatics are often hypertrophied and are "hyper-reactive" to constricting stimuli. Bronchitis and infections are frequent complications. Most cases of asthma are due to immediate hypersensitivity, and the bronchial mucosa contains increased numbers of eosinophils and $CD4^+$ T cells of the T_H2 subset. However, less frequently asthma may not be associated with atopy.

Systemic Immediate Hypersensitivity

In systemic immediate hypersensitivity, such as **anaphylactic shock,** vasodilation and vascular exudation of plasma occur in vascular beds throughout the body. This usually implies the systemic presence of antigen, either by injection, insect sting, or absorption across an epithelial surface, such as the skin. The decrease in vascular tone and leakage of plasma lead to a fall in blood pressure, or shock, that may be fatal. The cardiovascular effects are complicated by constriction of the upper and lower airways, hypersensitivity of the gut, outpouring of mucus in the gut and respiratory tree, and urticarial lesions (hives) in the skin. The most important mast cell mediators of anaphylactic shock are not fully known. The mainstay of treatment is systemic epinephrine, which can be life-saving, reversing the bronchoconstrictive and vasodilatory effects of the various mast cell mediators. Epinephrine also improves cardiac output, further aiding survival from threatened circulatory collapse. Antihistamines may also be beneficial in anaphylaxis, suggesting a role for histamine in this reaction. In some animal models, PAF receptor antagonists offer partial protection. It is also possible that TNF is an important mediator of anaphylactic shock, much as it is in septic shock (see Chapter 12).

Immunotherapy for Allergy

In addition to therapy aimed at the consequences of immediate hypersensitivity, clinical immunologists often try to limit the onset of allergic reactions by treatments aimed at reducing the quantity of IgE present in the individual. Despite the fact that the regulation of IgE synthesis and T_H2 cell development are not fully understood, several empirical protocols have been developed to diminish specific IgE synthesis. In one approach, called **desensitization,** small but increasing quantities of antigen are administered subcutaneously over a period of hours or more gradually over weeks or months. As a result of this treatment, specific IgE levels decrease and IgG titers often rise, perhaps further inhibiting IgE production by neutralizing the antigen and by antibody feedback (see Chapter 10). It is also possible that desensitization may work by inducing specific T cell tolerance or by changing the predominant phenotype of antigen-specific T cells from T_H2 to T_H1; however, there are few direct data to support these hypotheses. The beneficial effects of desensitization may occur in a matter of hours, much earlier than changes in IgE levels. Although the precise mechanism is unknown, this approach has been very successful in preventing acute anaphylactic responses to protein antigens (e.g., insect venoms) or vital drugs (e.g., penicillin). It is more variable in its effectiveness for chronic atopic conditions such as hay fever.

Several new approaches to therapy are in the experimental and trial stage. One approach is to promote T_H1 development by administration of interferons (IFNs). Another is to prevent T cell activation by treatment with peptides that compete with immunodominant peptides of natural allergens (e.g., ragweed or cat dander) for binding to specific class II MHC molecules.

SUMMARY

Binding of antigen to IgE attached to mast cells or basophils initiates an effector reaction that functions to protect the host against parasitic infection. The same reaction may be triggered by environmental antigens, called allergens, producing an injurious process called immediate hypersensitivity. Immediate hypersensitivity is characterized by rapid vascular leakage of plasma, vasodilation, bronchoconstriction, and, at later times, inflammation. The inflammatory infiltrates of this late phase reaction are enriched in eosinophils and T_H2 cells. In extreme cases (anaphylaxis), death may result from asphyxiation and circulatory collapse. Individuals prone to immediate hypersensitivity reactions are called atopic and often have more IgE and more IgE receptors per mast cell than do non-atopic individuals. IgE synthesis is regulated by heredity, exposure to antigen, and T cell cytokines. In particular, T_H2 cells, through secretion of IL-4 and IL-5, favor IgE production and eosinophil-rich inflammation. Mast cells are derived from bone marrow and mature in the tissues. In mice, mast cells can be classified as connective tissue type, maturing under the influence of fibroblast-derived factors, and mucosal type, responding to T cell–derived cytokines such as IL-3. Human mast cells may also consist of distinct subsets, but these are not as well defined. Basophils are granulocytes that accumulate at inflammatory sites. They are functionally similar to mast cells but appear to be a distinct cell lineage. Eosinophils are a special class of granulocytes that are recruited into inflammatory reactions by IL-4 and are activated by IL-5. Eosinophils are effector cells of IgE-initiated reactions. They mediate IgE-dependent ADCC to eradicate parasites. In allergic reactions, they are responsible for tissue injury.

Upon binding of antigen to IgE on the surface of mast cells or basophils, the high-affinity Fcϵ receptors become cross-linked and activate intracellular second messengers. Activated mast cells and basophils produce three important classes of mediators: biogenic amines, such as histamine; lipid mediators, such as prostaglandin D_2, leukotrienes C_4, D_4, and E_4, and platelet-activating factor; and cytokines such as TNF, IL-4, and IL-5. Biogenic amines and lipid mediators produce the rapid components of immediate hypersensitivity, such as vascular leakage, vasodilation, and bronchoconstriction. Cytokines mediate the late phase reaction.

Various organs show distinct forms of immediate hypersensitivity involving different mediators and target cell types. Drug therapy is aimed at inhibiting mast cell mediator production and at blocking the effects of mediators on target organs. The goal of immunotherapy is to prevent or reduce T cell responses and immediate hypersensitivity reactions to specific antigens.

SELECTED READINGS

Bochner, B. S., and L. M. Lichtenstein. Anaphylaxis. New England Journal of Medicine 324:1785–1790, 1991.

Corrigan, C. J., and A. B. Kay. T cells and eosinophils in the pathogenesis of asthma. Immunology Today 13:501–507, 1992.

Galli, S. J. New concepts about the mast cell. New England Journal of Medicine 328:257–265, 1993.

McFadden, E. R. Jr., and I. A. Gilbert. Asthma. New England Journal of Medicine 327:1928–1937, 1992.

O'Hehir, R. E., R. D. Garman, J. L. Greenstein, and J. R. Lamb. The specificity and regulation of T-cell responsiveness to allergens. Annual Review of Immunology 9:67–95, 1991.

Paul, W. E., R. A. Seder, and M. Plaut. Lymphokine and cytokine production by FcεRI⁺ cells. Advances in Immunology 53:1–29, 1993.

Romagnani, S. Regulation and deregulation of human IgE synthesis. Immunology Today 11:316–321, 1990.

Schwartz, L. B., and K. F. Austen. Structure and function of the chemical mediators of mast cells. Progress in Allergy 34:271–321, 1984.

Valent, P., and P. Bettelheim. Cell surface structures on human basophils and mast cells: biochemical and functional characterization. Advances in Immunology 52:333–423, 1992.

Weller, P. E. Immunobiology of eosinophils. New England Journal of Medicine 324:1110–1118, 1991.

CHAPTER · FIFTEEN

THE COMPLEMENT

SYSTEM

Soon after the discovery of humoral immunity, Charles Bordet demonstrated that if fresh serum containing an antibacterial antibody was added to the bacteria at physiologic temperature (37°C), the bacteria were lysed. If, however, the serum was heated to 56° C or more, it lost its lytic capacity. This was not because of decay of antibody activity, because antibodies are heat-stable and even heated serum was capable of agglutinating the bacteria. Bordet concluded that the serum must contain another heat-labile component that assists or "complements" the lytic function of antibodies. He called this heat-labile substance **complement**. We now know that *complement is not a single protein but a system of functionally linked proteins that interact with one another in a highly regulated manner to provide many of the effector functions of humoral immunity and inflammation.*

The principal biologic functions of the complement system are the following (Fig. 15–1):

1. Certain activated complement components mediate **cytolysis** by polymerizing on cell surfaces to form pores or by disrupting the integrity of the phospholipid bilayer in the membranes of these cells. In this way, foreign organisms that activate complement can be killed by osmotic lysis.

2. **Opsonization** of foreign organisms or particles occurs by the binding of complement proteins to their surfaces. These complement proteins are called **opsonins.** Phagocytic leukocytes express specific receptors for these opsonins. In this way, opsonins promote phagocytosis of particles or organisms.

3. **Activation of inflammation** occurs in response to the generation of certain proteolytic fragments of complement proteins. These complement-derived peptides act on several targets. They activate mast cells, causing reactions that resemble immediate hypersensitivity (see Chapter 14); in extreme cases, this reaction can mimic anaphylaxis, and these complement fragments are sometimes called **anaphylatoxins.** Other targets of these peptides include vascular endothelium and inflammatory leukocytes. Still other fragments of complement proteins can enhance B lymphocyte responses to antigen.

4. **Immune complexes** that could damage tissues are rendered innocuous by solubilization, limitation in size, and phagocytic clearance from the circulation as a result of binding complement proteins.

These functions will be discussed in detail later in the chapter. The complement system has a number of important properties that enable it to function efficiently in host defense against foreign invaders without injuring normal tissues:

1. The soluble serum complement components include multiple proteolytic enzymes, which become se-

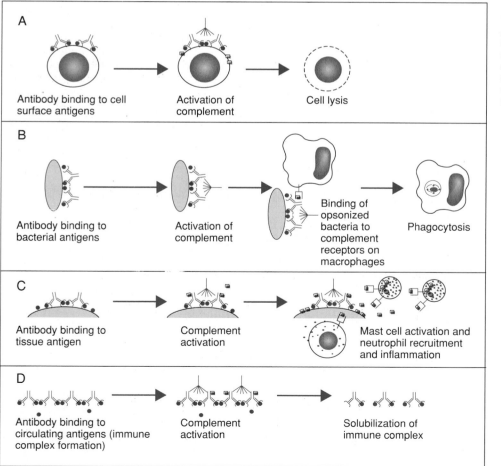

FIGURE 15–1. Biologic functions of the complement system. *Cell lysis, phagocytosis, and proinflammatory effects are depicted as a consequence of antibody-dependent activation of complement (A, B, and C), but these functions can also result after antibody-independent complement activation.*

A

Antibody binding to cell surface antigens → Activation of complement → Cell lysis

B

Antibody binding to bacterial antigens → Activation of complement → Binding of opsonized bacteria to complement receptors on macrophages → Phagocytosis

C

Antibody binding to tissue antigen → Complement activation → Mast cell activation and neutrophil recruitment and inflammation

D

Antibody binding to circulating antigens (immune complex formation) → Complement activation → Solubilization of immune complex

quentially activated only when they themselves are proteolytically cleaved by other previously activated complement system enzymes. Proteins that acquire proteolytic enzymatic activity by the action of other proteases are called zymogens. The process of sequential zymogen activation, i.e., an enzymatic cascade, is also characteristic of the coagulation and kinin systems. *The proteolytic cascades allow for tremendous amplification, since each individual enzyme molecule activated at one step can generate multiple activated enzyme molecules, or active fragments, at the next step.*

2. Although the proteins of the complement system are present in the blood, they are inactive or have only a low level of spontaneous activation in the circulation. Activation of the complement system normally occurs only at certain localized sites. First, immunoglobulin (Ig) molecules that have bound specific antigens can activate complement, and for this reason *complement serves as a major effector mechanism for specific humoral immunity.* The sequence of complement activation initiated by antibody-antigen complexes is called the **classical pathway.** Second, some complement components are directly activated by binding to the surfaces of infectious organisms. In this way *complement activation also participates in natural immunity.* The sequence of complement activation that occurs on microbial surfaces in the absence of antibody is called the **alternative pathway.** The name "alternative" comes from the fact that this pathway was discovered after the classical pathway. Despite its name, the alternative pathway is as important as the classical pathway in host defense against infectious organisms. As we shall see later, these two pathways differ in their initiation but share many late stages and effector functions.

3. The complement system is tightly regulated by several soluble and cell membrane–associated proteins that inhibit complement activation at multiple steps. These regulatory mechanisms have two main functions. First, they limit or stop complement activation in response to physiologic stimuli. Second, they prevent abnormal or constitutive complement activation in the absence of microbes and antibodies.

The various biologic functions of the complement system are mediated by (1) complexes of complement components bound to cell or viral surfaces or immune complexes where complement is activated, and by (2) soluble fragments of complement proteins that diffuse from the sites where they were generated and bind to specific receptors on other nearby cells.

This chapter describes the biochemistry, functions, and regulation of the complement system. The relationship of complement to other components of the immune system will be emphasized.

THE COMPLEMENT CASCADES

Before we describe the individual proteins of the complement system, it is useful to present an overview of complement activation (Fig. 15–2). The central com-

ponent of the complement system is a protein called **C3**, which is critical for the effector functions of this system. The biologically active forms of C3 are its proteolytic cleavage products. The classical and alternative pathways include distinct protein components that are activated in different ways to generate enzymes called **C3 convertases**, which cleave C3 to produce C3a and C3b. (By convention, lower case letter suffixes denote proteolytic products of each complement protein.) In the early steps of the *classical pathway*, antibody molecules that are complexed with specific antigen sequentially bind and proteolytically activate three complement proteins, called C1, C4, and C2, leading to the formation of a $\overline{C4b2a}$ complex, which functions as the **classical pathway C3 convertase.** (By convention, complement complexes with enzymatic activity are designated by a bar over the components.) In the *alternative pathway,* C3b generated spontaneously at low levels, or by the classical pathway, binds to a protein fragment called Bb, generated by proteolytic cleavage of a protein called Factor B. The $\overline{C3bBb}$ complex is the **alternative pathway C3 convertase**, functioning, like the classical pathway C3 convertase, to further break down C3 to generate more C3b. The next step in both pathways is the binding of C3b to the C3 convertase enzymes, changing them to **C5 convertases**, which catalyze the proteolytic cleavage of the C5 protein. Although the C5 convertases of the two pathways are molecularly distinct, they catalyze identical reactions and act on identical substrates. Once C5 is cleaved, both pathways share the same terminal steps. These terminal events do not involve proteolysis, but rather the sequential binding of several soluble complement proteins, called C6, C7, C8, and C9, to the activating surface. This leads to the formation of a lipid-soluble pore structure called the **membrane attack complex** (MAC), which causes osmotic lysis of cells.

Different effector functions are mediated by different proteins produced during complement activation. Cytolysis is mediated by the MAC. Opsonization is largely due to a fragment of C3 called C3b, specific receptors for which are expressed on many leukocytes and other cells. Inflammation, consisting of the recruitment and activation of leukocytes, is mediated by cleavage products of C3, C4, and C5, called C3a, C4a, C5a, respectively. Immune complexes are solubilized by binding of the classical pathway proteins to the Fc regions of antibody molecules. Each of these functions will be discussed in more detail later.

In the following discussion, we describe the various proteins that make up the complement system; these proteins are listed in Table 15–1.

The Classical Pathway

The classical pathway (Fig. 15–3) is one of the major effector mechanisms of humoral immunity. It is activated principally by the binding of the first classical pathway component, C1, to the Fc portions of antigen-complexed antibody molecules. There are stringent re-

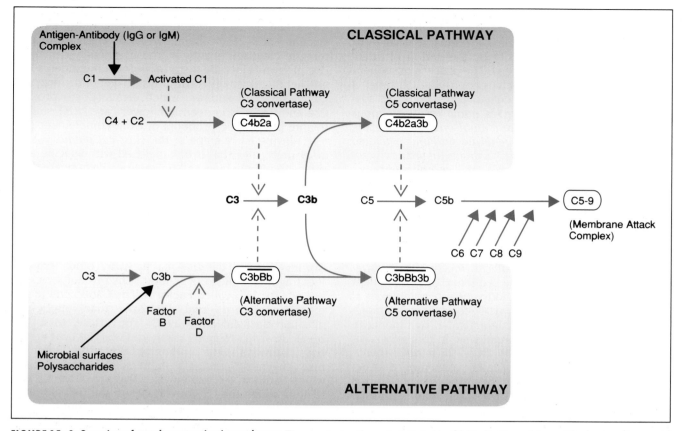

FIGURE 15–2. Overview of complement activation pathways. *The classical pathway is initiated by C1 binding to antigen-antibody complexes, and the alternative pathway is initiated by C3b binding to various activating surfaces, such as microbial cell walls. The C3b involved in alternative pathway initiation may be generated in several ways, including spontaneously, by the classical pathway, or by the alternative pathway itself (see text). Both pathways converge and lead to the formation of the membrane attack complex. In this and subsequent figures, bars over the letter designations of complement components indicate enzymatically active forms and dashed lines indicate proteolytic activities of various components.*

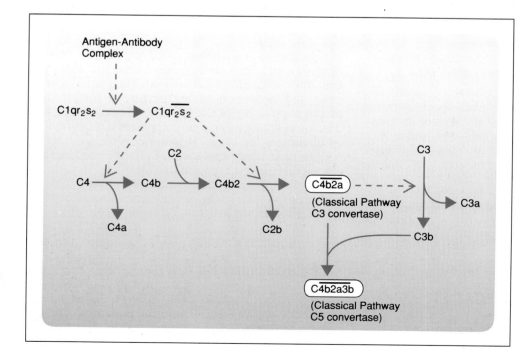

FIGURE 15–3. Classical pathway of complement activation. *Antigen-antibody complexes that activate the classical pathway may be soluble or fixed on the surface of cells or trapped in interstitial spaces. The C5 convertase formed by the classical pathway proteolytically cleaves C5 to begin the formation of the membrane attack complex.*

TABLE 15–1. Protein Components of the Complement Cascades

Component	Molecular Size (kD)	Serum Concentration (μg/ml)	Subunit Chains; Molecular Size of Each (kD)	Activation Products	Comments on Function
Classical Pathway					
C1	750				Initiates classical pathway
(C1qr₂s₂)					
C1q	410	75	6 of A;24 6 of B;23 6 of C;22		Binds to Fc portion of Ig
(C1r)₂	85	50	1	$\overline{C1r}$	$\overline{C1r}$ is a serine protease; cleaves $\overline{C1s}$
(C1s)₂	85	50	1	$\overline{C1s}$	$\overline{C1s}$ is a serine protease; cleaves C4 and C2
C4	210	200–500	1 of α;90 1 of β;78 1 of γ;33	C4a C4b	C4a is an anaphylatoxin C4b covalently binds to activating surfaces, where it acts as an opsonin and is part of C3 convertase
C2	110	20	1	$\overline{C2a}$ C2b	$\overline{C2a}$ is a serine protease, part of C3 and C5 convertases
C3 (Also part of alternative pathway)	195	550–1200	1 of α;110 1 of β; 85	C3a C3b	C3a is an anaphylatoxin C3b covalently binds to activating surfaces, where it is part of C3 and C5 convertases and also acts as opsonin
Alternative Pathway					
Factor B	93	200	1	$\underline{Ba}$ $\overline{Bb}$	$\overline{Bb}$ is a serine protease, part of C3 and C5 convertases
Factor D	25	1–2	1	$\overline{D}$	Protease that circulates in active state; cleaves Factor B bound to C3b
Properdin	220	25	4; 56		Stabilizes alternative pathway C3 convertase
Terminal Lytic Components					
C5	190	70	1 of α;115 1 of β;75	C5a C5b	C5a is an anaphylatoxin C5b initiates MAC assembly
C6	128	60	1		Component of MAC
C7	121	60	1		Component of MAC
C8	155	60	1 of α;64 1 of β;64 1 of γ;22		Component of MAC
C9	79	60	1		Component of MAC; polymerizes to form membrane pores

Abbreviations: kD, kilodalton; MAC, membrane attack complex; Ig, immunoglobulin.

quirements for antibody-mediated C1 activation that ensure that the classical pathway is activated only under certain conditions:

1. Activation of C1 occurs at significant levels only when it binds to the C_H3 domains of IgM or C_H2 domains of IgG molecules (see Chapter 3). Furthermore, only certain subclasses of IgG are effective C1 activators (human IgG1, IgG2, and IgG3, but not IgG4).

2. A single C1 molecule must bind simultaneously to at least two Fc portions of Ig, each Fc portion having a single C1 binding site (Fig. 15–4). This is required in order to induce a conformational change in the C1 molecule that turns on its enzymatic activity. Because secreted IgM is a pentamer containing five Fc regions, even a single IgM molecule can bind C1 and trigger the classical pathway. In contrast, since IgG is a monomer, multiple IgG molecules must be aggregated, bringing multiple Fc regions sufficiently close together, before C1 can be activated. Such aggregation typically occurs if the IgG antibody binds to a multideterminant antigen, such as on a bacterial cell surface. Because of these structural differences in the Ig isotypes, IgM is a much more efficient complement-binding (also called **complement-fixing**) antibody than IgG.

3. Only antigen-antibody complexes and not free or soluble antibodies activate complement. For IgG this is because of the requirement for aggregation mentioned above. Soluble IgM does not bind C1, even though it is pentameric, apparently because the Fc regions are inaccessible to C1 in solution. Binding of the IgM to an antigen or a cell surface induces a conformational change that exposes the Fc regions, allowing C1 to bind.

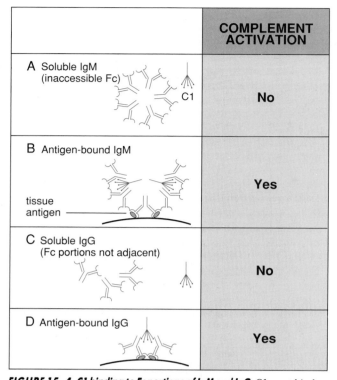

	COMPLEMENT ACTIVATION
A Soluble IgM (inaccessible Fc)	No
B Antigen-bound IgM tissue antigen	Yes
C Soluble IgG (Fc portions not adjacent)	No
D Antigen-bound IgG	Yes

FIGURE 15–4. C1 binding to Fc portions of IgM and IgG. *C1 must bind to two or more Fc portions in order to initiate the complement cascade. The Fc portions of soluble pentameric IgM are not accessible to C1 (A). After IgM binds to surface bound antigens, it undergoes a shape change that permits C1 binding and activation (B). Monomeric soluble Ig molecules will not activate C1 (C), but after binding to cell surface antigens, adjacent IgG Fc portions can bind and activate C1 (D).*

Experimental evidence indicates that the classical pathway may also be activated in the absence of Ig, on the surfaces of certain infectious organisms such as retroviruses and *Mycoplasma*, and by polyanionic molecules such as DNA. The mechanisms of activation in these cases and the significance of antibody-independent activation of the classical pathway *in vivo* are not known.

C1 is itself a large, multimeric molecular complex, approximately 750 kD, composed of one C1q subunit associated with two C1r and two C1s molecules. C1q is the subunit that actually binds to Ig molecules, and C1r and C1s are serine esterase zymogens required for the progression of the proteolytic cascade. C1q is a 410 kD protein complex composed of three different kinds of polypeptide chains that combine to form heterotrimeric rod-like structures with a collagen-like triple helix at the amino terminal end and a globular head at the carboxy terminus. Six of these rod-like structures (containing 18 separate polypeptides) combine to form one symmetric molecular complex with a central core composed of the triple helices at one end and a radial array of the globular heads at the other end (Fig. 15–5). C1r and C1s are both single-chain 85 kD proteins, which combine, in a calcium-dependent manner, to form a flexible linear tetramer composed of two molecules of each type, in the sequence C1s-C1r-C1r-C1s. One tetramer is associated with each C1q molecule. *Binding of*

two or more of the globular heads of C1q to IgM or IgG molecules induces a conformational change that leads to the enzymatic activation of the associated C1r. As a result, the C1r molecules cleave themselves, generating a 28 kD proteolytic fragment called C$\overline{1r}$, which has **serine esterase** activity. C$\overline{1r}$ then cleaves the associated C1s molecule to generate another 28 kD serine protease, C$\overline{1s}$, which in turns acts on the next two components of the classical pathway, C4 and C2. Recently, structural similarities have been identified between C1q and other proteins, including mannose-binding protein in the serum and lung surfactant proteins. Interestingly, after mannose-binding protein binds to mannose residues on cells surfaces, C1r, C1s, and the subsequent classical pathway are activated. It is possible that this may be a mechanism for classical pathway activation on some microbial surfaces in the absence of antibody.

C4 is the second distinct soluble serum protein to be activated in the classical pathway. It participates in the formation of the C3 convertase and is critical for

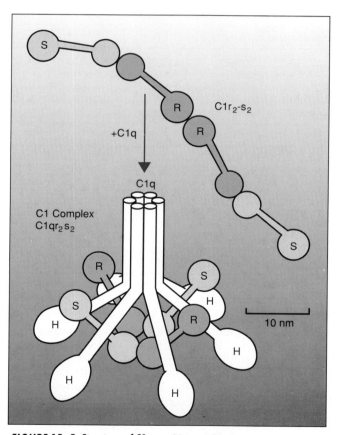

FIGURE 15–5. Structure of C1q,r,s. *C1r and C1s form a tetramer composed of two C1r and two C1s molecules. The larger balls at the ends of C1r and C1s, designated by the letters R and S, are the catalytic domains of these proteins. C1q consists of six identical subunits, arranged to form a central core and symmetrically projecting radial arms. The globular heads at the end of each arm, designated H, are the contact regions for immunoglobulin. One C1r$_2$s$_2$ tetramer wraps around the radial arms of the C1q complex in a manner that juxtaposes the catalytic domains of C1r and C1s. (Modified with permission form Arlaud, G. J., M. G. Colomb, and J. Gagnon. A functional model of the human C1 complex. Immunology Today 8:107–109, 1987.)*

keeping subsequent activation steps localized to the initial site where the antibody bound. C4 is a 210 kD heterotrimeric complex of polypeptide chains called α, β, and γ, and is homologous to the C3 protein. The α chain contains an unusual internal thioester bond between a cysteine residue and a nearby glutamate residue. This feature, which is also found in the C3 molecule, is important for the localizing role of C4 and C3, as discussed below (Fig. 15–6). C$\overline{1s}$ cleaves the α chain of C4, yielding an 8.6 kD fragment called C4a, and a large remaining molecule, called C4b. (C4a diffuses from the cell surface and has biologic effects discussed later in the chapter.) One C$\overline{1s}$ molecule can generate multiple C4b molecules. As a result of this proteolytic step, the thioester bond in the α chain of the C4b fragment is susceptible to nucleophilic attack by amine and hydroxyl groups and thus becomes highly unstable. This chemically reactive form of the molecule is called **metastable C4b**. Most of the C4b thioester bonds rapidly react with water molecules, generating a short-lived inactive intermediate, iC4b. However, some C4b thioester bonds undergo transesterification to form covalent amide or ester bonds with cell surface molecules (Fig. 15–6). There are two isoforms of C4, called C4A and C4B, encoded by adjacent genes, and there is evidence that C4A preferentially forms amide bonds with proteins, whereas C4B forms ester bonds with carbohydrates. *As a result, the C4b molecule becomes covalently attached to nearby cell surfaces, ensuring that complement activation occurs stably and efficiently at cell surfaces to which antibodies are bound.* C4b may also form covalent bonds with the Ig molecule itself.

C2 is the third soluble serum component of the classical pathway and is also involved in the formation of the C3 convertase. It is a 110 kD single-chain polypeptide that binds to cell surface–bound C4b molecules in the presence of Mg^{++}. Once complexed with C4b, C2 is cleaved by a nearby C$\overline{1s}$ molecule to generate a 35 kD C2b molecule, which may diffuse off the cell surface, and a 75 kD C2a fragment, which remains physically associated with C4b on the cell surface. *The resulting $\overline{C4b2a}$ complex is the* **classical pathway C3 convertase**, *having the ability to bind to and proteolytically cleave C3.* Binding to C3 is mediated by the C4b component, and proteolysis is catalyzed by the C2a component.

C3 is sequentially the fourth soluble serum component of the classical pathway. As mentioned earlier, it is also a central component of the alternative pathway. The serum concentration of C3, approximately 0.55 to 1.2 mg/ml, is higher than that of any other member of the complement system. C3 is a 195 kD disulfide-linked heterodimeric glycoprotein composed of α and β polypeptide chains. C3 contains the same type of internal thioester bond as the C4 molecule (Fig. 15–6). C3 convertase removes a 9 kD fragment, C3a, from the α chain of C3, leaving a molecule called **metastable C3b** with the thioester bond exposed to potential reactants. (C3a has several biologic activities initiated by binding to C3a receptors on other cells; these are discussed later in the chapter.) As with C4b, most of the metastable C3b thioester bonds react with water, yielding inac-

tive C3b by-products, which no longer participate in the complement cascade. Up to 10 per cent of C3b molecules, however, do form covalent bonds with cell surfaces or with the Ig to which the C4b2a is bound. This results in the formation of a new complex, C$\overline{4b2a3b}$, which functions as the **classical pathway C5 convertase**. As the name implies, this complex catalyzes the enzymatic cleavage of C5, which begins the formation of the MAC, described below.

The Alternative Pathway

The alternative pathway (Fig. 15–7) is activated in the absence of antibody and generates both soluble and membrane-bound forms of C3 convertase, which catalyze the proteolysis of C3. Because stable alternative pathway C3 convertase is formed on microbial cell surfaces but not on the surfaces of autologous cells or cells of the same species, the alternative pathway has a primitive capacity for discriminating between one's own cells and foreign microbes. In addition, there is a built-in amplification loop in the alternative pathway that can increase the magnitude of complement activation of both pathways. The alternative pathway includes five proteins—Factors, B, D, H, and I and properdin—which are distinct from the proteins of the classical pathway. A sixth alternative pathway protein is the same C3 that is part of the classical pathway.

C3 itself plays a critical role in both the initiation and the progression of the alternative pathway because this pathway is triggered by one of two altered forms of C3. The first is C3b, which is usually generated by the classical pathway. The second is called $C3(H_2O)$, and it is produced when the internal thioester bonds of circulating C3 undergo slow spontaneous hydrolysis (Fig. 15–7). C3b or C3 (H_2O) binds to the alternative pathway protein, **Factor B**, a single-chain 93 kD protein that is homologous to C2 of the classical pathway. After it is complexed with C3b or C3 (H_2O), Factor B becomes susceptible to proteolysis by another alternative pathway protein, **Factor D**. Factor D is a 25 kD serine protease that circulates at very low concentrations in the serum, probably in its enzymatically active form. Factor D proteolytically cleaves bound Factor B, releasing a 33 kD fragment (Ba) and leaving a 63 kD fragment, $\overline{Bb}$, attached to C3b or $C3(H_2O)$. The resulting complex, C$\overline{3bBb}$ or C$\overline{3(H_2O)Bb}$ is the **alternative pathway C3 convertase**, with the $\overline{Bb}$ fragment functioning as a serine protease capable of cleaving C3. This convertase may be in the fluid phase, if formed with $C3(H_2O)$, or cell surface–bound, if formed with surface-bound C3b. Even the C$\overline{3bBb}$ complex is unstable, however, and it rapidly decays unless another alternative pathway member, **properdin**, binds to the complex. Properdin is a 220 kD protein consisting of four identical, noncovalently linked subunits. This molecule binds to and stabilizes C$\overline{3bBb}$. In addition, a conformationally altered "active" form of properdin can bind C3b and enhance its association with Factor B. It should be noted that the formation of the classical and alternative pathway C3 convertases involves homologous proteins, and

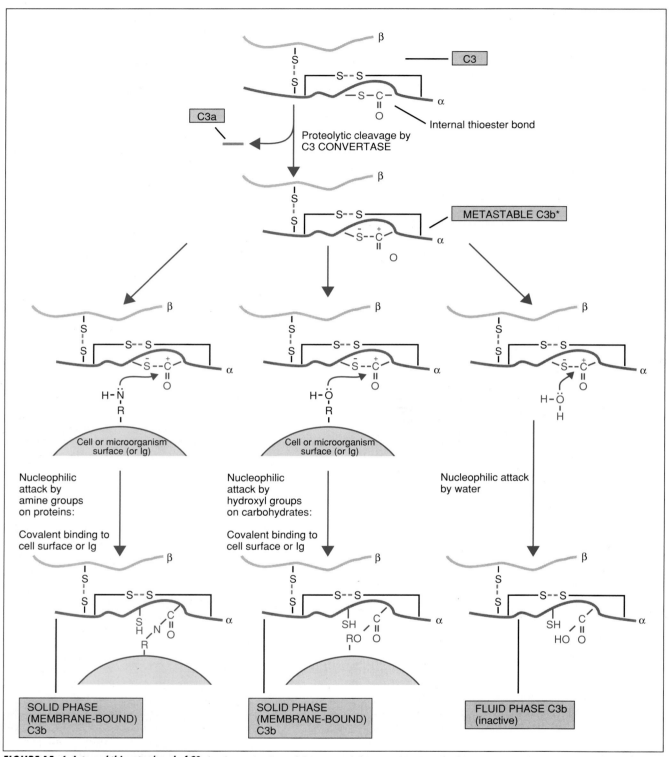

FIGURE 15–6. Internal thioester bond of C3. *A schematic view of the internal thioester bond in the C3 molecule and its role in forming covalent bonds with other molecules is shown. Proteolytic cleavage of the α chain converts the C3 molecule into a metastable form (C3b*) in which the internal thioester bond is susceptible to nucleophilic attack by oxygen or nitrogen atoms. The result is the formation of covalent bonds with proteins or carbohydrates on cell surfaces (solid phase C3b) or with a hydroxyl group donated by water molecules (fluid phase C3b). The C4 molecule has a similar internal thioester bond that is involved in covalent bonding of C4b to cell surfaces in the classical pathway of complement activation (not shown).*

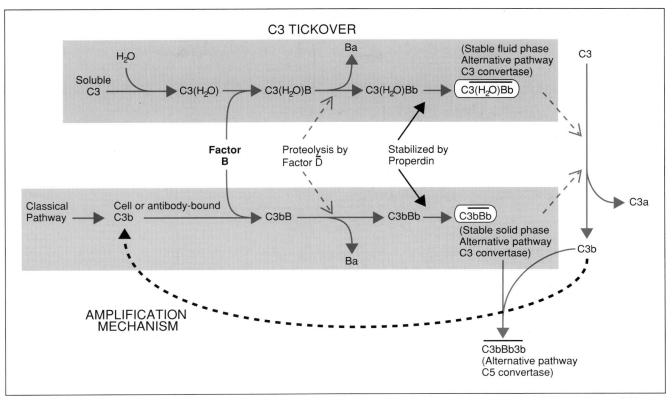

FIGURE 15–7. Alternative pathway of complement activation. *Soluble C3 in serum undergoes a slow spontaneous hydrolysis of its internal thioester bond, generating C3(H₂O), which binds Factor B and forms a fluid phase alternative pathway C3 convertase. The resulting continuous, low-level production of C3b by fluid phase C3 convertase is called C3 tickover. C3b can also be produced by the classical pathway. The C3b formed by either way can then participate in the formation of alternative pathway C3 convertase, which generates C3b from C3. The alternative pathway has a built-in amplification mechanism because the C3b generated by the alternative pathway C3 convertase is also a component of the convertase. The C3 convertase formed by the alternative pathway proteolytically cleaves C5, just as the classical pathway C5 convertase does, to begin the formation of the membrane attack complex.*

the events are fundamentally similar. For example, Factor B is structurally homologous to C2, and Factor B binding to C3b or C3(H₂O) is analogous to C2 binding to C4b.

The normal function of the alternative pathway is dependent on two important features of the activation and regulation of its components:

1. As discussed above, C3b is continuously generated by fluid phase alternative pathway C3 convertase, initiated by spontaneous hydrolysis of the internal thioester bond of C3. This is called **C3 tickover** and probably goes on at a low level all the time, even in the circulation. However, it has no deleterious effects because the C3b generated by the C3 tickover mechanism is usually hydrolyzed to an inactive form within a fraction of a second. As a result, significant complement activation does not occur in the fluid phase, i.e., in the circulation. Rare C3b molecules do form covalent bonds with particle surfaces in a random manner. It is at this stage of the alternative pathway that the rudimentary capacity for self/non-self discrimination is apparent. If the C3b is deposited on autologous cell surfaces, it is rapidly inactivated by the action of regulatory proteins, described later, thus stopping the cascade. In contrast, C3b binding to the surfaces of

many microbes (which lack the regulatory proteins) leads to the binding of Factor B and, as described above, to the formation of stable enzymatically active surface-bound alternative pathway C3 convertase or C3bBb.

2. The alternative pathway provides an intrinsic amplification mechanism for the complement system. The surface-bound C3bBb enzyme complex generates many more C3b molecules, and these, in turn, are deposited on the same surface, forming more C3 convertase. *Thus, C3b is both a component of the C3 convertase enzyme complex as well as a product generated by the action of C3 convertase. This situation allows for a positive feedback amplification of the alternate pathway* (Fig. 15–7). In fact, because C3b generated by the classical pathway can trigger the alternative pathway, the alternative pathway C3 convertase is also an amplification mechanism for complement activation initiated by the classical pathway.

Some of the C3b molecules generated by the alternative pathway C3 convertase bind to the C3 convertase to form a new complex, C3bBb3b. This is the **alternative pathway C5 convertase**, analogous to the classical pathway C5 convertase, C4b2a3b, and its function is to proteolytically cleave C5. After this step, the classical and alternative pathways converge, and the same terminal sequence of events occurs.

The Membrane Attack Complex

The C5 convertases, generated by either the classical or the alternative pathway, initiate the activation of the terminal components of the complement system, culminating in the formation of the cytocidal membrane attack complex (Fig. 15–8). This process begins with the cleavage of C5 by either of the C5 convertases. This is the last enzymatic step in the complement cascade; subsequent steps involve binding and polymerization of intact proteins. **C5** is a 190 kD disulfide–linked heterodimer with homology to C3 and C4, but without an internal thioester bond. C5 binds to the C3b molecule within either classical or alternative pathway C5 convertases. C5 is then cleaved into a small (11 kD) C5a fragment that is released and a two-chain 180 kd C5b fragment that remains bound to the cell surface. (C5a has potent biologic effects on several cells; these will be discussed later in the chapter.) C5b transiently maintains a conformation capable of binding the next protein in the cascade, **C6**, a 128 kD single-chain protein. The stable C5b,6 complex remains loosely associated with the cell surface until it binds **C7**, a 121 kD single-chain protein. One C7 molecule binds to each C5b,6 complex. The resulting C5b,6,7 complex is highly lipophilic, and it inserts into the hydrophobic lipid bilayer of cell or viral membranes, where it becomes a high-affinity integral membrane receptor for one **C8** molecule. The C8 protein is a 155 kD trimer composed of three distinct chains, including a 64 kD α chain that is disulfide linked to a 22 kD γ chain and a noncova-

valently linked 64 kD β chain. The γ chain inserts into the lipid bilayer of the membrane, and the C5b,6,7,8 complex (C5b-8) becomes stably attached to the cell surface. This complex has the ability to initiate lysis of some microorganisms and eukaryotic cells, and is considered to be one form of the MAC.

The lytic activity of the MAC is enhanced by binding of **C9**, the final component of the complement cascades, to the C5b-8 complex. C9 is a 79 kD monomeric serum protein that polymerizes at the site of the C5b-8. MACs with just four C9 molecules (C5b-8,9$_4$) have full lytic capabilities for many microorganisms and eukaryotic cells. When the MAC contains between 12 and 15 C9 molecules associated with one C5b-8 complex, it is called "poly-C9" and forms pores in plasma membranes with a characteristic electron microscopic appearance. The pores have an internal diameter of about 110 Å, a 115 Å stalk embedded in the lipid bilayer, and a 100 Å long projection above the membrane surface. Viewed *en face*, they appear as doughnuts (Fig. 15–9). This structure is similar to the membrane pores formed by the pore-forming protein, called perforin or cytolysin, found in cytolytic T lymphocytes (CTLs) and natural killer (NK) cells (see Chapter 13).

The pores formed by the MAC permit the passive exchange of small soluble molecules, ions, and water, but they are too small to allow large molecules, such as proteins, to escape from the cytoplasm. This situation results in influx of water into the cells, leading to osmotic lysis. As stated above, some degree of lysis can occur without full poly-C9 polymerization and pore formation. In part, this may be due to the reorientation of the normal lipid arrangement of the membrane as a consequence of the insertion of the hydrophobic portions of the C5b-9 complex, creating local areas of leaki-

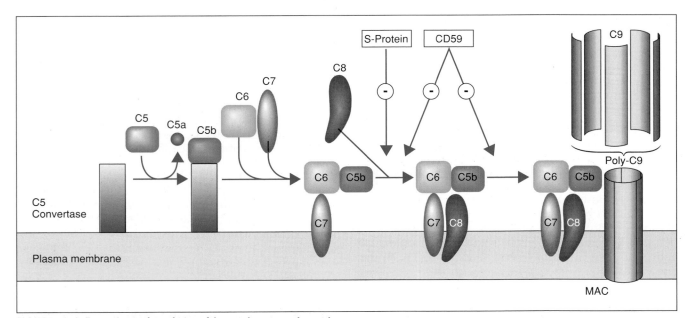

FIGURE 15–8. Formation and regulation of the membrane attack complex. *A schematic view of the cell surface events leading to the formation of the MAC is shown. Cell-associated C5 convertase cleaves C5, generating C5b, which becomes bound to the convertase. C6 and C7 bind sequentially, and the C5b,6,7 complex becomes directly inserted into the lipid bilayer of the plasma membrane, followed by stable insertion of C8. Up to 15 C9 molecules may then polymerize around the complex to form lytic pores in the membrane. The sites of action of regulatory proteins, including S-protein (vitronectin) and CD59 are shown.*

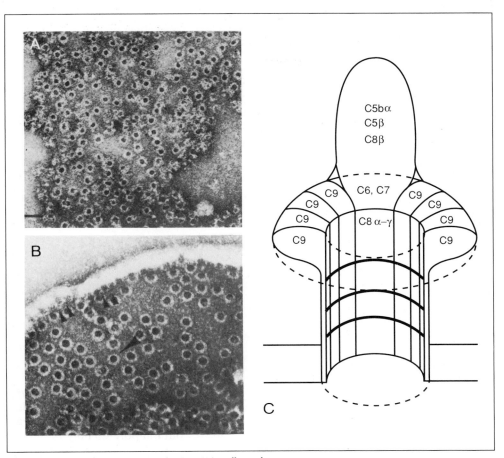

FIGURE 15–9. Structure of the membrane attack complex (MAC) in cell membranes.

A. *Complement lesions in erythrocyte membranes are shown in this electron micrograph. The lesions consist of holes approximately 100 Å in diameter and are formed by poly-C9 tubular complexes.*

B. *For comparison, membrane lesions induced on a target cell by a cloned cytolytic T lymphocyte (CTL) line are shown in this electron micrograph. The lesions have a morphology similar to that of complement-mediated lesions, except for a larger internal diameter (160 Å). In fact, CTL and natural killer (NK) cell–induced membrane lesions are formed by tubular complexes of a polymerized protein (perforin), which is homologous to C9 (see Chapter 13).*

C. *A model of the subunit arrangement in the MAC is shown. The transmembrane region consists of 12 to 15 C9 molecules arranged as a tubule, in addition to single molecules of C6, C7, and C8 α and β chains. The C5bα, C5β, and C8β chains form an appendage that projects above the transmembrane pore.*
(Reproduced from Podack, E. R. Molecular mechanisms of cytolysis by complement and cytolytic lymphocytes. Journal of Cellular Biochemistry 30:133–170, 1986. Copyright Alan R. Liss, Inc., 1986.)

ness. Furthermore, the insertion of the terminal complement components into a cell membrane may lead to cell death independent of osmotic lysis, by allowing a lethal amount of calcium to passively diffuse into the cell.

REGULATION OF THE COMPLEMENT CASCADES

Uncontrolled activation of complement can lead to formation of the MAC on self tissues and excessive generation of inflammatory mediators. This does not normally happen because both the classical and alternative complement cascades are tightly regulated by several fluid-phase and membrane proteins that interact in specific ways with the various components of the complement system. Furthermore, activation of com-

plement cascades does not occur spontaneously in the blood because the classical pathway is triggered by antigen-antibody complexes, particularly when formed on cell surfaces, and the alternative pathway C3b convertase is unstable unless it is bound to cell surfaces with particular biochemical characteristics. Because of these regulatory mechanisms, a delicate balance of activation and inhibition of the complement cascades is achieved that prevents damage to autologous cells and tissues but promotes the effective destruction of foreign organisms. The pathologic consequences of unregulated complement activation are apparent in various disease states in which the regulatory proteins are deficient. The major identified regulatory elements of the complement system, including individual regulatory proteins that work at various points in the cascades, are described next. The regulatory proteins are listed in Table 15–2.

TABLE 15–2. Soluble and Membrane Proteins That Regulate Complement Activation

Protein	Molecular Size (kD)/Molecular Characteristics	Serum Concentration (μg/ml) or Cellular Distribution	Specifically Interacts With	Function
Soluble Serum Proteins				
C1 inhibitor (C1 INH)	104 Serpin Heavily glycosylated	200	C$\overline{1}$r, C$\overline{1}$s	Serine protease inhibitor covalently binds to C$\overline{1}$r and C$\overline{1}$s and blocks their ability to participate in classical pathway Binds to inactive C1 and prevents spontaneous activation Also inhibits kallikrein, plasmin, and factors XIa and XIIa of coagulation system
C4bp	550 56 SCRs	250	C4b	Accelerates decay of classical pathway C3 convertase (C4b2a) Acts as cofactor for Factor I–mediated cleavage of C4b
Factor H	150 20 SCRs	480	C3b	Accelerates decay of alternative pathway C3 convertase (C3bBb) Acts as cofactor for Factor I–mediated cleavage of C3b
Factor I	88	35	C4b, C3b	Proteolytically cleaves and inactivates C4b and C3b, using C4bp, factor H, CR1, or MCP as cofactors
Anaphylatoxin inactivator	310 Carboxypeptidase N	35	C3a, C4a, C5a	Proteolytically removes terminal arginine residues and inactivates the anaphylatoxins
S protein	83 (Vitronectin)	505	C5b-7	Binds to C5b-7 complex and prevents membrane insertion of MAC
SP-40,40	80 Heterodimer	50	C5b-9	Modulates MAC formation
Integral Membrane Proteins				
Complement receptor type 1 (CR1) (CD35)	190–280 30 SCRs	Most blood cells, mast cells	C3b, C4b, iC3b	Accelerates dissociation of classical and alternative pathway C3 convertases Acts as cofactor for Factor I–mediated cleavage of C3b and C4b (Binds immune complexes and promotes their dissolution and phagocytosis)
Membrane cofactor protein (MCP) (CD46)	45–70 4 SCRs	Most blood cells (except erythrocytes), epithelial cells, endothelial cells, fibroblasts	C3b,C4b	Acts as cofactor for Factor I–mediated cleavage of C3b and C4b
Decay accelerating factor (DAF)	70 4 SCRs; Phosphatidylinositol linkage	Most blood cells, endothelial cells, epithelial cells	C4b2b C3bBb	Accelerates dissociation of classical and alternative pathway C3 convertases
Homologous restriction factor (HRF)	65 Phosphatidylinositol linkage	Erythrocytes, lymphocytes, monocytes, neutrophils, platelets	C8 C9	Inhibits lysis of bystander cells (reactive lysis) Blocks C8 or C9 binding to MAC of autologous cells and lysis; action restricted to C9, C8 of same species
CD59 (membrane inhibitor of reactive lysis [MIRL])	18 Phosphatidylinositol linkage	Erythrocytes, lymphocytes, monocytes, neutrophils, platelets, endothelial cells, epithelial cells	C7 C8	Inhibits lysis of bystander cells (reactive lysis) Blocks C9 binding to C8, preventing MAC formation and lysis; action restricted to C8, C9 of same species

Abbreviations: SCR, short consensus repeat; MAC, membrane attack complex.

Regulation of the Classical Pathway

Activation of the classical pathway is regulated at two stages:

1. The initiation of the classical pathway is inhibited by **C1 inhibitor (C1INH)**, a 104 kD serum glycoprotein that is a member of the serpin (serine protease inhibitor) family, which includes α_1-antitrypsin, antithrombin II, and α-1-antichymotrypsin. C1INH inhibits the ability of C1r and C1s to cleave their normal substrates. As with other serpins, C1INH accomplishes this by presenting a "bait" sequence that mimics the normal substrates of C1r and C1s. When C1INH is cleaved by C1r or C1s, it forms covalent stable ester linkages with these serine proteases, which effectively blocks their ability to cleave other substrates such as C4 and C2. C1INH also prevents spontaneous activation of C1, which can occur at a low but significant rate in the absence of antibody. Most of the C1 in the blood is bound to C1INH (which is present at seven times the molar concentration of C1), and this prevents the conformational changes that cause spontaneous activation. Once C1 binds to antigen-complexed antibody, via the C1q subunit, the C1INH is released and this allows the classical pathway to proceed.

2. The classical pathway is also regulated by proteins that interefere with C3 and C5 convertase formation and activity (Table 15–3). Regulation of these convertases is accomplished in two distinct ways. First, certain serum and plasma membrane proteins have **decay accelerating activity**, which is the ability to prevent the formation of, or to accelerate the dissociation of, components of the C3 convertase enzyme complex. In particular, the proteins with decay accelerating activity for the classical pathway include an abundant soluble serum glycoprotein called **C4 binding protein (C4bp)**, and two membrane proteins, **decay accelerating factor (DAF)**, and the **type 1 complement receptor (CR1)**. DAF is a phosphatidylinositol-linked glyco-

protein found on all peripheral blood cells, endothelium, and various mucosal epithelial cells. CR1 is an integral membrane protein expressed on a variety of cell types (CR1 will be discussed more thoroughly later in the chapter). C4bp, DAF, and CR1 are structurally homologous members of a family of proteins called **regulators of complement activity (RCA)** (described later). They work as classical pathway regulators by binding to C4b in competition with C2, thereby preventing the assembly of, and promoting the dissociation of, the C3 convertase, C4b2a (Fig. 15—10).

The second way in which classical pathway C3 convertase is inhibited is by proteins that provide **cofactor activity for Factor I–catalyzed proteolytic degradation of C4b**. Factor I is a disulfide-linked heterodimeric serum protein with serine esterase activity. It cleaves C4b to generate two fragments: C4c, which is released into the fluid phase, and a smaller C4d fragment, which remains bound to the original surface (Fig. 15–10). C4d is not able to contribute to C3 convertase formation. Factor I–mediated cleavage of C4b occurs efficiently only when a cofactor binds to the C4b molecule. Three different proteins serve as cofactors in this way. These include CR1 and C4bp, which, as mentioned above, also act as decay accelerators. In addition, another member of the RCA family that acts as a cofactor for Factor I–mediated inactivation of C4b is **membrane cofactor protein (MCP)**, or CD46. MCP is a 45 to 70 kD integral membrane glycoprotein widely distributed on most cell types. It does not possess decay accelerating activity. Factor I also cleaves C3b, which is generated by both classical and alternative pathways. Since C3b is a component of the alternative but not classical pathway C3 convertase, Factor I–mediated cleavage of C3b is best considered as a regulatory mechanism of the alternative pathway and is discussed below.

Regulation of the Alternative Pathway

The alternative pathway is also regulated by several circulating and membrane proteins, some of which function as regulators of the classical pathway as well. Like in the classical pathway, the major way these proteins function as regulators is by inhibiting C3 and C5 convertase activity, either by decay acceleration or by providing cofactor activity for Factor I (Table 15–3).

1. Proteins with decay accelerating activity for the alternative pathway competitively inhibit Bb binding to C3b, thus blocking the formation, and promoting the disassembly, of the alternative pathway C3 convertase (Fig. 15–11). In addition, these proteins may block binding of Factor B to C3b, leading to the same functional effect. A soluble serum protein with decay accelerating activity specifically for the alternative pathway is **Factor H**. In addition, the two membrane proteins mentioned above, CR1 and DAF, also have alternative pathway decay accelerating activity.

2. The formation of the alternative pathway C3 convertase, C3bBb, is inhibited by Factor I–mediated

---

TABLE 15–3.   Regulators of C3 Convertase Activity

Protein	Dissociation of C3 Convertases		Factor I Cofactors	
	Classical	Alternative	C4b	C3b
Factor H	−	+	−	+
C4bp	+	−	+	−
DAF	+	+	−	−
MCP	−	−	+	+
CR1	+	+	+	+

Abbreviations: C4bp, C4 binding protein; DAF, decay accelerating factor; MCP, membrane cofactor protein; CR1, complement receptor type 1.

Modified with permission from Weisman, H. F., T. Bartow, M. K. Leppo, H. C. Marsh, Jr., G. R. Carson, M. F. Concino, M. P. Boyle, K. H. Roux, M. L. Weisfeldt, and D. T. Fearon. Soluble human complement receptor type 1: in vivo inhibition of complement suppressing post-ischemic myocardial inflammation and necrosis. Science 249:146–151, 1990. Copyright 1990 by the AAAS.

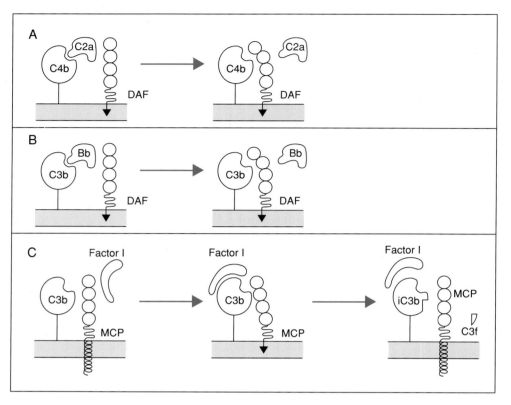

FIGURE 15–10. Membrane protein regulators of complement activation.

A. *Decay accelerating factor (DAF) interferes with the formation of the classical pathway C3 convertase. CR1 and soluble C4 binding protein (C4bp) have the same activity.*

B. *DAF interferes with the formation of the alternative pathway C3 convertase. CR1 and soluble Factor H have the same activity.*

C. *MCP is a cofactor for Factor I–mediated proteolysis of C3b. CR1 and Factor H have the same activity. Similarly, MCP, CR1, and C4bp, are cofactors for Factor I–mediated proteolysis of C4b.*

proteolysis of C3b. Factor I cleavage of C3b is promoted by at least three different cofactors, including Factor H, CR1, and MCP (Fig. 15–11). Factor I first cleaves C3b, releasing a 3 kD fragment and leaving an inactive C3b (iC3b) attached to the activating surface. iC3b cannot participate in C3 convertase formation. It is further cleaved by Factor I to yield a 41 kD fragment, C3dg, which remains bound to the activating surface, and a soluble C3c fragment. Factor H and CR1, but not MCP, serve as cofactors for this step. C3dg is susceptible to proteolysis by any one of several enzymes, including plasmin and trypsin, yielding a 33 kD surface-bound C3d molecule and a soluble 8 kD C3g fragment.

Different cells express different amounts of the regulatory proteins, MCP and CR1, thus controlling the site at which C3b and the alternative pathway C3 convertase are formed. This is particularly important because, as we mentioned earlier, the C3 tickover mechanism is capable of continuously generating C3b, with the potential to form more and more alternative pathway C3 convertase. Most normal cells express high levels of MCP, which protect these cells from complement-mediated injury. In contrast, infectious organisms lack MCP, so that C3b deposited on these surfaces is not inactivated and binds Factor B with higher affinity than Factor H. This promotes the formation of the C3bBb complex, leading to effective complement activation on these foreign surfaces. In addition, this relative preference for Factor B binding to microbial or heterologous

cell surfaces may be a function of other biochemical characteristics. For example, high sialic acid content favors Factor H binding over Factor B, and conversely, cell surfaces with reduced sialic acid content bind Factor B with greater affinity. Many bacteria contain low amounts of surface sialic acid compared with mammalian cells, and this is another reason why complement activation occurs preferentially on bacterial cell surfaces.

Regulation of Membrane Attack Complex Formation

Even after the classical or alternative pathway C3 convertase is formed, excessive complement-mediated cell lysis is prevented by a number of proteins that act at the level of the MAC.

1. The regulatory protein mainly responsible for inhibiting formation of the MAC is **CD59** (also called **membrane inhibitor of reactive lysis**, or **MIRL**). CD59 is widely distributed among different cell types and is inserted into the plasma membrane by phosphatidylinositol linkages. CD59 is probably the most important factor that protects normal bystander cells from being lysed when complement is activated on nearby bacteria or immune complexes. CD59 works by binding to C8

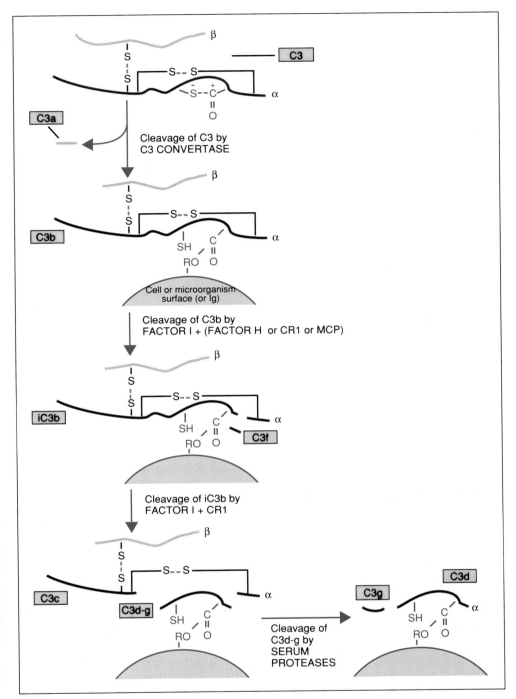

FIGURE 15–11. Sequential proteolytic cleavage of C3. *Each proteolytic step generates a soluble fragment and a membrane-bound fragment. Inactive C3b (iC3b), generated by the first Factor I–mediated cleavage, can no longer participate in the formation of C3 convertase. Many of the soluble fragments released in this sequence have biologic activities related to inflammation (see text). Factor I also proteolytically cleaves C4b generated by the classical pathway.*

and C9 during MAC formation, thereby inhibiting C9 membrane insertion and subsequent addition of C9 molecules.

2. The insertion of the terminal complement components into lipid membranes is inhibited by **S protein**, also called **vitronectin**, an 83 kD serum protein related to laminin and fibronectin. It functions by binding to the soluble C5b,6,7 complex and preventing the

complex from inserting into cell membranes near the site where the complement cascade was inhibited. In this way, S protein can diminish the potentially indiscriminate lysis of autologous cell surfaces.

3. The ability of the MAC to lyse cells may be modulated by a circulating protein called **SP-40,40**. SP-40,40 is a heterodimer that has been isolated from soluble C5-9 complexes. It may be a normal component of

the MAC whose principal function is to control the ability of the MAC to lyse cells. The mechanism of action of SP-40,40 is not known.

RECEPTORS FOR FRAGMENTS OF THE C3 COMPONENT OF COMPLEMENT

Many of the biologic activities of the complement system are mediated by the binding of complement fragments to specific integral membrane protein receptors expressed on various cell types. These complement receptors can be divided into three functional categories:

1. Receptors for fragments of C3 that are covalently bound to activating surfaces.
2. Receptors for soluble C3a and C5a fragments (anaphylatoxins), which mediate the inflammatory effects of complement activation.
3. Receptors that regulate the complement cascades by binding to specific complement proteins and inhibiting their functions.

Receptors for surface-bound C3 fragments are the most thoroughly characterized and will be considered in detail in this section of the chapter (Table 15–4). The molecular nature of the receptors for other complement fragments will be considered briefly in the discussion of the biologic activities of complement fragments later in this chapter. The regulatory activities of complement receptors have been described above.

COMPLEMENT RECEPTOR TYPE 1 (CR1, C3b RECEPTOR, CD35). This molecule is centrally involved in several biologic functions of the complement system, as well as in the regulation of complement activation. It is a single-chain integral membrane glycoprotein that serves as a high-affinity C3b and C4b receptor. CR1 is present on many cell types, including erythrocytes, neutrophils, monocytes, eosinophils, T and B lymphocytes, and follicular dendritic cells. There are at least four polymorphic forms of CR1 varying in molecular weight from 190 to 280 kD. An interesting feature of CR1 that is shared by all members of the RCA family of complement proteins is the presence of multiple, tandemly arranged repeated structures called **short consensus repeats** (SCRs). Each SCR is 65 to 70 amino acids long, with 11 to 14 conserved amino acid residues, including four highly conserved cysteine residues that form two intrachain disulfide-bonded loops. The most common form of CR1 has 30 tandem SCRs, 28 of which are arranged into four groups, each with seven SCRs. The C3b/C4b binding site of CR1 is located within the second SCR of each group. This repeating structural organization of CR1 ensures that ligand binding sites will be present at some distance from the surface of the CR1-expressing cell, where they may be most effective at binding C3b- or C4b-coated cells and particles. Other molecules of the complement system that contain SCRs include C4bp, CR2, DAF, MCP, Factor H, C1r, C1s, C6, C7, Factor B, and C2.

CR1 performs at least three important functions. First, CR1 is a regulator of complement activation by virtue of its ability to inhibit C3 convertase activity, discussed previously. Second, CR1 functions as an opsonin receptor that enhances the ability of phagocytic leukocytes to ingest C3b- or C4b-coated particles and microorganisms. Third, CR1 is important for the clearance of immune complexes from the circulation. These functions are described in detail later in the chapter. A genetically engineered, soluble form of CR1, lacking transmembrane and cytoplasmic domains, has been produced as an experimental therapeutic anti-inflammatory agent. This soluble CR1 markedly inhibits both alternative and classical pathway activation and limits tissue injury in an *in vivo* model of acute inflammation.

COMPLEMENT RECEPTOR TYPE 2 (CR2, C3d RECEPTOR, CD21). This receptor may play a role in humoral immune responses. It is a 145 kD, single-chain integral membrane glycoprotein present on B lymphocytes, follicular dendritic cells, and epithelial cells. CR2 specifically binds iC3b and C3dg, the Factor I–generated cleavage products of surface- or immune complex–bound C3b. The physiologic consequences of the binding of these fragments is not well understood. CR2 also specifically binds interferon α and Epstein-Barr virus (discussed later). CR2 on follicular dendritic cells may serve to trap antigen-antibody complexes in germinal centers, leading to the activation of memory B lymphocytes. On B cells, CR2 is expressed as part of a trimolecular complex that includes two other proteins called CD19 and target of antiproliferative antibody–1 (TAPA-1). Experiments with *in vitro* B cell lines suggest that this complex delivers signals to the B cell that significantly lower the threshold concentration of anti-Ig antibody required to induce certain responses of B cells. Furthermore, soluble CR2 receptors block humoral immune responses to protein antigens in mice, and deficiencies in complement activation are known to be associated with impaired antibody responses to antigens. However, there is no direct evidence yet that iC3b and C3dg binding to CR2 on B cells potentiates B cell responses to antigens, and the role of CR2 in physiologic responses of B cells to antigen *in vivo* is not clear.

CR2 is also the cell surface receptor for the **Epstein-Barr virus** (EBV). Ironically, more may be known about the role of CR2 in EBV-related pathology than about the role of this complement receptor in normal physiology. EBV is a human herpes virus that infects most people by adulthood and remains latent within B cells or pharyngeal epithelial cells for the duration of life. Infection may be subclinical or may cause infectious mononucleosis. In addition, EBV is linked to several human malignancies, including African Burkitt's lymphoma (a malignant B cell tumor), B cell lymphomas associated with therapeutic drug-induced or human immunodeficiency virus (HIV)–induced immunodeficiency, and nasopharyngeal carcinoma (a malignant tumor of nasopharyngeal epithelium) (see Chapter 18, Box 18–2). These tumors are derived from the only normal cells known to express CR2. EBV is a potent polyclonal B cell activator, and *in vitro* the virus can transform normal blood B lymphocytes into im-

TABLE 15–4. Receptors for Complement Fragments

Receptor	Molecular Weight (kD) Molecular Features	Ligand	Cell Distribution	Biologic Function
Complement Receptor Type 1 (CR1)	190–280 (Polymorphism) 30 SCRs form entire extra-cellular region	C3b, C4b, iC3b	Erythrocyte	Clearance of circulating immune complexes Accelerates dissociation of classical and alternative pathway C3 convertases Acts as cofactor for Factor I–mediated cleavage of C3b and C4b
			Neutrophils, monocytes, macro-phages	Enhances Fc receptor–mediated phagocytosis Mediates Fc receptor–independent phagocytosis
			Eosinophils	?
			B lymphocytes	?
			T lymphocytes	?
			Glomerular epithelial cells	?Solubilization of trapped immune complexes
			Follicular dendritic cells	?Binding of immune complexes
Complement Receptor Type 2 (CR2)	145 15 SCRs form entire extracellu-lar region	iC3b, C3dg, EBV	B lymphocytes	?B cell activation Mode of EBV infection
			Nasopharyngeal epithelial cells	Mode of EBV infection
			Follicular dendritic cells	?Binding of immune complexes, memory B cell activation
Mac-1 (complement receptor type 3, CR3, CD11bCD18)	α:165 β:95 Integrin, common β chain with CR4, LFA-1	iC3b (Cation-dependent)	Monocytes/macrophages, neutro-phils, natural killer cells	Cellular adhesion protein required for surface adhe-sion, chemotaxis, phagocyto-sis
			Splenic dendritic cells	?
Complement Receptor Type 4 (CR4, CD11cCD18, p150,95)	α:150 β:95 Integrin, common β chain with CR3, LFA-1	iC3b	Neutrophils, monocytes, plate-lets	Enhances Fc receptor–mediated phagocytosis Mediates Fc receptor–indepen-dent phagocytosis
C3a/C4a Receptor	?	C3a, C4a	Mast cells, basophils	Degranulation releasing hista-mine and other mediators of inflammation
			Smooth muscle cells	Contraction (?histamine-inde-pendent)
			Lymphocytes	?
C5a Receptor	40 G protein–linked seven trans-membrane segments	C5a, C5a-des arg	Mast cells, basophils	Degranulation releasing hista-mine and other mediators
			Endothelial cells	Increases vascular permeability
			Neutrophils, monocytes/macro-phages	Promotes chemotaxis

Abbreviations: SCR, short consensus repeat; LFA, leukocyte function–associated antigen; EBV, Epstein-Barr virus.

mortalized lymphoblastoid cell lines. These effects of the virus depend on CR2 expression on the B cells.

MAC-1 (COMPLEMENT RECEPTOR TYPE 3, CR3, CD11bCD18). This is a specific receptor for the iC3b fragment generated by Factor I–mediated cleavage of C3b and plays an important role in the elimination of microorganisms by leukocyte phagocytosis. Mac-1 is expressed on many different bone marrow–derived cells, including neutrophils, mononuclear phagocytes, mast cells, and NK cells. It is a member of the integrin family of cell surface receptors (see Chapter 7, Box 7–3). It consists of a 165 kD α chain (CD11b) noncovalently linked to a 95 kD β chain (CD18), which is identical to the β chains of two closely related integrin molecules, lymphocyte function–associated antigen (LFA-1) and p150, 95 (see below).

Mac-1 is thought to be important for phagocytosis of iC3b-coated microorganisms or particles. Furthermore, it has a specific carbohydrate-binding capacity (i.e., a lectin activity) that may be responsible for complement-independent binding of certain microorganisms to Mac-1 expressing phagocytic cells. In addition, Mac-1 on neutrophils and monocytes promotes the attachment of these cells to endothelium, even without complement activation, via binding to ICAM-1. This may be important for the accumulation of inflammatory cells at sites of tissue injury.

COMPLEMENT RECEPTOR TYPE 4 (**CR4, p150,95, CD11cCD18**). This is another integrin, with a 150 kD α chain and the same β chain as CR3. It has a similar cellular distribution as CR3 and can bind iC3b as well as C3dg. The function of this receptor may be similar to that of Mac-1.

BIOLOGIC FUNCTIONS OF COMPLEMENT PROTEINS

The functions of the complement system fall into two broad categories: (1) cell lysis by the MAC, and (2) biologic effects of proteolytic fragments of complement. We have previously described how complement activation on cell surfaces leads to the insertion of the MAC into lipid bilayers, causing osmotic lysis of the cell. The many other effects of complement in immunity and inflammation are mediated by the proteolytic fragments generated during complement activation. These biologically active fragments may remain bound to the same cell surfaces where complement has been activated, or they may be released into the fluid phase (e.g., blood or extracellular fluid). In either case, they mediate their effects by binding to specific receptors expressed on a variety of other cell types, including phagocytic leukocytes and endothelium. In this section of the chapter, we will discuss each of these functional roles of the complement system, with reference to the particular fragments and receptors that are involved (Table 15–5).

Complement-Mediated Cytolysis

Complement-mediated lysis of foreign organisms is an important defense mechanism against microbial infection. Specific humoral responses to microbes gen-erate antibodies that bind to the organisms; these antibodies activate complement on the surfaces of the microbes and lead to their lysis by the formation of the MAC. Some microorganisms may activate the alternative pathway or less frequently the classical pathway in the absence of antibody, also leading to lysis. This mechanism may be important for preventing bacteremia by *Neisseria* bacteria. Acquired resistance to complement-mediated lysis is a mechanism by which some microbes evade host immunity (see Chapter 16). In certain pathologic conditions, the complement system may cause lysis of host cells, leading to tissue injury and disease. For example, some autoimmune diseases are characterized by the production of autoantibodies specific for self proteins expressed on cell surfaces. These autoantibodies may fix complement, and subsequent formation of the MAC may lead to osmotic lysis of these normal cells (see Chapter 20).

Opsonization and Promotion of Phagocytosis of Microbes

As discussed previously, activation of both classical and alternative pathways leads to the generation of C3b and iC3b covalently bound to cell surfaces. Both C3b and iC3b act as opsonins by virtue of the fact that they specifically bind to receptors on neutrophils and macrophages. C3b binds to CR1, and iC3b (but not C3b) binds to Mac-1 and CR4. In addition, activation of the classical pathway leads to generation of C4b covalently bound to cell surfaces, and C4b is also a ligand for CR1. Thus, complement activation on the surface of a microbial cell promotes the adherence of the microbe to a phagocytic cell that is competent at phagocytosing and killing the microbe. *C3b- and iC3b-dependent phagocytosis of microorganisms is probably the major defense mechanism against systemic bacterial and fungal infections.*

Complement receptors and Fcγ receptors (see Chapter 3) cooperate to mediate binding and phagocytosis of opsonized particles. For example, if an unac-

TABLE 15–5. Biologic Functions of Complement

Function	Complement Components	Mechanisms
Lysis of cells	C5–C9	MAC formation kills microorganisms
Opsonization/phagocytosis	C3b,iC3b	C3b or iC3b on the surface of microorganisms binds to CR1 (and CR3, CR4) on neutrophils and macrophages, promoting phagocytosis
Immunization		
Vascular responses	C5a > C3a ≫ C4a	C5a, C3a, and C4a stimulate mast cell histamine release and smooth muscle contraction
Polymorphonuclear leukocyte activation	C5a	C5a is a chemoattractant for neutrophils and activates neutrophil oxidative metabolism
Immune complex removal	Classical pathway, C3b	Complement activation on Ig molecules inhibits immune complex formation; C3b on immune complexes binds to CR1 on erythrocytes, and the immune complexes are cleared from the circulation as the erythrocytes traverse the liver and spleen
B cell activation	?iC3b,C3dg	B cell responses to antigen may be enhanced by CR2/CD19 signalling; memory B cell activation is dependent on C3 and may require complement-dependent immune complex adherence to follicular dendritic cells

Abbreviations: MAC, membrane attack complex; Ig, immunoglobulin.

tivated neutrophil or monocyte encounters a particle coated with IgG, the particle is phagocytosed relatively slowly via the Fcγ receptors. If the same particle bears iC3b, so that it simultaneously binds to CR3 on the leukocyte, Fcγ receptor–mediated phagocytosis is also greatly enhanced. Similarly, binding of opsonized particles to Fcγ receptors augments CR1- and CR3-mediated phagocytosis. Such observations suggest that Fcγ and complement receptors on leukocytes function not only to bind opsonized particles but also to transduce signals that stimulate the phagocytic capacities of the leukocytes.

Anaphylatoxins and Inflammatory Responses

C3a, C4a, and C5a are called **anaphylatoxins** because they induce the release of mediators from mast cells, which cause rapid increases in vascular permeability characteristic of anaphylaxis (see Chapter 14). As described earlier, C3a is a 9 kD peptide fragment derived from proteolytic cleavage of the C3 α chain by either classical or alternative pathway C3 convertase. C4a is the 8.7 kD peptide released from the α chain of C4 by C2b-mediated cleavage in the classical pathway. C5a is the 11 kD peptide released from the α chain of C5 by the action of either classical or alternative pathway C5 convertase. C3a and C4a receptors are expressed on mast cells, basophils, smooth muscle cells, and lymphocytes. C5a receptors are expressed on mast cells, basophils, neutrophils, monocytes/macrophages, and endothelium (see Table 15–4). Ligand binding and functional response data indicate that these receptors are specific, saturable receptors with signal-transducing properties.

The major effects of anaphylatoxin binding to mast cells and basophils are granule exocytosis and release of vasoactive mediators, such as histamine (see Chapter 14). Histamine increases vascular permeability and stimulates the contraction of visceral smooth muscles. The anaphylatoxins also bind to smooth muscle and stimulate its contraction. C5a is the most potent mediator of these effects, C3a is 20-fold less potent, and C4a is 2500-fold less potent. C5a also stimulates TNF release from mast cells. C5a acts directly on vascular endothelial cells, stimulating contraction, causing vascular leak and exocytosis, and stimulating P-selectin expression, which promotes neutrophil binding. C5a has several direct effects on neutrophils *in vitro*, including stimulation of movement (**chemokinesis** and **chemotaxis**), increased Mac-1 adhesiveness for ICAM-1, and at high doses, stimulation of the respiratory burst and production of reactive oxygen intermediates. The combination of C5a actions on mast cells, endothelial cells, and neutrophils contributes to inflammation at sites of complement activation. The specificity of the response for foreign and not self tissues is imparted either by specific antibody activating the complement cascade at the appropriate location, i.e., where the foreign antigen is, or by the capacity of the alternative pathway to be activated on the surface of foreign organisms.

Solubilization and Phagocytic Clearance of Immune Complexes

Small numbers of immune complexes are constantly being formed in the circulation and may increase dramatically when an individual mounts a vigorous humoral immune response to an abundant circulating antigen. These immune complexes are potentially harmful because they may deposit in vessel walls, activate complement, and lead to inflammatory reactions that damage surrounding tissues. Formation of large, potentially harmful, immune complexes requires not only the multivalent binding of Ig Fab regions to antigens but also non-covalent interactions of Fc regions of juxtaposed Ig molecules (see Chapter 3). Complement binding to Ig can sterically block these Fc-Fc interactions, thereby inhibiting new formation of, or destabilizing already formed, immune complexes.

In addition to interfering with immune complex formation, the complement system can promote the clearance of immune complexes from the circulation by the mononuclear phagocyte system. In humans, this function is largely mediated by CR1 on the surface of erythrocytes, which, because of their number, account for the great majority of cell-associated CR1 molecules in the circulation. Circulating antigen-antibody complexes activate complement, and the C3b that is generated forms covalent bonds with the antibody. Such complexes may be adsorbed by CR1-expressing erythrocytes because of the high affinity of CR1 for C3b. *In vivo* primate studies have demonstrated that phagocytic cells in the liver (Kupffer cells) and spleen are responsible for removing the immune complexes along with CR1 molecules from the erythrocyte membranes as the erythrocytes traverse the sinusoids of these organs.

COMPLEMENT GENES AND BIOSYNTHESIS
Gene Families Represented by Complement Proteins

The complement system proteins can be categorized as members of various gene families on the basis of sequence homologies. Members of the same gene family often have similar functional characteristics that are dependent on their shared protein structures. Assignment of proteins to one or another gene family (usually based on the amino acid sequences predicted from the nucleotide sequences of the cloned genes) is often useful for studying the structural basis of function. Furthermore, the homologies among genes encoding various complement proteins suggested that members of each gene family may have arisen by duplication of an ancestral gene, followed by the structural diversification that imparts specialized functions to the individual proteins.

The most well-defined complement gene family is the regulators of complement activity (RCA) family mentioned earlier. All the members of this family share the ability to bind C3b and C4b; they include C4bp, Factor H, CR1, CR2, DAF, MCP, C1r, C1s, C2, and Factor B. Four of these proteins (C4bp, Factor H, CR1, and MCP) act as cofactors for Factor 1–catalyzed cleavage of C3b or C4b. The common genetic and structural feature of this family of proteins is the presence of SCRs, described in our discussion of CR1. SCRs constitute a significant part of the structure of all these proteins. For example, the amino acid sequence of Factor H is composed entirely of 20 SCRs, and the common form of CR1 has 30 SCRs making up the entire extracellular domain. The C3b/C4b binding regions of these molecules are formed, at least in part, by the SCRs. The presence of SCRs in other complement proteins, including Factor B and C2, reflects exon duplication and fusion with otherwise unrelated genes during evolution. Several non-complement proteins also contain SCRs, including the interleukin-2 receptor, the selectins (see Chapter 11, Box 11–1), and coagulation factor XIII. The structure-function relationships of SCRs in these molecules are not well understood.

Several proteins of the complement system are members of other gene families, sharing functions with other family members as well as the amino acid sequences that are critical for those functions. The five serine esterases of the complement system, including Factor I, Factor B, C1r, C1s, and C2, all have sequence homologies with one another and with non-complement serine esterases such as trypsin and chymotrypsin. The serine protease inhibitor, C1INH, is a member of the serpin family. C3 and C4 are members of a small family of proteins that also includes α_2-macroglobulin, characterized by the presence of internal thioester bonds. This feature allows the proteins to form covalent bonds with cell surfaces or Ig molecules. CR3 and CR4 are integrins sharing the same β-chain as LFA-1. The membrane pore-forming C9 is homologous to the pore-forming protein (cytolysin or perforin) found in CTLs and NK cells.

Chromosomal Linkage of Complement Genes

At least three groups of complement proteins can be defined by close chromosomal linkage of their respective members. The members of each of these groups probably arose by duplication from a common ancestral gene. The genes encoding several members of the RCA family, including CR1, CR2, C4bp, MCP, and DAF are all found in an 800 kb segment of DNA on the long arm of human chromosome 1. The genes encoding the MAC components C6, C7, C8, and C9 are also linked in another region on chromosome 1.

The close proximity of the genes encoding C2, Factor B, and C4 within the major histocompatibility complex (MHC) in humans, mice, and other species is the most thoroughly analyzed example of complement gene linkage. In humans, these complement protein genes are present between the class II HLA–DR and class I HLA–B loci on the chromosome 6 (Fig. 15–12; see also Chapter 5). MHC-linked complement genes are sometimes called class III genes. Interestingly, as is characteristic of the peptide-binding class I and class II MHC molecules, the class III complement genes are polymorphic. For example, there are over 35 alleles identified for the two closely linked loci that encode the C4 protein. Certain alleles of the C2, Factor B, and C4A and C4B genes are in linkage disequilibrium, so that they are often inherited *en bloc*.

Biosynthesis of Complement Proteins

Both hepatocytes and mononuclear phagocytes can synthesize most of the complement proteins present in the serum. The liver probably makes quantitatively more complement proteins, but mononuclear phagocyte synthesis may be significant at sites of inflammation. Various other cell types can make one or more complement proteins as well. Interestingly, interferon-γ induces the synthesis of a number of alternative pathway proteins in macrophages and vascular endothelial cells. The C1 proteins can also be synthesized by various types of epithelial cells other than hepatocytes. The regulation of synthesis of the various complement proteins is complicated, and incompletely characterized. Many complement proteins are "acute phase reactants" that are synthesized in response to circulating cytokines such as interleukin-1, interleukin-6, and tumor necrosis factor (see Chapter 12, Box 12–4). The C1 and C8 proteins are unusual, in that they are complexes of polypeptide products of more than one gene. The individual chains of each protein are secreted independently, and the mature proteins assemble extracellularly.

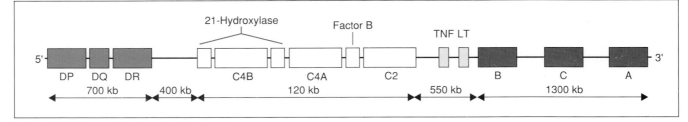

FIGURE 15–12. Complement genes in the human major histocompatibility complex (MHC). *The genes encoding C2, Factor B, and C4 are located between the DR locus and the class I MHC genes, 5' to genes encoding the cytokines tumor necrosis factor (TNF) and lymphotoxin (LT). Two genes encode the isoforms of C4 (C4A and C4B). Both the C2 and C4 genes are polymorphic.*

HUMAN DISEASES RELATED TO THE COMPLEMENT SYSTEM

The complement system is related to human disease in two general ways. First, deficiencies in any one of the protein components, usually due to abnormalities in gene structure, can lead to abnormal patterns of complement activation. If regulatory components are absent, too much complement activation may occur at the wrong time or wrong site. The absence of an integral component of the classical, alternative, or terminal pathways can result in too little complement activation and a lack of complement-mediated biologic functions. In either case, pathologic consequences may be severe. Second, an intact, normally functioning complement system may be activated in response to abnormal stimuli, such as a persistent microorganism or autoimmune humoral responses to self antigens. In these infectious or autoimmune diseases, the inflammatory or lytic effects of complement may contribute significantly to the pathology of the disease.

Complement Deficiencies

Deficiencies in many of the complement proteins have been described (Table 15–6), and these deficiencies are usually attributable to inherited or spontaneously mutated genes. Alternatively, acquired deficiencies in certain components can arise in individuals with normal complement genes. Deficiencies can be categorized on the basis of the functional type of protein that is lacking. Thus, there are deficiencies of the components of the classical, alternative, and terminal pathways and deficiencies in either soluble or membrane regulatory proteins. Beyond the significance to the affected individuals, an understanding of these diseases provides insights into the normal physiologic roles of the deficient proteins.

1. Genetic deficiencies in *classical and alternative pathway components,* including C1q, C1r, C4, C2, C3, properdin, and Factor D, all have been described; C2 deficiency is the most commonly identified human complement deficiency. C3 deficiency is associated with frequent serious pyogenic bacterial infections that may be fatal. The frequency of pyogenic infections in these patients illustrates the importance of C3 for opsonization, enhanced phagocytosis, and destruction of these organisms. Deficiencies in the early components of the classical pathway are associated with immune complex and/or autoimmune diseases, such as glomerulonephritis and systemic lupus erythematosus (SLE) (see Chapter 19, Box 19–1). More than 50 per cent of patients with C2 and C4 deficiencies have SLE. This association has been attributed to the requirement of the classical pathway for the clearance and solubilization of circulating immune complexes. If normally generated immune complexes are not cleared from the circulation, they may deposit in blood vessel walls and tissues, where they activate the complement cascade and produce local inflammation. Such inflammatory reactions may augment the antigen-presenting functions of mononuclear phagocytes, leading to the abnormal presentation of self antigens and autoimmunity. Other explanations for the association include genetic linkage of defective complement alleles in the MHC with certain

TABLE 15-6. Complement Deficiencies and Abnormalities

Protein	Resulting Complement Activation Abnormalities	Associated Diseases/Pathology
Classical Pathway		
C1q, C1r, C1s	Defective classical pathway activation	Systemic lupus erythematosus Pyogenic infections
C4	Defective classical pathway activation	Systemic lupus erythematosus Glomerulonephritis
C2	Defective classical pathway activation	Systemic lupus erythematosus Vasculitis Glomerulonephritis Pyogenic infections
C3	Defective classical/alternative pathway activation	Pyogenic infections Glomerulonephritis Immune complex disease
Alternative Pathway		
Properdin, Factor D	Defective alternative pathway activation	Neisserial infections Other pyogenic infections
Terminal Components		
C5, C6, C7, C8	Defective MAC formation	Disseminated Neisserial infections
C9	Defective MAC formation	None

Abbreviation: MAC, membrane attack complex.

pathogenic immune response genes (see Chapter 19). Somewhat surprisingly, C2 and C4 deficiencies are often not associated with increased infections. This suggests that the alternative pathway may be adequate for the elimination of most bacteria and that a key function of the classical pathway is to remove circulating immune complexes.

2. Deficiencies in members of the *terminal complement components,* including C5, C6, C7, C8, and C9, have also been described. These patients cannot generate the MAC and would therefore be expected to be inefficient in lysing foreign organisms. Interestingly, the only consistent clinical problem in these patients is a propensity for disseminated infections by the intracellular *Neisseria* bacteria, including *N. meningitidis* and *N. gonorrhoeae,* suggesting that complement-mediated bacteriolysis is particularly important for defense against these organisms. Interestingly, individuals with C9 deficiencies do not show the same susceptibility to infection, suggesting that poly-C9 formation is not necessary for *Neisseria* bacteriolysis.

3. Deficiencies in *soluble and membrane-bound complement regulatory proteins* are associated with abnormal complement activation and a variety of related clinical abnormalities (Table 15–7). The absences of classical, alternative, and terminal pathway regulatory proteins have each been described.

a. **Hereditary angioneurotic edema (HANE)** is an *autosomal dominant deficiency in C1INH.* Clinical manifestations of the disease include intermittent, acute accumulation of edema fluid in skin and mucosa, lasting from 24 to 72 hours. The skin of the face and

extremities and the laryngeal and intestinal mucosa are most frequently involved. Serious symptoms resulting from edema in these locations include abdominal pain, nausea and vomiting, diarrhea, and potentially life-threatening airway obstruction. Attacks have been associated with antecedent emotional stress and trauma; the physiologic basis for the association is not understood. The deficiency in C1INH in HANE patients may be caused either by an absolute reduction in C1INH protein due to inheritance of a nonfunctional gene or by synthesis of a normal amount of a dysfunctional protein due to mutations in the coding sequences of the gene. Although there is usually one normal allele of the C1INH gene in these patients, the plasma levels of the C1INH protein are sufficiently reduced (20 to 30 percent of normal) so that activation of C1 by immune complexes is not properly controlled. It is clear that during attacks there are elevated plasma levels of activated C1 and decreased levels of the substrates of activated C1, namely C2 and C4. The mediators of edema formation in HANE patients include a proteolytic fragment of C2, called C2 kinin, and bradykinin. C1INH is a major regulator of other plasma serine proteases besides C1, including kallikrein and coagulation factor XII, and both activated kallikrein and factor XII can promote increased formation of bradykinin, which can cause edema. Furthermore, C1INH deficiency can lead to increased plasmin generation, which in turn can proteolytically generate a fragment from C2 with kinin activity.

b. Deficiencies of the *soluble alternative pathway regulators* (Factor I and Factor H) are rare; the

TABLE 15–7. Abnormalities/Deficiencies of Regulatory Complement Proteins

Protein	Resulting Complement Activation Abnormalities	Associated Diseases/Pathology	Disease/Syndrome Name
Regulatory Proteins			
C1 inhibitor	Deregulated classical pathway activation, consumption of C3	Acute, intermittent attacks of skin and mucosal edema	Hereditary angioneurotic edema
		Systemic lupus erythematosus	Autosomal dominant
		Acute, intermittent attacks of skin and mucosal edema	Acquired angioneurotic edema
		Systemic lupus erythematosus	
		B cell lymphoproliferative diseases	
Factor I	Deregulated alternative pathway activation, consumption of C3	Pyogenic infections	
		Immune complex disease	
Factor H	Deregulated classical pathway activation, consumption of C3	Pyogenic infections	
		Glomerulonephritis	
Decay accelerating factor (DAF)	Deregulated C3 convertase activity	Complement-mediated intravascular hemolysis	Paroxysmal nocturnal hemoglobinuria
CD59 (MIRL)	Increased susceptibility of erythrocytes to MAC-mediated lysis	Complement-mediated intravascular hemolysis	Paroxysmal nocturnal hemoglobinuria
Complement Receptors			
CR1	Defective immune complex clearance	? Systemic lupus erythematosus	
CR3		Pyogenic infections	Leukocyte adhesion deficiency

Abbreviations: MIRL, membrane inhibitor of reactive lysis; MAC, membrane attack complex.

clinical consequences appear to include increased infections with pyogenic bacteria. These deficiencies have provided insights into the role of Factor I–mediated cleavage of C3b. Plasma C3 is completely consumed in these patients as a result of unregulated formation of fluid-phase C3 convertase (by the tickover mechanism). This is similar to the effects of an autoantibody called **C3 nephritic factor** (C3NeF), which is specific for alternative pathway C3 convertase (C3bBb). This antibody stabilizes C3bBb and protects the complex from Factor H–mediated dissociation, therefore causing unregulated consumption of C3. Patients with this antibody often have glomerulonephritis, possibly caused by inadequate clearing of circulating immune complexes.

   c. Deficiencies in *integral membrane protein regulators of complement activation* include the absence of DAF, and CD59. These proteins are normally bound to the plasma membrane of erythrocytes and other cell types by phosphatidylinositol linkages. **Paroxysmal nocturnal hemoglobinuria** (PNH) is a disease in which cells lack the ability to express phosphatidylinositol-linked membrane proteins, including DAF, HRF, and CD59. PNH is characterized by recurrent bouts of intravascular hemolysis, at least partially attributable to complement activation on the surface of erythrocytes. This is predictable, since DAF normally functions to inhibit C3 convertase formation on autologous cell surfaces, and HRF and CD59 normally serve to inhibit MAC formation on autologous cell membranes.

   4. Deficiencies in *complement receptors* include the absence of CR3 and CR4, both resulting from rare mutations in the β chain (CD18) gene common to the CD11CD18 family of integrin molecules. The congenital disease caused by this gene defect is called **leukocyte adhesion deficiency** (see Chapter 21). This disorder is characterized by recurrent pyogenic infections, probably due to a combination of impaired iC3b–dependent phagocytosis of bacteria and inadequate adherence of neutrophils to endothelium at tissue sites of infection.

Pathologic Effects of a Normal Complement System

   Even when it is properly regulated and appropriately activated, the complement system can cause significant tissue damage. In fact, much of the pathology associated with bacterial infections is attributable to the biologic effects of complement activation. These pathologic effects include the bystander destruction of normal host cells when acute inflammatory responses to infectious organisms take place. For example, a bacterial infection can stimulate a humoral immune response, and antibody bound to bacterial antigens can activate complement. Direct activation of the alternative pathway on bacterial surfaces may also occur, in the absence of antibody. The generation of C3a and C5a

stimulates the accumulation of neutrophils at the site of infection. The neutrophils adhere to and phagocytose the infecting organisms. In addition, neutrophils release free radicals and proteases that destroy microbes and may damage normal cells in the vicinity as well. Histamine released from mast cells in response to C5a may amplify the inflammatory response by increasing vascular permeability.

   Perhaps the clearest example of complement-mediated pathology occurs in immune complex diseases. Systemic vasculitis and immune complex glomerulonephritis may result from deposition of antigen-antibody complexes in the walls of vessels and kidney glomeruli (see Chapter 20). Complement activated by the Ig in these deposited immune complexes initiates the acute inflammatory responses that destroy the vessel walls or glomeruli, leading to thrombosis, ischemic damage to tissues, and scarring.

SUMMARY

   The complement system includes serum and membrane proteins that interact in a highly regulated manner to produce biologically active protein products. The system includes two convergent proteolytic pathways, composed of several different zymogens. The classical pathway is initiated by antigen-antibody complexes, and the alternative pathway is usually activated directly by the surfaces of infectious organisms. The two pathways converge, both utilizing the C3 protein to form enzymes that initiate the common terminal pathway leading to formation of a cytolytic protein complex called the membrane attack complex. These pathways are regulated by various soluble and membrane-bound proteins, which inhibit different steps in the cascades. The biologic functions of the complement system include cytolysis, opsonization of organisms and immune complexes for phagocytosis, production of inflammation, enhancement of humoral immune responses, and solubilization and clearance of immune complexes. Cytolysis is mediated by MAC formation on cell surfaces. Opsonization is largely mediated by proteolytic fragments of C3, as is immune complex clearance. Inflammation is promoted by proteolytic fragments of complement proteins called anaphylatoxins (C3a, C4a, C5a). Specific membrane receptors for complement fragments are required for the opsonin and anaphylatoxin effects. The complement proteins are members of several different gene families, reflecting the common usage of duplicated exons and genes encoding functionally significant domains during the evolution of the system. Many genetic deficiencies in one or more complement components have been described, with associated infections and autoimmune diseases.

SELECTED READINGS

Ahearn, J. M., and D. T. Fearon. Structure and function of the complement receptors, CR1 (CD35) and CR2 (CD21). Advances in Immunology 46:183–219, 1989.

Campbell, R. D., M. C. Carroll, and R. R. Porter. The molecular genetics of components of complement. Advances in Immunology 38:203–244, 1986.

Colten, H. R., and F. S. Rosen. Complement deficiencies. Annual Review of Immunology 10:809–834, 1992.

Holers, V. M., T. Kinoshita, and H. Molina. The evolution of mouse and human complement C3-binding proteins: divergence of form but conservation of function. Immunology Today 13:231–237, 1992.

Hourcade, D., M. Holers, and J. P. Atkinson. The regulators of complement activation (RCA) gene cluster. Advances in Immunology 45:381–416, 1989.

Lachman, P. J. The control of homologous lysis. Immunology Today 12:312–315, 1992.

Lubin, D. M., and J. P. Atkinson. Decay-accelerating factor: biochemistry, molecular biology, and function. Annual Review of Immunology 7:35–58, 1989.

Morgan, B. P., and M. J. Walport. Complement deficiency and disease. Immunology Today 12:301–306, 1991.

Muller-Eberhard, H. J. The membrane attack complex. Annual Review of Immunology 4:503–528, 1986.

Muller-Eberhard, H. J. Molecular organization and function of the complement system. Annual Review of Biochemistry 57:321–347, 1988.

Reid, K. B. M., and A. J. Day. Structure-function relationships of the complement components. Immunology Today 10:177–180, 1989.

Schumaker, V. N., P. Zavodszky, and P. H. Poon. Activation of the first component of complement. Annual Review of Immunology 5:21–42, 1987.

Sim, R. B., and K. B. M. Reid. C1: molecular interactions with activating systems. Immunology Today 12:307–311, 1991.

IMMUNITY
IN DEFENSE
AND
DISEASE

In this final section, we apply our knowledge of the fundamental mechanisms of specific immunity to understanding immunologic defenses against potential pathogens and tumors, immune reactions to transplants, and the principles of diseases that are caused by abnormalities in immune responses. We begin with a discussion of the role of specific immunity in combating microbial infections in Chapter 16. Chapter 17 is devoted to tissue transplantation, an increasingly promising therapy for a variety of diseases in which the major limitation is immunologic rejection. Chapter 18 describes immune responses to tumors as well as the mechanisms by which cancer cells evade elimination by the immune system. Chapter 19 deals with the mechanisms that maintain tolerance to self antigens and how self-tolerance may fail, leading to autoimmunity. Chapter 20 describes the effector mechanisms of immune-mediated tissue injury and disease. In Chapter 21 we discuss the cellular and molecular bases of congenital and acquired immunodeficiencies, including the acquired immunodeficiency syndrome (AIDS), and the pathologic complications of deficient immunity.

CHAPTER SIXTEEN

IMMUNITY TO

MICROBES

The principal physiologic function of the immune system is to protect the host against pathogenic microbes. Resistance to infections formed the basis for the original identification of acquired immunity. As our understanding of specific immune responses has increased, we are better able to explain the mechanisms of antimicrobial immunity. Throughout this book we have mentioned examples of specific immune responses to particular microbes, largely to illustrate the physiologic relevance of various aspects of lymphocyte function. In this chapter, we discuss in more detail the main features of immunity to different types of pathogenic microorganisms.

The evolution of an infectious disease in an individual involves a sequence of interactions between the microbe and the host. These include entry of the microbe, invasion and colonization of host tissues, evasion from host immunity, and tissue injury or functional impairment. Some microbes produce disease by liberating toxins, even without extensive colonization of host tissues. Many features of microorganisms determine their virulence, and many diverse mechanisms contribute to the pathogenesis of infectious diseases. These are largely beyond the scope of this book and will not be discussed in detail. Rather, our discussion will focus on the host immune response to pathogenic microorganisms. There are several important general features of immunity to microbes:

1. *Defense against microbes is mediated by both natural and acquired immunity.* Microbial infections provide clear demonstrations of the role of specific immunity in enhancing the protective mechanisms of natural immunity and in directing these mechanisms to sites where they are needed.

2. *Different types of microbes stimulate distinct lymphocyte responses and effector mechanisms.* Because microbes differ greatly in patterns of host invasion and colonization, their elimination requires diverse effector systems. Not surprisingly, the magnitude and type of immune response to an infectious agent often determine the course and outcome of the infection. Studies in humans and experimental models have led to reports of virtually every type of immune response to infections by different classes of microorganisms. Our subsequent discussions will attempt to highlight the principal mechanisms of specific immunity against different bacteria, viruses, and parasites.

3. *The survival and pathogenicity of microbes in a host are critically influenced by their ability to evade or resist protective immunity.* Microorganisms have developed a variety of strategies for surviving in the face of powerful immunologic defenses.

4. *Tissue injury and disease consequent to infections may be caused by the host response to the microbe and its products rather than by the microbe itself.* Immunity, like many other homeostatic mechanisms, is necessary for host survival but also has the potential of causing injury to the host.

This chapter considers four types of pathogenic microorganisms that illustrate the main features of immunity to microbes: (1) extracellular bacteria, (2) intracellular bacteria, (3) viruses, and (4) intracellular protozoan and multicellular parasites. (Fungal infections are not considered separately as these organisms elicit responses that are similar to a combination of responses to extracellular and intracellular bacteria.) In each group, selected examples will be used to highlight key points. As we shall see, these four groups of microbes illustrate the diversity of antimicrobial immunity and the physiologic significance of many of the responses and effector functions of lymphocytes discussed in earlier chapters.

IMMUNITY TO EXTRACELLULAR BACTERIA

Extracellular bacteria are capable of replicating outside host cells, e.g., in the circulation, in extracellular connective tissues, and in various tissue spaces such as the airways and intestinal lumens. These bacteria include gram-positive pus-forming, or pyogenic, cocci (*Staphylococcus, Streptococcus*), gram-negative cocci (meningococcus and gonococcus, two species of *Neisseria*), many gram-negative bacilli (including enteric organisms such as *Escherichia coli*), and some gram-positive bacilli (particularly anaerobes such as the *Clostridium* species).

Extracellular bacteria cause disease by two principal mechanisms. First, they induce inflammation, which results in tissue destruction at the site of infection. Pyogenic cocci are responsible for a large number of suppurative infections in humans. Second, many of these bacteria produce **toxins**, which have diverse pathologic effects. Such toxins may be **endotoxins**, which are components of bacterial cell walls, or **exotoxins**, which are actively secreted by the bacteria. The endotoxin of gram-negative bacteria, also called **lipopolysaccharide** (LPS), has been mentioned in earlier chapters as a potent stimulator of cytokine production by macrophages, and as an adjuvant. Many exotoxins are primarily cytotoxic, and they kill cells by poorly defined mechanisms. There are also many other examples of exotoxins whose mode of action is known in precise detail. For instance, diphtheria toxin inhibits protein synthesis by enzymatically modifying and thereby blocking the function of elongation factor-2, which is necessary for the synthesis of all polypeptides. Cholera toxin stimulates cyclic adenosine monophosphate production in intestinal epithelial cells, leading to active chloride secretion, water loss, and intractable diarrhea. Tetanus toxin is a neurotoxin that binds to motor end plates at neuromuscular junctions and causes persistent muscle contraction, which can be fatal if it affects the muscles involved in breathing. Clostridial toxins cause extensive tissue necrosis and lead to gas gangrene. *Immune responses against extracellular bacteria are aimed at eliminating the bacteria and at neutralizing the effects of their toxins.*

Natural Immunity to Extracellular Bacteria

Because extracellular microbes are rapidly killed by the microbicidal mechanisms of phagocytes, a principal mechanism of natural immunity to these microbes is phagocytosis by neutrophils, monocytes, and tissue macrophages. The resistance of bacteria to phagocytosis and digestion within macrophages is an important determinant of virulence. Activation of the complement system, in the absence of antibody, also plays an important role in the elimination of these bacteria. Gram-positive bacteria contain a peptidoglycan in their cell walls that activates the alternative pathway of complement by promoting the formation of the alternative pathway C3 convertase (see Chapter 15). LPS in the cell walls of gram-negative bacteria was one of the first agents shown to activate the alternative complement pathway, in the absence of antibody. Bacteria that express mannose on their surface may also bind a mannose-binding protein that is homologous to C1q, leading to complement activation by the classical pathway without the participation of antibody (see Chapter 15). One result of complement activation is the generation of C3b, which opsonizes bacteria and enhances phagocytosis. In addition, the membrane attack complex (MAC) lyses bacteria, and complement by-products participate in inflammatory responses by recruiting and activating leukocytes.

Endotoxins, such as LPS, stimulate the production of cytokines by macrophages and by other cells, e.g., vascular endothelium. These cytokines include tumor necrosis factor (TNF), interleukin-1 (IL-1), interleukin-6 (IL-6), and chemokines. The structure and functional effects of these cytokines have been discussed in Chapter 12. The principal physiologic functions of macrophage-derived cytokines are to stimulate inflammation. These cytokines induce the adhesion of neutrophils and monocytes to vascular endothelium at sites of infection, which is followed by migration, local accumulation, and activation of the inflammatory cells. The inflammatory cells serve to eliminate the bacteria; injury to adjacent normal tissues is a pathologic side effect of these defense mechanisms. Cytokines also induce fever and stimulate the synthesis of acute phase proteins (see Chapter 12, Box 12–4). Some of these cytokines may also stimulate T and B lymphocytes, providing amplification mechanisms for specific immunity.

Large amounts of cytokines or their uncontrolled production can be harmful and are responsible for some of the clinicopathologic manifestations of infections by extracellular bacteria. The most severe cytokine-induced pathologic consequence of infection by gram-negative bacteria is septic shock, a syndrome characterized by circulatory collapse and disseminated intravascular coagulation. As discussed in Chapter 12, TNF and IL-1 are the principal mediators of septic shock.

Specific Immune Responses to Extracellular Bacteria

Humoral immunity is the principal protective specific immune response against extracellular bacteria. Some of the most immunogenic components of the cell walls and capsules of these microbes are polysaccharides, which are prototypical thymus-independent antigens. Such antigens directly stimulate B cells, giving rise to strong specific IgM responses. In addition, other immunoglobulin (Ig) isotypes may be produced, probably as a result of the production of cytokines that promote heavy chain isotype switching (see Chapter 9). The best documented example of heavy chain class switching induced by a T cell–independent antigen is the humoral immune response to pneumococcal capsular polysaccharides in humans, which is dominated by IgG2 antibodies.

The principal T cell response to extracellular bacteria consists of CD4+ T cells responding to protein antigens in association with class II major histocompatibility complex (MHC) molecules. As discussed in Chapter 6, extracellular microbes and soluble antigens are phagocytosed by antigen-presenting cells (APCs), the antigens are processed, and fragments of the processed proteins preferentially associate with class II MHC molecules. It is not known whether macrophages, B cells, or other cell types are the most important APCs for such bacterial protein antigens *in vivo*.

Antibodies and T cells perform several functions that serve to eliminate bacteria. Both IgM and IgG antibodies against bacterial surface antigens and toxins stimulate three types of **effector mechanisms**:

1. *IgG antibodies opsonize bacteria and enhance phagocytosis* by binding to Fcγ receptors on monocytes, macrophages, and neutrophils (see Chapter 3). Both IgM and IgG antibodies activate complement, generating C3b and iC3b, which bind to specific type 1 and type 3 complement receptors, respectively, and further promote phagocytosis. Individuals deficient in C3 are extremely susceptible to pyogenic infections.

2. *Both IgG and IgM antibodies neutralize bacterial toxins* and prevent their binding to target cells. Passive immunization against tetanus toxin by injection of antibody is a potentially life-saving treatment in acute tetanus infections. IgA antibody present in various secretions, e.g., in the gastrointestinal and respiratory tracts, is important for neutralizing the toxins of bacteria in these organs and for preventing colonization of extraluminal tissues.

3. *Both IgM and IgG antibodies activate the complement system,* leading to the production of the microbicidal MAC and the liberation of by-products that are mediators of acute inflammation. It is likely, however, that the lytic function of the MAC is important for the elimination of only some microbes. As we mentioned in Chapter 15, deficiencies of the late components of complement, C5 to C8, which are involved in the formation of the MAC, are associated with increased susceptibility to *Neisseria* but not to other bacterial infections.

The effector functions of CD4+ T cells are mediated by secreted cytokines, which stimulate antibody production, induce local inflammation, and enhance the phagocytic and microbicidal activities of macrophages (Fig. 16–1). Interferon-γ (IFN-γ) and TNF are the principal cytokines responsible for macrophage activation and inflammation.

As mentioned earlier, acute inflammation and septic shock are two of the injurious consequences of defense against extracellular bacteria. Recently, it has been observed that some bacterial toxins stimulate large numbers of CD4+ T cells. Any one of these toxins can stimulate all the T cells in an individual that express a particular set or family of V_β T cell receptor genes. Such toxins have been called **super-antigens** (Box 16–1). Their importance lies in their ability to activate many T cells, resulting in large amounts of cytokine production and clinicopathologic abnormalities that may be similar in some respects to septic shock.

A late complication of the humoral immune response to bacterial infections may be the generation of disease-producing antibodies. The best-defined examples are two sequelae of streptococcal infections of the throat or skin, which are manifested weeks or even months after the infections are controlled. In **rheumatic fever,** pharyngeal infection with some serologic types of β-hemolytic streptococci leads to the production of antibodies against a bacterial cell wall protein (M protein). Some of these antibodies cross-react with myocardial sarcolemmal proteins and myosin, leading to antibody deposition in the heart and subsequent inflammation (carditis). In **post-streptococcal glomerulonephritis**, infection of the skin or throat with other serotypes of β-hemolytic streptococci leads to the formation of immune complexes of bacterial antigen and specific antibody. The complexes deposit in kidney glomeruli and produce nephritis. It is worth noting that thorough antibiotic therapy is recommended for "sore throats" caused by β-hemolytic streptococci, not because of the severity of the pharyngitis but to prevent the later development of rheumatic fever. Other bacterial infections may lead to different sequelae. The polyclonal lymphocyte activation induced by bacterial endotoxins and super-antigens may contribute to the development of autoimmunity. Such bacterial infections may lead to the stimulation of many lymphocytes, among which are self-reactive clones that are normally anergic to stimulation by self antigens. This concept, and other possible links between infections and autoimmune diseases, are discussed more fully in Chapter 19.

Evasion of Immune Mechanisms by Extracellular Bacteria

The virulence of extracellular bacteria has been linked to a number of mechanisms that favor tissue invasion and colonization. These include adhesive properties of bacterial surface proteins, anti-phagocytic mechanisms, and inhibition of complement or inactivation of complement products. For instance, the capsules of many gram-positive and gram-negative bacteria contain one or more sialic acid residues that inhibit complement activation by the alternative pathway. Encapsulated bacteria also resist phagocytosis and, therefore, are much more virulent than homologous strains lacking a capsule.

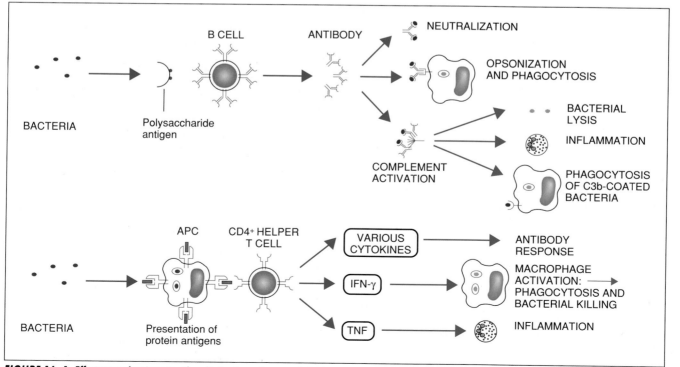

FIGURE 16–1. Effector mechanisms for the elimination of extracellular bacteria.

BOX 16–1.   BACTERIAL "SUPER-ANTIGENS"

Staphylococcal enterotoxins (SEs) are exotoxins produced by the gram-positive bacterium *Staphylococcus aureus*, and consist of five serologically distinct groups of proteins: SEA, SEB, SEC, SED, and SEE. These toxins are the most common cause of food poisoning in humans. A related toxin, TSST, causes a disease called the **toxic shock syndrome** (TSS), which is associated with tampon use. Pyrogenic exotoxins of streptococci and exotoxins produced by mycoplasma may be structurally and functionally related to these enterotoxins.

The immune response to staphylococcal enterotoxins and related proteins has a number of features that make these bacterial products quite unique in terms of biologic and pathologic effects:

1. *Staphylococcal enterotoxins are among the most potent naturally occurring T cell mitogens known.* They are capable of stimulating the proliferation of normal T lymphocytes at concentrations of 10^{-9} M or less. As many as one in five normal T cells in mouse lymphoid tissue or human peripheral blood may respond to a particular enterotoxin.

2. *The T cells that respond to each enterotoxin express a V_β gene from a particular V_β family in the antigen receptors.* Responsiveness is apparently not related to other components of the T cell receptor (TCR), i.e., V_α, J, or D segments. This is because enterotoxins bind directly to the β chains of TCR molecules outside the antigen binding regions. Different enterotoxins stimulate T cells expressing V_β genes from different families (see table). Because T cells expressing only certain TCRs recognize and respond to each enterotoxin, these proteins are called antigens and not polyclonal mitogens. However, since the frequency of enterotoxin-responsive T cells is much higher than the frequency of cells specific for conventional protein antigens, the enterotoxins have been named "**super-antigens**."

3. *Responses to staphylococcal enterotoxins require antigen-presenting cells that express class II MHC molecules.* Depletion of class II–bearing cells or addition of anti–class II antibody inhibits the T cell proliferative response to these toxins.

4. *Staphylococcal enterotoxins directly bind to class II MHC molecules on accessory cells.* This complex is then recognized by CD4$^+$ T cells expressing antigen receptors with a particular V_β. Enterotoxins bind to class II molecules outside the peptide-binding clefts, and do not need to be processed like other protein antigens. The same enterotoxin binds to class II molecules of different alleles, indicating that the polymorphism of the MHC does not influence presentation of these antigens.

The remarkably high frequency of staphylococcal enterotoxin–responding CD4$^+$ T cells has several functional implications. Acutely, exposure to high concentrations of enterotoxins leads to systemic reactions like fever, DIC, and cardiovascular shock. These abnormalities are probably mediated by cytokines, such as TNF, produced directly by the T cells or by macrophages that are activated by the T cells. This is the likely pathogenesis of the toxic shock syndrome, which is characterized by shock, skin exfoliation, conjunctivitis, and severe gastrointestinal upset, and can progress to renal and pulmonary failure and death. More prolonged administration of enterotoxins to mice results in wasting, thymic atrophy, and profound immunodeficiency, also probably secondary to chronic high levels of cytokine, e.g., TNF, production.

Staphylococcal enterotoxins are proving to be useful tools for analyzing T lymphocyte development. Administration of SEB to neonatal mice leads to intrathymic deletion of all T cells expressing $V_\beta3$ and $V_\beta8$ TCR genes. This mimics the postulated self antigen–induced clonal deletion of self-reactive T cells during thymic maturation.

Viral gene products may also function as super-antigens. In certain inbred strains of mice, different mouse mammary tumor virus genes have become incorporated into the genome. Viral antigens produced by the cells of one strain are capable of activating T lymphocytes from other strains that express particular V_βs in their antigen receptors. This is a form of "mixed lymphocyte reaction" that is not caused by MHC disparity. It was discovered long before viral super-antigens were identified, and the interstrain reactions were attributed to *Mls* (for minor lymphocyte stimulating) loci. We now know that *Mls* "loci" are actually different retroviral genes that are stably inherited in different inbred strains.

V_β Expression in Responding T Cells		
Enterotoxin	Mice	Humans
SEB	$V_\beta7$, 8.1–8.3, 17	$V_\beta3$, 12, 14, 15, 17, 20
SEC 2	$V_\beta8.2$, 10	$V_\beta12$, 13, 14, 15, 17, 20
SEE	$V_\beta11$, 15, 17	$V_\beta5.1$, 6.1–6.3, 8, 18
TSST-1	$V_\beta15$, 16	$V_\beta2$

Abbreviations: SE, staphylococcal enterotoxin; TSST, toxic shock syndrome toxin.

One mechanism utilized by bacteria to evade specific immunity is *genetic variation of surface antigens*. Surface antigens of many bacteria, such as gonococci and *Escherichia coli*, are contained in the pili, which are the structures primarily involved in bacterial adhesion to host cells. The major antigen of the pili is a protein of approximately 35 kilodaltons (kD) called pilin. The pilin genes of gonococci consist of one or two expression loci. In addition, there are ten to 20 silent loci, each containing six coding sequences, called "minicassettes." Antigenic variation results from a high rate of conversion between silent and expression loci. A gene conversion event replaces the minicassette on the expression locus with a duplicate of one of the minicassettes from one of the silent loci (Fig. 16–2). From ten

silent loci, each with six minicassettes, it is possible to create 10^6 combinations whose protein products are antigenically distinct. This mechanism helps the bacteria to escape specific antibody attack, although its principal significance for the bacteria may be to select for pili that are more adherent for host cells so that the bacteria are more virulent.

IMMUNITY TO INTRACELLULAR BACTERIA

A number of bacteria, and all viruses, survive and replicate within host cells. Among the bacteria, some of the most pathogenic are ones that are resistant to deg-

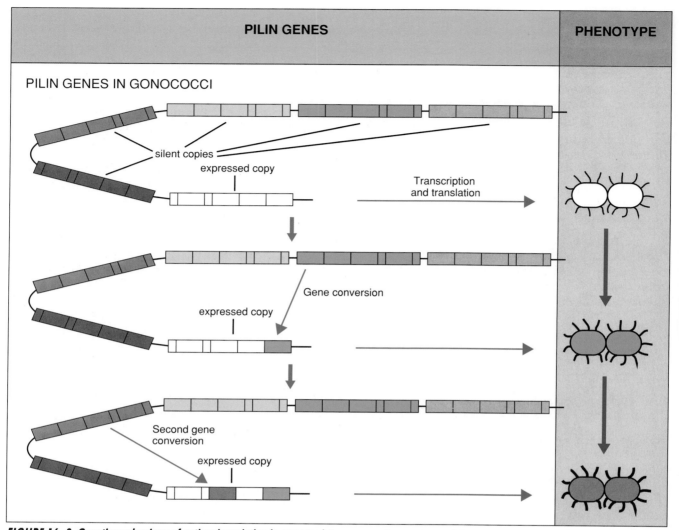

FIGURE 16–2. Genetic mechanisms of antigenic variation in gonococci. *In gonococci, a segment of the expressed pilin gene may be replaced by nucleotides from a DNA segment ("minicassette") in a silent pilin gene by a process of gene conversion, generating a new pilin gene and expressed protein. (Sizes of DNA segments are not to scale, and only five silent copies of the pilin gene are shown.)*

radation in macrophages and are therefore capable of surviving within phagocytes. Two of the best known examples are mycobacteria and *Listeria monocytogenes*. Since these microbes are able to find a niche where they are inaccessible to circulating antibodies, their elimination requires immune mechanisms that are very different from the mechanisms of defense against extracellular bacteria. Many fungi are also capable of surviving within host cells, and defense against them is mediated by mechanisms similar to those against intracellular bacteria.

Natural Immunity to Intracellular Bacteria

The principal mechanism of natural immunity against intracellular microbes is phagocytosis. However, pathogenic intracellular bacteria are relatively resistant to degradation within mononuclear phagocytes.

It is, therefore, not surprising that usually *natural immunity is quite ineffective in controlling colonization by and spread of these microorganisms.* Resistance to phagocytosis is also the reason why such bacteria tend to cause chronic infections that may last for years, often recur or recrudesce after apparent cures, and are difficult to eradicate.

Intracellular bacteria also activate natural killer (NK) cells, either directly or by stimulating macrophage production of interleukin-12 (IL-12), a powerful NK cell–activating cytokine. NK cells produce IFN-γ, which in turn activates macrophages and promotes killing of phagocytosed bacteria. Thus, NK cells provide an early defense against these microbes, prior to the development of specific immunity. In fact, T and B cell–deficient SCID mice are able to control infection by *L. monocytogenes*, at least temporarily, by NK cell–derived IFN-γ production. As we shall discuss later in this chapter, NK cells also provide initial defense against viral infections.

Specific Immune Responses to Intracellular Bacteria

The major protective immune response against intracellular bacteria is cell-mediated immunity. Individuals with deficient cell-mediated immunity, such as AIDS patients, are extremely susceptible to infections with intracellular bacteria (and viruses). Cell-mediated immunity was first identified by George Mackaness in the 1950s as protection against the intracellular bacterium *L. monocytogenes*. This form of immunity could be adoptively transferred to naive animals with lymphoid cells but not with serum from infected or immunized animals (Fig. 16–3).

Cell-mediated immunity consists of two types of reactions—killing of phagocytosed microbes as a result of macrophage activation by T cell–derived cytokines, particularly IFN-γ, and lysis of infected cells by CD8$^+$ cytolytic T lymphocytes (CTLs). Protein antigens of intracellular bacteria stimulate both CD4$^+$ and CD8$^+$ T cells. Presumably, CD4$^+$ T cells respond to released

antigens that are internalized and presented by class II MHC–expressing APCs; an example of such an antigen is the purified protein derivative (PPD) of *Mycobacterium tuberculosis*. Such microbes are potent inducers of the differentiation of CD4$^+$ helper T cells to the T$_H$1 phenotype, because intracellular bacteria stimulate IFN-γ production by NK cells and IL-12 production by macrophages, and both these cytokines promote the development of T$_H$1 cells (see Chapter 10). T$_H$1 cells secrete IFN-γ, which activates macrophages to produce reactive oxygen species and enzymes that kill phagocytosed bacteria. IFN-γ also stimulates the production of antibody isotypes (e.g., IgG2a in mice), which activate complement and opsonize bacteria for phagocytosis, thus aiding the effector functions of macrophages. T$_H$1 cells also produce TNF, which induces local inflammation. The importance of these cytokines in immunity to intracellular bacteria has been demonstrated in several experimental models. For instance, inhibitors of IFN-γ or TNF worsen the outcomes of such infections in mice. Furthermore, IFN-γ knockout mice and TNF receptor (p55) knockout mice are extremely susceptible to in-

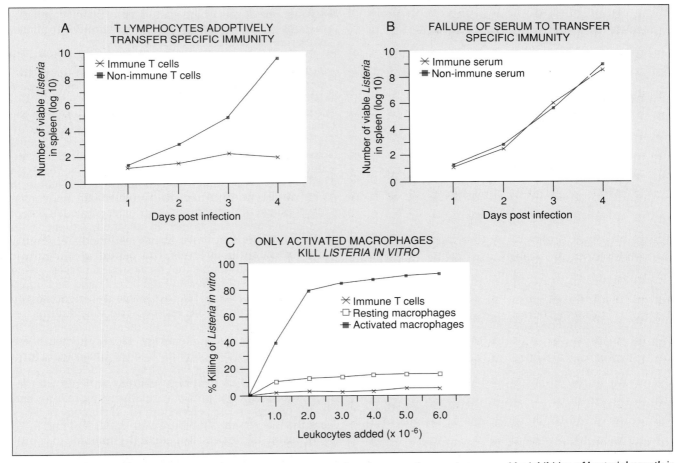

FIGURE 16–3. Cell-mediated immunity to Listeria monocytogenes. *Immunity to* L. monocytogenes *is measured by inhibition of bacterial growth in the spleens of animals inoculated with a known dose of viable bacteria. Such immunity can be transferred to normal mice by T lymphocytes (A) but not by serum (B) from syngeneic mice previously immunized with killed* L. monocytogenes. *In one form of cell-mediated immunity, the bacteria are actually killed by activated macrophages and not by T cells, even from immune animals (C). In another form of cell-mediated immunity, specific T lymphocytes kill infected cells (not shown).*

fections with intracellular bacteria (*M. tuberculosis* and *L. monocytogenes,* respectively).

If the bacteria survive within cells and release their antigens into the cytoplasm, they stimulate CD8$^+$ CTLs. CTLs produce IFN-γ, and are also capable of lysing infected cells. The two effectors of cell-mediated immunity, namely activated macrophages and CTLs, act in concert and may complement each other. For instance, by adoptively transferring CD4$^+$ or CD8$^+$ T cells from *L. monocytogenes*–infected mice to normal mice and challenging the recipients with the bacteria, it is possible to determine which effector population is responsible for specific immunity. Such experiments have shown that both CD4$^+$ and CD8$^+$ T cells are required to eliminate the infection. The CD4$^+$ cells produce IFN-γ, which activates macrophages to kill phagocytosed bacteria. However, *L. monocytogenes* produces a protein called hemolysin, which allows bacteria to escape from the phagolysosomes of macrophages into the cytoplasm. In their cytoplasmic haven, the bacteria are protected from the microbicidal mechanisms of macrophages, such as reactive oxygen species, which are produced mainly within phagolysosomes. CD8$^+$ T cells

function to kill any macrophages that may be harboring bacteria in their cytoplasm (Fig. 16–4). A mutant of *L. monocytogenes* that lacks hemolysin remains confined to phagolysosomes. Such mutant bacteria can be completely eradicated by macrophages that are activated by the IFN-γ produced by CD4$^+$ T cells.

The macrophage activation that occurs in response to intracellular microbes is also capable of causing tissue injury. This may be manifested as delayed type hypersensitivity (DTH) reactions to microbial protein antigens such as PPD (see Chapter 13). Since intracellular bacteria have evolved to resist phagocytes, they often persist for long periods, leading to chronic antigenic stimulation and T cell and macrophage activation. This may result in the formation of **granulomas** surrounding the microbes (see Chapter 13, Fig. 13–8). The histologic hallmark of infections with some intracellular bacteria and fungi is granulomatous inflammation. This type of inflammatory reaction may serve to localize and prevent the spread of the microbes, but is is also associated with severe functional impairment due to tissue necrosis and fibrosis. Thus, *the host immune response is the principal cause of tissue injury and disease in infections by some intracellular bacteria.* The concept that protective immunity and pathologic hypersensitivity may co-exist because they are manifestations of the same type of specific immune response is perhaps most clearly exemplified in mycobacterial infections (Box 16–2).

Differences among individuals in the patterns of immune responses to intracellular microbes are important determinants of disease progression and clinical outcome. An example of this is leprosy, caused by *Mycobacterium leprae.* There are two polar forms of the disease, although many patients fall into less clear intermediate groups. In lepromatous leprosy, patients have high specific antibody titers but weak cell-mediated responses to *M. leprae* antigens. Mycobacteria proliferate within macrophages and are detectable in large numbers. The bacterial growth and inadequate macrophage activation result in destructive lesions of skin and underlying bones. In contrast, patients with tuberculoid leprosy have strong cell-mediated immunity but low antibody levels. This pattern of immunity is reflected in granulomas that form around nerves, giving rise to sensory peripheral nerve defects and secondary traumatic skin lesions but less tissue destruction and a paucity of bacilli in the lesions. The mechanisms responsible for the defective cell-mediated immunity in lepromatous leprosy patients are not fully known. Some studies indicate that patients with the tuberculoid form of the disease produce IFN-γ and IL-2 in lesions (suggesting T$_H$1 cell activation), whereas patients with lepromatous leprosy produce relatively more IL-4 and IL-10 (typical of T$_H$2 cells). Both the deficiency of IFN-γ and the macrophage inhibitory effects of IL-4 and IL-10 may result in weak cell-mediated immunity in lepromatous leprosy. It is also possible that the lepromatous form of the disease is due to anergy in *M. leprae*–specific T cells. As one would expect, intradermal injection of IFN-γ has a beneficial effect on the skin lesions of lepromatous leprosy.

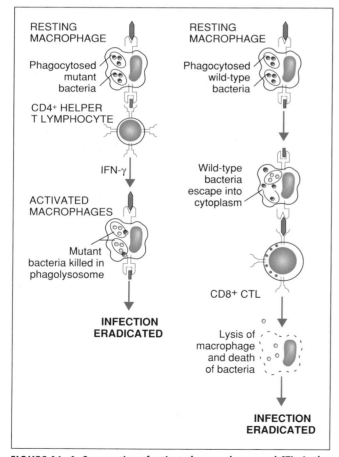

RESTING MACROPHAGE

Phagocytosed mutant bacteria

CD4$^+$ HELPER T LYMPHOCYTE

IFN-γ

ACTIVATED MACROPHAGES

Mutant bacteria killed in phagolysosome

INFECTION ERADICATED

RESTING MACROPHAGE

Phagocytosed wild-type bacteria

Wild-type bacteria escape into cytoplasm

CD8$^+$ CTL

Lysis of macrophage and death of bacteria

INFECTION ERADICATED

FIGURE 16–4. Cooperation of activated macrophages and CTLs in the elimination of an intracellular bacterium, L. monocytogenes. *L. monocytogenes–infected macrophages may stimulate CD4$^+$ and CD8$^+$ T cells. Infection by mutant bacteria can be eradicated by macrophages activated by IFN-γ produced by CD4$^+$ T cells, but wild-type bacteria are eradicated only after the colonized macrophages are lysed by CTLs.*

BOX 16—2.   IMMUNITY TO *MYCOBACTERIUM TUBERCULOSIS*

Mycobacteria are slow-growing, aerobic, facultative intracellular bacilli whose cell walls contain high concentrations of lipids. These lipids are responsible for the acid-resistant staining of the bacteria with the red dye, carbol fuchsin, because of which these organisms are also called acid-fast bacilli (AFB). The two common human pathogens in this class of bacteria are *M. tuberculosis* and *M. leprae*; in addition, atypical mycobacteria such as *M. avium–intracellulare* cause opportunistic infections in immunodeficient hosts, e.g., AIDS patients. *M. bovis* infects cattle and may infect humans, and bacillus Calmette-Guérin (BCG) is an attenuated, nonvirulent strain of *M. bovis* that is used in Europe as a prophylactic vaccine against tuberculosis.

Tuberculosis is an example of an infection with an intracellular bacterium in which protective immunity and pathologic hypersensitivity co-exist, and the lesions are caused mainly by the host response. *M. tuberculosis* does not produce any known exotoxin or endotoxin. Infection usually occurs by the respiratory route, and is transmitted from person to person. In a primary infection, bacilli multiply slowly in the lungs and cause only mild inflammation. The infection is contained by alveolar macrophages. Over 90 per cent of infected patients remain asymptomatic, but bacteria survive in lungs and can be reactivated. By 6 to 8 weeks after infection, regional lymph nodes are involved, and CD4$^+$ T cells are activated. These T cells produce IFN-γ, which activates macrophages and enhances their ability to kill phagocytosed bacilli. TNF produced by T cells and macrophages also plays a role in local inflammation and macrophage activation, and anti-TNF antibodies inhibit mycobacterial elimination in animal models. However, *M. tuberculosis* is capable of surviving within macrophages, because components of its cell wall inhibit the fusion of lysosomes with phagocytic vacuoles. Continuing T cell activation leads to the formation of granulomas, with central necrosis, called caseous necrosis, caused by macrophage products (lysosomal enzymes, reactive oxygen species). This is a form of DTH reaction to the bacilli. It is postulated that necrosis serves to eliminate infected macrophages, and provides an anoxic environment in which the bacilli cannot divide. Thus, even the tissue injury may serve a protective function. Caseating granulomas, and the fibrosis (scarring) that accompanies granulomatous inflammation, are the principal causes of tissue pathology and clinical disease in tuberculosis. Only a minority of infected individuals (probably less than 10 percent) develop clinical symptoms. Previously infected persons show cutaneous DTH reactions to skin challenge with a bacterial antigen preparation (PPD, or tuberculin). Bacilli may survive for many years even without overt

clinical manifestations, and may be reactivated at any time. This is the reason for treating individuals who convert from PPD-negative to PPD-positive with antibiotics such as isoniazid and rifampin, even though they may have no symptoms of the disease. Tuberculosis is becoming more prevalent, in part because of the increase in AIDS and the emergence of antibiotic-resistant strains. The efficacy of BCG as a prophylactic vaccine remains controversial. This might be predictable, given that the specific immune response mediates both protection against infection and tissue injury. In rare cases, *M. tuberculosis* may cause lesions in extrapulmonary sites. In chronic tuberculosis, sustained production of TNF leads to cachexia.

Different inbred strains of mice vary in their susceptibility to infection with *M. tuberculosis* (and with other intracellular microbes, such as the protozoan *Leishmania major*). Susceptibility or resistance maps to a single gene, called the *bcg* or *lsh* gene, which is expressed in macrophages. This gene has recently been shown to be homologous to genes encoding nitrate-transport membrane proteins, raising the possibility that susceptibility is related to defective production of microbicidal nitrate derivatives such as nitric oxide. However, neither the protein product of the *bch/lsh* gene nor its function is defined as yet.

Some studies have shown that both *in vivo* and *in vitro*, *M. tuberculosis* stimulates T cells expressing the $\gamma\delta$ form of the antigen receptor. These T cells may be reacting to mycobacterial antigens that are homologous to heat shock proteins. Heat shock proteins are evolutionarily conserved, being present in prokaryotes and eukaryotes. They are induced upon exposure to many kinds of stress, including heat, depletion of oxygen, nutrients and essential ions, and exposure to free radicals. In infected cells, heat shock proteins may be produced by the stressed cells or by the bacteria. It is postulated that the response of $\gamma\delta$ T cells to these proteins is a primitive defense mechanism against some microbes. However, neither the effector function nor the physiologic significance of this T cell population is known.

Atypical mycobacteria constitute a heterogeneous group of non-tuberculous mycobacteria that are widely distributed in the animal kingdom and in nature. They frequently infect humans but rarely cause disease, and usually only in individuals with deficiencies in T cell numbers or functions. The lesions caused by these bacteria may involve diverse tissues.

M. leprae is the cause of leprosy. The nature of the T cell response, and specifically the types of cytokines produced by activated T cells, is an important determinant of the lesions and clinical course of *M. leprae* infection (see text).

Evasion of Immune Mechanisms by Intracellular Bacteria

An important mechanism for survival of intracellular bacteria is their ability to resist elimination by phagocytes. Mycobacteria do this by inhibiting phagolysosome fusion, perhaps by interfering with lysosome movement. The phenolic glycolipid of *M. leprae* functions as a scavenger of reactive oxygen species. The hemolysin produced by virulent strains of *L. monocytogenes* blocks bacterial killing in macrophages, and may also inhibit antigen presentation by infected macrophages. *Legionella pneumophila* is an intracellular bacterium that is the causative organism of Legionnaires' disease. Mutants of these bacteria that lose their ability to inhibit phagolysosome fusion also lose their virulence. The outcome of infection by these organisms often depends on whether the microbicidal mechanisms of macrophages or microbial resistance to killing gain the upper hand.

IMMUNITY TO VIRUSES

Viruses are obligatory intracellular microorganisms that replicate within cells, often using the nucleic acid and protein synthetic machineries of the host.

Many viruses enter host cells by binding to physiologically important, normal cell surface molecules. Three well-known examples are (1) human immunodeficiency virus-1 (HIV-1), which binds to the CD4 molecule on human T cells; (2) Epstein-Barr virus (EBV), which binds to the type 2 complement receptor (CD21) on human B cells; and (3) rhinovirus, the agent of the common cold, which binds to intercellular adhesion molecule (ICAM-1, or CD54) expressed on a variety of cell types, including airway epithelium.

After entering cells, viruses can cause tissue injury and disease by any of several mechanisms. Viral replication interferes with normal cellular protein synthesis and function, leading to injury to and ultimately death of the infected cell. This is one type of **cytopathic effect of viruses**, and the infection is said to be "lytic" because the infected cell is lysed. Noncytopathic viruses may cause latent infections, during which they reside in host cells and produce proteins that are foreign to the host and stimulate specific immunity. As a result, infected cells are recognized and killed by viral antigen-specific CTLs. Released viral proteins may also stimulate DTH reactions. *In these situations, cell injury is a direct consequence of physiologic immune responses to the virus.* Relatively little is known about the pathogenic mechanisms in many viral infections. Human immunodeficiency virus is discussed in Chapter 21.

Natural Immunity to Viruses

There are two principal mechanisms of natural immunity against viruses:

1. *Viral infection directly stimulates the production of type I IFN by infected cells.* Type I IFNs function to inhibit viral replication. The characteristics of the cytokine-induced "antiviral state" have been described in Chapter 12.

2. *Natural killer (NK) cells lyse a wide variety of virally infected cells.* NK cells (see Chapter 13) may be one of the principal mechanisms of immunity against viruses early in the course of infection, before specific immune responses have developed (Fig. 16–5). Type I IFN can enhance the ability of NK cells to lyse infected target cells.

In addition, complement activation and phagocytosis serve to eliminate viruses from extracellular sites and from the circulation.

Specific Immune Responses to Viruses

Immunity against viral infections is mediated by a combination of humoral and cellular immune mechanisms. *Specific antibodies are important in defense against viruses early in the course of infection.* Neutralizing antiviral antibodies bind to envelope or capsid proteins and prevent viral attachment and entry into host cells. Opsonizing antibodies may enhance phagocytic clearance of viral particles. Somewhat perversely, however, opsonizing antibodies may actually enhance the invasion of Fc receptor–bearing cells by viruses; this has been postulated to be a mechanism for HIV-1 infection of mononuclear phagocytes. Secretory immunoglobulins of the IgA isotype may be important for neutralizing viruses that enter via the respiratory or intestinal tract. Oral immunization against poliomyelitis works by inducing secretory immunity. Complement activation may also participate in antibody-mediated viral immunity, mainly by promoting phagocytosis and possibly by direct lysis of viruses with lipid envelopes.

The success of prophylactic vaccination with attenuated or killed viruses is largely related to the ability of these vaccines to stimulate specific antibody responses. The importance of humoral immunity is suggested by the observation that resistance to a particular virus, induced by either infection or vaccination, is often specific for the serologic type of the virus and seems to correlate with antibody specificity. An example of this is influenza virus, in which exposure to one serologic type does not confer resistance to other serotypes of the virus. However, several points about the role of humoral immunity in protection against viruses should be emphasized. First, antibodies may be effective against viruses before the organisms enter cells, or may block spread from cell to cell, but intracellular viruses are inaccessible to antibodies. Second, it has generally proved difficult to transfer antiviral immunity to naive animals with purified antibodies. Third, the neutralizing capacity of an antibody *in vitro* often shows little or no correlation with its protective capacity *in vivo*. Taken together, these observations suggest that although antibodies are an important component

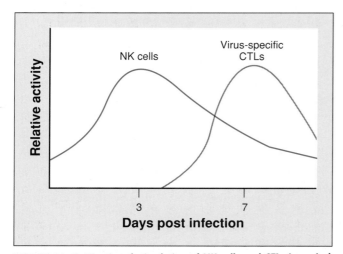

FIGURE 16–5. Kinetics of stimulation of NK cells and CTLs in a viral infection. *In an acute lymphocytic choriomeningitis virus infection of mice, NK activity in the spleen is increased prior to the development of virus-specific CTLs. Type I IFN production by spleen cells parallels NK activity. (Adapted from Welsh, R. M., H. Yang, and J. F. Bukowski. The role of interferon in the regulation of virus infections by cytotoxic lymphocytes. BioEssays 8:10–13, 1988, with permission of the publisher, ICSU Press.)*

of immunity to viruses, they may not be sufficient for eliminating many viral infections.

The principal mechanism of specific immunity against established viral infections is CTLs. The best defined virus-specific CTLs are CD8+ cells that recognize endogenously synthesized viral antigens in association with class I MHC molecules on virtually any cell type. A smaller but detectable proportion of virus-specific CTLs in humans and mice consists of CD4+ CTLs that recognize viral antigens presented in association with class II MHC molecules. CD4+ CTLs can be effective only against infected cells that express class II molecules, whereas CD8+ CTLs have a much broader range of cellular reactivity. The full differentiation of CD8+ CTLs requires cytokines produced by CD4+ helper cells, which recognize endogenously synthesized or shed viral antigens in association with class II molecules. As discussed in Chapter 13, the antiviral effects of CTLs are due to lysis of infected cells, stimulation of intracellular enzymes that degrade viral genomes, and secretion of cytokines with interferon activity.

The importance of CTLs in the outcome of viral infections has been demonstrated in many experimental systems. Mice can be protected against influenza virus by adoptive transfer of virus-specific, class I–restricted CTLs and by cloned lines of such T cells. Interestingly, a large proportion of influenza-specific CTLs are not serotype-specific because they recognize peptides derived from internal proteins (like matrix protein and nucleoprotein) rather than the envelope proteins (hemagglutinin, neuraminidase) that determine serotype. Nevertheless, as mentioned above, actively acquired immunity to influenza virus is serotype-specific. These findings support the view that both antibodies and CTLs cooperate to protect the host against viruses—the former act to block viral binding and entry into host cells, and the latter inhibit viral replication by killing infected cells.

In some infections with non-cytolytic viruses, CTLs may be responsible for tissue injury. The clearest example is lymphocytic choriomeningitis virus (LCMV) infection in mice, which induces inflammation of the spinal cord meninges. LCMV infects meningeal cells but does not injure them. It stimulates the development of specific CTLs that lyse meningeal cells during a physiologic attempt to eradicate the viral infection. T cell–deficient mice infected with LCMV become chronic carriers of the virus, but pathologic lesions do not develop; whereas in normal mice, meningitis develops. On face value, this observation appears to contradict the usual situation, in which immunodeficient individuals are more susceptible to infectious diseases than normal individuals. Hepatitis B virus infection in humans shows some similarities to murine LCMV, in that immunodeficient persons who become infected do not develop the disease, but become carriers who can transmit the infection to otherwise healthy persons. The livers of patients with acute and chronic active hepatitis contain large numbers of CD8+ T cells, and hepatitis virus–specific, class I MHC–restricted CTLs can be isolated from liver biopsies and propagated *in vitro*.

Viral infections, and immune responses to them, may be involved in producing disease in two other ways. First, a consequence of persistent infection with some viruses, such as hepatitis B, is the formation of circulating immune complexes composed of viral antigens and specific antibodies. These complexes deposit in blood vessels and lead to widespread, destructive vasculitis (see Chapter 20). Second, some viruses are known to contain amino acid sequences that are also present in some self antigens. It has been postulated that because of this "molecular mimicry" antiviral immunity can lead to immune responses against self antigens. There is, however, no proof that molecular mimicry participates in the development of any immune disease.

Evasion of Immune Mechanisms by Viruses

The intracellular persistence of viruses is the most obvious mechanism by which they can be hidden from immune effector cells and molecules. Viruses have evolved other mechanisms for evading host immunity:

1. *Many viruses are capable of great antigenic variation,* and large numbers of serologically distinct strains of these viruses have been identified. The influenza pandemics that occurred in 1918, 1957, and 1968 were all due to different strains of the virus, and subtler variants arise more frequently. As a result, the virus becomes insusceptible to immunity generated in the population by previous infections. There are so many existing serotypes of rhinovirus that specific immunization against the common cold may not be a feasible preventive strategy. HIV-1, the virus that causes AIDS, is also capable of tremendous antigenic variation (see Chapter 21). In these situations, prophylactic vaccination may have to be directed against invariant viral proteins, such as surface molecules that mediate virus entry into host cells.

2. *Viruses suppress immune responses by various mechanisms.* Some viruses may infect the cells of the immune system, impairing their function and resulting in inhibition of specific immunity. The most obvious example of this is, of course, HIV-1–induced acquired immunodeficiency syndrome (AIDS). Immune suppression has been described in infections with retroviruses, Epstein-Barr virus (EBV), measles virus, and numerous others, but the mechanisms are not well defined. One intriguing possibility has been suggested by the observation that an EBV gene is homologous to a mammalian gene that encodes the cytokine IL-10. IL-10 inhibits the accessory functions of macrophages, and the production of cytokines, including IL-1, TNF, and IL-12, by macrophages (see Chapter 12). The result is an inhibition of T_H1 responses to antigens presented by macrophages. Thus, pathogenic viruses may contain or may have acquired genes whose products inhibit antiviral immune responses.

IMMUNITY TO PARASITES

In infectious disease terminology, "parasitic infection" refers to infection with animal parasites, such as protozoa, helminths, and ectoparasites (e.g., ticks and mites). Such parasites currently account for greater morbidity and mortality than any other class of infectious organisms, particularly in developing countries. It is estimated that about 30 per cent of the world's population suffers from parasitic infestations. Malaria alone affects almost 250 million people worldwide, with about 2 million deaths annually. The magnitude of this public health problem is the principal reason for the great interest in immunity to parasites and for the development of immunoparasitology as a distinct branch of immunology.

Most parasites go through complex life cycles, part of which is in humans (or other vertebrates) and part of which is in intermediate hosts such as flies, ticks, and snails. Humans are infected usually by bites from infected intermediate hosts or by sharing a particular habitat with an intermediate host. For instance, malaria and trypanosomiasis are transmitted by insect bites, and schistosomiasis is transmitted by exposure to water in which infected snails reside.

A fundamental feature of most parasitic infections is their chronicity. There are many reasons for this, including weak natural immunity and the ability of parasites to evade or resist elimination by specific immune responses. Furthermore, many anti-parasite antibiotics are toxic and/or relatively ineffective. Individuals living in endemic areas require repeated chemotherapy because of continued exposure, and this is often not possible because of expense and logistical problems. Because of these reasons, the development of prophylactic vaccines for parasites has long been considered an important goal for developing countries. The persistence of parasites in human hosts also leads to immunologic reactions that are chronic and may result in pathologic tissue injury as well as abnormalities in immune regulation. Therefore, some of the clinicopathologic consequences of parasitic infestations are due to the host response and not the infection itself.

Natural Immunity to Parasites

Protozoan and helminthic parasites that enter the blood stream or tissues are often able to survive and replicate because they are well adapted to resisting natural host defenses. The invertebrate stages of many parasites, which are recovered from the nonhuman intermediate hosts, activate the alternative pathway of complement and are lysed by the MAC. However, parasites recovered from the vertebrate, e.g., human, host are usually resistant to lysis by complement. This may be due to many reasons, including loss of surface molecules that bind complement or the acquisition of host regulatory proteins such as decay accelerating factor (DAF). Macrophages can phagocytose protozoa, but many pathogenic organisms are resistant to phagocytic killing and may even replicate within macrophages. The tegument of helminthic parasites makes them resistant to the cytocidal mechanisms of both neutrophils and macrophages.

Specific Immune Responses to Parasites

Different protozoa and helminths vary greatly in their structural and biochemical properties. It is, therefore, not surprising that different parasites elicit quite distinct specific immune responses, which are also different from the responses to bacteria and viruses. Although virtually every type of response to parasites has been reported, the major patterns of specific immunity to protozoa and helminths are the following:

1. *Production of specific IgE antibody and eosinophilia are frequently observed in helminthic infections.* Helminths such as *Nippostrongylus,* filariae, *Ascaris,* and schistosomes induce high levels of IgE in the blood. These responses are attributed to the propensity of helminths to stimulate the T_H2 subset of $CD4^+$ helper T cells, which secrete IL-4 and IL-5. In mice infected with *Nippostrongylus brasiliensis,* the elevation in serum IgE is known to be due to IL-4 because it is blocked by injection of a neutralizing antibody specific for IL-4, and eosinophilia is due to IL-5 because it is inhibited by anti–IL-5 antibody. *In vitro* experiments suggest that IgE antibody–dependent cytotoxicity mediated by eosinophils may be effective at killing some helminths, because the major basic protein of eosinophil granules may be more toxic for helminths than the proteolytic enzymes and reactive oxygen species produced by neutrophils and macrophages. Thus, IgE antibody binds to helminths, eosinophils attach to these opsonized organisms by Fc receptors specific for IgE, the eosinophils are activated and secrete their granule contents, and the major basic protein lyses the parasites. However, a role for IgE and eosinophils in resistance *in vivo* has been established in very few helminthic infections. In fact, immunity to *Schistosoma* infection in mice is associated with activation of T_H1 cells and production of IFN-γ. *In vitro*, activated macrophages directly kill schistosome larvae through the action of nitric oxide and TNF.

2. *Some parasites and their products induce granulomatous responses with concomitant fibrosis. Schistosoma mansoni* eggs deposited in the liver stimulate $CD4^+$ T cells, which in turn activate macrophages and induce DTH reactions. This results in the formation of granulomas around the eggs. The granulomas serve to contain the schistosome eggs, but severe fibrosis associated with this chronic cell-mediated immune response leads to disruption of venous blood flow in the liver, portal hypertension, and cirrhosis. In lymphatic filariasis, the parasites lodge in lymphatic vessels, leading to chronic cell-mediated immune reactions without granulomatous inflammation and ultimately to fibrosis. This results in lymphatic obstruction and severe, chronic lymphedema.

3. *$CD4^+$ helper T cells and cytokines are involved in the resolution and exacerbation of some parasitic infections.* Perhaps the best-documented example of

this is infection of mice with *Leishmania major*, a protozoan that survives within macrophages. Resistance to the infection is associated with the production of IFN-γ and TNF by the T$_H$1 subset of CD4$^+$ T cells, whereas exacerbation of lesions is associated with stimulation of T$_H$2 cells and production of IL-4. Inbred strains of mice that are susceptible to fatal leishmaniasis produce more IL-4 in response to the infection than resistant strains, and the injection of anti–IL-4 antibody induces resistance in the susceptible strains. In contrast, resistant strains produce higher amounts of IFN-γ and TNF, and antibodies against these cytokines make the mice susceptible to the infection. IFN-γ presumably activates macrophages and enhances intracellular killing of leishmania. High levels of IL-4 (and other T$_H$2-derived cytokines) inhibit activation of macrophages by IFN-γ, and block the production of cytokines, such as TNF, by the macrophages. Such observations indicate that different parasites may stimulate unique patterns of specific T cell activation and cytokine production in different individuals. The reasons for these distinct response patterns are not well defined. Attempts to alter the outcome of these infections with cytokines or cytokine antagonists are going on in many laboratories at present.

4. *Protozoa that replicate inside cells may stimulate specific CTLs.* The CTL response to malaria is an important defense against the spread of this intracellular protozoan (Box 16–3). The poor efficacy of vaccination with malarial antigens is attributed to the inability of such immunizations to stimulate CTLs.

Specific immune responses to parasites can also contribute to tissue injury. Chronic and persistent parasitic infestations are often associated with the formation of complexes of parasite antigens and specific antibodies. The complexes can deposit in blood vessels and kidney glomeruli, producing vasculitis and nephritis, respectively (see Chapter 20). Immune complex disease has been described in schistosomiasis and malaria. Malaria infections and African trypanosomiasis are also associated with the production of autoantibodies reactive with many self tissues. The myocarditis and neuropathy seen in Chagas' disease, which is caused by *Trypanosoma cruzi*, are probably autoimmune reactions, because few or no parasites are present even in active lesions. Autoantibody production may also be secondary to polyclonal lymphocyte stimulation by the parasites (see Chapter 19). In contrast, in many cases of malaria and African trypanosomiasis, there is a severe and generalized suppression of the immune system. This may be secondary to the production of immunosuppressive cytokines by activated macrophages and/or T cells.

Evasion of Immune Mechanisms by Parasites

The ability of parasites to survive in vertebrate hosts reflects evolutionary adaptations that permit these organisms to evade or resist immune effector mechanisms. Different parasites have developed remarkably effective ways of resisting specific immunity. The most important of these fall into two categories: (1) parasites can reduce or alter their own antigenicity, and (2) they can actively inhibit host immune responses.

1. *Anatomic sequestration is commonly observed with protozoa.* Some (e.g., malaria parasites and *Toxoplasma*) survive and replicate inside cells, and others (like *Entamoeba* and *Trichinella*) develop cysts that are resistant to immune effectors. Some helminthic parasites reside in intestinal lumens and are sheltered from cell-mediated immune effector mechanisms.

2. *Antigen masking is an intriguing phenomenon in which a parasite, during its residence within a host, acquires on its surface a coat of host proteins.* The larvae of *S. mansoni* enter the skin and travel to the lungs and then into the circulation. By the time they enter the lungs, these larvae are coated with ABO blood group glycolipids and MHC molecules derived from the host. It is likely that many other host molecules attach to the surface of the schistosome larvae. It has been postulated that as a result of this coat of self proteins, parasite antigens are masked, and the organism is seen as self by the host immune system. Although this is an interesting hypothesis, the significance of antigen masking is not clear because schistosome larvae do elicit specific immunity in vertebrate hosts.

3. *Parasites become resistant to immune effector mechanisms during their residence in vertebrate hosts.* Lung stage schisotosome larvae develop a tegument that is resistant to damage by antibodies and complement or by CTLs directed against surface-bound antigens. This resistance is presumably due to a biochemical change in the surface coat. The structural complexity of the larval tegument has made it difficult to define the molecular alterations that are associated with acquired resistance. Infective forms of *T. cruzi* synthesize membrane glycoproteins similar to decay accelerating factor that inhibit complement activation. *L. major* promastigotes induce rapid breakdown or release of the membrane attack complex, thus reducing complement-mediated lysis. Parasites also evade macrophage killing by various mechanisms. *Toxoplasma gondii* inhibits phagolysosome fusion, and *T. cruzi* lyses the membranes of phagosomes and enters the cytoplasm before fusion with lysosomes can occur. Finally, some parasites express ectoenzymes that cleave bound antibody molecules and thus become resistant to antibody-dependent effector mechanisms.

4. *Parasites have developed effective mechanisms for varying their surface antigens during their life cycle in vertebrate hosts.* Two forms of antigenic variation are well defined.

a. The first is a stage-specific change in antigen expression, such that the mature tissue stages of parasites produce different antigens from the infective stages. For example, the infective sporozoite stage of malaria parasites is antigenically distinct from the merozoites that reside in the host and are responsible for chronic infection. By the time the immune system has responded to the infection, the parasite expresses

BOX 16-3.   IMMUNITY TO MALARIA

Malaria is a disease caused by a protozoan parasite (*Plasmodium*) that infects more than 250 million people and causes over two million deaths annually. Malaria, especially that caused by infection with *Plasmodium falciparum*, continues to be one of the most widespread and prevalent diseases today.

Infection is initiated when sporozoites are inoculated into the blood stream by the bite of an infected mosquito (*Anopheles*). The sporozoites rapidly disappear from the blood, in part because of phagocytic clearance by liver and spleen macrophages, and some invade the parenchymal cells of the liver. The interaction of *P. falciparum* sporozoites with hepatocytes may be mediated by an amino acid motif that is found in a region of a 44 kD coat protein called the circumsporozoite protein. In the hepatocyte, sporozoites develop into merozoites by a multiple fission process termed schizogony. One to two weeks after infection, the hepatocyte bursts, releasing thousands of merozoites, thereby initiating the erythrocytic stage of the life cycle. The merozoites invade red blood cells in an interaction that can be inhibited with certain O-linked oligosaccharides derived from glycophorin A. Merozoites develop sequentially into ring forms, trophozoites and schizonts, each of which expresses shared and unique antigens. The erythrocytic cycle continues when schizont-infected red blood cells burst and release merozoites that invade other erythrocytes. Sexual stage gametocytes develop in some cells and are taken up by mosquitoes during a blood meal, after which they fertilize and develop into oocysts. Immature sporozoites develop in the mosquitoes within 2 to 3 weeks and travel to the salivary glands, where they mature and become infective.

The clinical features of malaria caused by the four species of *Plasmodium* that infect humans include fever spikes, anemia, and splenomegaly. Many pathologic manifestations of malaria may be due to activation of T cells and macrophages and production of TNF. The development of cerebral malaria in a murine model is prevented by depletion of CD4$^+$ T lymphocytes or by injection of neutralizing anti-TNF antibody.

The immune response to malaria is complex and stage-specific, i.e., immunization with antigens derived from sporozoites, merozoites, or gametocytes protects only against the particular stage. Based on this observation, it is postulated that a vaccine consisting of combined immunogenic epitopes from each of these stages should stimulate more effective immunity than a vaccine that incorporates epitopes from only one stage. A synthetic multicomponent vaccine consisting of epitopes identified from erythrocytic and sporozoite stages has provided limited protection against *P. falciparum* infection in humans.

Vaccines effective against sporozoites are better characterized. Due to their stage-specific nature, such vaccines must provide sterilizing immunity to be effective. The protective immunity induced in humans by injection of irradiation-inactivated sporozoites is partially mediated by antibodies that inhibit sporozoite invasion of hepatoma cells *in vitro*. Such antibodies recognize the 44 kD circumsporozoite (CS) protein. The CS protein consists of an N-terminal signal sequence, a C-terminal hydrophobic membrane anchor, and a central region of about 40 tandem repeats of the sequence Asn-Ala-Asn-Pro (NANP)$_n$. This central region makes up the immunodominant B cell epitope of the CS protein, and anti-(NANP)$_n$ antibodies neutralize sporozoite infectivity. However, such antibodies provide only partial protection against infection. T cells are also important components of the immune response to sporozoites and sporozoite-infected hepatocytes. Most CS-specific T cells recognize epitopes that lie outside the NANP region, and some of these T cell epitopes correspond to the most variable residues of the CS protein. This suggests that variation or polymorphism of the antigens of the surface coat may have arisen as a result of selective pressures imposed by specific T cell responses.

CD8$^+$ T cells play a particularly important role in immunity to extra-erythrocytic stages of infection, e.g., sporozoites. If sporozoite-immunized mice are depleted of CD8$^+$ T cells by injection of anti-CD8 antibodies, they are unable to resist a challenge infection. Depletion of CD4$^+$ T cells does not abrogate resistance. However, a role for CD8$^+$ T cells in immunity to malaria has been demonstrated in some but not all inbred strains of mice, suggesting that host genetic factors influence the outcome of malaria infections. The protective effects of CD8$^+$ T cells may be mediated by direct lysis of sporozoite-infected hepatocytes or, indirectly, by the secretion of IFN-γ and activation of macrophages to produce nitric oxide and other agents that kill parasites. Resistance of *P. berghei* sporozoite–immunized mice to a challenge infection is abrogated by treatment with anti–IFN-γ antibodies. Other *P. falciparum* antigens that induce immunity include a sporozoite surface protein, CSP-2, which is unrelated to the CS protein, and a liver stage–specific antigen (LSA), which induces antibodies that block hepatocyte invasion and stimulates CTLs that react against infected hepatocytes.

Transmission blocking vaccines are being developed to act on stages of the parasite life cycle that are found in mosquitoes. Such vaccines provide no protection for the immunized individual, but act to reduce the number of parasites available for development in the mosquito vector. One such vaccine is an antigen, Pfs25, that is located on the surface of zygotes and ookinetes. These parasite stages are found only in the mosquito vector and would not be under the selective pressures imposed by specific T cell responses toward antigens found in the human intermediate host. Therefore, antigens that may be useful as transmission blocking vaccines are unlikely to show the high degree of variation that is characteristic of T cell epitopes of sporozoites.
(This Box is partly the courtesy of Dr. Peter Sayles, Trudeau Institute, Saranac Lake, NY.)

---

new antigens and is no longer a target for immune elimination.

b. The most remarkable antigenic variation in parasites is the continuous variation of major surface antigens seen in African trypanosomes such as *Trypanosoma brucei* and *Trypanosoma rhodesiense.* Infected individuals show waves of blood parasitemia, and each wave consists of one antigenically unique parasite. The same phenomenon can be reproduced in experimental animals infected with a single clone of a trypanosome (Fig. 16–6). Thus, by the time the host produces antibodies against the parasite, an antigenically different organism has replicated. Over a hundred such recrudescent waves of parasitemia can occur in an infection. The major surface antigen of African trypanosomes is a glycoprotein dimer of approximately 50 kD, called the **variable surface glycoprotein** (VSG), which is attached to the surface by a phosphatidylinositol linkage. Trypanosomes contain more than 1000 different VSG genes, which vary markedly in their se-

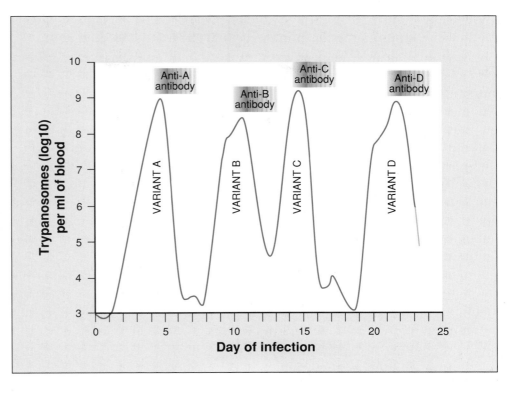

FIGURE 16–6. Parasitemia following trypanosome infections. *In a mouse infected experimentally with a single clone of* Trypanosoma rhodesiense, *the blood parasite counts show cyclical waves. Each wave is due to a new antigenic variant of the parasite (labeled A, B, C, and D) that expresses a new VSG, and each decline is a result of a specific antibody response to the variant. The durations of peak antibody production as shown are approximate. Similar waves of parasitemia are seen in natural infections in humans. (Courtesy of Dr. John Mansfield, University of Wisconsin, Madison.)*

quences except for the most C-terminal 50 amino acids (which are responsible for the surface linkage). Any one VSG gene is expressed in a particular clone at a particular stage of infection. Expression of a new gene may involve duplication and transposition of that gene to a more telomeric chromosomal site at which active transcription ensues (Fig. 16–7). In addition, gene conversion and activation of previously silent genes may also contribute to antigenic variation. Continuous antigenic variation in trypanosomes is neither induced by nor dependent on the specific antibody response and is probably due to a programmed variation in the expression of VSG genes. The molecular mechanisms that regulate this phenomenon are the focus of active investigation in many laboratories. One consequence of antigenic variation in parasites is that it is difficult to effectively vaccinate individuals against these infections.

5. *Parasites shed their antigenic coats, either spontaneously or after the binding of specific antibodies.* Examples of active membrane turnover and loss of surface antigens have been described with *Entamoeba histolytica*, schistosome larvae, and trypanosomes. Shedding of antigens and bound antibodies renders the parasites relatively resistant to immune effector mechanisms.

6. *Parasites alter host immune responses by multiple mechanisms.* Specific anergy to parasite antigens has been described in severe schistosomiasis involving the liver and spleen and in filarial infections. The mechanisms of immunologic unresponsiveness in these patients are not well understood. In lymphatic filariasis, infection of lymph nodes with subsequent architectural disruption may contribute to deficient immunity. More

nonspecific and generalized immunosuppression, e.g., in systemic leishmaniasis, has been mentioned earlier. It has been variously attributed to abnormalities in cytokine production, deficient T cell activation, immunosuppressive macrophages, and "suppressor cells." Better structural definition of parasite antigens and analysis of specific lymphocyte responses are now being done by many research groups.

The worldwide implications of parasitic infestations for health and economic development are well appreciated. Attempts to develop effective vaccines against these infections have been actively pursued for many years (Box 16–4). Although the progress has been slower than one would have hoped, elucidation of the fundamental mechanisms of immune responses to and immune evasion by parasites holds great promise for the future.

SUMMARY

The interaction of the immune system with infectious organisms is a dynamic interplay of host mechanisms aimed at eliminating infections and microbial strategies designed to permit survival in the face of powerful effector mechanisms. Different types of infectious agents stimulate distinct patterns of immune responses and have evolved unique mechanisms for evading specific immunity.

The principal protective immune response against extracellular bacteria consists of specific antibodies, which opsonize the bacteria for phagocytosis and activate the complement system. Toxins produced by such

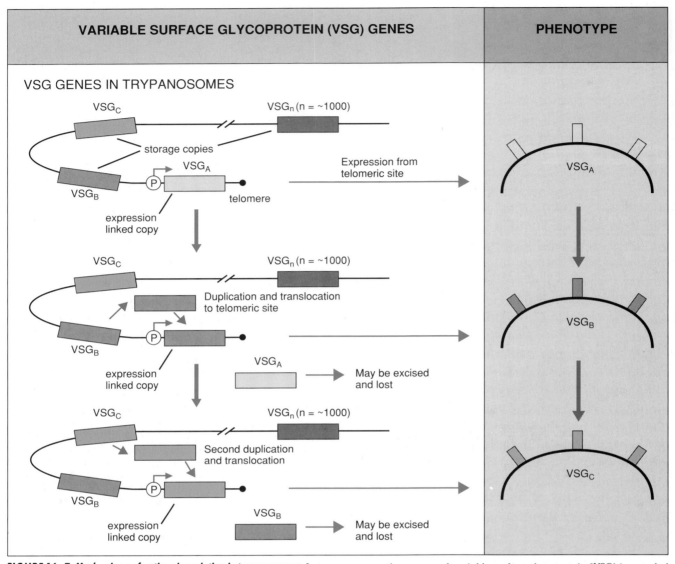

FIGURE 16–7. Mechanisms of antigenic variation in trypanosomes. *In trypanosomes, the expressed variable surface glycoprotein (VSG) is encoded by a gene located close to the telomere. Another VSG gene may be duplicated and translocated to this telomeric expression site, generating a new VSG. The fate of the previously expressed VSG gene is not known, but it may be excised and lost (as shown).* (P), *promoter.*

bacteria are also neutralized and eliminated by specific antibodies. Some bacterial toxins are powerful inducers of cytokine production, and cytokines account for much of the systemic pathology associated with severe, disseminated infections with these microbes.

Intracellular bacteria are capable of surviving and replicating within host cells, including phagocytes, because they have developed mechanisms for resisting lysosomal degradation. Immunity against these microbes is principally cell-mediated and consists of CD4$^+$ T cells activating macrophages (as in delayed type hypersensitivity) as well as CD8$^+$ cytolytic T lymphocytes. The characteristic pathologic response to infection by intracellular bacteria is granulomatous inflammation.

Viruses are obligatory intracellular microbes. Natural immunity against viruses is mediated by type I interferons and NK cells. Specific antibodies protect against viruses early in the course of infection. However, the major defense mechanism against established infections consists of specific CTLs. CTLs effectively lyse infected cells and may contribute to tissue injury even when the infectious virus is not cytopathic by itself.

Animal parasites, such as protozoa and helminths, give rise to chronic and persistent infections, because natural immunity against them is weak and because parasites have evolved multiple mechanisms for evading and resisting specific immunity. The structural and antigenic diversity of pathogenic parasites is reflected in the heterogeneity of the specific immune responses they elicit. Different parasites induce specific IgE antibodies and eosinophilia, granulomatous inflammation, cytokine production, and specific CTLs. Parasites evade the immune system by masking and shedding their surface antigens and by varying their antigens during resi-

BOX 16–4. STRATEGIES FOR VACCINE DEVELOPMENT

The birth of immunology as a science may be dated from Edward Jenner's successful vaccination against smallpox, which was reported in 1798. The importance of prophylactic immunization against infectious diseases is best illustrated by the fact that worldwide programs of vaccination have led to the complete or near complete eradication of many of these diseases in developed countries. Smallpox and polio are perhaps the two most impressive examples. The development of effective vaccines against viruses, bacteria, and parasites remains an important goal of immunologists worldwide.

The aim of all vaccination is to induce specific immunity that prevents microbial invasion, eliminates microbes that enter hosts, and neutralizes microbial toxins. Since effective vaccination as a public health measure requires long-lasting immunity, the ability of vaccines to stimulate memory T and B lymphocytes is an important consideration in vaccine design. The success of active immunization in eradicating infectious disease is dependent on numerous factors. For instance, infections that are limited to human hosts and are caused by poorly infectious agents whose antigens are relatively invariant are more likely to be controlled by vaccination. On the other hand, antigenic variation, the existence of animal or environmental reservoirs of infection, and high infectivity of microbes make it less likely that vaccination alone will eradicate a particular infectious disease.

Many types of infectious agents and their products have been used as vaccines.

ATTENUATED AND INACTIVATED BACTERIAL AND VIRAL VACCINES.

Live, attenuated bacteria were first shown by Louis Pasteur to confer specific immunity. Among the attenuated bacterial vaccines in use today are *Mycobacterium tuberculosis* bacille Calmette-Guérin (BCG), avirulent mutants of *Salmonella typhi*, inactivated *Vibrio cholerae*, and inactivated *Bordetella pertussis*. Many of these vaccines induce limited protection and are effective for relatively short periods. Live, attenuated viral vaccines are generally much more effective. The most frequently used approach for producing such vaccines is to derive attenuated viruses from long-term cell culture. More recently, temperature-sensitive and deletion mutants are being generated with the same goal in mind. Polio, measles, and yellow fever are three examples of effective attenuated viral vaccines. Inactivated viruses are also used as vaccines, e.g., in influenza, rabies, and Japanese encephalitis. Viral vaccines often induce long-lasting specific immunity, so that immunization of children is sufficient for life-long protection.

PURIFIED ANTIGEN (SUBUNIT) VACCINES.

One effective use of purified antigens as vaccines is for the prevention of diseases caused by bacterial toxins. Toxins can be rendered harmless without loss of immunogenicity, and such "toxoids" induce strong antibody responses. Diphtheria and tetanus are two infections that have been largely controlled because of immunization of children with toxoid preparations. Vaccines composed of bacterial polysaccharide antigens are used against pneumococcus and *Haemophilus influenzae*. They are effective in high-risk individuals, but they induce short-lived protection because polysaccharide antigens are inefficient at stimulating the development of memory cells. Subunit vaccines composed of purified peptides have been used for hepatitis B and influenza viruses and are in clinical trials for *Bordetella pertussis* and cholera.

SYNTHETIC ANTIGEN VACCINES.

Early approaches for developing synthetic antigens as vaccines relied on the synthesis of linear and branched polymers of three to ten amino acids based on the known sequences of microbial antigens. Such peptides are weakly immunogenic by themselves and need to be coupled to large proteins to induce antibody responses. This is much like generating antibody responses to hapten-carrier conjugates (see Chapter 9).

Two advances have revolutionized the development of synthetic peptide vaccines. First, it is now possible to deduce the protein sequences of microbial antigens from nucleotide sequence data and to prepare large quantities of proteins by recombinant DNA technology. Second, by testing overlapping peptides and by mutational analysis, it is possible to identify epitopes or even individual residues that are recognized by B or T cells or that bind to MHC molecules for presentation to MHC-restricted T lymphocytes. Empirical trial of peptides containing single or multiple amino acid substitutions has led to the construction of antigens with enhanced binding to MHC molecules or enhanced capacity to activate T cells. To date, such studies have been done largely in inbred mice. Because T cell antigen recognition is influenced by the polymorphism of MHC molecules, it is likely that in outbred human populations it will be much more difficult to "custom design" peptides with enhanced immunogenicity. Nevertheless, there is great potential in this approach for creating at will vaccines that are of high potency. Using recombinant DNA technology, synthetic peptide vaccines have been produced that correspond to immunogenic epitopes of hepatitis B virus, herpes simplex virus, and foot-and-mouth disease virus (a major pathogen for livestock). The same method is being explored in many other infectious diseases.

LIVE VIRAL VECTORS.

Perhaps the most exciting new approach to vaccine development is to introduce genes encoding microbial antigens into a nonpathogenic virus and infect individuals with this virus. Thus, the virus serves as a source of the antigen in the inoculated individual. This technique has been used most commonly with vaccinia virus vectors. The gene encoding the desired antigen is inserted by a process of homologous recombination into the vaccinia virus genome at the site of the nonessential viral thymidine kinase gene. Thymidine kinase–negative recombinant viruses are selected in culture medium containing bromodeoxyuridine (which kills all cells that produce thymidine kinase). At least 25,000 base pairs (bp) of foreign DNA can be inserted into the viral genome, and the upper limit of the size of the foreign gene may be much greater. With this method, recombinant vaccinia viruses producing hepatitis B surface antigen, herpes simplex virus proteins, influenza virus hemagglutinin and neuraminidase, malaria circumsporozoite protein, and many other microbial antigens have been generated. Inoculation of recombinant viruses into many species of animals induces both humoral and cell-mediated immunity against the antigen produced by the foreign gene (and, of course, against vaccinia virus antigens as well). Attempts are under way to improve the construction and efficiency of expression of viral vectors, to reduce the pathogenicity of the vaccinia virus, to enhance the immunogenicity of the expressed antigen, and to incorporate adjuvants or use delivery systems to maximize vaccine potency. Such live recombinant viruses have not been used in human trials to date because of safety concerns, but their enormous potential is undisputed.

PASSIVE IMMUNIZATION.

Finally, protective immunity can also be conferred by **passive immunization**, e.g., by transfer of specific antibodies. In the clinical situation, this is most commonly used for diseases caused by toxins, such as tetanus. Antibodies against snake venoms can be life-saving treatments for poisonous snake bites. Passive immunity is short-lived, because the host does not respond to the immunization and protection lasts only as long as the injected antibody persists. Moreover, passive immunization does not induce specific memory, so that the immunized individual is not protected against subsequent exposures to the toxin or microbe.

dence in vertebrate hosts. In addition, various parasites cause specific and generalized suppression of lymphocyte activation. The chronicity of parasitic infestations often leads to secondary immunopathologic consequences, including the formation of immune complexes and the development of autoimmunity.

SELECTED READINGS

Bloom, B. R., R. L. Modlin, and P. Salgame. Stigma variations: observations on suppressor T cells and leprosy. Annual Review of Immunology 10:453–488, 1992.

Dannenberg, A. H. Delayed-type hypersensitivity and cell-mediated immunity in the pathogenesis of tuberculosis. Immunology Today 12:228–233, 1991.

Doherty, P. C., W. Allan, P. Eichelberger, and S. R. Carding. Roles of $\alpha\beta$ and $\gamma\delta$ T cell subsets in viral immunity. Annual Review of Immunology 10:123–151, 1992.

Herman, A., J. W. Kappler, P. Marrack, and A. M. Pullen. Superantigens: mechanisms of T-cell stimulation and role in immune responses. Annual Review of Immunology 9:745–772, 1991.

Joiner, K. A. Complement evasion by bacteria and parasites. Annual Review of Microbiology 42:201–230, 1988.

Kaufman, S. H. E. Immunity to intracellular bacteria. Annual Review of Immunology 11:129–163, 1993.

Mahmoud, A. A. F. Parasitic protozoa and helminths: biological and immunological challenges. Science 246:1015–1022, 1989.

Morrison, D. C., and J. L. Ryan. Endotoxins and disease mechanisms. Annual Review of Medicine 38:417–432, 1987.

Nardin, E. H., and R. S. Nussenzweig. T cell responses to pre-erythrocytic stages of malaria: role in protection and vaccine development against pre-erythrocytic stages. Annual Review of Immunology 11:687–727, 1993.

Sher, A. Vaccination against parasites: special problems imposed by the adaptation of parasitic organisms to the host immune response. In P. T. Englund and A. Sher (eds.). The Biology of Parasitism: A Molecular and Immunologic Approach. Alan R. Liss, New York, 1988.

Sher, A., and R. L. Coffman. Regulation of immunity to parasites by T cells and T cell–derived cytokines. Annual Review of Immunology 10:385–409, 1992.

CHAPTER SEVENTEEN

IMMUNE RESPONSES

TO TISSUE

TRANSPLANTS

Transplantation is the process of taking cells, tissues, or organs, called a **graft**, from one individual and placing them into a (usually) different individual. The individual who provides the graft is referred to as the **donor**, and the individual who receives the graft is referred to as either the **recipient** or the **host**. If the graft is placed into its normal anatomic location, the procedure is called **orthotopic transplantation**; if the graft is placed in a different site, the procedure is called **heterotopic transplantation**. Transfusion is transplantation of circulating blood cells and/or plasma from one individual to another.

Although attempts at transplantation date back to ancient times, the impetus behind modern transplantation was World War II and the Battle of Britain. Royal Air Force pilots were often severely burned when their planes crashed. The mortality associated with burns corresponds to the size of the area of skin that has been injured, and survival can be improved if burned skin is replaced. For this reason, British doctors turned to skin transplantation from other human donors as a mode of therapy. However, attempts to replace damaged skin with skin from unrelated donors were uniformly unsuccessful. Over a matter of several days, the transplanted skin would undergo necrosis and fall off. This problem led many investigators, including Peter Medawar, to study skin transplantation in animal models. These experiments established that the failure of skin grafting was caused by an inflammatory reaction that was called **rejection**. More importantly, several features indicated that *rejection is a form of specific immunity*. The key experimental results may be summarized as follows (Table 17-1):

1. A skin graft transplanted between genetically unrelated individuals, e.g., from a strain A mouse to a strain B mouse, is rejected by a naive host in 7 to 10 days. This process is called **first set rejection** and is due to a primary immune response to the graft. A subsequent skin graft transplanted from the same donor to the same recipient is rejected more rapidly, i.e., in only 2 or 3 days. This accelerated response, called **second set rejection**, is due to a secondary immune response. Thus, genetically disparate grafts induce immunologic memory, one of the cardinal features of acquired immunity.

2. Second set rejection ensues if the first and second skin grafts are derived from the same donor or from genetically identical donors, e.g., strain A mice.

However, if the second graft is derived from an individual unrelated to the donor of the first graft, e.g., strain C, there is no second set rejection; the new graft elicits only a first set rejection. Thus, the phenomenon of second set rejection shows specificity, another cardinal feature of acquired immunity.

3. The ability to mount second set rejection against a graft from strain A mice can be adoptively transferred to a naive strain B recipient by immunocompetent lymphocytes taken from a strain B animal previously exposed to a graft from strain A mice. This experiment demonstrated that second set rejection is mediated by sensitized lymphocytes and provided the definitive evidence that rejection is a form of acquired immunity.

Transplant immunologists have developed a vocabulary to describe the kinds of cells and tissues encountered in the transplant setting. A graft transplanted from one individual to the same individual is called an **autologous graft** (shortened to **autograft**). A graft transplanted between two genetically identical or syngeneic individuals is called a **syngeneic graft** (or **syngraft**). A graft transplanted between two genetically different individuals of the same species is called an **allogeneic graft** (or **allograft**). A graft transplanted between individuals of different species is called a **xenogeneic graft** (or **xenograft**). The molecules that are recognized as foreign on allografts are called **alloantigens,** and those on xenografts are called **xenoantigens.** The lymphocytes or antibodies that react with alloantigens or xenoantigens are described as being **alloreactive** or **xenoreactive**, respectively.

Most of this chapter focuses on allogeneic transplantation because it is far more commonly practiced and better understood than xenogeneic transplantation, which is discussed briefly near the end of the chapter. We will consider both the basic immunology and some aspects of the clinical practice of transplantation. Transplantation of organs such as kidney, heart, lung, and liver is currently in widespread use, and the practice is growing. In addition, the transplantation of many other organs is now being attempted. The immunology of transplantation is important for two reasons. First, the immunologic rejection response is one of the major barriers to transplantation today. Second, although the encounter with alloantigens is unlikely in the normal life of an organism, the immune response to allogeneic molecules is very strong and has therefore

TABLE 17-1. First Set and Second Set Allograft Rejection

| Animal | Skin Graft Donor | Recipient | | Rejection |
		Strain	*Prior Treatment*	
1	Strain A	Strain B	None	Slow (first set)
2	Strain A	Strain B	Sensitized by previous graft from strain A donor	Rapid (second set); demonstration of immunologic memory
3	Strain A	Strain B	Injected with lymphocytes from animal No. 1	Rapid (second set); demonstration of role of lymphocytes in graft rejection
4	Strain C	Strain B	Sensitized by previous graft from strain A donor	Slow (first set); demonstration of immunologic specificity

been a useful model for elucidating the mechanisms of lymphocyte activation.

TRANSPLANTATION IMMUNOLOGY

The immune response to alloantigens can be either cell-mediated or humoral. In general, cell-mediated immune reactions are more important for rejection of transplanted organs, but antibodies may contribute. Most studies of the immune responses to tissue transplants have focused on T cell responses to allogeneic molecules. Three major questions are addressed by these studies:

1. What antigens in grafts stimulate alloreactivity?
2. What types of lymphocytes respond to transplants?
3. Why do individuals react so strongly against tissues that they do not encounter normally?

Molecular Basis of Allogeneic Recognition

In Chapter 5, we presented evidence that recognition of transplanted cells as self or foreign is determined by inheritance of co-dominant genes. This conclusion was based on the results of experimental transplantation between inbred strains of mice.

1. Cells or organs transplanted between individuals of the same inbred strain of mice are never rejected.
2. Cells or organs transplanted between individuals of different inbred strains of mice are almost always rejected.
3. The offspring of a mating between two different inbred strains will never reject grafts from either parent. In other words, an (A × B)F1 animal will not reject grafts from an A or B strain animal.
4. A graft derived from the offspring of a mating between two different inbred strains will almost always be rejected by either parent. In other words, a graft from an (A × B)F1 animal will be rejected by either an A or a B strain animal.

These genetic experiments led to the hypothesis that certain polymorphic gene products, co-dominantly expressed on a graft, are recognized by the immune system to identify a graft as self or foreign. Co-dominant expression means that an (A × B)F1 animal expresses both A strain and B strain alleles. This is why an (A × B)F1 animal is tolerant to both A and B strain grafts and why both A and B strain animals will recognize an (A × B)F1 graft as foreign. As described in Chapter 5, George Snell and colleagues were able to identify about 40 polymorphic genes that served as the molecular targets of rejection in mice. Specifically, they found that polymorphic molecules encoded by genes in histocompatibility locus 2 (H-2), now known as the

mouse major histocompatibility complex (MHC), were responsible for almost all strong (rapid) rejection reactions. *As many as 2 per cent of a host's T cells are capable of recognizing and responding to a single foreign MHC molecule.* This high frequency of T cells reactive with allogeneic MHC molecules is the reason why allograft rejection is a strong response *in vivo*.

At the time of these initial discoveries, immunologists were faced with two puzzles: (1) why do various cells express molecules that evoke such powerful responses from allogeneic T cells, and (2) why are so many T cells capable of recognizing alloantigens? As discussed in Chapters 5 and 6, the answer to the first question is that *MHC molecules are widely expressed because they play a critical role in the normal immune system,* namely the presentation of peptides derived from foreign protein antigens in a form that can be recognized by T cells. The role of MHC molecules as alloantigens is incidental. The answer to the second question is that *recognition of foreign MHC molecules is a cross-reaction of a normal T cell receptor that was selected to recognize self MHC plus foreign peptide.* Three kinds of experiments support this conclusion:

1. A T cell clone or hybridoma that contains one set of functionally rearranged T cell receptor (TCR) genes specific for self MHC plus a foreign peptide may also recognize one or more foreign MHC molecules in the absence of the specific foreign peptide.
2. Monoclonal antibodies reactive with idiotypic determinants on the TCR molecule of such a T cell clone or hybridoma may inhibit recognition of both self MHC–associated foreign peptide and foreign MHC molecules.
3. Transfection of rearranged α and β T cell receptor genes into a recipient T cell confers specificity both for self MHC plus foreign peptide and for foreign MHC molecules.

Because in these *in vitro* systems exogenously added foreign peptides were not necessary for allorecognition, the results initially seemed to support the conclusion that bound peptide does not contribute to the determinant formed by a foreign MHC molecule. However, it is now apparent that MHC molecules expressed on cell surfaces normally contain bound peptides. Even in artificial systems, such as lipid bilayers containing purified foreign MHC molecules, peptides remain associated with the MHC molecules through purification. Moreover, some alloreactive T cell clones have now been shown to be specific for foreign MHC plus a particular bound peptide. The peptides recognized in association with foreign MHC molecules may be self peptides because thymic education does not produce tolerance to self proteins plus foreign MHC.

It may seem surprising that many more mature T cells recognize a particular foreign MHC molecule than recognize a specific foreign peptide. The explanation of this phenomenon lies in a molecular analysis of the bases of alloantigen recognition (Fig. 17–1). The three-dimensional determinant recognized by a TCR includes amino acid residues present in the α-helices of the MHC molecule that form the sides of the peptide-binding

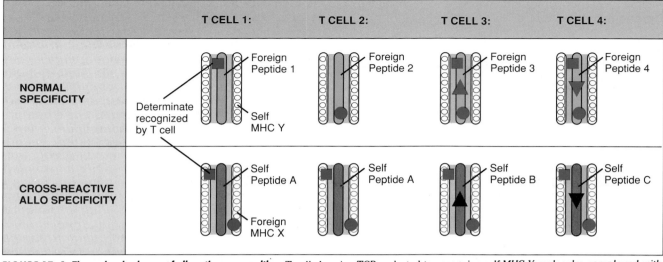

FIGURE 17–1. The molecular bases of alloantigen recognition. *T cells bearing TCRs selected to recognize self MHC Y molecules complexed with foreign peptides (1–4) may cross-react with foreign MHC X molecules complexed with self peptides (A–C). In this example, T cells 1 and 2, specific for amino acid residue determinants ■ and ● on foreign peptides 1 and 2, respectively, cross-react with the same determinants formed by polymorphic amino acids of the foreign MHC molecule. The amino acid determinants recognized by T cells 3 and 4 on foreign peptides 3 and 4 are formed by amino acid side chains contributed by both the foreign MHC molecule and bound self peptides B and C.*

cleft as well as amino acid residues in the bound peptide. As a consequence of thymic selectin, the TCR repertoire is poised to detect small differences between foreign peptides bound to self MHC molecules and self peptides bound to self MHC molecules. In the normal (autologous) situation, these differences arise entirely from amino acid residues of the foreign peptide. In the allogeneic situation, differences may be contributed by either the foreign MHC molecule, or the bound peptide, or both. The large numbers of TCRs that cross-react with each foreign MHC allelic molecule may be attributed to three factors.

1. *Foreign MHC molecules differ from self MHC molecules at multiple amino acid residues, each of which individually or in combination may produce a determinant recognized by a different cross-reactive T cell clone.* Thus, each foreign MHC molecule is recognized by multiple clones of T cells whose receptors are specific for different foreign peptides in association with self MHC molecules. For example, foreign MHC molecule X (with some bound self peptide A) may be recognized by T cell 1, which is specific for self MHC molecule Y plus foreign peptide 1, and by T cell 2, which is specific for self MHC molecule Y plus foreign peptide 2 (Fig. 17–1, T cells 1 and 2).

2. *Multiple bound peptides, in combination with one foreign MHC gene product, may produce determinants recognized by different cross-reactive T cells.* Any single foreign MHC molecule can bind only one peptide at a time, but on each foreign cell surface, there are many copies of each foreign MHC molecule, and each copy can form a complex with a different peptide. Each different complex may be recognized by a different T cell. For example, T cell 3, which is specific for self MHC Y plus foreign peptide 3, may recognize foreign MHC X plus self peptide B, whereas T cell 4, which is specific

for self MHC Y plus foreign peptide 4, may recognize foreign MHC X plus self peptide C (Fig. 17–1, T cells 3 and 4). In this example, peptides B and C could also be foreign peptides. The key point is that *self peptides can contribute to T cell recognition when bound to foreign MHC molecules because the TCRs that recognize determinants formed by foreign MHC plus self peptides were not eliminated during negative selection in the thymus.* Because many different self peptides form determinants with foreign MHC molecules that are recognized by different T cell clones, each allogeneic cell may be recognized by many different T cell clones, each with a distinct specificity for a different foreign peptide. This is the principal reason for the high frequency of alloreactive T cells.

3. *Allodeterminants may be expressed on foreign antigen-presenting cell (APC) surfaces at higher densities than are determinants formed by specific foreign peptides bound to self MHC molecules on self APC surfaces.* This is clearly true for allogeneic determinants that are formed wholly by the foreign MHC molecule since a specific foreign peptide probably never occupies more than 1 per cent of the total MHC molecules expressed by an APC. The high density of these allogeneic determinants on foreign APCs may allow activation of T cells with low specificity for the determinant, increasing the numbers of T cells that can respond.

Polymorphic alloantigens other than MHC molecules generally produce weak or slower (more gradual) rejection reactions and are called minor histocompatibility antigens. Most minor histocompatibility antigens are proteins that are processed and presented to host T cells in association with either self MHC or graft MHC molecules. In contrast, foreign MHC molecules can be recognized directly by host T cells without any requirement for processing or association with self MHC molecules.

Cellular Basis of Allogeneic Recognition

Vigorous rejection reactions of allografts generally result from recognition of the transplanted tissues by both CD4$^+$ and CD8$^+$ T cells. The **mixed leukocyte reaction** (MLR) has been a useful model for understanding the cellular basis of alloantigen recognition by different T cell subpopulations.

THE MIXED LEUKOCYTE REACTION

As we have discussed above, MHC genes were initially identified for their role in graft rejection, which is often a T cell–mediated process. The MLR is an *in vitro* model of T cell recognition of foreign MHC gene products and is used as a predictive test of cell-mediated graft rejection.

The MLR is induced by culturing mononuclear leukocytes (which include T cells, B cells, natural killer [NK] cells, mononuclear phagocytes, and dendritic cells), from one individual or inbred strain with mononuclear leukocytes derived from another individual or strain. In humans, these cells are typically isolated from peripheral blood; in the mouse or rat, mononuclear leukocytes are usually purified from spleen or lymph nodes. If there are differences in the alleles of the MHC genes between the two individuals, a large proportion of the mononuclear cells will proliferate over a period of 4 to 7 days. This proliferative response, usually measured by incorporation of ^{3}H-thymidine into DNA during cell replication, is called the **allogeneic MLR** (Fig. 17–2). In the experiment described above, the cells from each donor react and proliferate against the other, resulting in a "two-way MLR." To simplify the analysis, one of the two mononuclear leukocyte populations can be rendered incapable of proliferation, either by gamma irradiation or by treatment with mitomycin C, an antimitotic drug, prior to culture. In this "one-way MLR," the treated cells serve exclusively as **stimulators** and the untreated cells, still capable of proliferation, serve as the **responders**.

Two populations of alloreactive T cells are stimulated during an allogeneic MLR, and each responding T cell subset recognizes a different MHC gene product. One type of T cell expresses the CD8 but not the CD4 molecule, usually functions as a cytolytic T lymphocyte (CTL), and is indistinguishable from self class I MHC–restricted CTLs specific for foreign protein antigens. The CTLs generated during an allogeneic MLR lyse target cells derived from the same individual or strain as the original stimulator cell population. The molecules on stimulator and target cells that are recognized by CD8$^+$ CTLs are the class I MHC molecules, namely, HLA-A, -B, or -C in humans or H-2K, -D, or -L in mice. Several lines of evidence have indicated that foreign class I MHC gene products are the actual molecular targets recognized by the CD8$^+$ CTLs generated in the MLR:

1. If there are no differences in class I MHC alleles

between the stimulator and responder cell populations in the MLR, CD8$^+$ CTLs are not generated.

2. The CTLs generated against one stimulator cell population will lyse third-party target cells only if these targets share a class I MHC allele with the original stimulators.

3. Antibodies directed against class I MHC allelic gene products on the stimulator cells protect target cells against lysis.

4. Transfection and expression of an allelic class I MHC gene can render a cell susceptible to lysis by a CTL population specific for that allele.

The full differentiation of CTLs in the MLR requires stimulation by class I MHC molecules as well as help that is optimally provided by CD4$^+$ T cells present in the same culture (see Chapter 13).

Within the CD8$^+$ CTL population derived from an MLR, each individual CTL is specific for only one particular class I MHC gene product (usually involving a specific bound peptide). However, the bulk population contains CTLs directed against all class I MHC allelic differences between the original stimulator and responder populations. Furthermore, in an outbred individual, all the class I MHC alleles inherited from both parents are co-dominantly expressed on every class I–expressing cell, so that an individual target cell can be lysed by several different CTLs, each with a different class I MHC specificity.

The second type of T cell that is generated during the MLR was initially called a primed responder cell, because when such T cells are recultured with stimulator cells from the same donor individual (or strain) used in the original MLR, a secondary MLR ensues that is stronger and more rapid; i.e., peak proliferation occurs by 2 or 3 days. It is now appreciated that primed responder cells are cytokine-producing CD4$^+$ helper T cells, indistinguishable from CD4$^+$ helper T cells specific for foreign protein antigens. Alloreactive CD4$^+$ helper T cells are specific for allogeneic class II MHC molecules, i.e., HLA-DR, -DP, and -DQ in humans and I-A and I-E in mice. The class II MHC molecules have been established as the molecules seen by the CD4$^+$ helper cells by the same kind of evidence that established the class I MHC molecules as the targets of CD8$^+$ CTLs.

1. Alloreactive CD4$^+$ T cells are stimulated only if there are differences in class II MHC alleles between the original stimulator and responder cells in the primary MLR.

2. Alloreactive CD4$^+$ T cells respond to third-party stimulator cells only if they share class II MHC alleles with the original stimulator population.

3. Antibodies directed against class II MHC gene products prevent development of the secondary MLR.

4. Transfection of appropriate allelic class II MHC genes can convert a cell from a non-stimulator to a stimulator of a CD4$^+$ T cell population specific for that MHC allele.

Alloreactive CD4$^+$ T cells, like self MHC–restricted antigen-specific helper cells, can be stimulated only by cells that express class II MHC molecules associated

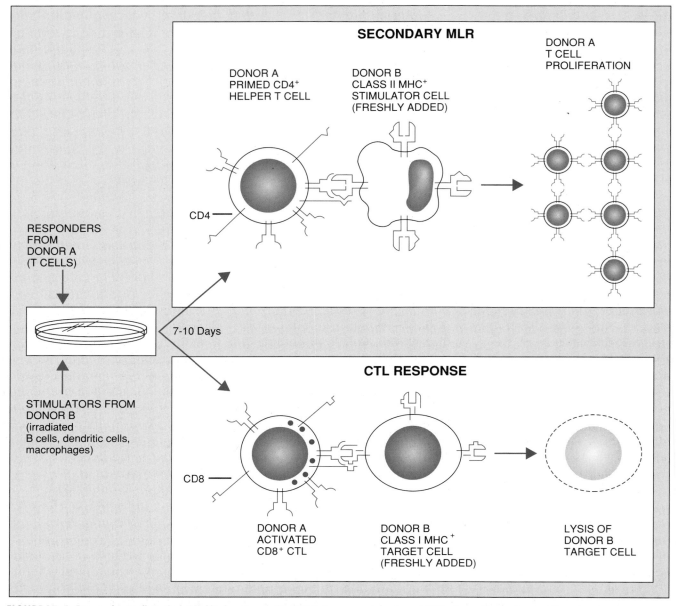

FIGURE 17–2. Responder T cells in the mixed leukocyte reaction (MLR). *In a one-way primary MLR, donor B stimulator cells activate and cause the expansion of two types of donor A responder T cells: CD4+ helper T cells, which can be detected in a secondary MLR by rapid proliferation to antigen-presenting cells (APCs) bearing donor B class II molecules; and CD8+ cytolytic T lymphocytes (CTLs), which can be detected in a specific killing assay using target cells bearing donor B class I molecules.*

with specific peptides and provide costimulatory signals. The most efficient stimulators are dendritic cells, although B lymphocytes, mononuclear phagocytes, and, in humans, vascular endothelial cells are also able to stimulate proliferative responses of alloreactive CD4+ T cells. Each individual CD4+ helper T cell is specific for one particular class II gene product (usually with a specific bound peptide). However, the bulk population contains helper cells reactive with all class II allelic differences between the original stimulator and helper cell population (and with many different peptides bound to each allelic MHC product). Furthermore,

since there is no allelic exclusion of class II genes on individual cells and all the parental alleles are co-dominantly expressed, one stimulator cell can activate several different helper T cells, each with a different class II MHC specificity.

The functional subdivision of CD4+ and CD8+ alloreactive T cells into helper cells and CTLs is not absolute. CD4+ class II specific CTLs can be detected in the MLR, particularly in humans. Moreover, at least some CD8+ T cells produce interleukin-2 (IL-2), interferon-γ (IFN-γ), tumor necrosis factor (TNF), and lymphotoxin (LT), which is similar to the cytokine profile of many

TABLE 17–2. Induction of Mixed Leukocyte Reaction by Class I and Class II Major Histocompatibility Complex (MHC) Mismatches

MHC Differences Between Stimulator and Responder Cells			Induction of	
Class I	Class II	Proliferation	Cytokine-Producing T Cells	CTLs
Yes	Yes	++++	++++ (CD4$^+$, class II–specific)	++++ (CD8$^+$, class I–specific)
Yes	No	+	+ (CD8$^+$, class I–specific)	+++ (CD8$^+$, class I–specific)
No	Yes	+++	+++ (CD4$^+$, class II–specific)	+ (CD4$^+$, class II–specific)

In a one-way MLR between stimulator and responder cells that differ at class I or class II MHC loci or both, the predominant phenotype (CD4$^+$ or CD8$^+$) and MHC specificity (class II or class I) of the cytokine-producing T cells and CTLs are different.

Abbreviations: CTL, cytolytic T lymphocyte; MLR, mixed leukocyte reactions.

CD4$^+$ cells. As discussed in Chapters 6 and 7, the same exceptions have been found for self MHC–restricted T cells specific for foreign protein antigens.

A more specific analysis of the role of class I and class II molecules in allogeneic immune responses has been performed by considering the one-way MLR when only isolated class I or class II differences exist between the stimulator and responder cell populations (Table 17–2). In the extreme case, this has been done by using cells from mouse strains that differ only by a small mutation in a single class I or class II gene product. Proliferation is strongest when stimulators and responders differ by a class II gene product and can directly stimulate CD4$^+$ T cells. Fewer CTLs arise in this instance, and many of these are CD4$^+$ class II–specific CTLs. When only class I differences exist between stimulator and responder cells, the proliferative response is small. Nevertheless, there is a proliferative response, and CD8$^+$ CTLs specific for the class I difference do arise. In this situation, proliferation and the development of CTLs may be mediated by cytokines produced by the CD8$^+$ T cells themselves responding to the foreign class I molecules. Alternatively, if class II MHC$^+$ accessory cells are present, they may take up, process, and present foreign class I molecules in the form of peptides associated with self class II molecules. In this setting, the foreign class I molecules behave like other foreign protein antigens that are recognized by CD4$^+$ T cells present in the responder population. This process, called **indirect presentation**, is far less efficient than direct presentation of foreign class II molecules. Therefore, stimulator cell populations that differ from the responders at both the class I and class II MHC loci induce many more allospecific CTLs than stimulators that differ at only class I loci.

The contributions of both class I and class II MHC molecules to the allogeneic response are the reason why graft survival improves when both class I and class II alleles are matched between donor and recipient.

Two additional points about the MLR should be noted:

1. *The MLR is the only* in vitro, *antigen-specific response of T cells that can be readily observed without prior immunization* in vivo. This is because T cells reactive with allogeneic MHC molecules are much more numerous in an unstimulated population than are the T cells specific for any single foreign protein antigen. In addition, an allogeneic stimulator cell may express a large number of foreign MHC molecules that are capable of stimulating alloreactive T cells. In contrast, on an APC that normally presents a foreign peptide antigen, a minor fraction of the MHC molecules may be complexed with the specific peptide. As a result, many more alloreactive than foreign antigen–specific, self MHC–restricted T cells are stimulated by such APCs.

2. Although the MLR is initiated by allogeneic stimulation, the majority of helper T cells and CTLs that proliferate in the primary MLR are actually not specific for the allogeneic MHC gene products on the stimulator cells. Rather, they are driven to proliferate by growth factors, such as IL-2, produced by a small number of specifically stimulated alloreactive cells. However, the specifically stimulated alloreactive cells preferentially increase in number, compared with any other T cell, and thus become the only cells sufficiently numerous to be detectable as CTLs or primed helper cells after the primary MLR.

STIMULATION OF ALLOREACTIVE T CELLS *IN VIVO*

In the case of allografts that differ from hosts at both class I and class II loci, both CD8$^+$ and CD4$^+$ T cells are activated by recognition of alloantigens of the grafts. CD8$^+$ cells recognize foreign class I MHC molecules, which are expressed by all the cells in the graft. The differentiation of these CTLs is largely dependent on CD4$^+$ T cells being stimulated by allogeneic class II molecules present on APCs in the allograft. Therefore, one can predict that tissue allografts that stimulate strong rejection contain class II–bearing APCs. It has more recently been appreciated that some CD8⁺ T cells can also provide sufficient help to allow CTLs to differentiate independent of CD4⁺ T cells. However, these CD8⁺ T cells appear to depend on the same professional APCs as those required by CD4⁺ T cells. The most important APCs stimulating an antigraft response may be dendritic cells resident in the interstitium of the graft. The key feature of these APCs is the presence of costimulators that contribute to the activation of CD8⁺ as well as CD4⁺ T cells.

The importance of professional APCs in stimulating an alloantigenic immune response *in vivo* has most clearly been demonstrated by experiments in rodents. If class II–bearing cells (which include professional APCs) are removed from a graft prior to transplantation, such grafts are usually rejected slowly or may even be accepted despite class I MHC differences. (Experimentally, APCs may be eliminated from such grafts by several treatments, including prolonged culture; treatment with anti–class II antibody plus complement; or, in some cases, extensive perfusion of graft blood vessels to "wash out" the APCs.) When rat kidney allografts are purged of APCs by perfusion, infusion of dendritic cells derived from the organ donor concomitant with transplantation restores allorecognition and leads to rapid rejection. These observations have led to several conclusions, collectively described as the **passenger leukocyte hypothesis**.

1. To stimulate a rejection reaction, host CD4⁺ helper T cells are activated by foreign cells that express allogeneic class II molecules and provide costimulators. The CD4⁺ T cells then stimulate the growth and differentiation of alloreactive CD8⁺ CTLs. Alternatively, these CD8⁺ T cells may be directly activated by foreign APCs, resulting in the production of cytokines that stimulate autocrine growth and differentiation into CTLs.

2. The cells that provide costimulatory functions are professional APCs and are usually present as "passenger leukocytes" carried along with the graft.

3. Elimination of passenger leukocytes reduces the incidence and severity of rejection by reducing the activation of T cells.

Although the role of passenger leukocytes is well documented in rodents, attempts to remove such cells have not been useful in human transplantation. The probable explanation is that human, but not rodent, endothelial cells provide costimulator functions, activate alloreactive T cells, and are sufficient to initiate rejection, even in the absence of passenger leukocytes.

In contrast to T cell alloreactivity, much less is known about the mechanisms that lead to the production of alloantibodies against foreign MHC molecules. Presumably, B cells specific for alloantigens are stimulated by mechanisms similar to those involved in stimulation of B cells reactive with other foreign proteins.

Before we conclude this section of the chapter, we should point out that many of the issues that arise in discussions of alloreactivity and graft rejection are also relevant to maternal-fetal interactions. The fetus expresses paternal MHC molecules and is therefore semiallogeneic to the mother. Nevertheless, the fetus is not rejected by the maternal immune system. Many possible mechanisms have been proposed to account for this, and it is not yet clear which of these mechanisms are the most significant (Box 17–1).

Effector Mechanisms in Allograft Rejection

So far, we have described the molecular basis of allogeneic recognition and the cells involved in the recognition of, and responses to, allografts. We now turn to a consideration of the effector mechanisms used by the immune system to reject allografts. In different experimental models, alloreactive CD4⁺ or CD8⁺ T cells or specific alloantibodies are all capable of mediating allograft rejection upon adoptive transfer. Furthermore, graft rejection can be inhibited by anti-CD4 or anti-CD8 antibodies. These different immune effectors cause graft rejection by different mechanisms.

1. Alloreactive T cells can recruit and activate macrophages, initiating graft injury by a delayed type hypersensitivity response (see Chapter 13).
2. Alloreactive CTLs directly lyse graft endothelial and parenchymal cells.
3. Alloantibodies bind to endothelium, activate the complement system, and injure graft blood vessels.

For historical reasons, graft rejection is usually classified on the basis of histopathology rather than on immune effector mechanisms. Based on the experience of renal transplantation, the histopathologic pattern is called hyperacute, acute, or chronic.

The names of the various forms of rejection imply a temporal sequence of events, but this is not strictly true. Although hyperacute rejection is always a very rapid process immediately following transplantation, acute and chronic rejection can occur at almost any time after transplantation. Indeed, acute and chronic rejection often co-exist in the same graft. Histology, rather than the length of time following transplantation, is the major criterion for classifying rejection reactions. However, in the current era of renal transplantation, in many centers biopsies are performed less frequently than in the past, and diagnosis is often made on the basis of clinical features and post-transplantation time without histologic confirmation.

HYPERACUTE REJECTION

Hyperacute rejection is characterized by rapid thrombotic occlusion of the graft vasculature that begins within minutes after host blood vessels are anastomosed to graft vessels (Fig. 17–3). Thrombosis occurs prior to the development of inflammation. *Hyperacute rejection is mediated by pre-existing antibodies that bind to endothelium and activate complement.* Antibody and complement induce a number of changes in the graft endothelium that promote intravascular thrombosis. The endothelial cells are stimulated to se-

BOX 17-1.   IMMUNITY TO AN ALLOGENEIC FETUS

The mammalian fetus, except in instances in which the mother and father are syngeneic, will express paternally inherited antigens that are allogeneic to the mother. Nevertheless, fetuses are not normally rejected by the mother. An understanding of how the fetus escapes the maternal immune system may be relevant for transplantation.

Three experimental observations indicate that the anatomic location of the fetus is a critical factor in the absence of rejection:

1. Wholly allogeneic fetal blastocysts that lack maternal genes can successfully develop in a pregnant or pseudopregnant mother. Thus, neither specific maternal nor paternal genes are necessary for survival of the fetus.

2. Hyperimmunization of the mother with cells bearing paternal antigens does not compromise placental and fetal growth.

3. Pregnant mothers are able to recognize and reject allografts syngeneic to the fetus placed at extrauterine sites without compromising fetal survival.

The failure to reject the fetus has focused attention on the region of physical contact between the mother and fetus. The fetal tissues of the placenta that most intimately contact the mother may be classified as vascular trophoblast, which is exposed to maternal blood for purposes of mediating nutrient exchange, and **implantation site trophoblast**, which diffusely infiltrates the uterine lining (decidua) for purposes of anchoring the placenta to the mother.

One simple explanation for fetal survival is that trophoblast cells fail to express paternal major histocompatibility complex (MHC) molecules. So far, class II molecules have not been detected on trophoblast. In mice, cells of implantation trophoblast, but not vascular trophoblast, do express paternal class I molecules. In humans, the situation may be more complex, in that trophoblast cells may express only a nonpolymorphic class I–like molecule. However, even if these cells do express classical MHC molecules, they may lack costimulator molecules and fail to act as antigen presenting cells.

A second explanation for lack of rejection is that the uterine decidua may be an immunologically privileged site that is not accessible to functional T cells. In support of this idea is the observation that mouse decidua is highly susceptible to infection by *Listeria monocytogenes* and cannot support a delayed type hypersensitivity response. The basis of immunologic privilege is clearly not a simple anatomic barrier because maternal blood is in extensive contact with trophoblast. Rather, the barrier is likely to be functional inhibition. Cultured decidual cells directly inhibit macrophage and T cell functions, perhaps by producing inhibitory cytokines, such as transforming growth factor-β (see Chapter 12). Some of these inhibitory decidual cells may be resident suppressor T cells, although the evidence for this proposal is not convincing.

crete high molecular weight forms of von Willebrand factor that mediate platelet adhesion and aggregation. Both endothelial cells and platelets undergo membrane vesiculation, leading to shedding of lipid particles that promote coagulation. Endothelial cells lose their cell surface heparan sulfate proteoglycans that normally interact with anti-thrombin III to inhibit coagulation. Complement activation also leads to endothelial cell injury and exposure of subendothelial basement membrane proteins that activate platelets. These processes contribute to thrombosis and vascular occlusion, and the organ suffers irreversible ischemic damage.

In the early days of transplantation, hyperacute rejection was often mediated by pre-existing IgM antibodies which were present at high titer prior to any exposure to alloantigens. Such "natural antibodies" are believed to arise in response to carbohydrate antigens expressed by the bacteria that normally colonize the bowel. The best known examples of such antibodies are those directed against the ABO blood group antigens expressed on red blood cells (Box 17–2). ABO antigens are also expressed on vascular endothelial cells. Today, hyperacute rejection by anti-ABO antibodies is not a clinical problem, because all graft donors and recipients are selected so that they have the same ABO type. However, hyperacute rejection caused by less well-characterized natural antibodies has become the major barrier to xenotransplantation, limiting the use of animal organs for human transplantation.

In more recent clinical experience, hyperacute rejection of allografts is usually mediated by antibodies directed against protein alloantigens, such as foreign MHC molecules, or against less well-described alloantigens expressed on vascular endothelial cells. Such antibodies generally arise as a result of prior exposure to alloantigens through blood transfusion, prior transplantation, or multiple pregnancies. These alloantibodies are often of the IgG isotype. By testing recipients for the presence of such antibodies reactive with the cells of potential donors, hyperacute rejection has been virtually eliminated from clinical transplantation.

ACUTE REJECTION

ACUTE VASCULAR REJECTION. Acute vascular rejection is characterized by necrosis of individual cells of the graft blood vessels. The histologic pattern is one of vasculitis (Fig. 17–4) rather than of the bland thrombotic occlusion seen in hyperacute rejection. *Acute vascular rejection is often mediated by IgG antibodies against endothelial cell alloantigens (either MHC molecules or other antigens) and involves activation of complement.* In addition, T cells contribute to vascular injury by responding to alloantigens present on vascular endothelial cells, leading to direct lysis of these cells, or the production of cytokines that recruit and activate inflammatory cells, causing endothelial necrosis.

ACUTE CELLULAR REJECTION. This type of rejection is characterized by necrosis of parenchymal cells and is usually accompanied by lymphocyte and macrophage infiltrates (Fig. 17–5). These infiltrating leukocytes are responsible for the lysis of the graft parenchymal cells.

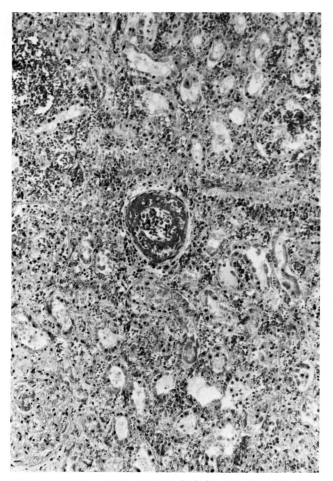

FIGURE 17–3. Hyperacute rejection in the kidney. *Pre-formed antibodies reactive with vascular endothelium of a kidney allograft activate complement and trigger rapid intravascular thrombosis and necrosis of the vessel wall, often preceding the development of an inflammatory reaction. (Courtesy of Dr. Helmut Rennke, Department of Pathology, Brigham and Women's Hospital, Boston.)*

Several different effector mechanisms may be involved in acute cellular rejection including CTL-mediated lysis, activated macrophage–mediated lysis (as in delayed type hypersensitivity [DTH]), and natural killer (NK) cell–mediated lysis (see Chapter 13). Several lines of evidence suggest that recognition and lysis of foreign cells by alloreactive CD8$^+$ CTLs is probably the most important mechanism of acute cellular rejection. First, the cellular infiltrates present in grafts undergoing acute cellular rejection are markedly enriched for CD8$^+$ CTLs specific for graft alloantigens. Second, cloned lines of alloreactive CD8$^+$ CTLs can be used to adoptively transfer acute cellular graft rejection. And third, most vascular and parenchymal cells express class I MHC molecules and are susceptible to lysis by CD8$^+$ CTLs but are usually resistant to killing by activated macrophages and NK cells.

The identification of both antibody and CTLs as important effector mechanisms in acute graft rejection suggests that this process is similar to normal antiviral immune responses (see Chapter 16). The basis of this similarity probably arises from the fact that the foreign class I MHC molecules present in the graft are recognized as if they were self MHC molecules associated with endogenously synthesized foreign (e.g., viral) peptides.

CHRONIC REJECTION

Chronic rejection is characterized by fibrosis with loss of normal organ structures (Fig. 17–6). The pathogenesis of chronic rejection is less well understood than is that of acute rejection. The fibrosis of chronic rejection may represent wound healing following the cellular necrosis of acute rejection. However, in many instances, chronic rejection develops without evidence that acute rejection ever occurred. Two other possible explanations of the fibrosis are that chronic rejection represents a form of chronic DTH in which activated macrophages secrete mesenchymal cell growth factors, such as platelet-derived growth factor or, alternatively, that chronic rejection is a response to chronic ischemia caused by injury to blood vessels. Vascular injury could result from repeated bouts of antibody-mediated

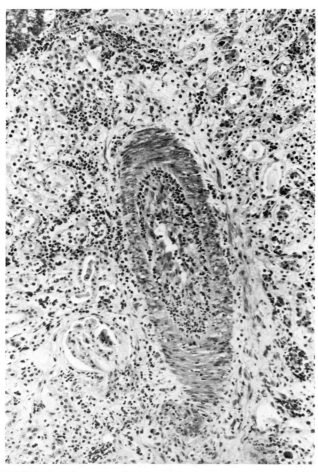

FIGURE 17–4. Acute vascular rejection in the kidney. *Antibodies reactive with graft endothelial cells arise in a transplant recipient and cause a destructive inflammatory reaction in the vessel wall. T lymphocytes reactive with graft alloantigens may also participate in vascular injury. (Courtesy of Dr. Helmut Rennke, Department of Pathology, Brigham and Women's Hospital, Boston.)*

BOX 17–2.   ABO BLOOD GROUP ANTIGENS

The first alloantigen system to be defined was a family of red blood cell surface antigens called ABO. Differences in the ABO system between donors and recipients limit blood transfusions by causing antibody and complement-dependent lysis of the foreign red blood cells (transfusion reactions). IgM antibodies to these red blood cell antigens pre-exist in a naive host prior to transfusion, and it has been speculated that they arise as responses to cross-reactive microbial antigens. The red blood cell antigen responsible for these transfusion reactions is expressed as a cell surface glycosphingolipid. All normal individuals synthesize a common core glycan, called the O antigen, that is attached to a sphingholipid. A single genetic locus encodes three common alleles of a glycosyl transferase enzyme. The O allele gene product is devoid of enzymatic activity, whereas the A allele gene product transfers a terminal *N*-acetylgalactosamine moiety and the B allele gene product transfers a terminal galactose moiety. Individuals who are homozygous O cannot attach terminal sugars to the O antigen and express only the O antigen. In contrast, individuals who possess an A allele (AA homozygotes, AO heterozygotes, or AB heterozygotes) form the A antigen by adding terminal *N*-acetylgalactosamine to some of their O antigens. Similarly, individuals who express a B allele (BB homozygotes, BO heterozygotes, or AB heterozygotes) form the B antigen by adding terminal galactose to some of their O antigens. AB heterozygotes form both A and B antigens from some of their O antigens. Because all individuals express the O antigen, all individuals are tolerant to the O antigen. Individuals with A or B glycosyltransferase alleles are also tolerant to A or B antigens, respectively.

However, OO and AO individuals form anti-B IgM antibodies, whereas OO and BO individuals form anti-A IgM antibodies. If a patient receives a transfusion of red blood cells from a donor who expresses a form of the antigen not expressed on self red blood cells, massive red cell lysis will result. It follows that AB individuals can tolerate transfusions from all potential donors and are therefore called **universal recipients**; similarly, OO individuals can tolerate transfusions only from OO donors but can provide blood to all recipients and are therefore called **universal donors**. The terminology has been simplified so that OO individuals are said to be blood type O; AA and AO individuals are blood type A; BB and BO individuals are blood type B; and AB individuals are blood type AB.

The same glycosphingolipid that carries the ABO determinants can be modified by other glycosyltransferases to generate minor blood group antigens that elicit milder transfusion reactions. In general, differences in minor blood groups lead to red cell lysis only after repeated transfusions produce a secondary antibody response. Almost all individuals possess a fucosyl transferase that adds a fucose moiety to a side branch of the ABO glycosphingolipid. After fucosylation, the O antigen is technically called the H antigen, and the whole antigenic system is often called ABH rather than ABO. Addition of fucose moieties at other side branch positions can be catalyzed by different fucosyl transferases and results in epitopes of the Lewis antigen system. Lewis antigens have received much recent attention from immunologists because these carbohydrate groups serve as ligands for E-selectin and P-selectin.

---

acute humoral rejection, or it may result from cell-mediated injury of microvascular endothelial cells.

More commonly, however, vascular occlusion is due to proliferation of intimal smooth muscle cells, called **accelerated** or **graft arteriosclerosis**, that may occur without overt vascular injury (Fig. 17–7). This lesion has been described in renal and cardiac transplants. It may develop within a few months after transplantation and is the major cause of late graft failure. The smooth muscle cell proliferation in the vascular intima may represent a specialized form of chronic DTH, in which lymphocytes activated by alloantigens in the graft vessel wall induce macrophages to secrete smooth muscle cell growth factors. The risk of developing graft arteriosclerosis is increased in patients with cytomegalovirus infection (see below), suggesting that viral antigens may also contribute to the immune reaction. This model is similar to that proposed for chronic rejection as a form of chronic DTH, except that in the vessel wall, smooth muscle cells rather than fibroblasts proliferate and produce collagen.

Prevention and Treatment of Allograft Rejection

If the recipient of an allograft has a fully functional immune system, transplantation almost invariably results in some form of rejection. Two approaches have

been used in clinical practice and in experimental models to avoid or delay rejection:

1. *The graft recipient's immune system may be suppressed.* Immunosuppression is the major approach to prevention and management of transplant rejection. Several methods of immunosuppression are commonly used.

a. *T cells may be inhibited or lysed by various immunosuppressive treatments. Immunosuppressive drugs are the principal treatment regimen for graft rejection.* Commonly used immunosuppressive therapies include corticosteroids; metabolic toxins, such as azathioprine and cyclophosphamide; irradiation of lymphoid organs; specific immunosuppressive drugs, the prototype of which is cyclosporin A (also known as cyclosporine); and antibodies reactive with T cell surface molecules.

Corticosteroids have two proposed mechanisms of action. First, they may cause selective lysis of T cells. Corticosteroids are known to cause lysis of immature cortical thymocytes as well as certain T cell lines by activating endogenous nucleases that cleave DNA. However, corticosteroids do not lyse mature medullary thymocytes or mature T cells isolated from blood or peripheral lymphoid organs. A second and more likely proposed mechanism is that corticosteroids act by blocking cytokine gene transcription in and cytokine secretion from mononuclear phagocytes. Inhibition of IL-1, IL-6 and TNF synthesis by corticosteroids has

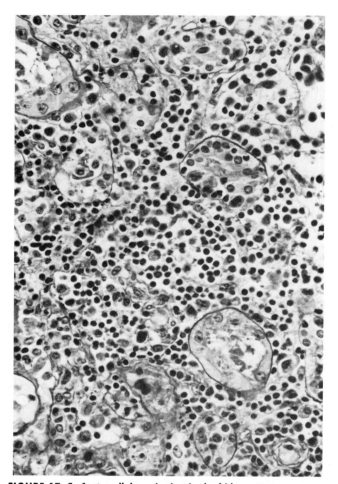

FIGURE 17–5. Acute cellular rejection in the kidney. *T lymphocytes reactive with alloantigens in a kidney graft mediate necrosis of tubular epithelial cells as well as of interstitial cells and microvascular endothelial cells. (Courtesy of Dr. Helmut Rennke, Department of Pathology, Brigham and Women's Hospital, Boston.)*

been demonstrated both *in vitro* and *in vivo*. Lack of IL-1 and TNF will limit the development of inflammatory reactions. Corticosteroids may also impair IL-2 production by antigen-activated T cells, but this effect may not occur at the doses commonly used in immunosuppressive therapy.

The metabolic toxins in clinical use, namely azathioprine and cyclophosphamide, inhibit the growth of lymphocytes (and other leukocytes) from hematopoietic precursors and may cause preferential lysis of T cells. Irradiation was similarly used as an immunosuppressive agent because T cells are radiosensitive.

The most important immunosuppressive agent in current clinical use is cyclosporin A. Cyclosporin A is a cyclic peptide that is a natural metabolite in a species of fungus. The major action of cyclosporin A on T cells is to inhibit transcription of certain genes, most notably the IL-2 gene. Cyclosporin A binds with high affinity to a ubiquitous small molecular size (approximately 12 kD) cellular protein called cyclophilin. As we discussed in Chapter 7 (see Box 7–5), the complex of cyclosporin A and cyclophilin, but not either component alone, binds

to and inhibits the enzymatic activity of the calcium/calmodulin–activated protein phosphatase, calcineurin. Since calcium/calmodulin–activated calcineurin function is required to activate the cytoplasmic component of the transcription factor NFAT, cyclosporin A blocks NFAT activation and the transcription of IL-2 and other cytokine genes. The net result of this action is that *cyclosporin A blocks the IL-2–dependent growth and differentiation of T cells.*

The introduction of cyclosporin A into clinical practice opened the modern era of transplantation. Prior to the use of cyclosporin A, the majority of transplanted hearts and livers were rejected. Nevertheless, cyclosporin A is not a panacea for transplantation. Drug levels needed for optimal immunosuppression cause kidney damage. For this reason, there was much excitement about a recently characterized fungal metabolite called FK506. FK506 is structurally unrelated to cyclosporin A, but the complex of FK506 and its binding protein (called FKBP) share with the cyclosporin A–cyclophilin complex the ability to bind calcineurin and inhibit its action. Another recently introduced immuno-

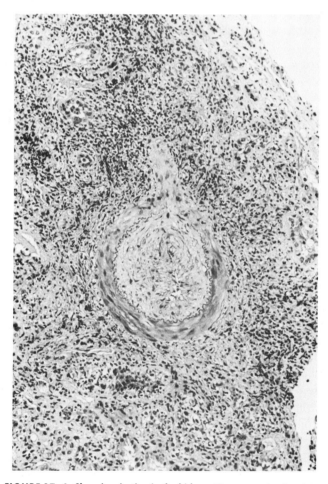

FIGURE 17–6. Chronic rejection in the kidney. *The normal cells of the renal interstitium and tubules are replaced by fibrous tissue. As described in the text, this reaction may represent healing of acute rejection, chronic delayed type hypersensitivity to graft alloantigens, or chronic ischemia. (Courtesy of Dr. Helmut Rennke, Department of Pathology, Brigham and Women's Hospital, Boston.)*

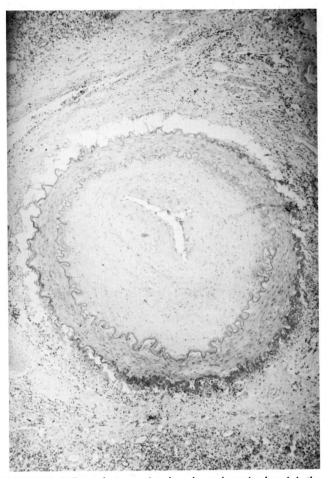

FIGURE 17–7. Transplant-associated accelerated arteriosclerosis in the kidney. In this variant of chronic rejection, the vascular lumen is replaced by accumulation of smooth muscle cells and connective tissue in the vessel intima.

suppressive agent is the antibiotic rapamycin. Rapamycin binds to FKBP and competes with FK506 for binding. Surprisingly, the rapamycin-FKBP complex does not inhibit calcineurin. The principal effect of rapamycin is to block T cell growth in response to IL-2. Combinations of cyclosporin A (which blocks IL-2 synthesis) and rapamycin (which blocks IL-2–driven proliferation) are particularly potent inhibitors of T cell responses.

Antibodies reactive with T cell surface structures are important agents for treating acute rejection episodes. In the 1960s, commonly used agents for this purpose were polyclonal horse antisera reactive with human lymphocytes or thymocytes. Since the 1980s, mouse monoclonal antibodies to specific T cell surface markers have been more commonly used. The most widely used antibody is OKT3, the first anti-CD3 antibody. It may seem surprising that one would use a potential polyclonal activator such as anti-CD3 to reduce T cell reactivity. *In vivo*, however, OKT3 either acts as a lytic antibody, activating the complement system to eliminate T cells, or opsonizes T cells for phagocytosis. T cells that escape probably do so by capping and endocytosing ("modulating") CD3 off their surface, but these may be rendered transiently nonfunctional.

Newer antibodies are being tested for immunosuppressive effects without causing T cell elimination. For example, antibodies to the α subunit of the IL-2 receptor are in clinical trial because these antibodies can prevent T cell activation by blocking IL-2 binding to activated T cells. Other antibodies in clinical trial block T cell adhesion molecules, such as LFA-1 or VLA-4, or their endothelial cell ligands, such as ICAM-1 and VCAM-1, respectively. These antibodies prevent T cells from homing into the allograft. The major limitation on the use of mouse monoclonal antibodies is that human recipients rapidly develop anti–mouse Ig antibodies that eliminate the injected mouse Ig. For this reason, attempts are being made to produce human monoclonal antibodies or human-mouse chimeric antibodies that may be less immunogenic.

b. *B cells may be inhibited and pre-formed antibodies, such as those that mediate hyperacute rejection, can be removed.* Several new immunosuppressive agents, such as rapamycin, brequinar, and 15-deoxyspergualin, effectively inhibit antibody synthesis. However, since pre-formed antibodies can persist in the plasma for days to weeks, use of these agents may be preceded by plasmaphoresis to remove antibodies and other plasma proteins. In allogeneic transplantation, these modalities are reserved for patients with high levels of pre-formed antibodies against a wide variety of donor alloantigens.

c. *The graft recipient may be made tolerant to the allograft.* The original strategy for inducing tolerance was based on the observation that patients who received multiple allogeneic blood transfusions prior to renal transplantation had a better acceptance rate of their grafts than patients who had not received transfusions. Subsequently, patients were intentionally given multiple transfusions to induce "tolerance." The mechanisms of this form of tolerance are not fully known. Several new strategies to induce tolerance (see Chapter 10) are now in pre-clinical or clinical trial. For example, recipients may be treated with high doses of peptides derived from polymorphic regions of donor MHC molecules or with soluble donor MHC molecules to induce specific T cell tolerance. Alternatively, attempts are being made to induce specific T cell clonal anergy by preventing T cells from receiving costimulatory signals during their initial encounter with graft alloantigens. In particular, soluble forms of CTLA-4 have been administered to prevent interactions of graft cell B7 molecules with host T cell CD28 (see Chapter 7). Under these circumstances, inadequate IL-2 will be produced, so that alloantigen-activated T cells should become anergic.

2. *The graft may be made less immunogenic.*

a. In human transplantation, the major strategy to reduce graft immunogenicity has been to minimize alloantigenic differences between the donor and recipient by selection. For example, to avoid hyperacute rejection, the ABO blood group antigens of the donor and recipient are always compatible. In addition, MHC molecule allelic differences are also considered at both class I and class II loci. For kidney transplantation, all potential donors and recipients are "tissue-typed" to

BOX 17-3. TISSUE TYPING

Tissue typing, also called HLA typing, is the determination of the particular MHC alleles expressed by an individual. The classical approach to tissue or HLA typing is testing whether sera collected from certain donors mediate complement-dependent lysis of an individual's lymphocytes. The sera used for this purpose are obtained from donors who have been inadvertently immunized with foreign cells bearing MHC molecules by transfusion, transplantation, or multiple pregnancies. Such sera characteristically have a low specific antibody titer and react with multiple foreign MHC molecules encoded by several loci. To determine whether an individual expresses HLA-A2, for example, lymphocytes would be tested with a panel of sera, each of which can recognize HLA-A2–bearing cells but may differ in the other specificities they recognize. Only if all of the appropriate sera react and cause lysis is the individual "typed" as HLA-A2 positive. Naturally, well-characterized human sera are in short supply. Therefore, the assays have been honed to a microscale, where 1 μl of serum plus 1 μl of complement can be tested against 50 target cells in 3 μl of solution in the bottom of a tiny well, kept from evaporating by an overlaid oil drop! In general, tissue typing is still performed this way, using standarized sera that have been tested and characterized by many different laboratories. It is hoped that conventional typing sera will be replaced by monoclonal antibodies reactive with specific HLA molecules. Unfortunately, these reagents are not yet available for most specificities.

The HLA types defined by serologic methods are not necessarily single alleles. Some common HLA types contain several different closely related alleles that may be "split" as new reagents become available that can distinguish among them. Typing with antibodies for class II alleles is especially imprecise.

Alloreactive T cells often recognize some but not all of the cells that are said to share a D-related (DR) specificity. The information from secondary mixed leukocyte reactions (MLRs) can thus be useful at splitting class II types. Interestingly, some of the T cell responses that are used to split DR types are actually directed against DQ molecules present in linkage disequilibrium with a subset of the DR molecules within a type.

Recently, two new approaches have been introduced that should permit more precise typing of the class II loci, replacing both serology and secondary MLRs. The first approach takes advantage of the fact that serologically similar MHC allelic products may be biochemically quite different and can be separated by an analytical technique, such as two-dimensional gel electrophoresis combining isoelectric focusing and sodium dodecyl sulfate–polyacrylamide gel electrophoresis (SDS-PAGE) (see Box 3–3, Chapter 3). The position of a "spot" on a two-dimensional gel can thus be used to split a serologic type. The second method is even more precise. The polymorphic residues of class II MHC molecules are largely located within exon 2 of both the α and β chains (i.e., within the $\alpha 1$ and $\beta 1$ polypeptide regions; see Chapter 5). This entire region of the gene can be amplified by **polymerase chain reaction (PCR)** methods using primers that bind to conserved sequences within the 5' and 3' ends of these exons. The amplified segment of DNA can then be readily sequenced. Thus the actual predicted amino acid sequence can be directly determined for the HLA-DR, -DQ, and -DP alleles of any cell, providing precise molecular tissue typing. Indeed, it is exactly for this purpose that the method of polymerase chain reaction was initially developed (see Chapter 5, Box 5–2).

---

determine the identity of the HLA molecules that are expressed (Box 17–3). Good matches, involving identity at three or four alleles of four HLA-A and -B loci, are favored. Matching is possible because donor kidneys can be stored in organ banks prior to transplantation until a well-matched recipient can be identified and because, with dialysis, patients needing a kidney allograft can be clinically treated until a well-matched organ is available. In the case of heart and liver transplantation, organ preservation is more difficult, and potential recipients are often in critical condition. For these reasons, HLA typing is simply not considered in pairing of potential donors and recipients.

b. In rodents, as discussed above, grafts may be made less immunogenic by elimination of passenger leukocytes, an approach that has not worked for vascularized grafts in humans and other primates. Nevertheless, depletion of professional APCs may prove useful for transplanting non-vascularized grafts, such as pancreatic islets.

CLINICAL ORGAN TRANSPLANTATION

We now turn our attention to some of the important clinical issues that have arisen in the practice of solid organ transplantation. Kidney transplants have

been successfully performed for the longest period (since the 1950s), and the renal allograft experience has formed the basis of considering transplantation of other organs. For this reason, our discussion focuses on the kidney, but refers to other organs for comparison when appropriate.

Selection of donor and recipient matches in renal transplantation is based on blood group (ABO) matching, absence of pre-formed antibodies against donor cells in the blood of the recipient (called cross-matching), and HLA typing. Analysis of the results of graft survival as a function of HLA type has led to four conclusions:

1. The larger the number of HLA-A and -B alleles that are matched between donor and recipient (e.g., three or four of four loci), the better is graft survival, especially in the first year following transplantation. (HLA-C is not routinely matched and is believed to be a less important target of T cell recognition.)

2. Matches at HLA-DR alleles are important, independent of the number of HLA-A or -B matches. Because HLA-DR and -DQ are in strong linkage disequilibrium, matching at the DR locus often also matches at the DQ locus. DP typing is not in common use, and its importance is unknown.

3. Matching is more predictive of outcome in Europe, where populations are more inbred, than in the

United States, where extensive outbreeding has probably diminished linkage disequilibrium among HLA loci.

4. The recipient HLA-DR types influence graft survival independent of the degree of matching. This effect of HLA-DR type of the recipient has been interpreted as an "immune response" gene effect, presumably because host HLA-DR molecules were involved in selecting the mature T cell repertoire. Thus, in recipients who express particular DR alleles, the T cell repertoire may not contain cells specific for some alloantigens, so that grafts bearing these antigens would fail to induce immune responses and would be accepted.

In renal transplantation, immunosuppression with corticosteroids, azathioprine, and anti–T cell antibodies was sufficient to allow survival of unrelated cadaveric donor grafts of 50 to 60 per cent at 1 year and survival of living related donor grafts of 90 per cent at one year. Since cyclosporin A was introduced, survival of unrelated cadaveric donor grafts has approached about 80 per cent.

In the early years of renal transplantation, rejection was often assessed by biopsy. In the 1970s, biopsy was used less commonly in many transplant centers, and rejection severity was usually assessed by following renal function, e.g., as measured by plasma creatinine levels. However, cyclosporin A, which is now universally used in kidney transplantation, is itself a cause of renal injury and can elevate plasma creatinine levels. Thus, a common clinical dilemma is to distinguish declining renal function caused by rejection from that caused by cyclosporin A toxicity. This distinction is usually made by histopathologic examination of biopsy specimens of the transplanted kidney. A useful distinction may be made by examining kidney cells collected by needle biopsy or fine needle aspiration biopsy with an immunocytochemical stain for class II MHC molecule expression. If renal tubular cells express HLA-DR molecules, one may infer that IFN-γ is being produced locally by activated T cells and that renal failure is likely due to rejection. If, on the other hand, HLA-DR is not expressed by tubular cells, the kidney is apparently failing in the absence of local T cell cytokine production, and the likely cause is cyclosporin A toxicity. (The functional role or consequence of class II MHC molecule expression on renal tubular cells is unknown.)

Monitoring the rejection of other transplanted organs is somewhat different. Liver allograft rejection can often be measured by assessing liver function; cyclosporin A is not as toxic to the liver, and failure of bile excretion is a good measure of rejection. Needle biopsies may be used if the clinical pattern is confusing, and expression of HLA-DR molecules by biliary epithelial cells may be indicative of rejection. In the case of heart allografts, functional impairment usually indicates that the rejection process is already quite severe and potentially irreversible. For this reason, cardiac allograft biopsies are performed on regular schedules to assess rejection regardless of cardiac function. (Such biopsy specimens are obtained through a catheter passed into the right ventricle via the venous circulation. Biopsies of the intraventricular septum may be taken with little risk to the patient, since even punctures of the septum will likely scar without sequelae.) Rejection is assessed by histologic examination evaluating myocyte necrosis and T cell infiltration. Studies are currently in progress to learn whether these histologic and functional tests may be supplemented or replaced by serologic assays of T cell activation, such as the presence of shed α subunit of the IL-2 receptor in the blood. In addition, serum can be assayed for the presence of shed endothelial cell adhesion molecules, such as ICAM-1 (see Chapter 13), that are induced by cytokines during rejection episodes.

Acute rejection, when present, is often managed by rapidly intensifying immunosuppressive therapy. This may involve a large "pulse" of corticosteroids or administration of an antibody such as OKT3. Cyclosporin A doses can also be increased. Although acute rejection can cause loss of a graft, most rejection episodes can be reversed by such therapeutic intervention. In modern transplantation, chronic rejection has become a more common cause of allograft failure, especially in cardiac transplantation. Chronic rejection is more insidious than acute rejection, and it is much less reversible. It is likely that prevention rather than treatment will be the best approach to this problem, but successful intervention will probably require a better understanding of pathogenesis.

Graft survival is dependent on adequate immunosuppression. This has introduced a clinical dilemma because transplant patients often manifest two other clinical problems caused by immunosuppressive therapy. First, they are particularly susceptible to infections, especially by viruses. Infection by cytomegalovirus, a herpes family virus, is particularly common and may be fatal in the immunosuppressed patient. As noted earlier, cytomegalovirus infection may contribute to graft arteriosclerosis and chronic rejection. Second, transplant patients have an increased proclivity to the development of certain tumors (see Chapter 18). The three malignancies commonly seen in these patients are B cell lymphomas, squamous cell carcinoma of the skin, and Kaposi's sarcoma. The B cell lymphomas are thought to be sequelae of unchecked infection by Epstein-Barr virus, another herpes family virus (see Chapter 18, Box 18–1). The squamous cell carcinomas of the skin are associated with human papilloma virus and probably also represent virally induced malignancies. Kaposi's sarcoma is now well known for its prevalence in patients with the acquired immunodeficiency syndrome (see Chapter 21) and may be yet another example of a virally induced or provoked malignancy.

In patients receiving immunosuppression for transplantation, clinical problems related to viral infection and virally induced or virally potentiated malignancies are not coincidental. The major thrust of transplant-related immunosuppression is to reduce CTL function, the key effector mechanism of acute cellular rejection. It should thus be no surprise that defense against viruses, the physiologic function of CTLs, is preferentially undermined.

Xenogeneic Transplantation

A major barrier to increased use of solid organ transplantation as a clinical therapy is the availability of donor organs. For this reason, many transplant immunologists have become interested in the possibility of transplantation of organs from other mammals, such as pigs, into human recipients. The principal obstacle to xenogeneic transplantation is the presence of natural antibodies. As discussed earlier, many individuals develop natural IgM antibodies to non-self carbohydrate determinants of the ABO blood group system. Similarly, most individuals (over 95 per cent) develop natural antibodies that are reactive with carbohydrate determinants expressed by the cells of members of species that are evolutionarily distant, such as humans and pig. Such species combinations that give rise to reactive natural antibodies are said to be **discordant**. Natural antibodies are rarely produced against carbohydrate determinants of closely related, concordant species, such as human and chimpanzee or mouse and rat. Thus, chimpanzee or other higher primates technically can and have been used as organ donors to humans. However, both ethical and logistical concerns have limited such operations. For reasons of anatomic compatibility, pigs are the preferred species for organ donation to humans. To date, the carbohydrate structures that are recognized by human natural antibodies on pig cells are not defined. Some immunologists hope that when these structures are known, transgenic pigs might be produced that express human rather than pig carbohydrate–synthesizing enzymes so that pigs will become concordant with humans.

The consequence of high titers of natural IgM antibodies on xenogeneic organ grafts are the same as were seen in ABO-incompatible human allogeneic transplantation, namely hyperacute rejection. This reaction depends on complement proteins and involves the same basic mechanisms seen in humans, namely generation of endothelial cell procoagulants and platelet-aggregating substances coupled with loss of endothelial anticoagulant mechanisms, such as heparan sulfates. A strategy under exploration for reducing hyperacute rejection is prevention or reversal of complement activation with agents such as soluble complement receptor type 1 (CR1) or decay accelerating factor, or CD59 (see Chapter 15).

Cell-mediated rejection of xenografts may occur if hyperacute rejection is avoided. Surprisingly, T cell responses to xenoantigens are often weaker than responses to alloantigens. This has been especially striking when murine responses to pig MHC molecules have been examined. There are several possible reasons for the weak responses to xenoantigens. T cells specific for foreign peptides and self MHC, which are responsible for allorecognition, may fail to cross-react with xenoantigens. Instead, xenoantigens may need to be processed and presented in association with self MHC molecules, just like any other foreign protein antigens. In addition, adhesion molecules and costimulation may be species specific, so that T cells from one species are not efficiently activated by APCs from another. It is not yet clear if human T cells will react weakly or strongly to xenoantigens from different species. Indeed, initial reports suggest that the human response to pig MHC molecules is actually stronger than the response to allogeneic human MHC molecules. Nevertheless, immunosuppressive strategies developed for allogeneic transplantation may well prove adequate for reducing xenogeneic cell-mediated rejection.

BONE MARROW TRANSPLANTATION

Bone marrow transplantation is actually the transplantation of pluripotent hematopoietic stem cells (see Chapter 2). After transplantation, these cells then repopulate the recipient's bone marrow with their differentiating progeny. Clinically, allogeneic bone marrow transplantation may be used to remedy acquired defects in the hematopoietic system or in the immune system, since both types of cells develop from a common stem cell. It has also been proposed as a means of correcting inherited enzyme deficiencies, by providing a self-renewing source of enzyme-producing cells. In addition, allogeneic bone marrow transplantation may be used as part of the treatment of bone marrow malignancies, i.e., leukemias. In this case, the chemotherapeutic agents needed to destroy leukemia cells also destroy normal marrow elements, and bone marrow transplantation is used to "rescue" the patient from the side effects of chemotherapy. For other malignancies, when the marrow is not involved by tumor or when it can be purged of tumor cells, the patient's own bone marrow may be harvested and reinfused after chemotherapy. This procedure, called autologous bone marrow transplantation, lacks the immunologic problems associated with allogeneic bone marrow transplantation and will not be discussed further.

Several unique problems that are associated with bone marrow transplantation lead us to consider it separately from solid organ transplantation:

1. The transplanted stem cells must "home" to establish themselves in the appropriate environment; surgeons cannot place the stem cells in a particular location in the bone marrow. Moreover, experimental and clinical experience suggests that there are only a limited number of "niches" within marrow cavities, and if these are occupied at the time of transplantation, the graft cells cannot establish themselves. The recipient often must be prepared with intense radiation and chemotherapy prior to transplantation to deplete his or her own marrow cells and vacate these sites.

2. Allogeneic stem cells are readily rejected by even a minimally immunocompetent host. The mechanisms of rejection are not completely known, but in addition to specific immune mechanisms, hematopoietic stem cells may also be rejected by NK cells. The recipient's immune system must be nearly ablated to permit successful bone marrow transplantation. Again, this is accomplished by intense preparation of the recipient with radiation and chemotherapy.

3. Graft cells may mount a rejection response against the host. This response, called the **graft-versus-host reaction**, can injure the host and cause graft-versus-host disease (GVHD) (see below). The graft-versus-host reaction arises only after extreme injury to the host immune system, a consequence of the preparation necessary to avoid stem cell rejection.

4. Recipients of allogeneic bone marrow transplants often show prolonged and profound immunodeficiencies. In human bone marrow transplantation, this consequence is a major cause of morbidity and mortality.

Graft-versus-Host Disease

Graft-versus-host disease is the principal limitation on the use of bone marrow transplantation. As in solid organ transplantation, GVHD may be classified on the basis of histologic patterns into acute and chronic categories.

Acute GVHD involves epithelial cell necrosis in three principal target organs: skin, liver, and the gastrointestinal tract (Fig. 17–8). In the liver, the biliary epithelial cells but not the hepatocytes are involved. Clinically, acute GVHD is characterized by skin rash, jaundice, and diarrhea. When the epithelial necrosis is

extensive, the skin or lining of the gut may simply slough off. In this circumstance, acute GVHD may be fatal.

Chronic GVHD is characterized by fibrosis and atrophy of one or more of the same organs, without evidence of acute cell necrosis (Fig. 17–8). Occasionally, necrosis and fibrosis can be present at the same time, leading to a diagnosis of acute and chronic GVHD. When severe, chronic GVHD leads to complete dysfunction of the affected organ and may also be fatal.

In animal models, acute GVHD is initiated by mature T cells present in the bone marrow inoculum. Elimination of mature donor T cells from the graft can prevent development of GVHD. Efforts to eliminate T cells from human marrow inoculum have reduced the incidence of GVHD but also appear to reduce the efficiency of engraftment; mature T cells, perhaps through production of colony-stimulating factors (CSFs), significantly improve stem cell repopulation. Since failure to engraft is even more lethal than GVHD, it is not yet clear whether the removal of T cells will be clinically beneficial. An alternative approach is to combine removal of T cells with supplemental granulocyte-macrophage colony-stimulating factor to promote engraftment.

Although GVHD is initiated by T cell recognition of host alloantigens, the effector cells that produce epi-

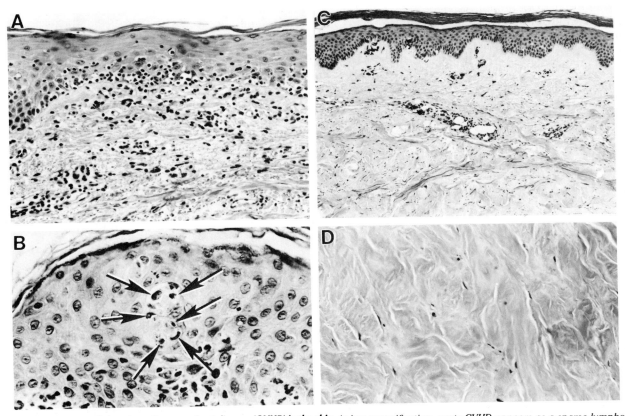

FIGURE 17–8. Acute and chronic graft-versus-host disease (GVHD) in the skin. *At low magnification, acute GVHD appears as a sparse lymphocytic infiltrate at the dermal-epidermal junction (A); at higher magnification (B), lymphocytes can be identified in the epidermis adjacent to injured epithelial cells (arrows). In contrast, chronic GVHD (C) shows fibrosis of the dermis and epidermal thinning. At higher magnification (D), dermal appendages can be seen to be trapped in the dense fibrosis. (Courtesy of Dr. George Murphy, Departments of Dermatology and Pathology, University of Pennsylvania, Philadelphia.)*

thelial cell necrosis are less well defined. Histologically, NK cells are often attached to the dying epithelial cells, suggesting that NK cells are the effector cells of acute GVHD. This hypothesis has raised the issue of how NK cells lyse normal epithelial cells, since they do not recognize alloantigens and cannot lyse epithelial cells *in vitro*. It has been proposed that the NK cells are activated by locally produced IL-2 to differentiate into lymphokine-activated killer (LAK) cells. As was discussed in Chapter 13, LAK cells can lyse normal cell types, including epithelium, and are not restricted by MHC molecules.

The relationship of chronic GVHD to acute GVHD is unknown and raises issues similar to those of relating chronic allograft rejection to acute allograft rejection. For example, chronic GVHD may represent the fibrosis of wound healing secondary to epithelial cell necrosis. However, chronic GVHD can arise without evidence of prior acute GVHD. An alternative explanation is that chronic GVHD represents a response to ischemia caused by vascular injury.

Both acute and chronic GVHD are commonly treated with intense immunosuppression. It is not clear that either condition responds very well. A possible explanation is that conventional immunosuppression is targeted against T lymphocytes, especially CTLs. This works well in allogeneic rejection of solid organs but is less efficacious for NK cell–mediated or LAK cell–mediated responses. TNF and perhaps IL-1 appear to be important mediators of acute GVHD. Agents that suppress cytokine production or antagonize cytokine action have been effective at treating GVHD in preclinical and early clinical trials. Much effort has focused on prevention of GVHD. HLA typing is very important for preventing GVHD. Indeed, most human bone marrow transplants are performed between siblings who are completely identical at all HLA loci, and clinical GVHD is due to differences at minor histocompatibility loci. Transplantation between parent and child may be performed when necessary, but only after stringent elimination of mature T cells from the marrow inoculum.

Immunodeficiency Following Bone Marrow Transplantation

As noted above, bone marrow transplantation is often accompanied by clinical immunodeficiency. Several factors may contribute to defective immune responses in recipients:

1. Bone marrow transplant recipients may be unable to regenerate a completely new T cell repertoire. The transplanted bone marrow may not contain a sufficient number and variety of self-renewing lymphoid progenitors, and the thymus gland of the recipient may have undergone irreversible changes during or after involution in early childhood.

2. The ablation of the specific immune system in preparation for bone marrow transplantation unmasks a "natural suppression" system that prevents adequate regeneration of a specific immune system. Some immunologists have referred to specific populations of natural suppressor cells, observed after whole body irradiation. Such natural suppressor cells may be identical or related in lineage to NK cells.

3. The allogeneic host environment may overwhelm the developing immune system with alloantigenic stimuli that prevent development of a normal repertoire. An alternative statement of this explanation is that the graft-versus-host reaction pre-empts normal immunity. Many immunologists regard immunodeficiency as part of GVHD. However, immunodeficiency may well exist in bone marrow transplant recipients who lack clinically overt or histologically detectable GVHD.

The consequence of immunodeficiency is that bone marrow transplant recipients are very susceptible to viral infections, especially cytomegalovirus. They are also susceptible to Epstein-Barr virus–provoked B cell lymphomas. However, the incidence of other malignancies, namely squamous cell carcinoma of the skin and Kaposi's sarcoma, has not increased as in solid organ transplant recipients. The basis for this difference is unclear.

Paradoxically, bone marrow transplant recipients also suffer from autoimmunity (see Chapter 19). Two factors may contribute to autoimmunity in the face of immunodeficiency. First, graft CD4$^+$ T cells respond to alloantigens on residual host B cells, leading to inappropriate antibody (and autoantibody) production. Second, inadequate thymic development of the repopulating T cells not only may cause deficiencies in positive selection but may also lead to defects in negative selection, allowing emergence of autoreactive T cells.

Summary

Transplantation of tissues from one individual to a genetically nonidentical recipient leads to a specific immune response, called rejection, that can destroy the graft. The major molecular targets in transplant rejection are non-self allelic forms of class I and class II MHC molecules complexed to self peptides.

The reaction to foreign class I and class II molecules can be analyzed *in vitro* in the MLR. In general, foreign class I molecules stimulate alloreactive CD8$^+$ CTLs, whereas foreign class II molecules stimulate alloreactive CD4$^+$ helper T lymphocytes, although the largest reactions occur when there are differences at both class I and class II loci.

In vivo rejection is mediated by T cells, including CTLs and helper T cells that cause DTH, and by antibodies. Alloreactive T cells may be stimulated by professional APCs, such as dendritic cells, in the graft.

Several patterns of rejection can occur in solid organ transplants. Pre-existing antibodies, often IgM directed against ABO antigens on endothelial cells, can cause hyperacute rejection characterized by thrombosis of graft vessels. Antibodies produced in response to the graft cause blood vessel cell necrosis, called acute vascular rejection. Infiltrating alloreactive CTLs cause parenchymal cell necrosis, called acute cellular rejection. Chronic rejection, characterized by fibrosis, may represent healing of acute rejection or may represent a chronic delayed type hypersensitivity reaction in the walls of muscular arteries, producing accelerated arteriosclerosis and ischemic injury of the graft.

Rejection may be prevented or treated by host immunosuppression, by minimizing the immunogenicity of the graft (e.g., by limiting MHC allelic differences), or by induction of tolerance. Most immunosuppression is directed at T cell responses, using glucocorticoids, cytotoxic drugs, specific immunosuppressive agents, or anti–T cell antibodies. The prototypic specific immunosuppressive agent is cyclosporin A, which blocks IL-2 synthesis. Induction of specific tolerance is the goal of much current experimental therapy.

Patients receiving solid organ transplants may experience complications related to their therapy, including viral infections, especially with cytomegalovirus, and virus-related malignancies, such as B cell lymphoma, squamous cell carcinoma of the skin, and Kaposi's sarcoma. Xenogeneic transplantation of solid organs is a major goal of current research. It is limited by the existence of natural antibodies to surface glycans on cells of discordant species that cause hyperacute rejection. The cell-mediated immune response to xenogeneic MHC molecules is less well characterized than the response to allogeneic molecules.

Bone marrow transplant recipients are very susceptible to graft rejection and require intense preparatory immunosuppression. In addition, two unique problems not seen with solid organ transplants may develop. First, lymphocytes in the bone marrow graft may respond to alloantigens of the host, producing GVHD. Acute GVHD is characterized by epithelial cell necrosis in the skin, liver, and gut, causing a rash, jaundice, and diarrhea, respectively. When severe, acute GVHD may be fatal. Chronic GVHD is characterized by fibrosis and atrophy of one or more of these same target organs and may also be fatal. Second, bone marrow transplant recipients often have immunodeficiencies, rendering them susceptible to infections.

SELECTED READINGS

Clift, R. A., and R. Storb. Histoincompatible bone marrow transplants in humans. Annual Review of Immunology 5:43–64, 1987.

Ferrara, J. L. M., and H. J. Deeg. Graft-versus-host disease. New England Journal of Medicine 324:667–674, 1991.

Krensky, A. M., A. Weiss, G. Crabtree, M. M. Davis, and P. Parham. T-lymphocyte-antigen interactions in transplant rejection. New England Journal of Medicine 322:510–517, 1990.

Mason, D. W., and P. J. Morris. Effector mechanisms in allograft rejection. Annual Review of Immunology 4:119–145, 1986.

Platt, J. L., G. M. Vercellotti, A. P. Dalmasso, A. J. Matas, R. M. Bolman, J. S. Najarian, and F. H. Bach. Transplantation of discordant xenografts: a review of progress. Immunology Today 11:450–456, 1991.

Rosenberg, A. S., and A. Singer. Cellular basis of skin allograft rejection: an in vivo model of immune-mediated tissue destruction. Annual Review of Immunology 10:333–358, 1992.

Sherman, L. A., and S. Chattopadhyay. The molecular basis of allorecognition. Annual Review of Immunology 11:385–402, 1993.

Sigal, N. H., and F. J. Dumont. Cyclosporin A, FK-506 and rapamycin: pharmacologic probes of lymphocyte signal transduction. Annual Review of Immunology 10:519–560, 1992.

CHAPTER EIGHTEEN

IMMUNITY TO TUMORS

Malignant tumors, or cancers, grow in an uncontrolled manner, invade normal tissues, and often metastasize and grow at sites distant from the tissue of origin. In general, cancers are derived from only one or a few normal cells that have undergone a poorly defined process called malignant transformation. Cancers can arise from almost any tissue in the body. Those derived from epithelial cells, called carcinomas, are the most common kinds of cancers. Sarcomas are malignant tumors of mesenchymal tissues, arising from cells such as fibroblasts, muscle cells, and fat cells. Solid malignant tumors of lymphoid tissues are called lymphomas, and marrow and blood-borne malignant tumors of lymphocytes or other hematopoietic cells are called leukemias.

Although tumors are derived from self tissues, the process of malignant transformation may be associated with the expression of molecules on the tumor cells that are recognized as foreign by the specific immune system. Such molecules, called **tumor antigens,** may induce immune responses directed at the tumor cells that express them. In fact, *several clinical and experimental observations suggest that tumors can stimulate immune responses in their hosts.*

A common histologic observation that suggests that tumors may be immunogenic is the presence of mononuclear infiltrates, composed of T cells, natural killer (NK) cells, and macrophages, surrounding many tumors. Such infiltrates may develop at any site of tissue injury, but they are more frequently present around certain types of tumors, including testicular seminomas, thymomas, medullary breast carcinomas, and malignant melanomas in the skin, independent of the presence of other inflammatory stimuli, such as infection or tissue necrosis. Another histopathologic indication that tumors stimulate immune responses is the frequent finding of lymphocytic proliferation (hyperplasia) in lymph nodes draining sites of tumor growth. Furthermore, there is often evidence of cytokine effects in tumors, such as increased expression of class II major histocompatibility complex (MHC) molecules and intercellular adhesion molecule–1 (ICAM-1), suggesting an active immune response at the site of the tumor.

If cancer cells often express molecules that act as antigens in the host, it is possible that the immune system could recognize and destroy these abnormal cells before they grow into tumors, or could kill tumors after they are formed. This theoretical role for the immune system is often called **immunosurveillance.** It was originally articulated by Paul Ehrlich early in this century and was expanded in the 1950s and 1960s by Macfarlane Burnet and Lewis Thomas. If the concept of immunosurveillance is valid, then immune effector cells, such as B cells, helper T cells, cytolytic T lymphocytes (CTLs), and NK cells, must be able to recognize tumor antigens and mediate the killing of tumor cells. Although there still is no direct evidence that immunosurveillance actually protects individuals from tumors, certain observations support the validity of the concept. For example, immunodeficient individuals are more likely to develop certain types of tumors than normal individuals. Clinicopathologic correlations

show that the presence of lymphocytic infiltrates in some tumors (e.g., medullary breast carcinomas and malignant melanomas) is associated with a better prognosis compared with histologically similar tumors without infiltrates. There is also abundant experimental evidence that tumors can stimulate specific T cell–mediated immune responses. Recently, several tumor antigens that are recognized by class I MHC–restricted CTLs *in vivo* have been identified as mutant forms of normal cellular proteins. This finding further supports the idea that a function of CTLs is surveillance for and destruction of cells harboring mutated genes that could lead to, or be associated with, malignant transformation.

Immunosurveillance for tumors is often ineffective, as indicated by the fact that lethal cancers arise in immunocompetent individuals. It is therefore likely that immune responses to tumors are often weak, and the possible reasons for this are discussed later in this chapter. A major current focus of immunology and oncology research is the development of ways to augment host immune responses to tumors. This research is part of a broad field called **tumor immunology,** which encompasses the study of specific acquired immune responses to tumors, the antigens on tumor cells that induce immune responses, immunologic effector mechanisms that kill tumor cells, and immunologic approaches to detecting, diagnosing, and treating cancers. The great progress we have made over the last decade in understanding the physiology of normal immune responses is already being applied to the important practical problems of prevention and treatment of tumors. In this chapter, we discuss these different aspects of tumor immunology, referring to the basic principles of the cognitive and effector arms of the immune response that we have already described in detail in previous chapters.

TUMOR ANTIGENS

The abnormal growth behaviors of malignant tumors are the reflection of complex abnormalities in physiology that result from expression of mutated or viral genes and/or deregulated expression of normal genes. It is a reasonable assumption, therefore, that cancer cells express proteins that either are not expressed at all or are present in much lower quantities in normal cells. These proteins may appear foreign to a tumor host because they were never expressed on self tissues prior to tumor development, or were expressed at sufficiently low levels that they did not induce tolerance. Such proteins can therefore stimulate specific immune responses to tumor cells. In addition, surface proteins peculiar to tumors may serve as targets for effectors of natural immunity, such as NK cells.

The fact that tumor cells express antigens that can stimulate immune responses in the host has been clearly demonstrated in both experimental animal models and in human cancer patients. Tumor antigens can be classified into two main groups based on the types of immunologic probes used to detect them. First, many tumor antigens are molecules that are recognized by T lymphocytes, and in some experimental cases, these antigens may stimulate T cell–mediated rejection of tumor transplants in animals previously immunized with the tumor. These tumor antigens are cell proteins that have been processed and presented as peptide-MHC complexes to either CD4$^+$ or CD8$^+$ T lymphocytes. Some tumor antigens recognized by T cells are unique to particular tumors, whereas others are present on many or all cancers of a specific type. The use of T lymphocytes as sensitive probes for tumor antigens holds promise for new approaches to tumor therapy. Second, some tumor antigens can be detected by antibodies produced by immunizing an animal of one species with tumor cells from another species. These antibodies can then be used to identify different molecules expressed on the tumor cell surface. Such molecules do not necessarily stimulate immune responses in the tumor host, but the antibodies that bind to them are potentially valuable in diagnosis and therapy of tumors. This portion of the chapter describes different types of tumor antigens and their roles in the biology of tumor-host interactions.

Tumor Antigens Recognized by T Lymphocytes

Tumor antigens recognized by T lymphocytes include a wide variety of cellular and viral proteins, and they have been defined by different analytical techniques. The major categories of these antigens are discussed below, and are listed in Table 18–1.

TABLE 18–1. Tumor Antigens that Stimulate T Cell Responses

Category	Examples
Tumor-specific transplantation antigens on chemically induced rodent sarcomas	No examples defined molecularly
Products of random point mutations in cellular genes not involved in tumor pathogenesis	p91A mutation in mutagenized murine mastocytoma
Products of silent genes normally not expressed in adults	MAGE-1 (50% of human melanomas, 25% of human breast carcinomas)
Oncogene products activated by mutations or rearrangements of normal genes	p21^{ras} proteins with point mutation at position 12 (10% of human carcinomas)
	p210 product of *bcr/abl* rearrangements (chronic myelogenous leukemias)
Mutated tumor-suppressor gene products	p53 (>50% of human tumors)
Viral gene products in virus-associated malignancies	SV40 T antigen (SV40-induced rat tumors)
	Human papillomavirus E6 and E7 gene products (human cervical carcinoma)
	Epstein-Barr virus EBNA-1 gene product (Burkitt's, lymphoma and nasopharyngeal carcinoma)

Abbreviations: SV, simian virus; EBNA, Epstein-Barr nuclear antigen. Adapted from Pardoll, D. M. Cancer vaccines. *Immunology Today* 14:310–316, 1993.

TUMOR-SPECIFIC TRANSPLANTATION ANTIGENS (TSTAs) ON CARCINOGEN- OR RADIATION-INDUCED RODENT TUMORS

Studies in the 1950s with rodent tumors induced by chemical carcinogens or radiation provided the first clear evidence that tumor cells can express antigens that induce specific and protective immune responses. In a typical study of this kind, a sarcoma is induced in an inbred mouse by painting its skin with the chemical carcinogen methylcholanthrene (MCA). These MCA-induced sarcomas can be excised from the original host mouse and introduced into other mice, or back into the original animal. Transplantation of these tumors into other syngeneic mice is usually successful, and the tumors grow and eventually kill the new host. In contrast, reintroduction of the tumor into the original host results in a specific immunologic rejection of the tumor. Adoptive transfer experiments show that rejection is mediated mainly by tumor-specific CTLs. Alternatively, the cells of a tumor from one mouse can be killed by irradiation and used to immunize a second syngeneic mouse. Subsequent introduction of live cells from the original tumor into the immunized mouse will result in immunologic rejection of the tumor transplant (Fig. 18–1). These experiments demonstrate that the *rejection of the transplanted tumors displays the cardinal features of specific immune responses, namely specificity and memory.* In addition, they suggest that CTLs are an important effector mechanism for anti-tumor immunity. Since the tumor antigens in this experimental system are detected by rejection of transplanted tumor cells, they are called **tumor rejection antigens** or **tumor transplantation antigens.** A remarkable property of tumor rejection antigens on these rodent tumors is their enormous diversity, reflected by the specificity of the immune responses to each individual tumor. For example, one MCA-induced sarcoma will not induce protective immunity against another MCA-induced sarcoma, even if both tumors are derived from the same mouse (Table 18–2). For this reason, such antigens are called **tumor-specific transplantation antigens (TSTAs).**

The relevence of TSTAs to human cancers has not been established but is under active investigation. Obviously, the syngeneic transplantation protocols used to define TSTAs on experimentally induced tumors cannot be performed on human subjects. There is now indirect evidence in animal studies, however, that many tumors may express specific antigens that can be recognized by T cells, but these antigens may be difficult to detect because they do not induce effective immune responses. When the immunogenicity of these tumors is increased by ways discussed later in this chapter, specific rejection of the modified tumors can be observed. A concern about the significance of TSTAs on carcinogen- or radiation-induced rodent tumors is that although these antigens were described over 30 years ago, their molecular nature is unknown. For many years, investigators tried without success to raise monoclonal antibodies specific for these antigens. The

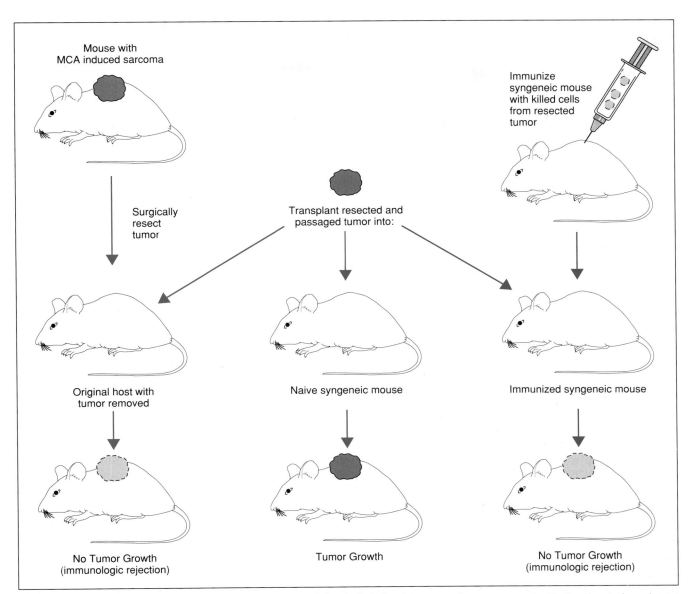

FIGURE 18–1. Tumor-specific transplantation antigens (TSTAs) of chemically induced sarcomas. *A mouse treated with the chemical carcinogen methylcholanthrene (MCA) develops a sarcoma. If this tumor is resected and transplanted into a normal syngeneic mouse, the tumor will grow. In contrast, the original tumor-bearing animal that was cured by surgical resection will reject a subsequent transplant of the same tumor. Injection of killed cells from the same tumor into a syngeneic mouse induces the same type of protective immunity.*

TABLE 18–2.   Transplantation Antigens on Chemically and Virally Induced Tumors

| | Treatment of Mouse | | | |
Experiment	*Immunization with Killed Tumor Cells from*	*Challenge with Live Tumors Cells from*	Result	Conclusion
1	Chemically induced sarcoma A	Chemically induced sarcoma A	No growth	Immunity to chemically induced tumors is specific for individual tumors.
	Chemically induced sarcoma A	Chemically induced sarcoma B	Growth of chemically induced sarcoma B	
2	MSV-induced sarcoma A	MSV-induced sarcoma A	No growth	Immunity to virus-induced tumors is virus-specific.
	MSV-induced sarcoma A	MSV-induced sarcoma B	No growth of sarcoma B	
	MSV-induced sarcoma A	Chemically induced sarcoma C	Growth of chemically induced sarcoma C	
	MSV-induced sarcoma A	MuLV-induced sarcoma D	Growth of MuLV-induced sarcoma D	

Abbreviations: MSV, murine sarcoma virus; MuLV, murine leukemia virus.

failure of this approach is not surprising, since TSTAs are recognizable by T cells, which means they are expressed on the cell surface only in the form of processed peptides bound in the clefts of MHC molecules; peptides within MHC clefts do not generally elicit antibodies. Furthermore, the enormous diversity of TSTAs, unique for each individual tumor, has been hard to understand. This diversity may reflect the possibility that TSTAs include various unrelated cellular proteins that carry random mutations resulting from the carcinogenic treatments used to induce the tumors. This basis for diversity has in fact been demonstrated in another experimental tumor system, described next.

TUMOR ANTIGENS EXPRESSED ON *IN VITRO* MUTAGENIZED TUMOR CELLS

Some tumor antigens expressed on experimental tumors are mutant cellular proteins with single amino acid substitutions. This has been shown by a method in which tumor-specific CTL clones were used to isolate genes encoding tumor antigens. The strategy was to artificially mutagenize a tumorigenic mouse cell line *in vitro* and isolate non-tumorigenic variant cell lines that were immunologically rejected when transplanted into syngeneic mice. (Note that the tumorigenic cell line does not express tumor rejection antigens, but the mutagenized cell line does. That is why the mutagenized tumor is rejected.) **Mixed lymphocyte-tumor cultures** were then prepared in which spleen cells from mice that had rejected one of these tumors were mixed with cells from the same non-tumorigenic variant line. Active CTLs that specifically recognized and lysed the variant tumor grew out of the cultures, and cloned lines of these CTLs, each derived from a single lymphocyte, were propagated. These clones are powerful tools for the identification of tumor antigens. For example, analysis of the ability of each of these CTL clones to lyse different tumor variants indicated that the antigens the CTLs recognize are highly diverse and restricted to individual tumors, similar to the TSTAs described previously. Furthermore, by culturing the non-tumorigenic variants of the mouse tumor with the different tumor-specific CTL clones, secondary variants could be selected that resisted lysis by these CTLs. These secondary variants presumably lost the expression of the antigens that the CTLs recognized. When these secondary variants were injected into syngeneic mice, they formed tumors, suggesting that the antigens recognized by the CTL clones were required for immune rejection of the tumor (Fig. 18–2). Thus, these antigens recognized by the CTLs may be considered to be tumor rejection antigens.

Tumor-specific CTL clones have been used to isolate genes that encode tumor antigens (Fig. 18–3). In one such study, a cosmid library of genes was derived from the non-tumorigenic line described above, and these genes were transfected into the parental tumorigenic line. The transfectants were then screened for their sensitivity to lysis by the tumor-specific CTL clones. The genes identified in this manner are a sample of cellular genes with point mutations. They are unrelated to one another and have unknown functions; they are not involved in the malignant phenotype of the tumor cell. The proteins produced by these mutated genes are endogenously synthesized, processed, and presented to the host immune system, usually in association with class I MHC molecules. The processing and presentation of endogenously synthesized proteins occurs normally in many or all cells (see Chapter 6). If the proteins are normal self proteins, they do not induce immune responses because of the absence of self-reactive T cells. If, however, the proteins are altered forms of normal proteins, they will be recognized by specific CTLs and will serve as targets for cell lysis and rejection. Peptides encoded by the mutated portion of the isolated tumor antigen genes can bind self MHC molecules and activate CTLs, whereas the corresponding unmutated peptides either do not bind self MHC or are not recognized by the self-tolerant T cell repertoire. These observations are consistent with the idea that CTLs monitor cells for the presence of genetic mutations in a wide variety of endogenously synthesized or cytosolic proteins. Although initially the number of cells expressing the mutated gene product might be too small to elicit an immune response, an expanding clone of malignant cells may eventually present enough of the mutant protein to induce T cell stimulation.

TUMOR ANTIGENS ENCODED BY NORMALLY SILENT CELLULAR GENES IN SPONTANEOUS TUMORS

Some genes are usually not expressed in normal tissues or are expressed only early during development, before the mechanisms of self-tolerance are operative. When these genes are dysregulated as a consequence of malignant transformation of a cell and are expressed inappropriately in the wrong tissues at the wrong time of life, they may behave as tumor antigens and evoke immune responses. These tumor antigens may be shared by many different tumors. Mouse and human genes that encode these types of tumor antigens recognized by T cells have recently been identified. The strategy for isolating these genes employed tumor antigen–specific CTL clones and antigen-loss variants of tumors, as described above. The function of the proteins encoded by these genes are unknown, but they are not required for the malignant phenotype of the cells, and their sequences are identical to genes in normal cells, i.e., they are not mutated. One of the mouse genes identified in this way is expressed on mast cell tumors and perhaps on some immature normal mast cells but not on other cells, and its protein product behaves as a tumor rejection antigen *in vivo*. A human gene, called *MAGE-1* (for melanoma antigen–1) was isolated from a malignant melanoma cell line and encodes an antigen recognized by a melanoma-specific CTL clone derived from the melanoma-bearing patient. The MAGE-1 protein is expressed on up to 50 per cent of melanomas and 25 per cent of breast carcinomas, but it is not detectable on most normal tissues. Al-

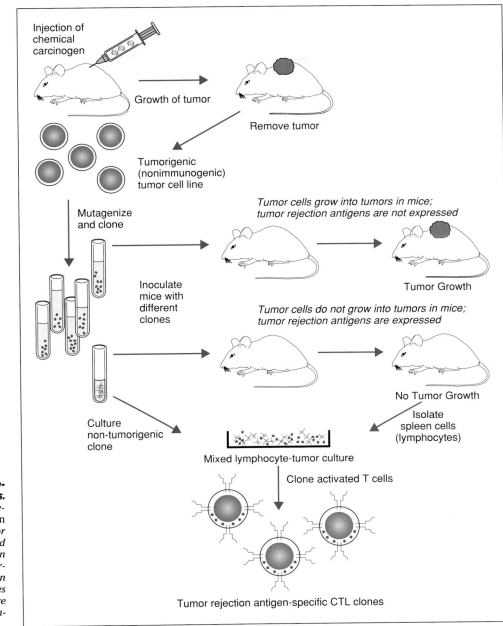

FIGURE 18–2. Cloning of CTLs specific for tumor rejection antigens. *Splenic CTLs specific for tumor rejection antigens are stimulated in vitro in mixed lymphocyte tumor cultures, analogous to the mixed leukocyte reactions described in Chapter 17. Cloned lines of tumor-specific CTLs can be used to screen for tumor antigen encoding genes (see Fig. 18–3). These clones are also potentially useful in the immunotherapy of tumors.*

Labels within figure:
- Injection of chemical carcinogen
- Growth of tumor
- Remove tumor
- Tumorigenic (nonimmunogenic) tumor cell line
- Mutagenize and clone
- Inoculate mice with different clones
- Tumor cells grow into tumors in mice; tumor rejection antigens are not expressed
- Tumor Growth
- Tumor cells do not grow into tumors in mice; tumor rejection antigens are expressed
- No Tumor Growth
- Culture non-tumorigenic clone
- Isolate spleen cells (lymphocytes)
- Mixed lymphocyte-tumor culture
- Clone activated T cells
- Tumor rejection antigen-specific CTL clones

though there is no evidence that MAGE-1 expression induces a tumor rejection response, it is clear that melanoma patients do have memory CTLs that are specific for MAGE-1. There is currently great enthusiasm for developing the use of such CTL clones as therapeutic tools for cancers, as we will discuss later in the chapter.

TUMOR ANTIGENS ENCODED BY ONCOGENES OR TUMOR-SUPPRESSOR GENES

Virtually all tumors express genes whose products are required for malignant transformation or maintenance of the malignant phenotype. In many instances, these genes have been identified, and often they are altered forms of normal cellular genes that control cell proliferation and differentiation. Cellular proto-onco-genes may be altered by carcinogen-induced point mutations, deletions, or chromosomal translocations to form oncogenes whose products have transforming activity. In addition, viral integration into normal cellular proto-oncogenes can result in structurally abnormal products that have oncogenic activity. Tumor-suppressor genes also encode proteins required for normal cellular growth and differentiation, and point mutations in these genes that render their products inactive can result in nonfunctional products and malignant transformation. The altered forms of proto-oncogene and tumor-suppressor gene products expressed in tumors may stimulate immune responses in the host. These proteins are usually intracellular molecules that are likely to be processed and presented as peptides in association with class I MHC molecules, but phagocyto-

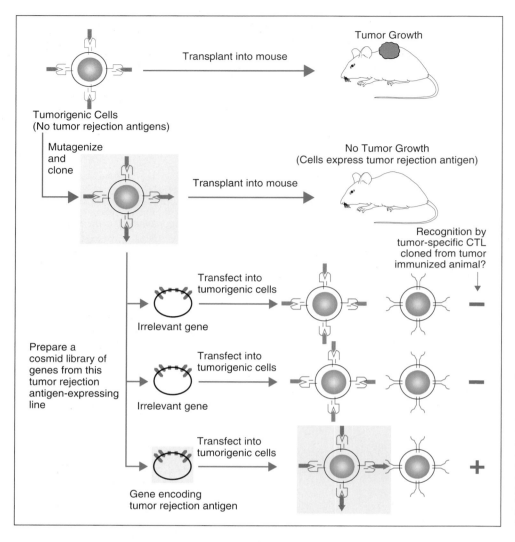

FIGURE 18-3. Identification of genes encoding tumor rejection antigens recognized by CTLs. Cells expressing tumor rejection antigens and genes encoding tumor rejection antigens are shown in shaded boxes. The genes identified by this approach encode a variety of unrelated endogenous cellular proteins with random point mutations, resulting in one or a few amino acid differences from normal proteins. These mutated proteins are processed and presented in association with class I MHC molecules and stimulate CD8+ CTL responses against the tumor cells.

sis or internalization of tumor cells or shed antigens may also result in class II MHC–associated presentation.

The mutations in some oncogenes are remarkably consistent among many different tumors, such as position 12 mutations in $p21^{ras}$ proteins, probably because only selected mutations impart a growth advantage to the cell. Furthermore, relatively few mutations appear in a wide variety of tumors. Significantly, these mutant gene products can act as tumor antigens. T cell responses specific for products of several of these genes, including mutated ras, p53, and bcr-abl proteins, have been demonstrated in mice and humans. Oncogene or tumor suppressor gene products are potential targets for cancer immunotherapy because their amino acid sequences are known and they are widely distributed on many different tumors.

TUMOR ANTIGENS ENCODED BY GENOMES OF ONCOGENIC VIRUSES

Both RNA and DNA viruses are implicated in the development of tumors in both experimental animals and humans. Virally induced tumors usually contain integrated proviral genomes in their cellular genomes and often express viral genome-encoded proteins. These endogenously synthesized proteins can be processed, and complexes of processed viral peptides with MHC molecules (usually class I) may be expressed on the tumor cell surfaces. Thus, tumor cells expressing viral proteins can stimulate and/or become the targets of specific T cell immune responses. Structurally and biologically distinct antigens are produced by various DNA and RNA tumor viruses.

DNA viruses are probably involved in the development of several different tumors. The papovaviruses (including polyoma virus and simian virus [SV]40) and the adenoviruses induce malignant tumors in neonatal or immunodeficient adult rodents. Several genes in these viruses cooperate to cause malignant transformation of infected cells. In humans, DNA viruses are associated with the development of several different tumor types. For example, the Epstein-Barr virus (EBV) is associated with B cell lymphomas, Hodgkin's lymphoma and nasopharyngeal carcinoma (Box 18–1). Human papilloma virus (HPV) is associated with most human cervical carcinomas. The viral genes responsible for pro-

Epstein-Barr virus (EBV) is a double-stranded DNA virus of the herpesvirus family. The virus is transmitted by saliva, infects nasopharyngeal epithelial cells and B lymphocytes, and is ubiquitous in human populations worldwide. It infects human B cells by binding specifically to the complement receptor type 2 (CD21), followed by receptor-mediated endocytosis. Two types of cellular infections can occur. In a lytic infection, viral DNA, RNA and protein synthesis begin, followed by assembly of viral particles and lysis of the host cell. Alternatively, a latent non-lytic infection can occur, in which the viral DNA is incorporated into the host genome indefinitely. Various virally encoded antigens are detectable in infected cells. Epstein-Barr nuclear antigens (EBNAs) include at least four nuclear proteins that are expressed early in lytic infections and may also be expressed by some latently infected cells. EBNAs are the only well-characterized EBV antigens that have been shown to be targets for specific cytolytic T lymphocytes (CTLs). Other viral structural protein antigens are expressed within infected cells and on released viral particles during lytic infections, including viral capsid antigens (VCAs). Antibodies specific for VCAs are present in acutely infected, recovering, and remotely infected individuals. EBV has profound effects on B lymphocyte growth characteristics in vitro. First, the virus is a potent, T cell–independent polyclonal activator of B cell proliferation. Second, EBV can immortalize normal human B cells so that they will proliferate in culture indefinitely. The resulting long-term B lymphoblastoid cell lines are latently infected with the virus and may express EBNA proteins, but they do not have a malignant phenotype. The molecular basis for these effects of EBV on B cells is presently unknown.

There is a wide spectrum of sequelae to infection by EBV. Most people are infected during childhood, they do not experience any symptoms, and viral replication is apparently controlled by humoral and T cell–mediated immune responses. In previously uninfected young adults, infectious mononucleosis typically develops during EBV infection. This disease is characterized by sore throat, fever, and generalized lymphadenopathy. Large morphologically atypical T cells are abundant in the peripheral blood of infectious mononucleosis patients. These cells are activated CTLs with specificity for EBV-encoded antigens. Previously infected, healthy individuals harbor the virus for the rest of their lives in latently infected B cells and, perhaps, in nasopharyngeal epithelium. An estimated one of every million B cells in a previously infected individual is latently infected. EBV infection is also strongly implicated as one of the etiologic factors for the development of certain malignancies, including nasopharyngeal carcinoma in Chinese populations, Burkitt's lymphoma in equatorial Africa, and histologically variable B cell lymphomas in immunosuppressed patients.

There is compelling evidence that T cell–mediated immunity is required for control of EBV infections and, in particular, for the killing of EBV-infected B cells. First, individuals with deficiencies in T cell–mediated immunity often have uncontrolled, widely disseminated, and perhaps lethal acute EBV infections. Second, EBV-infected B cells isolated from patients with infectious mononucleosis can be propagated in vitro indefinitely, but only if the patient's T cells are thoroughly removed or inactivated by drugs such as cyclosporin A. In fact, immortalization of normal peripheral blood B cells by in vitro infection with EBV is usually successful only if the donor's T cells are removed or inactivated. Third, CTLs specific for EBV-encoded antigens are present in acutely infected and completely recovered infectious mononucleosis patients. Cloned CTL lines have been established in vitro that spe-

cifically lyse EBV-infected B cells, and these CTLs most often recognize peptide fragments of EBNA proteins in association with class I MHC molecules. It is possible that EBV-specific T cells are required in vivo to limit the polyclonal proliferation of infected B cells as well as to kill potentially immortalized clones of latently infected B cells. A loss of normal T cell–mediated immunity may allow latently infected B cells to progress toward malignant transformation. We discuss this hypothesis below.

The epidemiology and molecular genetics of Burkitt's lymphoma and other EBV-associated lymphomas have been the subject of intense investigation, and they offer fascinating insights into various aspects of viral oncogenesis and tumor immunity. Burkitt's lymphoma refers to a histologic type of malignant B cell tumor composed of monotonous small malignant B cells. The African form of the disease is endemic in regions where both EBV and malarial infection are common. In these regions, the tumor occurs frequently in young children, often beginning in the jaw. Virtually 100 per cent of African Burkitt's lymphoma patients have evidence of prior EBV infection, and their tumors almost all carry the EBV genome and express EBV-encoded antigens. Malarial infections in this population are known to cause T cell immunodeficiencies, and this may be the link between EBV infection and the development of lymphoma. Sporadic Burkitt's lymphoma occurs less frequently in other parts of the world, and although these B cell tumors are histologically similar to the endemic form, only approximately 20 per cent carry the EBV genome. Both endemic and sporadic Burkitt's lymphoma cells have reciprocal chromosomal translocations involving immunoglobulin gene loci and the cellular myc gene on chromosome 8 (see Box 4–5, Chapter 4).

B cell lymphomas occur at a high frequency in T cell–immunodeficient individuals, including individuals with congenital immunodeficiencies, AIDS patients, and kidney or heart allograft recipients receiving immunosuppressive drugs. Only some of these tumors can be called Burkitt's lymphomas, based on histologic appearance. Regardless of histologic appearance, most of these tumors share with Burkitt's lymphoma one or both of the features described above, namely myc translocations to Ig loci and latent infection with EBV.

These observations can be synthesized into a hypothesis about the pathogenesis of EBV-associated B cell tumors. African children with malaria, allograft recipients, congenitally immunodeficient children, and AIDS patients all have deficiencies in normal T cell function. EBV infection proceeds unchecked in these individuals, and EBV-induced polyclonal proliferation of B cells is uncontrolled. This rapid, exuberant proliferation of B cells increases the chances of errors made by recombinases or isotype-switching enzymes, resulting in a relatively high frequency of genetic translocations to Ig loci. If the translocation involves the myc gene, this gene becomes transcriptionally deregulated. The resulting abnormal expression of myc may be causally related to malignant transformation and outgrowth of a neoplastic clone of cells. Other genetic events may be required as well. For example, the integrated EBV genome may contribute to the malignant phenotype in EBV-positive lymphomas. This proposed scheme predicts that early in their course, EBV-associated B cell tumors may be polyclonal, since they arise from a polyclonally stimulated population of normal B cells. Later, one or a few clones may obtain selective growth advantages, perhaps because of deregulation of myc. As a result, the polyclonal proliferation evolves into a monoclonal or oligoclonal tumor. In fact, this has been shown to be the case by Southern blot analysis of Ig gene rearrangements in EBV-positive B cell tumors from immunosuppressed patients.

ducing the malignant phenotype in these human tumors are only partially defined.

In most cases, DNA virus–induced tumor cells are latently infected with virus and do not produce viral particles. Virally encoded protein antigens that are not components of infectious viral particles may be found in the nucleus, cytoplasm, or plasma membrane of the tumor cells. Specific immunity to DNA virus–encoded nuclear antigens protects against tumor development in animals. For example, SV40-induced tumors in mice express antigens that induce specific protective immunity against subsequent challenge with other SV40-induced tumors, but not against tumors induced by other viruses. Because these antigens are targets for tumor transplant rejection, they are functionally defined as tumor rejection antigens. The viral tumor rejection antigens, however, are not unique for each tumor but are shared by all tumors induced by the same type of virus (see Table 18–2).

Although both humoral and T cell–mediated immune responses to DNA virus–encoded tumor antigens occur, only T cells specific for these antigens have been shown to mediate tumor rejection *in vivo.* One such virally encoded tumor rejection antigen is the T antigen, a nuclear protein in SV40-transformed cells. The T antigen is required to produce the malignant phenotype, and it is not part of infectious virus particles. Immunization of experimental animals with SV40 virus induces protective immunity against the development of SV40-induced tumors, and this immunity is mediated by T antigen–specific class I MHC–restricted CTLs. Human adenovirus–induced rodent tumors express a virally encoded protein called E1A, which is found largely in the nucleus and is the principal determinant of the transformed phenotype of the infected cells. E1A is not part of infectious adenovirus particles. When class I–restricted CTLs specific for a processed peptide derivative of the E1A protein are adoptively transferred into mice with adenovirus-induced tumors, these CTLs kill the tumors (Fig. 18–4). No comparably well-charac-

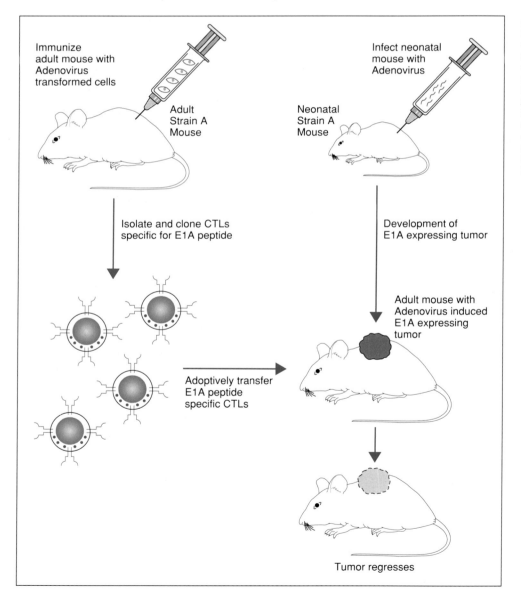

FIGURE 18–4. Viral antigen–specific cytolytic T lymphocytes (CTLs) kill virally infected tumors in vivo. *If neonatal mice are infected with adenovirus, they develop malignant tumors as adults, and these tumors express the virally encoded E1A protein. The CTL clones isolated from a syngeneic mouse immunized with E1A-expressing cells can kill these E1A-expressing tumors when the CTLs are adoptively transferred to the tumor-bearing animal.*

Immunize adult mouse with Adenovirus transformed cells

Adult Strain A Mouse

Isolate and clone CTLs specific for E1A peptide

Adoptively transfer E1A peptide specific CTLs

Infect neonatal mouse with Adenovirus

Neonatal Strain A Mouse

Development of E1A expressing tumor

Adult mouse with Adenovirus induced E1A expressing tumor

Tumor regresses

terized DNA virus–encoded tumor antigen is known to induce protective immunity in human tumors.

A protective role of the immune system in controlling the growth of DNA virus–induced tumors is suggested by the higher frequency of these tumors in immunodeficient individuals. In humans, EBV-associated lymphomas and HPV-associated skin cancers arise much more frequently in immunosuppressed individuals, such as allograft recipients receiving immunosuppressive therapy and acquired immunodeficiency syndrome (AIDS) patients, than in normal individuals. Adenovirus infection induces tumors much more frequently in neonatal or nude (congenitally T cell–deficient) mice, compared with normal adult mice. *Thus, a competent immune system may play a role in tumor immunosurveillance because of its ability to recognize and kill virally infected cells.*

One of the clearest examples of viral oncogenesis is the development of tumors in animals infected with certain types of retroviruses (RNA tumor viruses). Some of these viruses carry well-defined oncogenes, induce tumors in days to weeks after infection, and are called **acute transforming retroviruses.** Examples of these acute transforming retroviruses include Rous sarcoma virus (carrying the *src* oncogene), avian myelocytomatosis virus (carrying the *myc* oncogene), and Kirsten murine sarcoma virus (carrying the K-*ras* oncogene). Other retroviruses, such as the murine leukemia viruses, cause tumors months after infection and do not carry any well-defined oncogenes. These slow-transforming retroviruses may cause tumors by inserting near, and dysregulating transcription of, cellular genes that are responsible for growth control and differentiation.

The genomes of retroviruses are small, and they may express a limited number of potentially immunogenic proteins in their host tumor cells. These proteins include products of the envelope (*env*) gene; core protein (*gag*) gene; and, in the case of acute transforming retroviruses, the oncogene. Retroviral oncogene products theoretically have the same potential antigenic properties as mutated cellular oncogenes, but they generally do not evoke strong immune responses *in vivo*. In contrast, humoral and cell-mediated immune responses to the *env* and *gag* products on tumor cells can be observed experimentally. Furthermore, *env* and *gag* products behave as tumor rejection antigens, stimulating CTL-mediated rejection of transplanted tumors. These antigens are shared by all tumors induced by the same type of retrovirus.

The only well-established human RNA tumor virus is human T cell lymphotropic virus–1 (HTLV-1), which is the etiologic agent for adult T cell leukemia/lymphoma (ATL), an aggressive malignant tumor of CD4+ T cells. Although immune responses specific for HTLV-1 encoded antigens have been demonstrated, it is not clear whether they play any role in protective immunity against development of tumors in virally infected people. Furthermore, ATL patients are often profoundly immunosuppressed, perhaps because of an effect of the virus on CD4+ T cells, which the virus preferentially infects.

Tumor Antigens Defined by Xenogeneic Antibodies

Many cell surface molecules on tumors that have been identified by antibodies raised in other species after immunization with the tumor are called "tumor antigens." Almost all of these tumor antigens are shared by different tumors arising from the same types of cells, and most, if not all, may also be found on some normal cells or benign tumor cells. It is not surprising, therefore, that many of these molecules do not stimulate immune responses in tumor hosts. In cases in which antibodies or T cells specific for these molecules are found in tumor hosts, there is no evidence that such responses are protective. Such antigens are often called **tumor-associated antigens (TAAs).** Several classes of these antigens exist, and many different ones may be expressed on the same tumor. Despite the fact that they may not play a role in protective immune reactions in the host, these TAAs are important for diagnosis and possible treatment of cancers.

ONCOFETAL ANTIGENS

Oncofetal antigens are proteins normally expressed on developing (fetal) but not adult tissues. They are expressed on tumor cells as a result of the depression of genes by unknown mechanisms. The importance of oncofetal antigens is that they provide markers that aid in tumor diagnosis. As techniques for detecting these antigens have improved, it has become clear that their expression in adults is not strictly limited to tumors. The proteins can be found in tissues in various inflammatory conditions, and even in small quantities in normal tissues. Furthermore, oncofetal antigens are not antigenic in the host, since they are expressed as self proteins during development. Nonetheless, the study of oncofetal antigens has proved useful for diagnostic purposes and has provided some insights into tumor biology. The two most thoroughly characterized oncofetal antigens are **alpha-fetoprotein (AFP)** and **carcinoembryonic antigen (CEA).**

AFP is a 70 kD α-globulin glycoprotein normally synthesized and secreted in fetal life by the yolk sac and liver. Fetal serum concentrations can be as high as 2 to 3 mg/ml, but in adult life the protein is replaced by albumin, and only low levels are present in the serum. Serum levels of AFP can be significantly elevated in patients with hepatocellular carcinoma, germ cell tumors, and occasionally, gastric and pancreatic cancers. An elevated serum AFP level is a useful indicator of advanced liver or germ cell tumors, or of recurrence of these tumors after treatment. Furthermore, the detection of AFP in tissue sections by immunohistochemical techniques can help in the pathologic identification of tumor cells. The diagnostic value of AFP as a tumor marker is limited by the fact that elevated serum levels are also found in non-neoplastic liver diseases, such as cirrhosis.

CEA is a highly glycosylated 180 kD integral membrane protein that is a member of the Ig superfamily.

CEA is also released into the extracellular fluid. Normally, high CEA expression is restricted to the gut, pancreas, and liver during the first two trimesters of gestation, and reduced expression is found in normal adult colonic mucosa and lactating breast. CEA expression is greatly increased in colonic carcinomas, resulting in a rise in serum levels. Serum CEA is accordingly used to monitor the occurrence or recurrence of metastatic colon carcinoma after primary treatment. Recent studies have demonstrated that CEA functions as an intercellular adhesion molecule, promoting the binding of tumor cells to one another. Thus, CEA may play a role in the way tumor cells interact with one another and with the tissues in which they are growing.

ALTERED GLYCOPROTEIN AND GLYCOLIPID ANTIGENS

Most human and experimental tumors express abnormal surface glycoproteins or glycolipids as a result of defects in the sequential addition of carbohydrate moieties to core protein or lipid molecules. Examples include abnormal gangliosides, such as GD3 on human melanomas, and aberrantly high expression of blood group antigens, such as group A and Lewis Y (see Box 17–2, Chapter 17), on many human carcinomas. Some aspects of the malignant phenotype of tumors, including tissue invasion and metastatic behavior, may in part be a function of altered cell surface properties that result from abnormal glycolipid and glycoprotein synthesis. Many antibodies have been raised in animals that recognize carbohydrate groups or abnormally exposed mucin cores of these molecules. Although none of the epitopes recognized by these antibodies is specifically expressed on tumors, there is a relative abundance on cancer cells. This class of TAAs continues to be a preferred target for antibody-based approaches to cancer therapy.

TISSUE-SPECIFIC (DIFFERENTIATION) ANTIGENS ON TUMOR CELLS

Tissue-specific antigens or differentiation antigens are present on the surfaces of normal cells and are characteristic of a particular tissue type at a particular stage of normal differentiation of that tissue. Tumors arising from a certain tissue often express the differentiation antigens of that tissue. Since these antigens are part of normal cells, they do not stimulate immune responses against the tumors on which they are expressed. The clinical significance of differentiation antigens on tumors relates to their use as targets for immunotherapy, discussed later, and also as diagnostic markers of the tissue of origin of tumors. The histologic appearance of a tumor may not be characteristic enough to permit a diagnosis of the type of normal tissue from which the tumor arose. Therefore, antibody probes for the expression of tissue-specific antigens may be required. For example, malignant lymphomas arising from the malignant transformation of a developing B cell may often be diagnosed as B cell lineage

TABLE 18–3. Examples of Tissue-Specific Tumor Antigens Used in Clinicopathologic Analysis of Tumors

Tissue of Origin	Tumor	Antigens
B lymphocytes	B cell leukemias and lymphomas	CD10 (CALLA) Immunoglobulin
T lymphocytes	T cell leukemias and lymphomas	Interleukin-2 receptor (α chain) T cell receptor CD45R CD4/CD8
Prostate	Prostatic carcinoma	Prostate-specific antigen Prostatic acid–phosphatase
Neural crest–derived	Melanomas	S-100
Epithelial cells	Carcinomas	Cytokeratins

Abbreviations: CALLA, common acute lymphocytic leukemia antigen.

tumors by the detection of a surface marker characteristic of normal pre–B cells, called CD10 (previously called common acute lymphoblastic leukemia antigen, or CALLA). Tumors arising from more mature B cells can be characterized by the presence of surface immunoglobulin. Examples of tissue-specific antigens expressed on tumors are listed in Table 18–3.

EFFECTOR MECHANISMS IN ANTI-TUMOR IMMUNITY

Both humoral and cell-mediated immune responses to tumor antigens have been demonstrated *in vivo*, and many immunologic effector mechanisms have been shown to kill tumor cells *in vitro*. The challenge for tumor immunologists is to determine which, if any, of these effector mechanisms are important in protective immune responses to spontaneously arising (nonexperimental) tumors. In this section, we briefly review the evidence for tumor killing by these various effector mechanisms and discuss which are the most likely to be relevant to human tumors.

T Lymphocytes

CTLs provide effective anti-tumor immunity *in vivo*, as demonstrated by the experimental tumor transplantation studies discussed earlier. In fact, CTL-mediated rejection of transplanted tumors is the only established example of specific anti-tumor immunity *in vivo*. In these cases, the effector cells are predominantly CD8$^+$ CTLs, which are phenotypically and functionally identical to the CTLs responsible for killing virus-infected or allogeneic cells described in Chapters 13 and 17. As discussed previously, CTLs may perform a surveillance function by recognizing and killing potentially malignant cells that express peptides that are derived from mutant cellular proteins and are presented in association with class I MHC molecules. The importance of this form of immunosurveillance for common, non–virally induced tumors is uncertain, since such tumors do not arise more frequently in T cell–deficient animals or people, or in patients with suppressed T cell immunity due to therapeutic drugs or human immunodeficiency virus infection. On the other hand, as discussed earlier, tumor-specific CTLs can be isolated from animals and humans with already established tumors. For example, peripheral blood lymphocytes from patients with advanced carcinomas and melanomas contain CTLs that can lyse explanted tumors from the same patients. Furthermore, mononuclear cells derived from the inflammatory infiltrate in human solid tumors, called **tumor-infiltrating lymphocytes (TILs),** also include CTLs with the capacity to lyse the tumor from which they were derived. Although these CTL responses may not be effective in eradicating most tumors on their own, enhancement of CTL responses may be a target for anti-tumor therapy in the near future. CTL-mediated surveillance against cells infected with oncogenic viruses probably does occur naturally, as suggested by the fact that tumors associated with viral infections occur more frequently in immunosuppressed patients.

Although CD4$^+$ helper T cells are not generally cytotoxic to tumors, they may play a role in anti-tumor responses by providing cytokines for effective CTL development (see Chapter 13). In addition, helper T cells that are activated by tumor antigens may secrete tumor necrosis factor (TNF) and interferon-γ (IFN-γ), which can increase tumor cell class I MHC expression and sensitivity to lysis by CTLs. A minority of tumors that express class II MHC molecules may directly activate tumor-specific CD4$^+$ helper T cells. More commonly, class II–expressing professional antigen-presenting cells (APCs) process and present internalized proteins derived from dying or phagocytosed tumor cells. CD4$^+$ helper T cells from some tumor-bearing individuals are specific for oncogene products, such as mutated ras protein, but a thorough analysis of other antigens that tumor-specific helper T cells may recognize has not been accomplished.

Natural Killer Cells

NK cells may be effector cells of natural and acquired immune responses to tumors. They use the same lytic mechanisms as CTLs to kill cells, but they do not express T cell antigen receptors, and they kill targets in an MHC-unrestricted manner (see Chapter 13). NK cells can lyse both virally infected cells and certain tumor cell lines, especially hematopoietic tumors, *in vitro*. In fact, lysis of such lines serves as the major bioassay for NK activity. There appears to be a degree of specificity to NK killing, since many virally infected cells or tumor cells and most normal cells are not susceptible to NK lysis *in vitro*. The basis of this specificity is not understood. In addition, NK cells can be targeted to antibody-coated cells because they express low-affinity Fc receptors (FcγRIII or CD16) for IgG molecules. The tumoricidal capacity of NK cells is increased by cytokines, including interferons, TNF, interleukin-2 (IL-2), and interleukin-12. Therefore, their role in anti-tumor immunity may depend on the concurrent stimulation of T cells and macrophages that produce these cytokines. There is great interest in the role of IL-2–activated NK cells in tumor killing. These cells, called **lymphokine-activated killer (LAK) cells,** are derived *in vitro* by culture of peripheral blood cells or TILs from tumor patients with high doses of IL-2 (see Chapter 13). LAK cells exhibit a markedly enhanced and nonspecific capacity to lyse other cells, including tumor cells. The use of LAK cells in adoptive immunotherapy of tumors will be discussed later.

A role for NK cells in tumor immunity *in vivo* is suggested by a variety of indirect evidence. For example, the incidence of tumors in different strains of inbred mice, or in mice of different ages, correlates inversely with the functional capacity of NK cells in these mice. Interestingly, T cell–deficient nude mice have normal or elevated numbers of NK cells, and they do not have a high incidence of spontaneous tumors. NK cells may play a role in immunosurveillance against developing tumors, especially those expressing viral antigens. However, a high level of NK activity is not present in the cellular infiltrates associated with solid human tumors, before *in vitro* expansion with IL-2.

Macrophages

Macrophages are potentially important cellular mediators of anti-tumor immunity. Their role is largely inferred from the demonstration that activated macrophages can preferentially lyse tumor cells, and not normal cells, *in vitro*. Like NK cells, macrophages express Fcγ receptors, and they can be targeted to tumor cells coated with antibody. There are probably several mechanisms of macrophage killing of tumor target cells which are essentially the same as the mechanisms of macrophage killing of infectious organisms. These mechanisms include the release of lysosomal enzymes, reactive oxygen metabolites, and, in mice, nitric oxide.

Activated macrophages also secrete the cytokine **tumor necrosis factor (TNF),** which, as its name implies, was first characterized as an agent that can kill tumors but not normal cells. The various actions of TNF were discussed in Chapter 12. There is convincing evidence that a major component of macrophage-mediated killing of tumors is due to TNF secretion. For example, tumor cells selected *in vitro* for resistance to killing by TNF are often also resistant to killing by macrophages. Killing by both mechanisms is slow (24 to 48 hours), can be augmented by protein or RNA synthesis inhibitors, and involves nuclear DNA fragmentation rather than osmotic lysis.

TNF kills tumors by at least two different mechanisms. First, *binding of TNF to high-affinity cell surface receptors is directly toxic to tumor cells*. The toxicity may be a result of the production of free radicals. Normal cells respond to TNF by synthesizing superoxide dismutase, an enzyme that participates in the inactivation of free radicals. In contrast, many tumor cells fail to make superoxide dismutase in response to TNF. Thus, part of the explanation of selective tumor cell killing by TNF may be loss of responses in these cells, which serve to protect normal cells. Direct toxic effects of TNF may also involve disruption of cytoskeletal proteins, or interference with gap junction formation. Second, *TNF can cause tumor necrosis by mobilizing various host responses in vivo*. In fact, even tumor cells lacking TNF receptors can be eradicated in mice by treatment with TNF. A key observation is that TNF selectively eradicates vascularized tumors and is much less effective in killing avascular implants. Histologically, the response to TNF, described as hemorrhagic necrosis, looks very much like the localized Shwartzman reaction described in Chapter 12. This resemblance has led to the suggestion that TNF acts selectively on tumor vessels to produce a Shwartzman-like reaction causing thrombosis of the vessels and ischemic necrosis of tumors. Tumor vessels may be already "primed" to trigger the Shwartzman response once they encounter TNF. Some tumor-derived angiogenic factors, such as vascular endothelial growth factor, potentiate endothelial cell responses to TNF.

Antibodies

Although T cells are probably more important than antibodies in mediating effective anti-tumor immune responses, tumor-bearing hosts do produce antibodies against tumor antigens. The antigens that stimulate these immune responses are predictably limited to molecules that have not been expressed on normal tissues in a way that would induce tolerance. In some instances, these antibody responses are specific for viral antigens. For example, patients with EBV-associated lymphomas have serum antibodies against EBV-encoded antigens expressed on the surface of their tumor cells. In other cases, human cancer patients produce antibodies against their own tumors that can be used for *in vitro* "autologous typing" to identify tumor antigens. In these cases, the antigens recognized are almost always present on normal tissues as well. No evidence exists for a protective role of such humoral responses against tumor development or growth. Hybridomas have been prepared from the B cells of tumor patients that produce monoclonal antibodies reactive with antigens on the patients' tumors. Again, these antibodies are not specific for antigens expressed exclusively on tumor cells. The potential for antibody-mediated destruction of tumor cells has largely been demonstrated *in vitro* and is attributable to complement activation, or to antibody-dependent cell-mediated cytotoxicity in which Fc receptor–bearing macrophages or NK cells mediate the killing. Whether or not these Ig-dependent mechanisms of tumor killing play a role *in vivo* remains unknown.

Mechanisms of Evasion of the Immune System by Tumors

Although malignant tumors may express protein antigens that are recognized as foreign by the tumor host, and although immunosurveillance may limit the

outgrowth of some tumors, it is unfortunately clear that the immune system does not prevent the frequent occurrence of lethal human cancers. A major focus of tumor immunology is to understand the ways in which tumor cells may evade immune destruction, with the hope that interventions can be designed to increase the immunogenicity of tumors. The process of evasion, often called **tumor escape,** may be a result of several mechanisms.

1. *Class I MHC expression may be down-regulated on tumor cells so that they cannot form complexes of processed tumor antigen peptides and MHC molecules required for CTL recognition.* There are clear demonstrations that increasing class I MHC expression on tumor cells results in increased susceptibility of these cells to CTL lysis *in vitro* and decreased tumorigenicity *in vivo* (Fig. 18–5). Furthermore, transfecting class I MHC genes into murine tumor cells often decreases their ability to form tumors when they are reintroduced into healthy animals. However, when the level of MHC expression on a broad range of experimental or human tumor cells is compared with the *in vivo* growth of those cells, no clear correlation exists. For example, metastatic tumors, which presumably have evaded immune attack, do not on the average express any more or any fewer MHC proteins than non-metastatic tumors.

2. Because most human tumor cells do not express class II MHC molecules, they cannot directly activate tumor-specific $CD4^+$ helper T cells. Anti-tumor CTL activity is likely to be partly dependent on signals provided by helper T cells (see Chapter 13). If professional APCs do not adequately infiltrate these tumors, take up and present tumor antigens, and activate helper T cells, then maximal anti-tumor CTL differentiation will not occur.

3. Even in cases in which tumors express peptide-MHC complexes that are recognized by host T cells, a lack of costimulators on tumor cells may impair T cell activation. Most tumors are derived from tissues that do not express costimulators that provide second signals for helper T cell activation (see Chapter 7). Furthermore, CTL activation may require costimulation by cell surface molecules, such as B7, that are lacking on tumor cells. Tumor cell antigen presentation to T cells in the absence of costimulators may induce peripheral tolerance (clonal anergy) in tumor-specific T lymphocytes (see Chapter 10).

4. Tumor products may suppress anti-tumor immune responses. An example of an immunosuppressive tumor product is transforming growth factor–β (TGF-β), which is secreted in large quantities by many tumors and which inhibits a wide variety of lymphocyte and macrophage functions (see Chapter 12).

5. A host may be tolerant to some tumor antigens because of neonatal exposure to such antigens or because the tumor cell may present its antigens to the immune system in a tolerogenic form. Neonatally induced tolerance has been demonstrated for tumors caused by the murine mammary tumor virus. This virus causes breast tumors in adult mice that have acquired the viral infection during neonatal life by nursing. Although these tumors are not seen as foreign in these

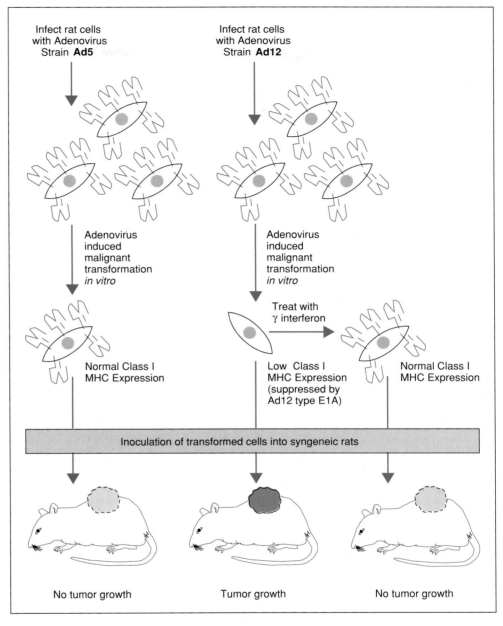

Infect rat cells
with Adenovirus
Strain **Ad5**

Infect rat cells
with Adenovirus
Strain **Ad12**

Adenovirus
induced
malignant
transformation
in vitro

Adenovirus
induced
malignant
transformation
in vitro

Treat with
γ interferon

Normal Class I
MHC Expression

Low Class I
MHC Expression
(suppressed by
Ad12 type E1A)

Normal Class I
MHC Expression

Inoculation of transformed cells into syngeneic rats

No tumor growth

Tumor growth

No tumor growth

FIGURE 18–5. Relationship between class I MHC expression and tumorigenicity in adenovirus-induced tumors. *Rat cells that are malignantly transformed in vitro by infection with the Ad5 strain of adenovirus express normal levels of class I MHC molecules and are not tumorigenic in syngeneic rats. In contrast, rat cells that are malignantly transformed in vitro by infection with the Ad12 strain of adenovirus express low levels of class I MHC molecules and are tumorigenic. Ad12-infected tumors can be induced to express higher levels of class I MHC molecules by interferon-γ, and this treatment renders them non-tumorigenic. An interpretation of this experiment is that class I MHC expression on a virally induced tumor permits the host animal to mount a protective immune response, presumably against a virally encoded antigen presented by the tumor cell in association with class I MHC molecules.*

mice and do not stimulate an immune response (because of neonatal tolerance), they are highly immunogenic when transplanted to syngeneic, virus-free adult mice. Another example of the relationship between neonatally induced tolerance to virally encoded tumor antigens and the growth of virally induced tumors is seen in SV40-transgenic mice. Strains of these transgenic mice that express SV40 genes during early development and have a high incidence of tumors do not mount immune responses against SV40 T antigen (again because of neonatal tolerance). In contrast, other SV40-transgenic mice in which expression of the transgene is delayed until later in life have a low incidence of tumors and are not tolerant to the SV40 T antigen.

6. Anti-tumor immunity may result in selection of mutant tumor cells that no longer express immunogenic peptide–MHC complexes. This could occur as a result of mutations or deletions in the genes encoding the tumor antigens, especially if the protein products of such genes are not critical for the malignant phenotype of the tumor. Alternatively, immunoselection may favor the growth of tumor cells with mutations or deletions in MHC genes whose products are needed to present antigenic peptides. Given the generally high mitotic rate of tumor cells and their relative genetic instability, such mutations or deletions are theoretically likely. Analysis of tumors that are serially transplanted from one animal to another has shown that the loss of antigens recognized by tumor-specific CTL clones correlates with increased growth and metastatic potential.

7. The loss of surface expression of tumor antigens as a result of antibody binding, called antigenic modulation, leads to acquired resistance to immune effector mechanisms. Antigenic modulation is due to endocytosis or shedding of the antigen-antibody com-

plexes. If antigenic modulation is caused by an anti-tumor antibody that does not fix complement, it may protect tumor cells from other complement-activating antibodies. Antigenic modulation is perhaps most relevant as a problem that complicates attempted passive immunotherapy with anti-tumor antibodies.

8. The kinetics of tumor growth may allow for the establishment of immunologically resistant tumors before an effective immune response develops. This phenomenon, called "sneaking through," has been experimentally modeled by transplantation studies. Transplantation of small numbers of tumor cells can lead to establishment of lethal tumors (i.e., lack of rejection), whereas larger transplants of the same tumor are rejected. One presumed reason for this apparent contradiction is that small doses of tumor antigens are not sufficiently stimulatory to the immune system, and by the time many tumor cells grow in the transplant recipient, mutations in tumor antigen genes may have occurred that reduce the chance of immune recognition.

9. Antigens shed by tumors, and complexes of antibodies with shed tumor antigens, have been postulated in the past to act as blocking factors that interfere with immune responses to tumors. The mechanisms of action of blocking factors remain obscure but could involve functional blockade of NK cell Fcγ receptors or induction of "suppressor cells" that specifically downregulate the function of tumor antigen–specific helper T cells.

10. Tumor cell surface antigens can be hidden from the immune system by glycocalyx molecules, including sialic acid–containing mucopolysaccharides. This process is called antigen masking, and may be a consequence of the fact that tumor cells often express more of these glycocalyx molecules than do normal cells. Similarly, some tumors may shield themselves from the immune system by activating the coagulation system, thereby investing themselves in a "fibrin cocoon."

IMMUNOTHERAPY OF TUMORS

The potential for treating cancer patients by immunologic approaches has held great promise for immunologists and cancer biologists over much of this century. Recent advances in our understanding of the immune system and advances in defining T cell antigens on tumor cells have encouraged many new strategies. Several of these new approaches are aimed at augmenting weak host immune responses to tumor antigens. In this section, we describe some of the modes of tumor immunotherapy that have been tried in the past or are currently being investigated.

Nonspecific Stimulation of the Immune System

Nonspecific immune stimulation of tumor patients with adjuvants, such as the bacille Calmette-Guérin (BCG) mycobacterium, injected at the sites of tumor growth has been tried for many years. This treatment serves mainly to activate macrophages. Oncologists are still assessing the potential of local BCG administration in bladder carcinomas and melanomas. An experimental approach to nonspecific immune stimulation is the administration of low doses of anti-CD3 antibodies to mice with transplanted fibrosarcomas. This treatment results in polyclonal activation of T cells and, concomitantly, prevention of tumor growth. Cytokine therapies, discussed below, represent another method of enhancing immune responses in a nonspecific manner.

Active Immunization Against Tumors

Induction of protective immunity to tumors can theoretically be accomplished by active immunization procedures. One method is to inject killed or irradiated tumor cells together with nonspecific adjuvants. The rationale for this approach is that antigen-bearing tumor cells may be able to induce a strong immune response if they are delivered to the immune system under artificial conditions that favor lymphocyte activation. Memory T cells expanded by such immunizations would hopefully limit the growth of already established tumors. The protocols used have been varied extensively, and the efforts have been largely unsuccessful, probably because the tumor cell vaccines do not effectively activate specific T cell responses. Two experimental areas that may help to make tumor vaccinations more specific and effective are the introduction of genes into tumor cells, which renders the cells more immunogenic, and the identification of tumor-specific antigens recognized by T lymphocytes. Various therapeutic approaches are being considered based on this research.

There is ample evidence, discussed previously in this chapter, that cancers express tumor-specific antigens and that hosts have T cells that can respond to these antigens. On the other hand, it is also likely that tumor cells may be poor APCs because they do not provide second signals needed for full T cell activation. Recent experiments demonstrate that when exogenous genes that encode either cytokines or costimulators are introduced into animal tumor cells, and these cells are reintroduced into the host from which they were derived, significant anti-tumor responses do occur (Fig. 18–6). For instance, when rodent tumors transfected with IL-2, IL-4, IFN-γ, or GM-CSF genes are injected into animals, the tumors are rejected or regress. In some cases, intense inflammatory infiltrates accumulate around the cytokine-secreting tumors, and the nature of the infiltrate varies with the cytokine (Table 18–4). Eosinophils and macrophages accumulate around IL-4–producing tumors, macrophages dominate infiltrates around IFN-γ–secreting tumors, and IL-2–producing tumors are surrounded by massive lymphocytic infiltrates. The importance of these findings is that the type of inflammatory cells recruited by different cytokines may provide different effector functions as well as accessory cell functions required for optimal activation of T cells. Importantly, in several of these studies, the

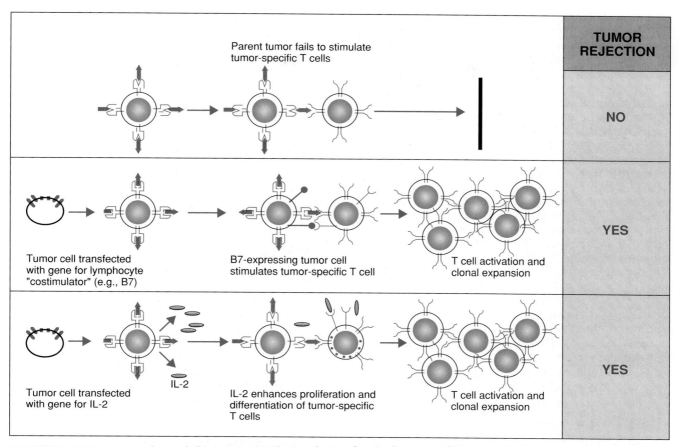

FIGURE 18–6. Enhancement of tumor cell immunogenicity by transfection of costimulator or cytokine genes. *Tumor cells that do not adequately stimulate T cells when transplanted into an animal will not be rejected and therefore will grow into tumors. Transfection of these tumor cells with constitutively active genes encoding costimulators or cytokines can lead to enhanced immunogenicity of the tumors, T cell–mediated rejection, and therefore no tumor growth. In addition, after rejection of these modified tumor cells, the animals retain specific immunity to subsequent challenges by the parent (untransfected) tumor cells.*

TABLE 18–4. Modification of Mouse Tumors by Transfected Cytokine Genes

Cytokine	Enhanced Rejection of Transfected Tumor	Inflammatory Infiltrate	Distant Immunity Against Parental Tumor
Interleukin-2	Yes (dependent on CD8$^+$ and not CD4$^+$ T cells)	Lymphocytes	Sometimes
Interleukin-4	Yes	Macrophages and eosinophils	Sometimes (dependent on both CD8$^+$ and CD4$^+$ T cells)
Interferon-γ	Sometimes (varies from tumor to tumor)	Variable	Sometimes
Tumor necrosis factor	Sometimes	Mixed neutrophils and lymphocytes	No
GM-CSF	Yes	Lymphocytes	Yes (long-lived immunity; dependent on both CD8$^+$ and CD4$^+$ T cells)
Monocyte chemotactic protein-1	No	Macrophages	No

Abbreviations: GM-CSF, granulocyte-macrophage colony-stimulating factor.
Adapted from Pardoll, D. M. Cancer vaccines. Immunology Today 14:310–316, 1993.

injection of cytokine-secreting tumors induced specific, T cell–dependent immunity to subsequent challenges by unmodified tumor cells. Thus, the local production of cytokines may augment specific T cell responses to tumor antigens.

A related approach is the transfection of tumor cells with genes that encode costimulatory molecules that are required for full T cell responses to antigens (see Chapter 7). For example, tumor cells transfected with the gene encoding the B7 costimulatory molecule are potent stimulators of anti-tumor immune responses compared with unmodified tumor cells (Fig. 18–6). These B7-expressing tumor cells are rejected in syngeneic hosts, whereas unmodified tumor cells are not. In addition, B7 expression on the injected tumor induces protective immunity against unmodified tumor cells injected at a distant site. As for cytokines, costimulation augments specific T cell responses to tumor antigens. These successes with experimental tumor models may lead to therapeutic trials in which a sample of a patient's tumor is propagated *in vitro*, transfected with cytokine or costimulator genes, irradiated, and reintroduced into the patient. Such approaches may succeed even if the rejection antigens expressed on tumors are not defined.

The identification of genes that encode tumor-specific antigens recognized by CTLs, described earlier, has provided a theoretical basis for another form of active anti-tumor immunization, namely the introduction of a large amount of the antigen into the tumor patient. This process could be accomplished by linking the genes encoding the antigens to active promoters, transfecting the constructs into host tumor cells or other cell types *ex vivo,* and reintroducing the transfected cells into the patient. Alternatively, recombinant vaccinia virus vaccines with tumor antigen gene inserts can be used to achieve expression of tumor antigens in the patient. Infection of animals with recombinant vaccinia virus–containing tumor antigen genes has already been shown to establish protective immunity to subsequent challenges with tumors expressing those antigens. It is also possible that direct immunization with purified tumor antigen peptides may be effective. For unique tumor antigens, such as may occur with random point mutations in cellular genes, such immunization protocols may be impractical because they would require initial identification of these antigens from individual tumors by use of T cell probes. On the other hand, tumor antigens shared by many tumors, such as the MAGE-1 antigen on melanomas or position 12–mutated ras proteins, are potentially useful immunogens for many different cancer patients. It would be possible to determine if a patient's tumor expresses a particular common tumor antigen by use of polymerase chain reaction (PCR)–based detection of the relevant mutated gene, and human leukocyte antigen (HLA) typing could be used to determine if the patient can express MHC molecules that bind the immunodominant peptide from that antigen. Although immunization against tumors would likely be used in patients with already established tumors, "vaccinations" against commonly expressed tumor antigens could conceivably be performed prophylactically in populations at high risk for certain cancers.

The development of virally induced tumors can be blocked by vaccination with viral antigens. This approach has been successful in reducing the incidence of feline leukemia virus–induced hematologic malignancies in cats and in preventing the herpesvirus-induced lymphoma called Marek's disease in chickens. In humans, the ongoing vaccination program against the hepatitis B virus (HBV) may reduce the incidence of hepatocellular carcinoma, a cancer associated with HBV infection of the liver.

Adoptive Cellular Therapy

Adoptive cellular immunotherapy refers to the transfer of cultured immune cells that have anti-tumor reactivity into a tumor-bearing host. Two variations to this approach have been tested in clinical trials.

1. **Lymphokine activated killer (LAK) cell therapy** involves the *in vitro* generation of LAK cells by culturing peripheral blood leukocytes removed from tumor patients in high concentrations of IL-2. The LAK cells are then injected back into the cancer patients. As discussed previously, LAK cells are predominantly derived from NK cells. Adoptive therapy with autologous LAK cells, in conjunction with *in vivo* administration of IL-2 or chemotherapeutic drugs, has yielded impressive results in mice, with regression of solid tumors. Human LAK cell therapy trials have so far been largely restricted to advanced cases of metastatic tumors, and the efficacy of this approach appears to be highly variable from patient to patient.

2. **Tumor infiltrating lymphocyte (TIL) therapy** involves the generation of LAK cells from mononuclear cells originally derived from the inflammatory infiltrate present in and around solid tumors, obtained from surgical resection specimens. The rationale for this approach is that TILs may be enriched for tumor-specific killer cells. In fact, TILs include activated NK cells and CTLs, but the specificity of these mixed populations of cells for tumors is not clearly established. Human trials with TIL therapy are ongoing. One approach for local delivery of cytokines to tumors is transfection of TILs with cytokine genes; this has been attempted with TNF in a small number of patients.

Passive Therapy with Anti-tumor Antibodies

Many variations on the use of passively administered antibodies in cancer therapy have been tried. One approach is to use antibodies that bind to antigens on tumor cell surfaces to carry toxic agents to the tumor and selectively kill tumor cells. The theoretical potential of using antibodies as "magic bullets" has been alluring to investigators for many years and is still a very active area of research. In addition, *in vivo* administration of antibodies specific for T cells may be employed to nonselectively augment cellular responses or to target immune effector cells to tumors. Several types of these antibody treatments are described below.

1. *Anti-tumor antibodies coupled to toxic molecules, radioisotopes, and drugs* have all been used in immunotherapy trials in cancer patients or in experimental animals (Table 18–5). Toxins such as ricin or diphtheria toxin are highly potent inhibitors of protein synthesis and can be theoretically useful at extremely low doses if they are bound to antibodies to form **immunotoxins**. This approach requires the covalent attachment of the toxin (lacking its cell-binding component) to an anti-tumor antibody molecule without loss of toxicity or antibody specificity. The systemically injected immunotoxin must be endocytosed by tumor cells and delivered to the appropriate intracellular site of action. Another approach is to covalently attach anti-neoplastic drugs or cytocidal radioisotopes to anti-tumor antibodies.

Several practical difficulties must be overcome for this technique to be successful. The specificity of the antibody must be such that it does not significantly bind to non-tumor cells. As we have discussed, there are few truly tumor-specific antigens to select when an antibody-based immunotherapy approach is designed. Most antibodies used in this way are directed at cell surface TAAs which are more highly expressed on tumor cells than on normal tissues. It is difficult to ensure that a sufficient amount of antibody reaches the appropriate target before clearance of the antibody from the blood by Fc receptor–bearing phagocytic cells. Such clearance may not only reduce anti-tumor effectiveness but may also damage phagocytic cells. The toxins, drugs, or radioisotopes attached to the antibody may have systemic effects as the result of circulation through normal tissues. For example, hepatotoxicity and vascular leak syndromes are common problems with immunotoxin reagents. Since the anti-human tumor antibodies used in clinical trials are usually made

in other species, as are conjugated plant or bacterial toxins, there is frequently an immune response resulting in anti-antibodies or anti-toxins that may cause increased clearance rates or block binding of the therapeutic reagent to its target. One way to diminish this problem is to use recombinant, "humanized" antibodies comprising the variable regions of a mouse monoclonal antibody specific for the tumor antigen combined with human Fc portions (see Box 3–1, Chapter 3). Another problem is the outgrowth of mutant tumor cells that no longer express the antigens that the antibody recognizes. This is particularly likely to happen if the target molecules are not required for the malignant phenotype. One way to avoid this problem is to use cocktails of antibodies with specificities for different TAAs expressed on the same tumor.

The results of clinical trials with anti-tumor antibody conjugates are variable (Table 18–5). Toxin- and radionuclide-conjugated antibodies with specificities for various TAAs on melanomas and carcinoma have been tried. In addition, antibody conjugates specific for CD19, CD22, and CD30 have been used to treat lymphomas. Several clinical trials have used antibodies specific for the human interleukin-2 receptor α (IL-2Rα) chain for treatment of adult T cell leukemias which usually express high levels of IL-2Rα. Mouse and humanized anti–IL-2Rα antibodies have been used in unconjugated forms. The rationale of this approach is that IL-2 may serve to stimulate the growth of these tumor cells, and such antibodies may cause modulation or functional blockade of IL-2 receptors (IL-2Rs). Alternatively, such antibodies could cause complement-mediated lysis of IL-2R–expressing tumor cells. Anti–IL-2 antibodies have also been conjugated to various agents, including diphtheria toxin and the radionuclide yttrium 90. In a related strategy, a chimeric protein in which IL-2 itself is linked to the effector chain of *Pseudomonas* toxin has been used to treat T cell lymphomas. Anti–IL-2R therapy is not tumor-specific and may be immunosuppressive because normal, activated

TABLE 18–5.   Examples of Immunotherapy with Anti-tumor Antibodies

Approach	Examples	Tumors	Current Status
Free antibody	Anti-Ig idiotype	B cell lymphomas	Human trials
	Anti–IL-2R	T cell lymphomas	Human trials
	Anti-ganglioside	Melanoma	Human trials
Ig-toxin conjugates	Ricin A–anti-CD5	T cell lymphomas	Human trials
	Ricin A–anti-CD19	B cell lymphomas	Human trials
	Ricin A–anti-gp72	Colon carcinoma	Human trials
Ig-drug conjugates	Chlorambucil–anti-melanoma	Melanoma	Human trials
	Doxarubin–anti-Le^y	Carcinomas	Mouse trials
Ig-radioisotope conjugates	^{90}Y-anti-IL-2R	T cells	Human trials
Dual-specificity heteroconjugate Ig	Anti-CD3: Anti-TAA	Sarcoma	*In vitro*
Ig-hormone heteroconjugate	Anti-CD3: Melanocyte-stimulating hormone	Melanoma	*In vitro*

Abbreviations: Ig, immunoglobulin; IL-2R, interleukin-2 receptor; TAA, tumor-associated antigen; Le^y, Lewis y antigen.

T cells would be rendered nonfunctional. In general, the efficacy of these various agents is limited, and only a small percentage of patients show significant reductions in tumor burden. Nonetheless, intermittent successes have encouraged further refinement of the reagents. Furthermore, trials of these reagents in immunodeficient mice with xenografted human tumors continue to generate new candidates for human trials. For example, a recent study showed that a monoclonal antibody specific for a Lewis Y–related antigen conjugated to the chemotherapeutic agent doxorubicin could cure widely metastatic human carcinomas in athymic mice.

2. *Anti-idiotypic antibodies* have been used in the treatment of B cell lymphomas that express surface Ig with particular idiotypes. The idiotype is a highly specific tumor antigen since it is expressed only on the neoplastic clone of B cells. (Anti-idiotype antibodies are raised by immunizing rabbits with a patient's B cell tumor and depleting the serum of reactivity against all other human immunoglobulins). This strategy relies on complement fixation or antibody-dependent cell-mediated toxicity (ADCC) to kill the lymphoma cells. The approach has not proved generally successful, and there are many theoretical reasons why it may not work. Because surface Ig expression is not functionally related to the malignant phenotype of the cell, selective outgrowth of non-Ig expressing tumor cells can occur. Alternatively, the high degree of somatic mutation known to occur in Ig genes could result in the selective outgrowth of tumor cells with altered idiotypes no longer reactive with the anti-idiotypic antibody. Furthermore, since rabbit antibodies are foreign proteins, the tumor patient may develop anti-rabbit Ig antibodies, and these may interfere with the efficacy of the rabbit anti-tumor antibodies. Attempts to circumvent these problems with cocktails of several different antibodies have also not proved successful.

3. *Heteroconjugate antibodies* may allow targeting of cytotoxic effector cells onto tumor cells. In this approach, an antibody specific for a tumor antigen is covalently coupled to an antibody directed against a surface protein on cytotoxic effector cells, such as NK cells or CTLs. Such heteroconjugates can promote binding of these effector cells to tumor cells. A heteroconjugate consisting of an anti-CD3 antibody coupled to an antibody against a cell surface protein has been used to enhance CTL-mediated lysis of the target cell. In this case, the anti-CD3 antibody not only served to bring the CTL into contact with the target cell, but it also activated the CTL. A related approach is to use conjugates of antibodies specific for effector cells with hormones whose receptors are expressed on tumor cells. For example, anti-CD3 antibodies coupled to melanocyte-stimulating hormone enhance *in vitro* destruction of human melanoma cells by CTLs. These types of antibody therapies have so far been tried only in experimental animal studies.

4. *In vitro depletion of bone marrow tumor cells by antibody plus complement–mediated lysis* is useful for autologous bone marrow transplants in B cell lymphoma patients. In this protocol, some of the patient's bone marrow is removed, and the patient is given lethal doses of radiation and chemotherapy, which destroy tumor cells and the remaining normal marrow cells in the patient. The bone marrow removed from the patient is then treated with antibodies directed against B lymphocyte–specific antigens, which are known to be expressed on the B cell–derived lymphoma cells. Complement is then added to promote lysis of the lymphoma cells that have bound antibody. The treated marrow, having been purged of lymphoma cells, is transplanted back into the patient and can reconstitute the hematopoietic system destroyed by irradiation and chemotherapy.

Cytokines

Cytokines have been used for the treatment of various tumors. This type of experimental therapy has become feasible only recently, as highly purified or recombinant cytokines have become available in sufficient quantities. The rationale for using cytokines is based on their ability to enhance one or more components of cellular immune function; the effects of the cytokines are not specific for anti-tumor–directed immune effector cells, although transfection of tumor cells with cytokine genes, mentioned previously, can increase the specificity of their effects.

1. IL-2, administered in high doses, is used alone or in conjunction with adoptive cellular immunotherapy. After administration of IL-2, there is an increased number of blood lymphocytes and NK cells, an increase in NK and LAK cell activity, and increases in serum TNF, IL-1, and IFN-γ. Presumably, the IL-2 works by stimulating the anti-tumor activity of NK cells and/or CTLs, i.e., by inducing LAK cell differentiation *in vivo*. The treatment can be highly toxic, causing fever, pulmonary edema, and often shock. These effects occur because the IL-2 stimulates production of other cytokines by T cells, which have deleterious effects at high doses. This treatment has been effective in inducing measurable tumor regression responses in about 10 to 15 per cent of patients with advanced melanoma and renal cell carcinoma and is currently approved by the United States Food and Drug Administration for treatment of these cancers.

2. TNF clearly has potent anti-tumor effects *in vitro*, and clinical trials of TNF in advanced cancer patients have been performed. Unfortunately, high doses of TNF produce many undesirable pathologic effects (see Chapter 12) and can be highly toxic at the doses required for tumor killing *in vivo*.

3. Alpha-interferon (IFN-α) is a type I interferon, produced largely by leukocytes (see Chapter 12). It has antiproliferative effects on cells *in vitro*, increases the lytic potential of NK cells, and increases class I MHC expression on various cell types. Clinical trials of this cytokine indicate that it is potentially useful. Objective tumor regression responses occurred in 10 to 15 per cent of renal carcinomas, melanomas, and Kaposi sarcomas; in 40 to 50 per cent of various lymphomas; and in 80 to 90 per cent of hairy cell leukemias (a B cell

lineage tumor). In fact, IFN-α treatment of hairy cell leukemia was used routinely in many medical centers until a new and successful chemotherapeutic drug was recently introduced.

4. IFN-γ treatment of various hematopoietic and solid tumors is intermittently successful. The rationale for using IFN-γ is that the macrophage- and NK-activating properties of this cytokine, as well as its ability to upregulate MHC molecule expression, would help to enhance anti-tumor immunity. Intraperitoneal administration of IFN-γ for the treatment of ovarian carcinomas is currently being evaluated.

5. Hematopoietic growth factors, including granulocyte-macrophage colony-stimulating factor (GM-CSF) and granulocyte colony-stimulating factor (G-CSF), are used in cancer treatment protocols, although not strictly to enhance immune responses against tumors. Rather, they shorten periods of neutropenia after chemotherapy or autologous bone marrow transplantation by stimulating maturation of granulocyte precursors.

SUMMARY

Malignant tumors express antigens that may stimulate and serve as targets for anti-tumor immunity. Protective anti-tumor immune responses have been convincingly demonstrated in experimental animal models. However, it has been more difficult to demonstrate that natural or acquired immune responses can protect humans against tumor growth. The development of virally induced tumors, which express virally encoded antigens, may be inhibited by specific immune responses. Antigens unique to individual tumors, which stimulate specific rejection of transplanted tumors, have been demonstrated only in experimental animals. Other tumor antigens that can stimulate immune responses are shared by different tumors, and these include viral antigens, products of mutated or rearranged oncogenes or tumor suppressor genes, and products of derepressed genes. Tumors may also express tissue differentiation antigens or embryonic antigens to which the host is tolerant; these molecules are useful diagnostic markers. Many immunologic effector mechanisms can destroy tumor cells *in vitro*. One or more of these mechanisms may work on tumor cells *in vivo*, and different mechanisms may be effective on different tumors. CTLs are probably the most important effectors of anti-tumor immunity *in vivo*, although NK cells and macrophages

may also be involved. There is no evidence that antibody responses to tumor antigens are beneficial to the host. Various mechanisms have been proposed to explain how antigen-expressing tumors escape destruction by the immune system. These mechanisms include poor immunogenicity of tumors due to lack of costimulators and/or inability to stimulate MHC class II–restricted helper T cells, down-regulation of MHC molecules, induction of tolerance to tumor antigens, loss of expression of immunogenic proteins due to mutations, modulation of tumor antigens by anti-tumor antibodies, and immunosuppression of the host. Treatment of tumors by immunologic approaches has not yet succeeded on a large scale, but new techniques are actively being tested. Strategies to enhance T cell–mediated anti-tumor immunity, adoptive cellular immunotherapy, and cytokine treatment all continue to be investigated.

SELECTED READINGS

Boon, T. Toward a genetic analysis of human tumor rejection antigens. Advances in Cancer Research 58:177–210, 1992.

Burnet, F. M. The concept of immunological surveillance. Progress in Experimental Tumor Research 13:1–27, 1970.

Hanto D. W., G. Frizzera, K. J. Gajl-Peczalska, and R. L. Simmons. Epstein-Barr virus, immunodeficiency, and B cell lymphoproliferation. Transplantation 39:461–472, 1985.

Herlyn, M., and H. Koprowski. Melanoma antigens: immunological and biological characterization and clinical significance. Annual Review of Immunology 6:283–308, 1988.

Klein, G., and E. Klein. Evolution of tumors and the impact of molecular biology. Nature 315:190–195, 1985.

Lanzavecchia, A. Identifying strategies for immune intervention. Science 260:937–944, 1993.

Prehn, R. T., and M. J. Main. Immunity to methylcholanthrene-induced sarcomas. Journal of the National Cancer Institute 18:769–778, 1957.

Purtilo, D. T. Defective immune surveillance in viral carcinogenesis. Laboratory Investigation 51:373–385, 1984.

Rosenberg, S. A., and M. T. Lotze. Cancer immunotherapy using interleukin-2 and interleukin-2 activated lymphocytes. Annual Review of Immunology 4:681–709, 1986.

Rosenberg, S. A., P. Spiess, and R. Lafreniere. A new approach to the adoptive immunotherapy of cancer with tumor-infiltrating lymphocytes. Science 233:1318–1321, 1986.

Tonaka K., T. Yoshioka, C. Bieberich, and G. Jay. The role of the major histocompatibility complex class I antigens in tumor growth and metastasis. Annual Review of Immunology 6:359–380, 1988.

Urban, J. L., and H. Schreiber. Tumor antigens. Annual Review of Immunology 10:617–644, 1992.

Vitetta, E. S., P. E. Thorpe, and J. Uhr. Immunotoxins: magic bullets or misguided missiles. Immunology Today 14:253–259, 1993.

CHAPTER NINETEEN

SELF-TOLERANCE

AND

AUTOIMMUNITY

One of the cardinal properties of the immune system is its ability to discriminate between self and non-self antigens. Thus, mature functionally competent lymphocytes are able to recognize and respond to foreign antigens but cannot recognize and/or respond to self antigens. This remarkable property is unique to the specific immune system; as all other cells and molecules involved in homeostasis, host defense, and inflammation do not distinguish between self and non-self.

The unresponsiveness of the immune system to antigenic stimulation is called **immunologic tolerance.** The phenomenon of tolerance was introduced in Chapter 10, when the mechanisms by which foreign antigens may inhibit the development of specific immune responses were discussed. The necessity for maintaining tolerance to self antigens, which is referred to as **self-tolerance,** was appreciated from the early days of modern immunology. Loss of self-tolerance results in immune reactions against one's own, or autologous, antigens. Such reactions are called **autoimmunity,** and the diseases they cause are called **autoimmune diseases.**

In this chapter we will first review the mechanisms of self-tolerance in T and B lymphocytes. We will then discuss the factors that contribute to the development of autoimmunity. These topics have been important areas of investigation for several decades. Recent advances in techniques for studying the immune system are providing many new insights into self-tolerance and autoimmunity. Examples of diseases caused by autoimmunity and other abnormal immunologic reactions are described in Chapter 20.

MAINTENANCE OF TOLERANCE TO SELF ANTIGENS

Potentially immunogenic antigens are present on the cells and in the circulation and connective tissues of every individual. Such antigens are freely accessible to each individual's lymphocytes, yet normally one's lymphocytes do not react against one's own antigens. Unresponsiveness to self antigens, or self-tolerance, is maintained by mechanisms that actively prevent the maturation or stimulation of potentially self-reactive lymphocytes. Several fundamental concepts are relevant to our understanding of self-tolerance.

1. *Tolerance to self antigens is an actively acquired, or learned, process (rather than an inherited property), in which potentially self-reactive lymphocytes either are prevented from becoming functionally responsive to self antigens or are inactivated after encountering these antigens.* All individuals inherit roughly the same antigen receptor genes, and these genes recombine and are expressed in lymphocytes as the lymphocytes arise from stem cells. The recombinases that generate antigen receptors act independently of the antigens, self or non-self, that the receptors can recognize. As a result, some of these immature lymphocytes express receptors capable of recognizing various self antigens. Tolerance to self is induced after

antigen receptors are expressed, and is actually a consequence of the recognition of self antigens by specific lymphocytes under special conditions.

2. *During their maturation, all lymphocytes go through a stage in which encounter with antigen leads to tolerance rather than activation.* The concept that immature lymphocytes are more sensitive to tolerance induction than mature cells was introduced in Chapter 10. The tolerance-sensitive stages of lymphocyte maturation are largely anatomically confined to the generative lymphoid organs—the thymus for T cells, and the bone marrow for B lymphocytes. The antigens normally present in these organs are self antigens because foreign antigens that enter from the external environment are captured and transported to peripheral lymphoid organs, such as the lymph nodes and spleen (see Chapter 11). Therefore, immature lymphocytes normally encounter only self antigens, and clones of lymphocytes whose receptors may be specific for these self antigens are rendered tolerant. This process has also been called "central tolerance." Thus, self-tolerance is a process of selection of the lymphocyte repertoire based on recognition of self-antigens. It ensures that the lymphocytes that attain functional maturity, leave the generative lymphoid organs, and populate peripheral tissues have been largely depleted of clones that can respond to self antigens (Fig. 19–1). Self-reactive lymphocytes that escape this selection process and proceed to maturity may subsequently be inactivated as a result of encounter with self antigens under conditions that favor tolerance rather than activation. This process occurs in peripheral tissues and is therefore also called "peripheral tolerance." The biochemical basis for the tolerance susceptibility of immature lymphocytes and the reasons why these cells respond differently than mature lymphocytes to antigen encounter are not known.

3. *The principal mechanisms of tolerance in self antigen–specific clones of lymphocytes are **clonal deletion**, by a process of activation-dependent cell death, and **clonal anergy.*** Both deletion and anergy are induced by the binding of antigens to specific receptors. As we shall discuss below, deletion and anergy may occur under different conditions of antigen exposure. The intracellular biochemical signals that result in deletion or anergy, and how these are different from the signals that lead to lymphocyte activation, are largely unknown (see Chapter 10). In some situations, clones of lymphocytes specific for self antigens may survive and remain functionally competent, but do not respond to the self antigens and do not cause autoimmune reactions. This form of unresponsiveness has been called **clonal ignorance.** The reason why some self-reactive lymphocytes co-exist with self antigens without reacting in any detectable way is not known.

4. *Tolerance to self proteins is mainly due to deletion or anergy of self antigen–reactive T lymphocytes.* Since antibody responses to protein antigens are helper T cell–dependent, T cell tolerance may be sufficient to prevent autoantibody production. B cells specific for self protein antigens may survive if the antigens are present at low concentrations, but these B cells will

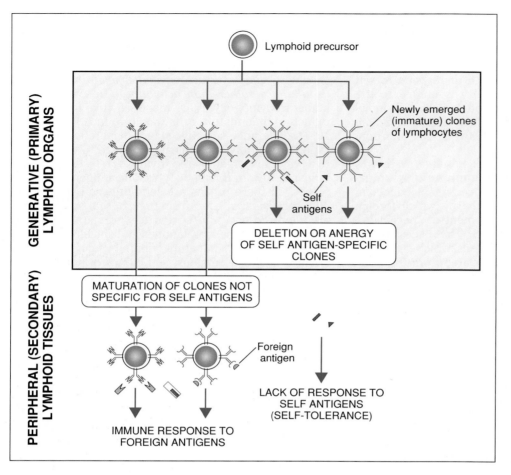

GENERATIVE (PRIMARY) LYMPHOID ORGANS

PERIPHERAL (SECONDARY) LYMPHOID TISSUES

Lymphoid precursor

Newly emerged (immature) clones of lymphocytes

Self antigens

DELETION OR ANERGY OF SELF ANTIGEN-SPECIFIC CLONES

MATURATION OF CLONES NOT SPECIFIC FOR SELF ANTIGENS

Foreign antigen

LACK OF RESPONSE TO SELF ANTIGENS (SELF-TOLERANCE)

IMMUNE RESPONSE TO FOREIGN ANTIGENS

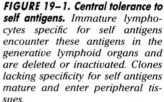

FIGURE 19–1. Central tolerance to self antigens. *Immature lymphocytes specific for self antigens encounter these antigens in the generative lymphoid organs and are deleted or inactivated. Clones lacking specificity for self antigens mature and enter peripheral tissues.*

remain incapable of producing high-affinity antibodies if specific helper T cells are deleted or anergic. Self proteins, however, are capable of inducing B cell tolerance if the proteins are present at high concentrations. Furthermore, *T cell–independent self antigens, such as polysaccharides and glycolipids, must directly induce B cell tolerance.*

Historically, studying self-tolerance has been difficult because lymphocytes specific for self antigens are either not present in a particular individual or experimental animal or are functionally silent. In either case, one cannot identify these cells by examining their responses to a self antigen. Technical developments, especially the creation of transgenic mice, have provided more opportunities to analyze self-tolerance, as is discussed later.

Mechanisms of T Lymphocyte Tolerance to Self Antigens

The induction of self-tolerance in immature T lymphocytes (a form of central tolerance) was described in Chapter 8, when the maturation of T cells in the thymus was discussed. To reiterate the key points, self proteins are processed and presented in association with self major histocompatibility complex (MHC) molecules on

thymic antigen-presenting cells (APCs). Among the T cells that develop in the thymus are some whose receptors specifically recognize self peptide–MHC complexes. If clones of immature T cells that are specific for self antigens encounter these antigens in the thymus, the result is deletion or anergy of the clones. This process is called **negative selection** and is responsible for the fact that the repertoire of T cells that continue to maturity, leave the thymus, and populate peripheral lymphoid tissues is self-tolerant. Illustrative experimental approaches that have established the importance of negative selection in the thymus as a mechanism for the maintenance of tolerance to self proteins were discussed in Chapter 8.

Several questions about thymic selection are unanswered. First it is not known why self-reactive T cells are negatively selected whereas other T cells that recognize self MHC molecules, presumably with some bound antigens, are positively selected and proceed to maturity to constitute the foreign antigen–specific, self MHC–restricted T cell pool (see Chapter 8). One possibility is that T cells that bind self peptide–MHC complexes with high avidity undergo negative selection; this process could occur in T cells whose antigen receptors have high affinities for self peptide–MHC complexes, especially if the self peptides bind avidly to self MHC and are present in the thymus at high concentrations. In contrast, cells that do not recognize antigens in the thymus with high avidity mature to CD4$^+$ or CD8$^+$ T lymphocytes; presumably, these cells have the capacity to recognize and respond to non-self, or foreign, antigens. An alternative possibility for negative selection is that antigens presented by some thymic APCs will induce negative selection, whereas antigens presented by other APCs may lead to positive selection. This hypothesis implies that certain types of APCs may preferentially present self antigens or may deliver negative signals to developing T cells, but no formal proof exists for either possibility. Second, how self-tolerance is maintained as individuals age is not known, because the thymus involutes after puberty and is virtually undetectable in adults. T lymphocytes continue to arise from bone marrow stem cells in adults, and they must continue to be negatively selected because normal individuals remain self-tolerant throughout their lives. In postpubertal humans, negative selection of T cells may occur in extrathymic tissues, or the thymic remnants that persist in adults may be sufficient to serve this function. Third, it is not known how many self proteins are continuously available in the thymus to interact with developing clones of T cells. Antigens common to all cells may be processed and presented in the thymus to induce negative selection, but this is unlikely to be true for tissue-specific self antigens that are normally expressed only in particular extrathymic tissues.

The second mechanism for self-tolerance in T cells is peripheral (extrathymic) tolerance. Peripheral tolerance is postulated to be a "fail-safe" mechanism that maintains self-tolerance even if some self-reactive T cells escape negative selection in the thymus, mature, and enter peripheral tissues. Peripheral tolerance may also be the principal mechanism for T cell tolerance to tissue-specific antigens that are not present in the thymus. The mechanisms of peripheral tolerance to self antigens are probably similar to those of peripheral tolerance to foreign antigens (see Chapter 10). One likely mechanism is that self antigens induce T cell clonal anergy because they are presented to T cells by costimulator-deficient APCs. Tissue injury and inflammation may activate resident APCs, leading to increased expression of costimulators, loss of self-tolerance, and local autoimmune reactions. According to this concept, the activation status of tissue APCs is an important determinant of whether peripheral tolerance or autoimmunity occurs. Other postulated mechanisms for tolerance in mature lymphocytes were discussed in Chapter 10.

Some self-reactive T cells may be neither deleted nor rendered anergic, but their activities may be inhibited by other cells. For instance, one hypothesis states that the T cells with the greatest potential for causing tissue injury are T$_H$1 cells, the mediators of delayed type hypersensitivity reactions. The injurious effects of self-reactive T$_H$1 cells may be blocked and kept in check by the concomitant activation of T$_H$2 cells specific for the same self antigens because the cytokines produced by the T$_H$2 subset inhibit both the production and the effector functions of T$_H$1-derived cytokines (see Chapters 10 and 12). Although this hypothesis is intriguing, its physiologic importance is not clearly estab-

lished. Moreover, T$_H$2 cells are capable of mediating inflammatory reactions under some conditions (see Chapter 14).

Mechanisms of B Lymphocyte Tolerance to Self Antigens

As B cells develop from committed precursors in the bone marrow, the first antigen receptor they express is IgM (see Chapter 4, Fig. 4–1). At this stage in their maturation, interaction of a specific clone of B cells with antigen (or of any B cell with anti-IgM antibody, an analog of antigen) leads to clonal deletion or clonal anergy. Thus, among developing B cells in the bone marrow, any self antigen–reactive clones that are exposed to self antigens are prevented from maturing or responding to the antigens (also a form of central tolerance). The B cell clones that do not encounter antigens in the bone marrow continue to mature, express both IgM and IgD, and enter peripheral lymphoid tissues, where interactions with antigens initiate humoral immune responses. The observation that IgM-expressing B cells are tolerance-sensitive whereas mature IgM- and IgD-bearing cells are activated by antigen has led to the hypothesis that membrane IgM on B cells delivers lethal or inhibitory signal(s), whereas IgD delivers signals that are stimulatory. However, consistent differences in the biochemical effects of antigen binding to membrane IgM and IgD have not been found, and deletion of the δ heavy chain gene in mice by homologous recombination does not prevent B cell maturation and subsequent activation by antigen.

Little is known about peripheral tolerance in mature, self-reactive B lymphocytes. Based on experiments with mice injected with polysaccharides, if B cells specifically recognize multivalent antigens with high avidity in the absence of T cell help, the result is tolerance (see Chapter 10). This mechanism is likely to be important for maintaining tolerance to T cell–independent self antigens.

Two transgenic mouse models have provided valuable information about the induction and maintenance of B cell tolerance to self antigens. In the first model, two sets of transgenic mice were created (Fig. 19–2). One expressed a transgene encoding a foreign protein, hen egg lysozyme (HEL); because this protein was present throughout the development of the mice, in effect it became a "self" protein. The other line of transgenic mice expressed functionally rearranged Ig heavy and light chain genes that coded for an anti-HEL antibody. These Ig transgenic mice had high serum levels of the anti-HEL antibody, and most of their B cells produced this Ig (endogenous Ig gene rearrangement being blocked by allelic exclusion, as described in Chapter 4). The two sets of mice were mated, so that in the first-generation (F1) offspring, the B cells that were producing HEL-specific Ig were exposed from their earliest developmental stage to the self antigen HEL. In these F1 mice, no detectable anti-HEL antibody was produced, even after immunization with HEL by itself or

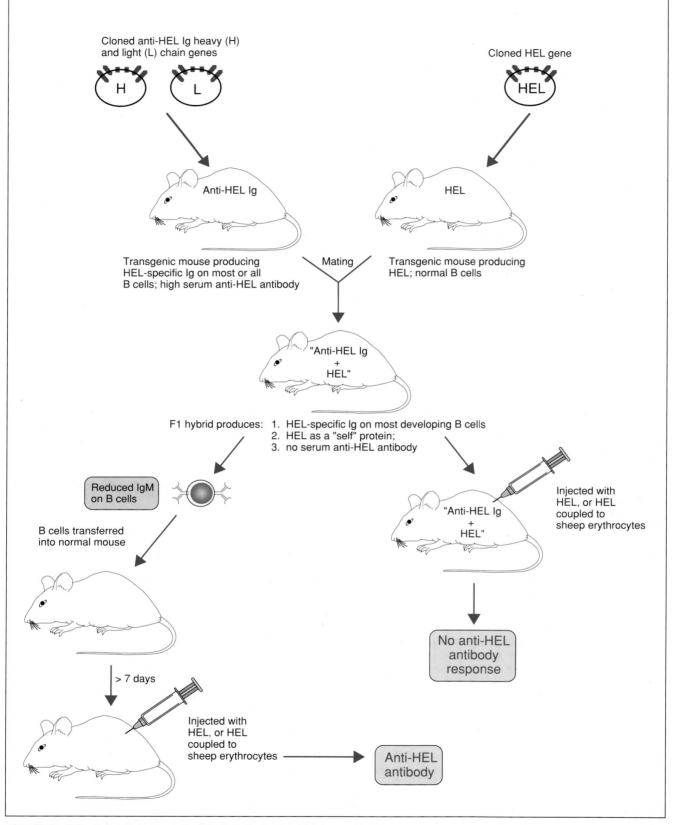

FIGURE 19–2. B cell clonal anergy to a "self" antigen in transgenic mice. *A transgenic mouse expressing anti-HEL Ig is bred with another transgenic mouse that produces HEL. In the "double transgenic" F1 hybrid mouse, most B cells express HEL-specific Ig, and HEL is a "self" antigen. Such mice do not produce anti-HEL antibody and fail to respond to immunization with HEL or HEL coupled to another antigen, sheep red blood cells (SRBC); in the latter case, unresponsiveness must be due to tolerance of HEL-specific B cells, because SRBC-specific T cells can provide help, yet there is no antibody response. Transfer of B cells into normal syngeneic recipients leads to gradual recovery of function. HEL, hen egg lysozyme; Ig, immunoglobulin.*

HEL conjugated to other proteins (to stimulate helper T cells). The B cells survived and even left the bone marrow and populated the spleen, but they expressed reduced levels of membrane IgM and remained anergic, or incapable of responding to antigenic stimulation. If the B cells from the F1 transgenic mice were transferred into normal syngeneic recipients, they gradually regained responsiveness to immunization with HEL. Therefore, in this model, self-tolerance is due to reversible clonal anergy and not deletion of B cells. The maintenance of clonal anergy requires continuous exposure to antigen, and it is short-lived, since the cells recover after they are removed from the self antigen. The reduced expression of membrane IgM is probably not the sole explanation for anergy, because IgD is expressed at normal levels on anergic, HEL-specific B cells. It is likely, therefore, that anergy is due to functional "silencing" of the B cells, such that they fail to respond to antigen; the biochemical basis of this unresponsiveness is not known. Interestingly, some B cells that bind HEL with low affinity may escape anergy in the F1 transgenic mice and may produce anti-HEL antibody. However, this antibody is of such low affinity that it does not cause autoimmune disease.

Subsequent experiments have shown that if the HEL is produced as a secreted protein it induces clonal anergy, but if it is expressed as a cell membrane–associated protein it causes deletion of specific B cell clones. Membrane antigens may provide a multivalent array that binds with high avidity to B cell antigen receptors, and the strength of antigen binding or extent of receptor cross-linking may determine whether a self antigen will cause clonal deletion or anergy. Moreover, by expressing different amounts of soluble HEL in transgenic mice by use of regulatable promoters, it has been shown that at very low levels of antigen, self-reactive T cells become tolerant, and B cell tolerance develops at 10 to 100 times higher antigen concentrations. Finally, even mature, HEL-specific B cells can be rendered anergic by transferring them into mice expressing the HEL transgene (instead of using mating to ensure an encounter of developing B cells with the antigen). In this case, tolerance probably develops because the B cells encounter antigen, the first signal, in the absence of T cell help, the second signal (see Chapter 10).

A second experimental model for B cell tolerance also uses transgenic mice and supports many of the conclusions described earlier. In these studies, transgenic mice were made to express Ig heavy and light chain genes coding for an antibody specific for a class I MHC molecule, the H-2K^k molecule (Fig. 19–3). If this Ig was expressed in mice of an H-2 haplotype other than H-2^k, the B cells matured normally and produced the transgenic Ig. However, if the transgenes were expressed in mice of the H-2^k haplotype, the peripheral lymphoid tissues contained reduced numbers of B cells, and none of the surviving B cells produced the transgenic Ig. Thus, as with membrane-bound HEL, interaction of developing B lymphocytes with a cell membrane–associated MHC antigen also leads to clonal deletion. A small proportion of the self-reactive B

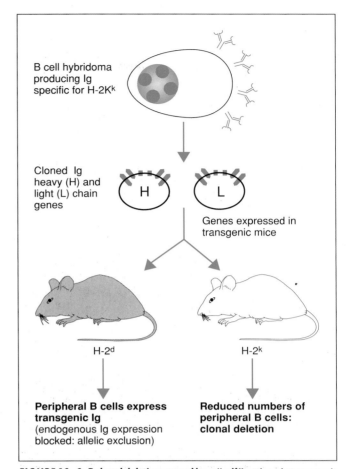

FIGURE 19–3. B clonal deletion caused by a "self" antigen in transgenic mice. *If an antibody specific for a class I MHC allele is expressed as a transgene in mice with that allele, B cells fail to develop and enter peripheral lymphoid tissues.*

cells may escape deletion by rearranging and expressing an endogenous Ig gene, thus generating antigen receptors that no longer recognize the self antigen. In this case, the B cells "overcome" allelic exclusion, since they initially express the transgenic Ig but are able to reactivate DNA rearrangement to "edit" their receptors and lose their specificity for the self antigen.

Both experimental models described above have focused on B cell tolerance to self proteins. As mentioned earlier, under normal conditions, tolerance to self proteins is probably most effectively maintained in T lymphocytes. B cells themselves must be tolerant to self T-independent antigens. For instance, individuals with a particular ABO blood group type do not produce antibodies against their own ABO antigens, which are glycolipids and behave as T cell–independent antigens. Establishing experimental models for analyzing B cell tolerance to self polysaccharides and lipids has proved difficult. It is, however, likely that the general principles and mechanisms are much like those previously described for protein antigens.

Finally, some self antigen–reactive B cells may be neither deleted nor anergic, but instead may mature and survive in normal animals. However, these cells may not produce high-affinity pathogenic autoanti-

TABLE 19–1. Self-Tolerance in T and B Lymphocytes

	T Lymphocytes	B Lymphocytes
Principal sites of tolerance induction	Thymus (cortex); periphery	Bone marrow; periphery?
Tolerance-sensitive stage of maturation	$CD4^+CD8^+$, low TCR : CD3–expressing (double-positive) thymoycte	Membrane IgM^+ IgD^- B lymphocyte
"Stimuli" for tolerance induction	Central (thymic): high-affinity antigen recognition, perhaps on bone marrow–derived thymic APCs Peripheral (extrathymic): antigen presentation by APCs lacking costimulators	High-affinity antigen recognition, especially of multivalent antigen, without T cell help
Mechanism of tolerance*	Clonal deletion: cell death (apoptosis) Clonal anergy: block in IL-2 gene transcription	Clonal deletion: cell death (apoptosis) Clonal anergy: reduced membrane Ig; block in signal transduction (undefined mechanism)
Duration of tolerance	Long-lived	Relatively short-lived
Tolerogenic concentration of antigen	Relatively low	Relatively high

* Intracellular biochemical alterations induced by tolerogenic antigens are not fully known.
Abbreviations: APC, antigen-presenting cell; Ig, immunoglobulin; IL, interleukin.

bodies because of self-tolerance in the helper T cell compartment.

The mechanisms of self-tolerance in T and B lymphocytes are clearly similar in some respects, but important differences also exist (Table 19–1). In the past few years, there has been remarkable progress in our understanding of self-tolerance in the immune system, even though important gaps in our knowledge remain. The most significant application of our current concepts of self-tolerance will undoubtedly be in elucidating the mechanisms of autoimmunity.

MECHANISMS OF AUTOIMMUNITY: GENERAL PRINCIPLES

The possibility that an individual's immune system will react against autologous antigens and cause tissue injury was appreciated by immunologists from the time that the specificity of the immune system for foreign antigens was recognized. In the early 1900s, Paul Ehrlich coined the rather melodramatic phrase "horror autotoxicus" for immunity against self. When Macfarlane Burnet proposed the clonal selection hypothesis about 50 years later, he added the corollary that clones of autoreactive lymphocytes were deleted during development to prevent autoimmune reactions. We now know that this postulate is partly correct, although it has been modified and expanded in many ways.

Autoimmunity is an important cause of disease in humans, estimated to affect 1 to 2 per cent of the United States population. The clinical designation of autoimmunity is often erroneous or unsubstantiated. Many diseases in which immune reactions accompany tissue injury have been called "autoimmune," but this appellation may not be correct. For example, tissue injury that occurs during normal immune responses against foreign antigens is not a type of autoimmune disease. Furthermore, the presence of antibodies or T cells reactive with self antigens may be the consequence and not the cause of tissue injury. For instance, some patients with myocardial infarction develop antibodies against their own myocardial antigens that were previously concealed from the immune system. Obviously, in this case, the autoantibodies are not the cause of the infarction. Despite these caveats, true autoimmune diseases are clearly serious health concerns worldwide.

Autoimmunity results from a failure or breakdown of the mechanisms normally responsible for maintaining self-tolerance. The potential for autoimmunity exists in all individuals because all individuals inherit genes that code for lymphocyte receptors that may recognize self antigens. As discussed earlier, autoimmunity is normally prevented by selection processes that act on developing lymphocytes and ensure that the repertoire of mature lymphocytes is self-tolerant, and by mechanisms that inactivate any self-reactive lymphocytes that do mature. Loss of self-tolerance may result from abnormal selection of self-reactive clones, abnormal stimulation of lymphocytes that are normally anergic to self antigens, or release of self antigens that are normally inaccessible to the immune system. Several important general concepts have emerged from the analyses of autoimmunity during the past 20 years.

1. *Multiple interacting factors contribute to the development of autoimmune diseases.* These factors may include immunologic abnormalities, genetic backgrounds that predispose to autoimmunity, local tissue alterations, and microbial infections. Because combinations of these factors may be operative in different disorders, it is not surprising that autoimmune diseases comprise a heterogeneous group of clinical and pathologic abnormalities.

2. *Autoimmune diseases may be systemic or organ-specific, and they may be caused by different types*

of antigens and different immunologic abnormalities. For instance, immune responses to widely disseminated antigens and the formation of circulating immune complexes (see Chapter 20) typically produce systemic diseases. In contrast, autoimmune responses against antigens with restricted tissue distribution lead to organ-specific or tissue-specific injury. Systemic diseases characterized by multiple autoimmune phenomena may be due to aberrant regulation or polyclonal activation of numerous clones of lymphocytes. In contrast, organ-specific autoimmune diseases may be due to failure or self-tolerance in lymphocytes specific for one or a few tissue antigens, or abnormal activation of lymphocyte clones reactive with a limited number of antigens, perhaps secondary to local tissue alterations.

3. *Various effector mechanisms are responsible for tissue injury in different autoimmune diseases.* These mechanisms including circulating autoantibodies, immune complexes, and autoreactive T lymphocytes, and are discussed in Chapter 20.

4. *Low levels of autoantibodies are produced in normal individuals during immune responses to foreign antigens.* The detection of such "natural autoantibodies" in healthy individuals supports the idea that the potential for autoreactivity exists normally. Natural autoantibodies are usually low-affinity antibodies of the IgM class that may be generated without T cell help and do not produce tissue injury. Pathologic autoimmunity may develop if larger amounts of high-affinity autoantibodies are produced.

A major difficulty in defining the mechanisms of many human autoimmune diseases has been the inability to identify the antigens that initiate autoimmune responses. As a result, the specific etiologies of most autoimmune diseases are not known. In the remainder of this chapter, we describe the general principles of the pathogenesis of autoimmune diseases, with an emphasis on the immunologic, genetic, and other factors that contribute to the development of autoimmunity.

LYMPHOCYTE ABNORMALITIES CAUSING AUTOIMMUNITY

Autoimmunity may result from primary abnormalities of B cells, T cells, or both. Much recent attention has focused on the role of T cells in autoimmunity for two main reasons: (1) helper T cells are critical regulators of all immune responses to proteins, and (2) several autoimmune diseases are genetically linked to the MHC (the human leukocyte antigen [HLA] complex in humans), and the function of MHC molecules is the presentation of peptide antigens to T cells. Failure of self-tolerance in T lymphocytes may result in autoimmune diseases in which the lesions are caused by cell-mediated immune reactions. Helper T cell abnormalities may also lead to autoantibody production because helper T cells are necessary for the production of high-affinity antibodies against protein antigens.

Abnormalities in lymphocytes that may result in autoimmunity could affect any of the mechanisms that normally maintain self-tolerance. Different aberrations may give rise to systemic or organ-specific autoimmunity. In the following discussion, we will consider immunologic abnormalities that have the potential for causing autoimmunity, using examples of animal and human diseases to illustrate key points.

Failure of Central Tolerance (Negative Selection of Lymphocytes)

It is often hypothesized that autoimmunity results from a failure of the selection processes that normally delete or inactivate clones of self antigen–specific lymphocytes during their maturation. However, little formal evidence supports this hypothesis in any human or experimental autoimmune disease. In fact, because the cellular and biochemical mechanisms of lymphocyte selection are not known, it is difficult to postulate how self-reactive lymphocytes may escape this process.

Since MHC molecules play an important role in the selection of developing T lymphocytes (see Chapter 8), one mechanism by which MHC genes influence autoimmunity may be by altering thymic selection. This idea is discussed later in the chapter.

Mechanisms that Overcome Peripheral Tolerance (Clonal Anergy)

Earlier in this chapter, we discussed the idea that resting, costimulator-deficient tissue APCs may induce peripheral T cell tolerance and thus provide a mechanism for controlling tissue-specific autoimmune reactions. It follows that conditions that promote the expression of costimulators on these APCs may overcome T cell anergy and lead to autoimmune reactions. These conditions include infections and local inflammation. Many experimental autoimmune diseases, such as thyroiditis and encephalomyelitis, develop only if the self antigens (thyroglobulin and myelin basic protein, respectively) are administered with strong adjuvants. Such adjuvants may activate macrophages to express costimulators, resulting in loss of T cell tolerance. Furthermore, experiments with T cell clones suggest that anergic cells can be "rescued," i.e., their responsiveness restored, by culture with the growth factor interleukin-2 (IL-2). Over-expression of IL-2 in mice, by infection with a retrovirus containing an IL-2 gene, leads to a breakdown of peripheral T cell anergy and multiple lesions that may be autoimmune. Such experiments suggest that local production of IL-2, e.g., during T cell responses to antigens in tissues, may overcome peripheral tolerance in self-reactive T cells present in the microenvironment. This could be another mechanism by which local inflammation leads to autoimmunity.

Peripheral tolerance may fail due to mechanisms unrelated to costimulation. One interesting possibility has emerged from the study of a mouse strain called MRL/*lpr*, which develops a systemic autoimmune disease resembling human systemic lupus erythematosus (SLE, Box 19–1). The MRL strain is prone to autoimmunity; MRL mice that are homozygous for the *lpr* gene (introduced by breeding) develop a greatly accelerated and severe form of autoimmunity. The *lpr* gene has been mapped to a gene called *fas* and shown to be a transposon insertion in the *fas* gene that prevents normal transcription and leads to a failure to express this protein in *lpr/lpr* homozygous mice. The product of the normal *fas* gene, i.e. the Fas protein, was originally identified as a surface molecule that plays a role in the induction of apoptosis in various cells, including lymphocytes. The Fas protein is structurally homologous to TNF receptors, which also mediate apoptosis in some cell types, and to the B cell surface molecule CD40, which promotes cell growth and is postulated to prevent programmed cell death. Defective Fas expression in homozygous MRL/*lpr* mice may result in a failure to induce apoptosis, which is a mechanism of clonal deletion of self antigen–specific lymphocytes. This may lead to a persistence of autoreactive lymphocytes

of many specificities, stimulation of numerous clones of autoreactive B cells, production of multiple autoantibodies, and systemic autoimmune disease. Interestingly, MRL/*lpr* mice appear to have normal thymic selection. The cellular and biochemical consequences of defective Fas expression are not yet known. There is also no evidence that abnormal Fas expression is associated with human SLE.

In B lymphocytes, clonal anergy is induced by antigen recognition in the absence of T cell help. Therefore, stimulation of helper T cells that can interact with potentially autoreactive but anergic B cells may overcome B cell tolerance. There are other situations in which autoreactive B cells are neither deleted nor anergic but fail to produce autoantibodies because of helper T cell tolerance. In these cases also, the provision of T cell help may lead to autoantibody production. One possible mechanism by which helper T cells may stimulate autoreactive B cells is exposure to a multideterminant antigen in which one epitope binds to the autoreactive B cells (and is, therefore, a self antigen epitope) but another linked epitope is foreign. For example, rats and mice immunized with rabbit thyroglobulin develop an-

---

BOX 19–1. SYSTEMIC LUPUS ERYTHEMATOSUS

Systemic lupus erythematosus (SLE) is a chronic, remitting and relapsing, multisystem autoimmune disease that affects predominantly women, with an incidence of one in 700 among women between the ages of 20 and 60 (about one in 250 among black women) and a female : male ratio of 10 : 1. The principal clinical manifestations are skin rashes, arthritis, and glomerulonephritis, but hemolytic anemia, thrombocytopenia, and central nervous system involvement are also common. Many different autoantibodies are found in patients with SLE. The most frequent are antinuclear, particularly anti-DNA, antibodies, and others include antibodies against ribonucleoproteins, histones, and nucleolar antigens. Immune complexes formed of these autoantibodies and their specific antigens are thought to be responsible for glomerulonephritis, arthritis, and vasculitis involving small arteries throughout the body. Hemolytic anemia and thrombocytopenia are due to autoantibodies against erythrocytes and platelets, respectively. The principal diagnostic test for the disease is the presence of antinuclear antibodies; antibodies against double-stranded native DNA are quite specific for SLE. The presence of so many distinct autoantibodies suggest that SLE is due to polyclonal lymphocyte stimulation and/or abnormalities in lymphocyte regulation rather than antigen-specific activation of an abnormal clone(s) of autoreactive lymphocytes. Genetic factors also contribute to the disease. The relative risk for individuals with HLA-DR2 or -DR3 is 2 to 3, and if both haplotypes are present, the relative risk is about 5. (The mechanisms of autoimmunity and the roles of immunologic abnormalities and genetic factors are discussed elsewhere in Chapter 19.) Deficiency of the complement protein C4 occurs in about 10 per cent of SLE patients but in only 1 per cent of the normal population.

Animal models of lupus provide valuable experimental systems for analyzing the pathogenesis of this disease. Several inbred mouse strains have been discovered to spontaneously develop autoimmune diseases that resemble human SLE to varying degrees.

The first to be described, and the one most like SLE, is the NZB strain and the (NZB × NZW)F1. Female mice develop kidney lesions and hemolytic anemia and produce anti-DNA autoantibodies spontaneously. Extensive breeding studies have shown that non-MHC genes in the F1 that are inherited from both parental strains contribute to the evolution of the disease. The B cells of (NZB × NZW)F1 mice are hyper-responsive to foreign antigens as well as to polyclonal activators and cytokines, and this may be the primary immunologic abnormality in these mice. The biochemical basis of the B cell hyperresponsiveness is unknown.

A second model of lupus is the MRL congenic strain called MRL-*lpr/lpr*, referring to an MRL mouse into a which a gene for "lymphoproliferation" has been bred. The MRL-*lpr/lpr* (also called MRL/*lpr*) strain develops massive lymphadenopathy due to the accumulation of an unusual population of CD3+CD4−CD8− T cells that also express a CD45 isoform called B220 that is normally found on B cells. MRL/*lpr* mice also contain high numbers of autoreactive CD4+ T cells. These mice produce autoantibodies and develop arthritis and kidney lesions. MRL mice are prone to developing autoimmunity, and the *lpr* gene greatly accelerates the disease. Autoantibody production may occur because the autoreactive T cells stimulate the growth and differentiation of many B cells, including autoreactive cells. A role for T cells is further supported by the observation that neonatal thymectomy prevents the development of lymphoproliferation and autoimmunity in MRL/*lpr* mice. The *lpr* gene has been identified as the *fas* gene, whose protein product may be required for a mechanism of cell death (apoptosis) that has been implicated in the clonal deletion of self-reactive lymphocytes (see text). The disease of MRL/*lpr* mice is not sex-related.

A third inbred strain that develops a lupus-like disease is a recombinant called BXSB, in which disease susceptibility is linked to the Y chromosome, and only the males are affected. These mice produce anti-DNA antibodies and develop severe nephritis and vasculitis.

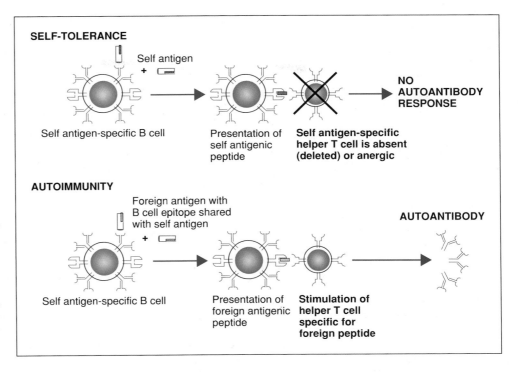

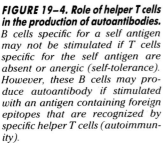

FIGURE 19–4. Role of helper T cells in the production of autoantibodies. *B cells specific for a self antigen may not be stimulated if T cells specific for the self antigen are absent or anergic (self-tolerance). However, these B cells may produce autoantibody if stimulated with an antigen containing foreign epitopes that are recognized by specific helper T cells (autoimmunity).*

tibodies against their own thyroglobulin and, subsequently, thyroiditis. The rabbit thyroglobulin may have some epitope(s) that are homologous to self thyroglobulin and bind to specific autoreactive B cells. Other determinants of the rabbit protein are foreign and stimulate specific helper T cells (which are specific for the foreign antigen and therefore not tolerant). These helper cells cooperate with the self thyroglobulin–specific B cells, leading to the production of autoantibodies (Fig. 19–4). Normally, i.e., without immunization, any mature thyroglobulin-specific B cells that are present do not make autoantibodies because helper T cells specific for autologous thyroglobulin are deleted or anergic.

Polyclonal Lymphocyte Activation

Autoimmunity may result from antigen-independent stimulation of self-reactive lymphocytes that are not deleted during development. Polyclonal activators stimulate many T or B lymphocyte clones, irrespective of antigenic specificity and, in some cases, by interacting with surface molecules other than antigen receptors. A good example is bacterial lipopolysaccharide (LPS), which functions as a polyclonal B cell activator in mice. Exposure to LPS may stimulate many clones of B lymphocytes, including self-reactive B cells that are anergic. Such anergic B cells are incapable of responding to the specific self antigens, but they may have retained their ability to proliferate and differentiate in response to antigen receptor–independent stimuli, such as LPS (Fig. 19–5). In fact, mice injected with LPS produce multiple autoantibodies (although in the ab-

sence of T cell help, most of these are low-affinity antibodies that do not cause disease). Polyclonal B cell activation may be induced by microbial products that act like LPS, and this may be one link between infections and autoimmunity. Polyclonal T cell activation by bacterial "super-antigens" is also a postulated mechanism for autoimmunity. Unlike the interaction of LPS with B cells, these super-antigens stimulate T cells by binding to the V regions of antigen receptors (see Chapter 15, Box 15–1). We do not know how, or even if, such agents overcome anergy in T cells.

Multiple autoimmune phenomena are associated with graft-versus-host disease, which develops after the transplantation of bone marrow containing allogeneic T cells (see Chapter 17). In recipients of such transplants, grafted helper T cells may recognize host B lymphocytes as foreign (a form of alloreactivity), leading to polyclonal B cell activation and autoantibody production in the absence of specific antigenic stimulation (see Fig. 19–4).

Predictably, in autoimmune diseases attributed to polyclonal lymphocyte activation, multiple autoantibodies are produced, giving rise to systemic rather than organ-specific lesions.

Immunologic Cross-reactions of Self and Foreign Antigens

Some autoimmune diseases are initiated by quite normal immune responses to foreign antigens, such as microbes, but the antibodies or T cells that are stimulated happen to recognize a similar (cross-reactive) self protein. One example is rheumatic fever, which develops after streptococcal infections and is caused by

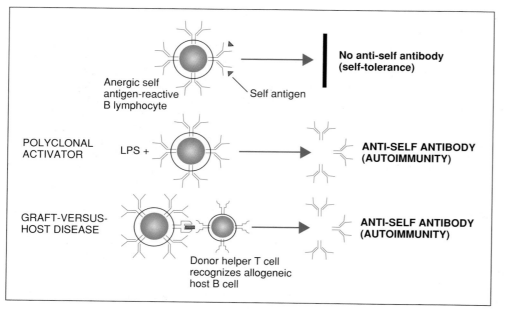

FIGURE 19-5. Polyclonal lymphocyte activation and autoantibody production. *Self antigen–reactive B cells fail to respond to self antigens, but may be stimulated by polyclonal activators such as LPS or by alloreactive T cells, as in graft-versus-host disease.*

anti-streptococcal antibodies that cross-react with human myocardial proteins, resulting in myocarditis. Strictly speaking, such diseases are not truly autoimmune but are sequelae of immune responses against foreign antigens. In some respects, the example of foreign antigen in which some epitopes are shared with self antigens (see Fig. 19–4) is also a form of cross-reaction between self and foreign proteins that leads to autoimmunity. Molecular sequencing techniques have revealed numerous short stretches of homology between various microbial and self antigens, particularly self MHC molecules. This homology is called **molecular mimicry,** and it is postulated to be one reason why immune responses against foreign antigens can lead to reactivity against self. However, the significance of such limited sequence homologies is unknown, and there is no clear evidence to support a role of molecular mimicry in autoimmune diseases.

Abnormal Lymphocyte Regulation

Various regulatory abnormalities have been associated with autoimmune diseases, particularly in animal models. Excessive or unbalanced cytokine production may be a mechanism for abnormal stimulation of multiple lymphocytes, including autoreactive cells. Some experimental models support a role for cytokines in "breaking" T cell tolerance. Other cytokines may serve as the effectors of tissue injury. However, there are no convincing examples of cytokine abnormalities being the initiating cause of spontaneous autoimmune diseases.

Deficiencies in the numbers and functions of suppressor or regulatory T cells are also postulated to be a mechanism of autoimmunity. If autoreactive T_H2 cells function normally to control autoreactive T_H1 cells, as has been suggested, then a change in the balance of these subsets, i.e., a relative deficiency of T_H2 cells or an excess of T_H1 cells, may result in pathologic autoimmunity. However, no evidence exists of suppressor cell deficiency or an imbalance of $CD4^+$ T cell subsets causing an autoimmune disease.

Finally, in some autoimmune diseases, lymphocytes may respond excessively to antigens or other stimuli. In an inbred mouse strain called (NZB × NZW)F1, which develops a disease resembling human SLE (see Box 19–1), the B cells are hyper-responsive, i.e., they produce much higher than normal amounts of antibodies not only against self antigens but also in response to foreign antigens and polyclonal activators. Neither the biochemical basis of this abnormality nor its relation to autoantibody production is known.

The Nature of Autoreactive Lymphocytes: Analysis of Antigen Receptor V Genes in Autoimmune Diseases

One approach for better defining the nature of the abnormal lymphocytes in autoimmune diseases is to analyze the patterns of antigen receptors expressed by disease-producing lymphocytes. Sensitive molecular techniques, such as the polymerase chain reaction (see Chapter 5, Box 5–2), have made it feasible to examine the expression of variable (V) genes of antigen receptors in cells isolated from the lesions or circulation of patients. Although such analyses cannot yet establish the actual specificities of autoreactive cells, they can provide valuable information. For instance, they can tell us if autoimmunity is due to the inheritance of particular antigen receptor genes (an unlikely possibility, given that all individuals inherit roughly the same antigen receptor genes). It is also possible to determine if lymphocytes expressing particular V genes are deleted from the mature repertoires of normal individuals but escape negative selection in individuals who develop autoimmunity. If, on the other hand, autoimmunity is due to aberrant activation or regulation of lymphocytes that are present normally, there may be no difference in V gene expression between autoimmune and normal individuals. Finally, sequencing of antigen receptor V regions could show if autoreactive lymphocytes arise as a result of abnormal somatic mutations in receptors that normally recognize foreign antigens, making these receptors reactive with self antigens.

Such considerations have spurred many studies aimed at defining the patterns of V gene expression in the circulation and lesional T and B lymphocytes of individuals with autoimmune diseases. In addition, one can compare the Ig and T cell receptor (TCR) V genes in the germlines of inbred strains of mice that do and those that do not develop spontaneous autoimmunity. Other studies have focused on the detailed structures of self-reactive antigen receptors or antibodies and have compared these with receptors and antibodies produced by normal, foreign antigen–specific lymphocytes in the same individual. Although the available results do not provide definitive clues about the mechanisms of autoimmunity, they do lead to certain conclusions.

1. *In individual patients with certain organ-specific autoimmune diseases, lymphocytes present in the lesions express limited numbers of V genes, whereas circulating lymphocytes from these patients usually show normal diverse patterns of V gene expression.* This finding suggests that the disease-producing cells may have arisen from one or a few clones of lymphocytes and recognize and respond to one or a few antigenic determinants. (Such responses are called "oligoclonal.") For example, most T lymphocytes isolated from the cerebrospinal fluid of an individual patient with multiple sclerosis express only a few TCR genes. Similarly, T cell clones isolated from the synovial (joint) fluid of individuals with rheumatoid arthritis are oligoclonal. However, different patients with the same disease express different V genes in their lesional lymphocytes. Therefore, restricted V gene expression in the autoreactive lymphocytes of individuals probably reflects the fact that these cells are specific for one or a few antigens. This is predictable in diseases restricted to one tissue or organ (such as multiple sclerosis or rheumatoid arthritis). These findings do not establish an association between a particular pattern of V gene usage and an autoimmune disease and do not reveal much about the mechanisms responsible for autoimmunity. The identification of V genes expressed by autoreactive lymphocytes may have some practical applications. It may be feasible to kill these cells by injecting antibodies specific for particular V regions, sparing lymphocytes that are not pathogenic. This kind of therapy has shown promise in inbred mouse strains responding to defined autoantigens. Doing the same for humans would require identifying the dominant V gene(s) expressed in disease-producing lymphocytes in each patient, and it is not yet clear if such an approach is realistic for large numbers of patients.

2. *Autoreactive B and T lymphocytes express the same antigen receptor gene segments as are present in lymphocytes specific for foreign antigens.* For instance, autoantibody-producing B cell clones from mice that develop SLE-like diseases (see Box 19–1) contain Ig V, D, and J gene segments that are also found in various combinations in B cells that secrete antibodies specific for foreign antigens. In other words, no unique pattern of somatic recombination of antigen receptor genes results in the production of receptors specific for self antigens. The Ig genes of autoantibody-producing B cells also show somatic mutations in V regions that are similar to mutations found in normal B cells. Therefore, autoantibodies are produced by the same cellular responses to antigenic stimulation that are seen in lymphocytes responding normally to foreign antigens.

3. *Autoimmunity is not due to a specific Ig or TCR repertoire, and is not associated with a specific V gene polymorphism.* Comparisons of restriction fragment length polymorphism (see Chapter 4, Box 4–2) in humans that do have autoimmune diseases and those that do not indicate no specific associations of the diseases with particular Ig or TCR gene loci. The Ig germline genes in strains of mice that develop SLE-like syndromes also reveal no consistent differences from non-autoimmune strains. These findings support the concept mentioned earlier, that autoimmunity is not attributable to the inheritance of particular disease-associated antigen receptor genes.

The general conclusions of these studies are that (1) organ-specific autoimmune diseases are usually caused by lymphocytes specific for a limited number of antigens, and (2) the molecular mechanisms leading to the production of autoreactive antibodies (and probably T cells) are similar to the mechanisms responsible for the generation of foreign antigen–specific antibodies (and T cells). These studies have not revealed whether autoreactive clones are abnormal cells that have escaped the process of self-tolerance or are normally present cells whose aberrant stimulation or regulation leads to pathologic autoimmunity. In the final analysis, studies of antigen receptor V gene expression have not yet provided much information about the mechanisms of autoimmunity.

GENETIC FACTORS IN AUTOIMMUNITY

From the earliest studies of patients with autoimmune disorders, it has been known that some of these diseases "run in families" and that there is a high rate of concordance in monozygotic twins. Genetic analyses of inbred mice with autoimmunity, mostly done by breeding with other strains, also indicate that heredity plays an important role in the development of autoimmunity. The inheritance patterns of these diseases are often complex—for instance, breeding of inbred mouse strains that spontaneously develop certain autoimmune diseases indicate that up to 20 genes may influence the time of onset and severity of the diseases.

Much of the recent interest in the genetic basis of autoimmunity has focused on MHC genes because of their critical role in the maturation of T cells and in the induction of immune responses to all protein antigens.

Role of MHC Genes in Autoimmunity

HLA typing of large groups of patients with various autoimmune diseases has shown that some HLA alleles occur at higher frequency in these patients than in the general population. From such studies, the relative risk of developing a disease in individuals who inherit various HLA alleles can be estimated (Table 19–2). The strongest such association is between ankylosing spondylitis, an inflammatory, presumed autoimmune, disease of vertebral joints, and the class I HLA allele B27. Individuals who are HLA-B27–positive have a 90 to 100 times greater chance of developing ankylosing spondylitis than individuals lacking B27. Neither the mechanism of this disease nor the basis of its association with HLA-B27 is known. Recently, much more work has been done on the polymorphic class II loci HLA-DR and HLA-DQ in autoimmune diseases because of the realization that class II MHC molecules are involved in the selection and activation of CD4$^+$ T cells, and because CD4$^+$ T cells regulate both humoral and cell-mediated immune responses to protein antigens.

Several issues about HLA-disease associations are worth emphasizing:

1. An HLA-disease association may be identified by serologic typing of one HLA locus, but the actual association may be with other alleles that are linked to the typed allele and inherited together. For instance, individuals with a particular HLA-DR allele (hypothetically, DR1) may show an increased inheritance of a particular HLA-DQ allele, hypothetically DQ2. This is an example of "linkage disequilibrium." Thus, a disease may be found to be DR1-associated, but the causal association may be with the co-inherited DQ2. This realization has emphasized the concept of "extended HLA

haplotypes," which refers to sets of linked genes, both classical HLA and adjacent non-HLA genes, that tend to be inherited together as a single unit (see Chapter 5).

2. HLA typing based on serology, using panels of antibodies that identify different alleles, may not identify the MHC molecules that are truly disease-associated. The reason for this is that a single serologically defined allele may actually consist of a family of related HLA alleles that differ slightly from one another in their polymorphic residues (see Chapter 5). Such differences can be identified only by more detailed molecular studies, such as nucleotide sequencing. In fact, the polymerase chain reaction was originally developed for studying disease-associated HLA molecules. Detailed structural studies of HLA genes in patients with autoimmunity have shown that some HLA-disease associations are much stronger than they appeared to be when calculations were based on less precise serologic typing. Furthermore, sequencing of HLA genes indicates that in many autoimmune diseases, the HLA molecules that show increased frequencies differ only in the peptide-binding clefts from HLA molecules that are not disease-associated. In some ways, this finding is not surprising, because polymorphic residues of MHC molecules are located within and adjacent to the clefts (see Chapter 5). Nevertheless, because the structure of the cleft is the key determinant of both functions of MHC molecules, namely antigen presentation and recognition by T cells (see Chapter 6), these results support the general concept that *MHC molecules influence the development of autoimmunity by controlling T cell selection and activation.*

3. The inheritance of some HLA genes may predispose to particular autoimmune diseases, whereas others may be protective, i.e., their absence may be associated with increased incidence of disease. Examples of both are described below.

4. Although some diseases show strong associations with certain HLA alleles (Table 19–2), there are also many reports of weak associations, with relative risks ranging from 1.5 to 2. In fact, studying HLA-disease associations has become a popular exercise in clinical and research laboratories. The significance of these weak associations is uncertain, at best.

The example of *insulin-dependent diabetes mellitus* (IDDM, Box 19–2) illustrates many of these features of HLA-disease associations. Ninety to 95 per cent of Caucasians with IDDM have HLA-DR3, or DR4, or both, in contrast to about 40 per cent of normal subjects, and 40 to 50 per cent of patients are DR3/DR4 heterozygotes, in contrast to 5 per cent of normal subjects. Interestingly, susceptibility to IDDM is actually associated with a linked DQ allele called DQ3.2 that is often in linkage disequilibrium with DR4. Sequencing of DQ molecules showed initially that all DQβ chains that are more common in IDDM patients than in control subjects have one of three amino acids (alanine, valine, or serine) at position 57 near the peptide-binding cleft, whereas the DQβ chains present at lower frequencies in IDDM patients than in control subjects have aspartic acid (Asp) at this position. The diabetes-prone NOD

TABLE 19–2. Examples of Human Leukocyte Antigen (HLA)–Linked Immunologic Diseases

Disease	HLA Allele	Relative Risk*
Rheumatoid arthritis	DR4	6
Insulin-dependent diabetes mellitus	DR3	5
	DR4	6–7
	DR3/DR4	20
	DR3, DQw8/DQw2	30
	DR2	0.25
Pemphigus vulgaris	DR4	24
Chronic active hepatitis	DR3	14
Sjögren's syndrome	DR3	10
Celiac disease	DR3	12
Ankylosing spondylitis	B27	90

* Relative risk defines the chance of individuals with a particular HLA allele(s) of developing a disease compared with individuals lacking that HLA allele(s).

BOX 19-2.   INSULIN-DEPENDENT DIABETES MELLITUS

Diabetes mellitus is a metabolic disease due to a deficiency of insulin or its inadequate function, leading to abnormalities in glucose metabolism that result in ketoacidosis, thirst, and increased urine production. The late stage of the disease is characterized by progressive atherosclerotic vascular lesions, which can lead to gangrene of extremities due to arterial obstruction, renal failure due to glomerular and arterial injury, and blindness due to arterial aneurysms and increased fragility of proliferating vessels in the retina. The relationship of abnormal glucose metabolism and vascular lesions is not known. Insulin-dependent diabetes mellitus (IDDM, also called juvenile or type I diabetes) affects about 0.2 per cent of the United States population, with a peak age of onset of 11 to 12 years. These patients have a deficiency of insulin resulting from destruction of the insulin-producing β cells of the islets of Langerhans in the pancreas, and continuous hormone replacement therapy is needed.

Several mechanisms may contribute to β cell destruction, including cytolytic T lymphocyte (CTL)–mediated lysis of islet cells, local cytokine (IFN-γ, TNF, and IL-1) production, and autoantibodies against islet cells. In the rare cases in which the pancreatic lesions have been examined at the early active stages of the disease, the islets show cellular necrosis and lymphocytic infiltrations. This lesion is also called **insulitis**. The infiltrates consist of both CD8$^+$ and CD4$^+$ T cells. Surviving islet cells often express class II MHC molecules. This aberrant expression of MHC molecules is probably an effect of local production of IFN-γ and other cytokines by the T cells. It has been suggested that abnormally high expression of MHC molecules may amplify T cell responses and worsen islet cell injury, but there is no evidence proving that islet cells can function as competent APCs. Autoantibodies against islet cells and insulin are also detected in the blood of these patients. These antibodies may participate in causing the disease or may be a result of T cell–mediated injury and release of normally sequestered antigens. In fact, in susceptible children who have not developed diabetes (such as relatives of patients), the presence of antibodies against islet cells is predictive of the development of IDDM. This suggests that the anti-islet cell antibodies contribute to injury to the islets. Multiple genes are involved in this disease. Recently, a great deal of attention has been devoted to the role of HLA genes (see text). Non-HLA genes also contribute to the disease, but these are undefined. Furthermore, viral infections, particularly with coxsackievirus B-4, may precede the onset of IDDM, perhaps by initiating cell injury, altering self antigens, and triggering an autoimmune response. However, the nature of the antigens that initiate islet-specific immune responses is not known.

Animal models of spontaneous IDDM have been described. The inbred BB rat strain develops a T cell–mediated insulitis that is linked to both MHC and non-MHC genes. The non-obese diabetic (NOD) mouse strain also develops a spontaneous T cell–mediated insulitis. The linkage of this disease with the H-2 complex is remarkably similar to HLA-linked IDDM in humans. Interestingly, certain MHC genes are protective and prevent IDDM. The NOD mouse expresses I-A but not I-E class II MHC molecules, and breeding with I-E–positive strains or the expression of various transgenic I-A or I-E molecules in NOD mice reduces the incidence of the disease. A postulated mechanism for this protection is that the transgenic class II MHC molecules may bind the diabetogenic self peptide antigen, thus competitively inhibiting its binding to endogenous class II and presentation to self-reactive T cells. In NOD mice, disease is induced by diabetogenic T cells that recognize an islet antigen called glutamic acid decarboxylase. As the mice age, cells reacting against other islet antigens are detectable.

Several experimental models have been created by expressing transgenes in pancreatic islet cells by introducing these genes into mice under the control of insulin promoters. Four types of transgenic mice are particularly interesting. First, allogeneic class I and class II MHC molecules can be expressed in islet cells to test the hypothesis that this will create an endogenous "allograft" that should be attacked by the immune system. Surprisingly, insulitis does not develop in these mice, because T cells specific for the allogeneic MHC molecules become tolerant. This result may be because islet cells lack costimulators and induce clonal anergy, or because some of the transgene-derived MHC molecules enter the thymus and cause negative selection. Second, cytokine genes have been expressed in islet cells. Mice expressing IFN-γ in the islets develop insulitis and IDDM. In some models, if both allogeneic MHC molecules and IL-2 are expressed in islets, insulitis does develop, probably because local IL-2 production breaks T cell anergy and initiates an allogeneic reaction against the islets. Third, the costimulator B7 has also been overexpressed in islets. These transgenic mice usually do not develop insulitis by themselves but do develop T cell–mediated injury if an allogeneic MHC molecule is co-expressed. Again, this result indicates that over-expression of a costimulator can break peripheral tolerance (clonal anergy) in alloreactive T cells. Finally, if a T cell receptor specific for an islet cell antigen is expressed as a transgene in mice, the mice develop insulitis and diabetes. Interestingly, the transgene-expressing T cells are not deleted in the thymus, indicating that islet antigens do not cause central tolerance. In addition, insulitis develops many weeks before overt diabetes, but the factors responsible for disease progression are not known. These models are clearly valuable for studying T cell responses to tissue antigens, but their relevance to human IDDM is uncertain.

---

mouse strain has serine at position 57 in its I-Aβ chain (the murine homolog of DQβ). In contrast, most other (normal) mouse strains, including the closely related non-obese normal, have Asp at this position. These findings have led to the intriguing hypothesis that Asp57 in the DQβ chain protects against IDDM, and its absence increases susceptibility. However, several exceptions to this association of Asp57 with IDDM have emerged. For instance, Japanese patients with the disease frequently have Asp57 in their DQβ chains. Moreover, if I-A molecules containing either Ser or Asp at position 57 in the β chain are expressed as transgenes in NOD mice, the incidence of disease is reduced. It is likely, therefore, that the residue at position 57 is only one determinant of the function of the MHC molecule, since it is one of the residues forming the peptide-binding cleft. Development of IDDM may be influenced by the structure of the entire cleft, with residue 57 playing a significant but not exclusive role. The HLA linkage of IDDM is also unusual in that it is inherited as a recessive trait—DR3/4 heterozygotes have a higher relative risk of the disease than individuals with either allele.

The likely reason for this is that increased susceptibility is associated with the absence of certain residues in the class II MHC molecules, and the presence of these residues in either chain is protective. Finally, despite the high relative risk of IDDM in individuals with particular class II alleles, most persons who inherit these alleles do not develop the disease. For instance, the frequency of DQ3.2 in the general population is approximately 27 per cent, but only a very small fraction of these individuals develop IDDM.

The finding of HLA alleles associated with autoimmune diseases initially led to the simple hypothesis that disease-associated MHC molecules were structurally abnormal and capable of presenting self antigens to T cells, thus triggering autoimmune reactions. We now know that this hypothesis is probably not correct, because even normal MHC molecules in all individuals present self antigens, but autoimmunity does not occur because of self-tolerance (see Chapter 6). *Several mechanisms have been postulated to explain the association of autoimmune diseases with the inheritance of particular MHC sequences.*

1. The structures of MHC molecules may determine which clones of T lymphocytes are negatively selected during their maturation. For instance, if the MHC molecules in the thymus of an individual cannot bind a self protein with high affinity, immature T cells reactive with this self antigen may escape negative selection and mature to functional competence. Such a mechanism may explain the HLA-DQβ–associated resistance to IDDM—failure to inherit "protective" HLA alleles may result in the failure to negatively select autoreactive T cells. This hypothesis, however, raises an obvious problem. If the relevant MHC molecule is absent, how can autoreactive T cells that mature and enter peripheral tissues ever recognize the self antigen that must be presented in association with this MHC molecule? At present, there is no answer to this question.

2. Class II MHC molecules may influence the activation of regulatory T cells whose normal function is to prevent autoimmunity. For instance, in IDDM, disease-producing T cells may be specific for a self peptide presented in association with HLA-DQ molecules lacking Asp at position 57 of the β chain, whereas T cells that prevent tissue injury may be specific for a complex of the self peptide and HLA-DQ with Asp at position 57. However, no evidence exists to support a difference in the fine specificity of functionally distinct, self-reactive T cell subpopulations.

3. The disease-associated gene may not be an HLA allele itself but another gene located in the HLA complex. The genes for two cytokines, tumor necrosis factor and lymphotoxin, are located within the MHC, and different HLA alleles are associated with different alleles of the cytokine genes. Some of these cytokine variants may be more pathogenic than others, although this theory is not established. Another interesting hypothesis is that autoimmunity is associated with the proteasome or transporter in antigen processing genes whose products serve to degrade protein antigens and transport peptides to sites within cells where the peptides bind to MHC molecules (see Chapter 6). Polymorphisms in proteasomes or transporter molecules could lead to the presentation of peptides that are structurally different from the peptides presented normally. Although this idea is intriguing, there is no evidence that it accounts for autoimmunity.

4. Similarities between microbial antigens and self MHC molecules may result in autoimmune reactions following infections. Although examples of such molecular mimicry have been described, their pathogenic significance is uncertain.

Thus, the available data do not permit firm conclusions about the mechanisms by which inherited MHC genes contribute to autoimmunity. Disease-associated HLA sequences are found in healthy individuals. In fact, as stated previously, if all individuals bearing a particular disease-associated HLA allele are followed prospectively, the vast majority will never develop the disease. Therefore, *the expression of a particular HLA gene is not by itself the cause of any autoimmune disease, but may be one of several factors that contribute to autoimmunity.*

Association of Other Genes with Autoimmunity

The development of autoimmunity is also influenced by multiple non-MHC genes, many of which are not identified. This fact has been most clearly established by breeding analyses of inbred mice that develop autoimmune diseases, such as NOD mice and the (NZB × NZW)F1 strain mentioned previously. Some non-MHC genes are known to predispose to autoimmunity. Genetic deficiencies of two complement proteins, C2 and C4, or the type 1 complement receptor (see Chapter 15) lead to impaired phagocytosis of immune complexes, increased levels of such complexes in the circulation, and SLE-like syndromes. C2 and C4 are located within the MHC locus (see Chapter 5) and have limited polymorphism, but it is not known if particular alleles of these complement genes are in linkage disequilibrium with certain disease-associated HLA alleles. The role of the *fas* gene in a mouse model of SLE has been mentioned earlier, and we have also described the importance of antigen receptor genes in autoimmunity. However, known genes clearly do not completely account for the inheritance patterns of autoimmune diseases. It is hoped that because of the remarkable progress made in the past decade in identifying disease-associated genes and in mapping the human genome, the genetic basis of autoimmunity will be understood in increasingly precise terms in the near future.

INFECTIONS, ANATOMIC ALTERATIONS, AND OTHER FACTORS IN AUTOIMMUNITY

The development of autoimmunity is also related to many other factors.

1. *Viral and bacterial infections* are associated with autoimmunity, and infectious prodromes often precede the clinical manifestations of autoimmune diseases. In most of these cases, the infectious microorganism is not present in lesions and is not even detectable in the individual when autoimmunity develops. Therefore, the lesions of autoimmunity are not due to the infectious agent itself, but result from host immune responses that may be triggered or dysregulated by the microbe. The many possible effects of infections include polyclonal lymphocyte activation, local tissue inflammation leading to enhanced expression of costimulators, alterations of self antigens to create partially cross-reactive neo-antigens, and tissue injury leading to release of anatomically sequestered antigens.

2. *Anatomic alterations in tissues,* such as inflammation (possibly secondary to infections), ischemic injury, or trauma, may lead to the exposure of self antigens that are normally concealed from the immune system. Such sequestered antigens may not have induced self-tolerance. Therefore, if previously sequestered self antigens are released, they can interact with immunocompetent lymphocytes and induce specific immune responses. Examples of anatomically sequestered antigens include intraocular proteins and sperm. Post-traumatic uveitis and orchitis, and orchitis following vasectomy, are thought to be due to autoimmune responses to self antigens that are released from their normal location.

Tissue inflammation may also cause structural alterations in self antigens and the formation of new determinants capable of inducing autoimmune reactions. Inflammation may result in macrophage activation by locally produced cytokines, and if these cytokines stimulate the expression of costimulators, the result may be loss of peripheral tolerance.

3. *Hormonal influences* play a role in human and experimental autoimmune diseases. For instance, SLE affects females about ten times as frequently as males. The SLE-like disease of (NZBxNZW)F1 mice develops only in females and is retarded by androgen treatment.

Many other autoimmune diseases have a higher incidence in females. Whether this predominance results from the influence of sex hormones or other factors is not known.

In conclusion, autoimmunity may result from a combination of local and systemic alterations and is strongly influenced by inherited genes (Fig. 19–6). The current knowledge of operative mechanisms remains incomplete, so that theories and hypotheses continue to outnumber facts. Autoimmune diseases constitute one of the major challenges facing immunologists today. The application of new technical advances and the rapidly improving understanding of self-tolerance are likely to lead to clearer and more definitive answers to the enigmas of autoimmunity.

SUMMARY

The immune system responds to foreign antigens but is unresponsive (tolerant) to each individual's self antigens. Self-tolerance is maintained by selection processes that kill or block the maturation of potentially self-reactive lymphocytes and by mechanisms that inactivate self-reactive lymphocytes in peripheral tissues.

Autoimmunity develops as a result of multiple interacting factors, which collectively lead to a failure or breakdown of self-tolerance. The immunologic mechanisms that may contribute to autoimmunity include abnormalities in lymphocyte selection, mechanisms that overcome peripheral tolerance, polyclonal lymphocyte stimulation, cross-reactions between foreign and self antigens, and abnormal regulation of lymphocyte responses. The strongest genetic association of autoimmunity is with MHC genes, and multiple mechanisms have been proposed to account for such associations. Infections, injury to tissues, and hormonal factors may also contribute to the development of autoimmune diseases. Recent advances in the understanding of self-

FIGURE 19–6. Factors that may contribute to the development of autoimmunity.

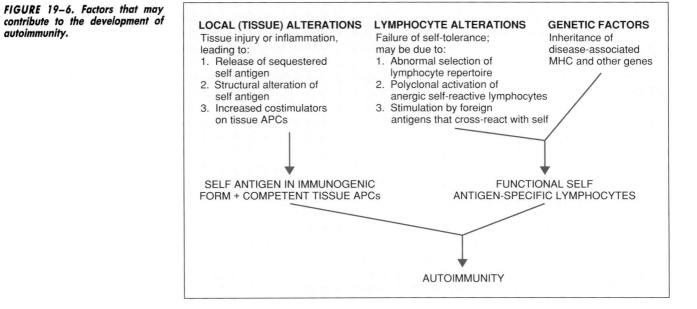

tolerance, and in techniques for analyzing antigen receptor and MHC genes, hold great promise for elucidating the mechanisms of autoimmunity, and for developing rational therapeutic strategies for this group of diseases.

SELECTED READINGS

Acha-Orbea, H. L., L. Steinman, and H. O. McDevitt. T cell receptors in murine autoimmune diseases. Annual Review of Immunology 7:371–405, 1989.

Castano, L., and G. S. Eisenbarth. Type I diabetes: a chronic autoimmune disease of human, mouse and rat. Annual Review of Immunology 8:647–679, 1990.

Cohen, P., and R. A. Eisenberg. *LPR* and *GLD*: single gene models of systemic autoimmunity and lymphoproliferative disease. Annual Review of Immunology 9:243–269, 1991.

Kikutani, H., and S. Makino. The murine autoimmune diabetes model: NOD and related strains. Advances in Immunology 51:285–322, 1992.

Kroemer, G., J. L. Andrew, J. A. Gonzalo, J. C. Gutierrez-Ramos, and C. Martinez. Interleukin-2, autotolerance, and autoimmunity. Advances in Immunology 50:147–235, 1991.

Nepom, G. T., and H. Erlich. MHC class II molecules and autoimmunity. Annual Review of Immunology 9:493–525, 1991.

Rose, N. R., and C. Bona. Defining criteria for autoimmune diseases (Witebsky's postulates revisited). Immunology Today 14:426–430, 1993.

Theofilopoulos, A. N., R. Kofler, P. A. Singer, and F. J. Dixon. Molecular genetics of murine lupus models. Advances in Immunology 46:61–110, 1989.

Todd, J. A. Genetic control of autoimmunity in type I diabetes. Immunology Today 11:122–129, 1990.

Zamvil, S. S., and L. Steinman. The T lymphocyte in experimental allergic encephalomyelitis. Annual Review of Immunology 8:579–621, 1990.

CHAPTER TWENTY

IMMUNE-MEDIATED

TISSUE INJURY

AND DISEASE

Specific immunity is a powerful homeostatic mechanism for eliminating pathogenic microbes and other foreign antigenic substances. The effector mechanisms of specific immunity, such as complement, phagocytes, inflammatory cells, and cytokines, are not themselves specific for foreign antigens. Therefore, immune responses and attendant inflammation are often accompanied by local and systemic injury to normal self tissues. Normally, however, such pathologic side effects are controlled and self-limited, and they abate as the foreign antigen is eliminated. Furthermore, normal individuals are tolerant of their own antigens and do not develop immune responses against autologous tissues. *Failure to control physiologic immune responses against foreign antigens or to maintain self-tolerance leads to diseases in which the primary pathogenic mechanism is immunologic.* Disorders that result from aberrant, excessive, or uncontrolled immune reactions are also called **hypersensitivity diseases.** This term arises from the clinical definition of immunity as "sensitivity," which is based on the observation that an individual who has been exposed to an antigen exhibits a detectable reaction to, or is "sensitive to," subsequent encounters with that antigen. As applied to the historical definition of immunity to microbes, such a "sensitive" individual, of course, would usually be resistant to infection by that microbe. Protective immunity and hypersensitivity may co-exist because both are manifestations of specific immune responses. Immunologic diseases that are thought to be due to immune responses against self antigens are called **autoimmune diseases** (see Chapter 19).

In this chapter we discuss the mechanisms by which humoral and cell-mediated immune responses lead to diseases, using examples of clinical and experimental disorders to illustrate the current understanding of their etiology and pathogenesis. We also touch on the principles of diagnosis and treatment of such diseases.

TYPES OF IMMUNOLOGIC DISEASES

Immunologic diseases comprise a clinically heterogeneous group of disorders. The two principal factors that determine the clinical and pathologic manifestations of such diseases are (1) the type of immune response that leads to tissue injury, and (2) the nature and location of the antigen that initiates or is the target of this response.

The most frequently used *classification of immunologic diseases is based on the principal pathogenic mechanism responsible for cell and tissue injury* (Table 20–1). Immediate hypersensitivity caused by IgE antibodies and mast cells, which is also called type I hypersensitivity, has been described in Chapter 14. Antibodies other than IgE can cause tissue injury by recruiting and activating inflammatory cells and the complement system (see Chapter 15). These antibodies may be specifically reactive with one's own antigens or with foreign antigens that are deposited in, or are antigenically cross-reactive with, self antigens. Such disease-producing antibodies may be detectable in two forms. Some can be found bound to their target antigens or in the circulation in a free form, and the diseases they cause are called type II hypersensitivity. Other antibodies may form immune complexes in the circulation, and the complexes subsequently deposit in tissues, particularly in blood vessels, and cause injury. Diseases caused by immune complexes are classified under type III hypersensitivity. Finally, tissue injury may be due to activated T lymphocytes and the effector cells of delayed type hypersensitivity (DTH), mainly activated macrophages; these are called type IV hypersensitivity disorders.

In our discussion, we use descriptions that identify the pathogenic mechanisms rather than the less informative numerical designations. This classification is useful because distinct types of pathogenic immune responses show quite different patterns of tissue injury and may vary in their tissue specificity. As a result, they produce disorders with distinct clinical and pathologic features. However, immunologic diseases in the clinical situation are often complex and are due to various combinations of humoral and cell-mediated immune responses and multiple effector mechanisms. This is not surprising, given that a single antigen may normally stimulate both humoral and cell-mediated immune responses.

Immunologic diseases can also be subdivided based on the source of the antigens against which the pathogenic immune responses are directed. Such a classification is often impractical in the clinical situation because in many immunologic disorders the target antigens have not been identified. Nevertheless, it is important to try to classify these diseases by the specificity of the immune response, because specificity may provide valuable insights into the etiologies of immunologic diseases.

1. *Immune responses to foreign antigens may be pathogenic in several situations.* First, some microbes persist for prolonged periods because they resist elimination by immune and inflammatory mechanisms. This leads to persistent antigenic stimulation, resulting in a response of increasing magnitude associated with severe tissue injury. Second, some foreign antigens may share antigenic determinants with self tissues and lead to immune responses that cross-react with self antigens. Third, the foreign antigen may be deposited, or "planted" in a particular tissue because of a physicochemical affinity with normal tissue components, so that an immune response directed against the foreign antigen becomes targeted to the tissue in which this antigen is fixed. Fourth, normal immune responses may become defective in their self-regulation, so that they continue unabated even after the initiating foreign antigen is eliminated. Examples of diseases caused by these different kinds of immune responses to foreign antigens are mentioned later in this chapter.

TABLE 20-1. Classification of Immunologic Diseases

Type of Hypersensitivity	Pathologic Immune Mechanisms	Mechanisms of Tissue Injury and Disease
Type I: immediate hypersensitivity	IgE antibody	Mast cells and their mediators (vasoactive amines, lipid mediators, cytokines)
Type II: antibody-mediated	IgM, IgG antibodies against tissue or cell surface antigen	1. Complement activation 2. Recruitment and activation of leukocytes (neutrophils, macrophages) 3. Abnormalities in receptor functions
Type III: immune complex–mediated	Immune complexes of circulating antigens and IgM or IgG antibodies	1. Complement activation 2. Recruitment and activation of leukocytes
Type IV: T cell–mediated	1. CD4$^+$ T cells (delayed type hypersensitivity) 2. CD8$^+$ CTLs (T cell-mediated cytolysis)	1. Activated macrophages, cytokines 2. Direct target cell lysis, cytokines

Abbreviations: Ig, immunoglobulin; CTL, cytolytic T lymphocyte.

2. Immune responses against self (autologous) antigens are usually abnormal. The mechanisms of autoimmunity have been described in Chapter 19.

DISEASES CAUSED BY ANTIBODIES

The first immunologic diseases in which the pathogenic mechanisms were identified were diseases caused by the deposition of antibodies in tissues. This discovery occurred largely because techniques for detecting abnormal circulating autoantibodies and immunoglobulins (Ig) deposited in tissues were developed well before methods for identifying and isolating T cells from lesions or from the blood of patients. Moreover, in experimental models of immunologic diseases, it was possible to cause tissue injury by transferring purified Ig before pure or clonal populations of tissue-reactive T cells became available. For historical reasons, therefore, many of the general principles of immunologic diseases are based on antibody-mediated disorders.

Antibody-mediated diseases are of two types, which differ in their clinicopathologic manifestations and are due to the deposition of antibodies in distinct forms (Fig. 20-1):

*1. Immunologic diseases may be produced by **immune complexes** composed of a soluble antigen and specific antibody; such complexes are formed in the circulation and may deposit in vessel walls virtually anywhere in the body.* This leads to local activation of leukocytes and the complement system, with resultant tissue injury. The antigens that induce the pathogenic humoral immune response can be foreign or self antigens, and the antibodies in the complexes are usually IgM or IgG because these isotypes are most efficient at activating complement and/or inflammatory cells. The pathologic features of such diseases reflect the site(s) of immune complex deposition and are not determined by the cellular source of the antigen. Therefore, immune complex–mediated diseases tend to be systemic, with little or no specificity for a particular antigen located in a particular tissue or organ.

2. Antibodies against circulating cells or fixed tissue antigens cause diseases that are specific for that cell or tissue. The lesions are due to the binding of specific antibodies and not to the deposition of immune complexes formed in the circulation. In most cases, such antibodies are autoantibodies, although occasionally they may be produced against a foreign antigen that is immunologically cross-reactive with a component of self tissues. Such antibodies are usually of the IgM or IgG class, and they cause disease by activating the same effector mechanisms as immune complexes. Some immunologic diseases are due to antibodies specific for cellular structures, such as hormone receptors, that are important for normal function. In these situations, diseases may occur because of interference with the normal functions of these structures and not because of antibody-mediated inflammation or complement activation leading to actual tissue injury.

To prove that a particular disease is caused by antibodies, one would need to demonstrate that the lesions can be induced in a normal animal by the adoptive transfer of Ig purified from the blood or affected tissues of individuals with the disease. An experiment of nature is occasionally seen in children of mothers suffering from antibody-mediated diseases. These infants may be born with transient expression of the diseases because of transplacental passage of antibodies. However, in the usual clinical situations it is not ethical or possible to experimentally transfer diseases with antibodies. Therefore, the *diagnosis* of antibody-mediated disease is usually based on the following criteria: (1) the demonstration of antibodies or immune complexes deposited in tissues, (2) the presence of anti-tissue antibodies or immune complexes in the circulation, and (3) clinicopathologic similarities with experimental diseases that are proved to be antibody-mediated by adoptive transfer.

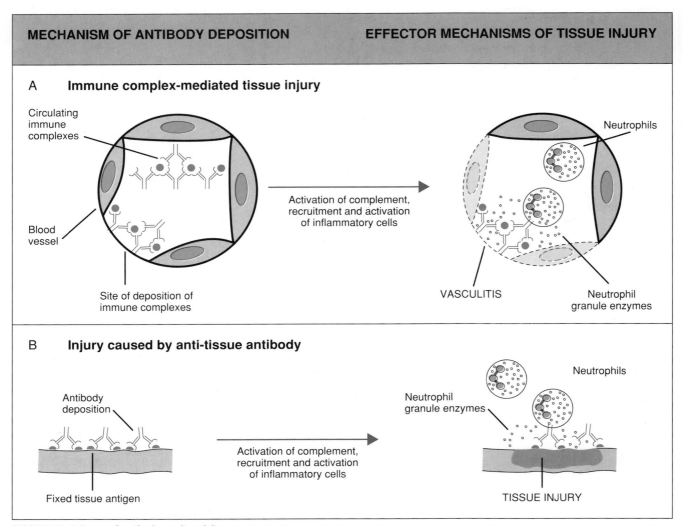

FIGURE 20–1. Types of antibody-mediated diseases. *Antibodies may be deposited as immune complexes that are formed in the circulation (A) or by binding specifically to tissue antigens (B). In both cases, similar effector mechanisms lead to tissue injury at the sites of antibody deposition.*

Mechanisms of Antibody-Mediated Tissue Injury and Functional Abnormalities

In normal immune responses, the protective functions of antibodies are mediated by neutralization of the antigen, activation of the complement system, and recruitment of host inflammatory cells. The same effector mechanisms are responsible for the pathologic consequences of antibody or immune complex deposition. Which effector systems are involved in mediating the protective functions or pathologic effects of different antibodies is determined largely by the isotype of the Ig and the nature of the target antigen:

1. *Complement-mediated lysis of cells* occurs after IgM and some classes of IgG antibodies bind to their specific antigens (see Chapter 15). Complement activa-tion leads to the generation of the membrane attack complex, which causes osmotic lysis of cells (Fig. 20–2A).

2. *Recruitment and activation of inflammatory cells,* mostly neutrophils and, to a lesser extent, monocytes, occur at sites of antibody deposition. This is largely in response to the local generation of complement by-products, particularly C5a, which is chemotactic for neutrophils (Fig. 20–2B). Cytokines, such as tumor necrosis factor (TNFα), and interleukin-1 (IL-1), which are produced by activated macrophages, may also play a role in the recruitment of leukocytes to sites of antibody deposition. Antagonists to these cytokines inhibit antibody and immune complex–mediated tissue injury in some experimental models. In addition, neutrophils and macrophages express surface receptors specific for the Fc portions of γ heavy chains and can therefore bind to and be activated by antigen-complexed IgG antibodies even in the absence of complement activation. Activated neutrophils and macrophages produce hydrolytic enzymes, reactive oxygen

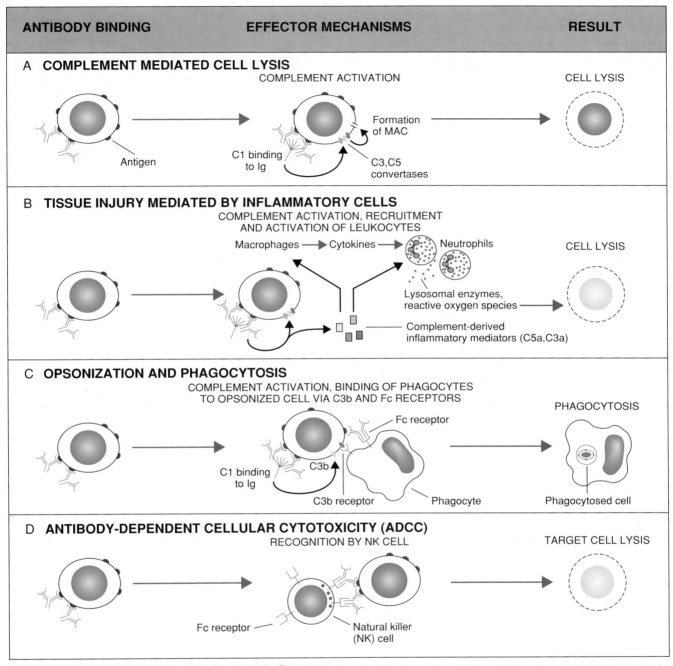

FIGURE 20–2. Effector mechanisms in antibody-mediated cell injury. *Binding of antibodies, such as IgG, to antigens on a cell may cause injury by different effector mechanisms (A–D).*
A. *Activation of complement and formation of the cytocidal membrane attack complex (MAC).*
B. *Recruitment and activation of neutrophils by complement by-products and by cytokines, followed by neutrophil degranulation and release of cytocidal substances.*
C. *Phagocytosis of opsonized cells by macrophages or neutrophils.*
D. *Cytolysis by natural killer (NK) cells and other leukocytes bearing Fcγ receptors.*

species, lipid mediators, and nitric oxide (in mice), which can all contribute to cell and tissue injury.

3. *Phagocytosis of antibody-coated cells* (Fig. 20–2C) may lead to selective depletion of the cells. For instance, in autoimmune hemolytic anemia, autoantibodies are produced against self erythrocytes. The opsonized erythrocytes are phagocytosed by macro-

phages in the liver and spleen. This leads to depletion of the erythrocytes and hence gives rise to anemia.

4. *Lysis of antibody-coated cells by natural killer (NK) cells* (Fig. 20–2D) has been postulated as a mechanism for tissue injury in some diseases, such as autoimmune thyroiditis.

5. *Antibodies can cause pathologic effects by bind-*

ing to functionally important molecules and altering cellular functions without causing tissue injury. Examples of such diseases are described later in the chapter.

Immune Complex–Mediated Diseases

The occurrence of diseases due to immune complexes was suspected as early as 1911 by an astute physician named Clemens von Pirquet. At that time, diphtheria infections were being treated with serum from horses immunized with the diphtheria toxin. This is an example of passive immunization against diphtheria toxin by the transfer of serum containing anti-toxin antibodies. Von Pirquet noted that patients injected with the anti-toxin–containing horse serum developed joint inflammation (arthritis), skin rash, and fever. Two clinical features of this reaction suggested that it was not due to the infection or a toxic component of the serum itself. First, these symptoms appeared even after the injection of horse serum not containing the anti-toxin, so that the lesions could not be attributed to the anti-diphtheria antibody. Second, the symptoms appeared at least a week after the first injection of the horse serum and more rapidly with each repeated injection. Von Pirquet concluded that this disease was due to a host response to some component of the serum. He suggested that the host made antibodies to horse serum proteins, these antibodies formed complexes with the injected proteins, and the disease was due to the antibodies or immune complexes. We now know that his conclusions were entirely accurate. He called this disease "serum disease"; it is now more commonly known as **serum sickness** and is the prototype for immune complex–mediated disorders.

EXPERIMENTAL MODELS OF SERUM SICKNESS

Much of our current knowledge of immune complex diseases is based on analysis of experimental models of serum sickness, performed in detail by Frank Dixon and his associates in the 1960s using techniques for accurately measuring the levels of antigens and antibodies in the blood and tissues. These investigators showed that if a rabbit is injected intravenously with a single dose (greater than 50 mg/kg of body weight) of a foreign protein antigen, bovine serum albumin (BSA), within a few days the rabbit begins to produce specific anti-BSA antibodies (Fig. 20–3). These antibodies complex with circulating BSA, leading to enhanced phagocytosis and clearance of the antigen by macrophages in the liver and spleen. Immune complexes are initially detected in the circulation and then deposit in tissues, where they activate complement, with a concomitant fall in serum complement levels. Complement activation leads to recruitment and activation of inflammatory cells, predominantly neutrophils, at the sites of immune complex deposition, and the neutrophils cause tissue injury. Since the complexes deposit mainly in arteries, renal glomeruli, and the synovia of joints, the clinical and pathologic manifestations are vasculitis, nephritis, and arthritis. The clinical symptoms are usually short-lived, and the lesions heal unless the antigen is injected again. This type of disease is an example of **acute serum sickness.** It is produced by the administration of a single large dose of a foreign antigen and is characterized by the deposition of large immune complexes. A more chronic disease, called **chronic serum**

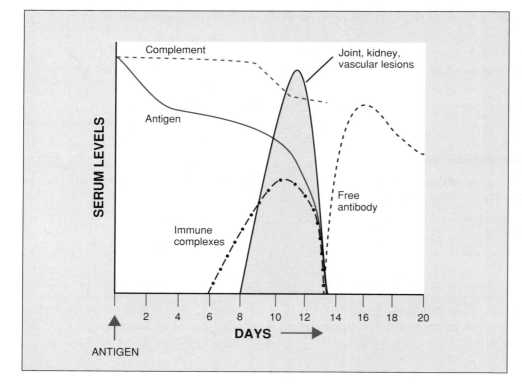

FIGURE 20–3. Sequence of immunologic responses in experimental acute serum sickness. *Injection of bovine serum albumin into a rabbit leads to the production of specific antibody and the formation of immune complexes. These complexes deposit in tissues, activate complement (leading to a fall in serum complement levels), and cause lesions, which resolve as the complexes as well as the remaining antigen are removed. (Adapted with permission from Cochrane, C. G. Immune complex-mediated tissue injury. In S. Cohen, P. A. Ward, and R. T. McCluskey (eds.). Mechanisms of Immunopathology. Werbel & Peck, New York, 1979, pp. 29–48.)*

sickness, is produced by multiple injections of antigen, which lead to the formation of smaller complexes that deposit most often in kidneys, arteries, and lungs.

A localized form of experimental immune complex–mediated vasculitis is called the **Arthus reaction.** It is induced by injecting an antigen subcutaneously into a previously immunized animal. In some models, immunization is passive, i.e., the animal is first given intravenous antibody specific for the antigen. Circulating antibodies rapidly bind to the injected antigen, forming immune complexes that deposit in the walls of small arteries at the injection site. This gives rise to a local cutaneous vasculitis with necrosis. A similar reaction can be elicited by injecting antibody into the tissue and antigen intravenously; this reaction is called a "reverse Arthus reaction." As we shall discuss later, various diseases in humans are believed to be the clinical counterparts of acute and chronic serum sickness and the Arthus reaction.

FACTORS THAT INFLUENCE IMMUNE COMPLEX DEPOSITION

From analyses of these experimental models of immune complex–mediated diseases, it is now known that several factors determine the extent of immune complex deposition.

1. The *size of circulating immune complexes* is a major factor, because very small complexes are not deposited, and large ones are phagocytosed by mononuclear phagocytes and cleared. Usually, small and intermediate-sized immune complexes are prone to tissue deposition, but this may vary with different combinations of antigens and antibodies.

2. The extent of immune complex deposition in tissues is inversely proportional to the *ability of the host to clear immune complexes from the circulation.* Removal of circulating immune complexes is determined by the functional integrity of the mononuclear phagocyte system and the binding of complement proteins, which enhance the clearance of the complexes. Defective phagocytosis may promote the persistence and subsequent tissue deposition of immune complexes. There is a high incidence of immune complex diseases in patients with genetic deficiencies of proteins of the classical complement pathway, such as C2 and C4 (see Chapter 15), because defective production of C3b by antigen-antibody reactions and the absence of complement receptor–mediated phagocytosis lead

to persistence of immune complexes in the blood. In this situation, immune complexes that deposit in tissues presumably recruit inflammatory cells by complement-independent mechanisms or by activation of the alternative complement pathway.

3. The *physicochemical properties of antigens and antibodies,* including charge, valence, avidity of interaction, and Ig isotype, may influence immune complex formation and deposition. For instance, complexes containing cationic antigens bind avidly to negatively charged components of the basement membranes of kidney glomeruli. Such complexes typically produce severe and long-lasting tissue injury.

4. *Anatomic and hemodynamic factors* are important determinants of the sites of immune complex deposition. Capillaries in renal glomeruli and synovia are vessels in which plasma is ultrafiltered (to form urine and synovial fluid, respectively) by passing through the capillary wall at high hydrostatic pressure, and these are among the most common sites of immune complex deposition.

5. Finally, immune complexes are thought to bind to inflammatory cells and stimulate *local secretion of cytokines and vasoactive mediators,* which cause increased adhesion of leukocytes to the endothelium, increased vascular permeability, and enhanced deposition of immune complexes in vessel walls by enlarging interendothelial spaces. This may lead to amplification of tissue injury and disease.

ROLE OF IMMUNE COMPLEXES IN TISSUE INJURY AND DISEASE

Antigen-antibody complexes are produced during many immune responses but are of pathologic significance only if the quantity, structure, or clearance of the complexes are such that abnormally large amounts are deposited in tissues. The *morphologic hallmarks of immune complex–mediated tissue injury are (1) necrosis,* which often contains fibrin because of leakage of plasma proteins and is also called *fibrinoid necrosis,* and *(2) cellular infiltrates composed predominantly of neutrophils.* Irregularly shaped (granular) deposits of antibody and complement components can be detected in these tissues by immunofluorescence, and if the antigen is known, it is possible to also identify antigen molecules in the deposits.

There is compelling evidence supporting a primary *pathogenic role of immune complexes in many human systemic immunologic diseases* (Table 20–2). **Systemic**

TABLE 20–2. **Examples of Human Immune Complex Diseases**

Disease	Antigen	Antibody	Clinicopathologic Manifestations
Post-streptococcal glomerulonephritis	Streptococcal cell wall antigen(s)	Anti-streptococcal antibody	Nephritis with glomerular lesions
Systemic lupus erythematosus	DNA, nucleoproteins, others	Autoantibodies (various)	Nephritis, arthritis, vasculitis (disseminated)
Polyarteritis nodosa	Hepatitis virus surface antigen (e.g., HBsAg)	Anti-HBs antibody	Arteritis (disseminated)

lupus erythematosus (SLE) (Box 19–1, Chapter 19) is an autoimmune disease in which numerous autoantibodies are produced. Its many clinical manifestations include glomerulonephritis and arthritis, which are attributed to the deposition of immune complexes composed of self DNA or nucleoprotein antigens and specific antibodies (Fig. 20–4). The glomerular lesions of SLE often resemble the lesions seen in chronic serum sickness. Some cases of a form of systemic vasculitis called **polyarteritis nodosa** occur as a late sequel of hepatitis B virus infection and are due to arterial deposition of immune complexes composed of hepatitis virus surface antigen and specific antibodies. **Post-streptococcal glomerulonephritis** is a kidney disease that develops 1 to 3 weeks after streptococcal skin and throat infections. It is thought to be due to glomerular deposits of immune complexes composed of strepto-

coccal antigen and anti-streptococcal antibodies. However, post-streptococcal glomerulonephritis differs from typical immune complex–mediated diseases because it involves only the kidneys and there are no systemic manifestations. Therefore, this disease may be due to initial binding of streptococcal antigen to glomeruli followed by deposition of the antibody, so that the pathogenic mechanism is not deposition of circulating complexes but free antibody against a "planted" bacterial antigen. Granular deposits of antibody and complement have been demonstrated in injured tissues in many other forms of cutaneous necrotizing vasculitis, arthritis, and glomerulonephritis. Some skin diseases associated with vasculitis are morphologically similar to experimental Arthus reactions. Such diseases are postulated to be due to immune complexes, but the nature of the antigens is unknown.

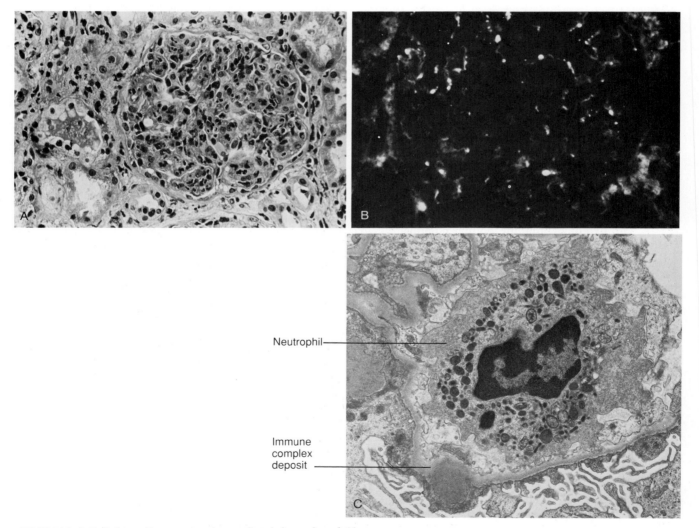

FIGURE 20–4. Pathology of immune complex–mediated glomerulonephritis.
A. Light micrograph of a kidney glomerulus, showing hypercellularity caused by infiltration of leukocytes.
B. Immunofluorescent stain for IgG showing granular deposits in a glomerulus. (Complement proteins, including C3b, would co-localize with the antibody.)
C. Electron micrograph of a glomerular capillary, showing an immune complex deposited in the wall and a neutrophil in the lumen.
(Courtesy of Dr. Helmut Rennke, Department of Pathology, Brigham and Women's Hospital, Boston; reproduced with permission from Brenner, B. M., F. L. Coe, and F. C. Rector. Clinical Nephrology. W. B. Saunders Co., Philadelphia, 1987.)

Diseases Mediated by Antibodies Against Fixed Cell and Tissue Antigens

As we mentioned earlier, antibodies produced against fixed cellular or tissue antigens are usually autoantibodies. Less frequently, the antibodies may be produced against extrinsic antigens but may bind to immunologically similar or cross-reactive antigens present in autologous cells or tissues.

Many tissue- or organ-specific immunologic diseases are associated with the production of, and are thought to be caused by, autoantibodies (Table 20–3). In most of these diseases, specific circulating antibodies can be found in the blood, but the mechanisms responsible for autoantibody production are not known. Autoimmune hemolytic anemia and immune thrombocytopenia are due to autoantibodies against erythrocytes and platelets, respectively. The antibodies cause complement-dependent lysis of the circulating cells and opsonize the cells, leading to enhanced phagocytosis by mononuclear phagocytes. Autoimmune hemolytic anemia and thrombocytopenia are usually idiopathic and may sometimes be associated with other immunologic abnormalities, e.g., in SLE. Similar diseases occur during idiosyncratic reactions to some drugs and may be due to binding of the drugs to cell surfaces, leading to the creation of neo-antigens that elicit specific antibody responses. **Goodpasture's syndrome** is a disease characterized by lung hemor-

rhages and severe glomerulonephritis. It is caused by an autoantibody that binds to a non-collagenous domain of type IV collagen found in the basement membranes of pulmonary alveoli and glomerular capillaries. Binding of this antibody leads to local activation of complement and neutrophils. On microscopic examination, necrosis, leukocytic infiltrates, and linear deposits of antibody and complement along basement membranes can be seen (Fig. 20–5). A number of skin diseases are due to antibodies against epidermal cells or basement membrane antigens. Many forms of **vasculitis** are associated with autoantibodies reactive with proteins, such as myeloperoxidase, in the granules of neutrophils. Such **anti-neutrophil cytoplasmic antigen (ANCA) antibodies** may react with neutrophils that have been partially activated, causing complete neutrophil degranulation and injury to surrounding blood vessels.

Autoantibodies against cell surface receptors may lead to functional abnormalities without the involvement of any other effector mechanisms. For instance, some antibodies against cell surface hormone receptors bind to these receptors and lead to aberrations in cellular physiology without inflammation or tissue injury. These functional abnormalities may result from receptor-mediated stimulation of target cells or inhibition due to interference with receptor function (Fig. 20–6).

One example of stimulation by an antibody mimicking a physiologic molecule is **Graves' disease,** an autoimmune disease of the thyroid gland characterized by hyperthyroidism. The clinical syndrome results from

TABLE 20–3. **Examples of Human Diseases Caused by Autoantibodies**

Disease	Principal Clinical Features	Effector Mechanisms	Autoantibody Detected: Specificity	Method of Detection
Glomerulonephritis (Goodpasture's syndrome)	Nephritis with proteinuria, renal failure; lung hemorrhages	Complement, neutrophils	Type IV collagen in basement membranes of kidney glomeruli and lung alveoli	Immunofluorescence
Autoimmune hemolytic anemia	Hemolysis, anemia	Complement-dependent phagocytosis, lysis	Erythrocyte membrane proteins	Hemagglutination
Autoimmune thrombocytopenic purpura	Platelet deficiency (thrombocytopenia), bleeding disorders	Complement-dependent phagocytosis	Platelet membrane proteins (e.g., gp IIb/IIIa)	Immunofluorescence
Pemphigus vulgaris	Decreased adhesions between keratinocytes; skin vesicles (bullae)	Antibodies stimulate epithelial proteases, leading to disruption of intercellular adhesions	Intercellular junctions of epidermal cells	Immunofluorescence
Bullous pemphigoid	Detachment of epidermal cells; skin vesicles	Disruption of dermal-epidermal junction	Epidermal basement membrane proteins	Immunofluorescence
Myasthenia gravis	Muscle weakness	Blocking and down-modulation of acetylcholine receptor; local inflammation?	Acetylcholine receptor	Immunoprecipitation
Graves' disease (hyperthyroidism)	Hyperthyroidism due to increased production of thyroid hormones	Stimulation of TSH receptor	Thyroid-stimulating hormone receptor on thyroid follicular epithelial cells	Bioassay
Insulin-resistant diabetes mellitus	Diabetes unresponsive to insulin therapy	Inhibition of insulin binding to receptor; down-modulation of receptor?	Insulin receptor	Inhibition of insulin binding to cultured cells
Pernicious anemia	Abnormal erythropoiesis due to vitamin B_{12} deficiency	Neutralization of intrinsic factor	Intrinsic factor; gastric parietal cells	Bioassay; immunofluorescence

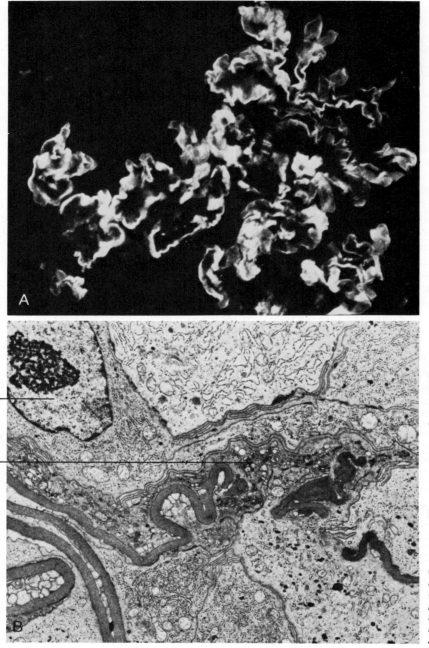

Monocyte

Disrupted
basement
membrane

FIGURE 20–5. Pathology of glomerulonephritis induced by an antibody against the glomerular basement membrane (Goodpasture's syndrome).
A. *Immunofluorescent stain for IgG, showing linear deposition of antibody along the capillary basement membrane of a glomerulus. (This pattern is very different from that of immune complex–mediated diseases; see Fig. 20–4B.)*
B. *Electron micrograph of a glomerular capillary, showing destruction of the basement membrane without evidence of immune complex deposition.*
(Courtesy of Dr. Helmut Rennke, Department of Pathology, Brigham and Women's Hospital, Boston; reproduced with permission from Brenner, B. M., F. L. Coe, and F. C. Rector. Clinical Nephrology. W. B. Saunders Co., Philadelphia, 1987.)

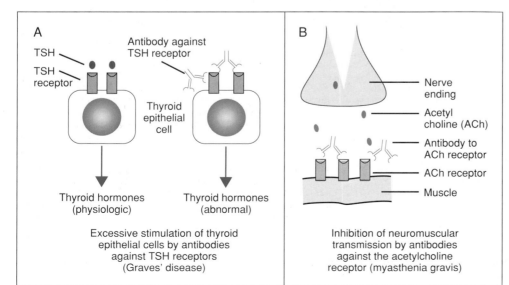

A

TSH

TSH receptor

Antibody against TSH receptor

Thyroid epithelial cell

Thyroid hormones (physiologic)

Thyroid hormones (abnormal)

Excessive stimulation of thyroid epithelial cells by antibodies against TSH receptors (Graves' disease)

B

Nerve ending

Acetyl choline (ACh)

Antibody to ACh receptor

ACh receptor

Muscle

Inhibition of neuromuscular transmission by antibodies against the acetylcholine receptor (myasthenia gravis)

FIGURE 20–6. Effector mechanisms in antibody-mediated diseases: functional abnormalities induced by antibodies against hormone receptors.
A. *Antibodies against thyroid-stimulating hormone (TSH) receptors stimulate thyroid epithelial cells by binding to the receptor and by mimicking the effects of TSH, the physiologic ligand.*
B. *Antibodies against the acetylcholine (ACh) receptor inhibit neuromuscular transmission by binding to the ACh receptor, leading to down-modulation of receptors and competitive inhibition of ACh binding.*

excessive production of thyroid hormones such as thyroxine. This disease is usually caused by an autoantibody specific for the receptor for thyroid-stimulating hormone (TSH) on thyroid epithelial cells. TSH is a pituitary hormone whose normal function is to stimulate the production of thyroid hormones by thyroid epithelial cells. Binding of antibody to the TSH receptor has the same effect as TSH itself, leading to unregulated stimulation of thyroid epithelial cells and excess thyroid hormone production, even in the absence of TSH.

An example of anti-receptor antibody-mediated functional inhibition is **myasthenia gravis,** a disease of progressive muscle weakness caused by autoantibodies reactive with acetylcholine receptors in the motor end plates of neuromuscular junctions. Binding of the antibodies interferes with acetylcholine-mediated neuromuscular transmission and may lead to a reduction in receptor numbers as a consequence of endocytosis and intracellular degradation ("down-modulation") of the receptors. The result is a failure of muscle to respond to normal neural impulses, leading to progressive muscle weakness. Experimentally, a disease resembling myasthenia gravis can be produced in rats and mice by immunizing them with purified acetylcholine receptors. The experimental disease can be adoptively transferred to normal animals by antibodies against the acetylcholine receptor. Interestingly, in some of these experimental models, the disease can

also be transferred to normal animals with acetylcholine receptor–specific CD4+ T cells. This illustrates a concept introduced in Chapter 19, that helper T cells may play a key role even in diseases caused by autoantibodies, and conversely, that tolerance in helper T cells may prevent the production of autoantibodies. Some patients with diabetes mellitus who are unresponsive to insulin have autoantibodies against insulin receptors that block the binding and the physiologic effects of the hormone.

Autoantibodies against physiologically important circulating molecules, such as hormones, may also lead to functional abnormalities and disease in the absence of cell or tissue destruction. Some cases of **pernicious anemia** are associated with autoantibodies against intrinsic factor, which is a cofactor for the intestinal absorption of vitamin B_{12}. The antibodies are thought to bind to and inhibit the function of intrinsic factor, resulting in vitamin B_{12} deficiency. This causes abnormal hematopoiesis and megaloblastic anemia.

Some human diseases are also due to antibodies produced against foreign antigens that cross-react with self proteins. Perhaps the best example is **acute rheumatic fever,** which, like post-streptococcal glomerulonephritis, is a late sequela of throat infection caused by streptococci. The bacterial strains associated with rheumatic fever are usually different from those that lead to glomerulonephritis. Rheumatic fever is charac-

BOX 20–1. RHEUMATOID ARTHRITIS

Rheumatoid arthritis is a destructive disease involving primarily the joints of the extremities, particularly of the fingers. As the disease progresses, more of the large joints are affected. Rheumatoid arthritis is characterized by destruction of the joint cartilage and inflammation of the synovium, with a morphologic picture suggestive of a local immune response. Both cell-mediated and humoral immune responses may contribute to development of lesions. CD4+ T cells, activated B lymphocytes, and plasma cells are found in the inflamed synovium, and in severe cases, well-formed lymphoid follicles with germinal centers may be present. Numerous cytokines, including interleukin-1 (IL-1), IL-8, TNFα, and IFN-γ, have been detected in the synovial (joint) fluid. Cytokines are believed to activate resident synovial cells to produce hydrolytic enzymes, such as collagenase, that mediate destruction of the cartilage, ligaments, and tendons of the joints. Many of the cytokines thought to play a role in initiating joint destruction are probably produced as a result of local T cell and macrophage activation. The specificity of the T cells that may cause arthritis, and the nature of the initiating antigen(s) are not known. Significant numbers of T cells expressing the γδ antigen receptor have also been detected in the synovial fluid of patients with rheumatoid arthritis. However, the pathogenic role of this subset of T cells, like their physiologic function, is obscure.

Systemic complications of rheumatoid arthritis include vasculitis, presumably caused by immune complexes, and lung injury. The nature of the antigen or the antibodies in these complexes is not known. Patients with the adult form of rheumatoid arthritis frequently have circulating antibodies, which may be IgM or IgG, reactive with the Fc (and rarely Fab) portions of their

own IgG molecules. These autoantibodies are called **rheumatoid factors,** and their presence is used as a diagnostic test for rheumatoid arthritis. Rheumatoid factors seem to play no role in the joint pathology or in the formation of injurious immune complexes. Although activated B cells and plasma cells are often present in the synovia of affected joints, the specificities of the antibodies produced by these cells or their roles in causing joint lesions are not known. Susceptibility to rheumatoid arthritis is linked to the HLA-DR4 haplotype and less so with DRI and DRW1D. In all these alleles, the amino acid sequences from positions 65 to 75 of the β chain are nearly identical. These residues are located in or close to the peptide-binding clefts of the HLA molecules, suggesting that they influence antigen presentation or T cell recognition. However, their precise role in rheumatoid arthritis is not yet known (see Chapter 19).

There are several experimental models of arthritis. MRL/*lpr* mice develop spontaneous arthritis and have high serum levels of rheumatoid factors. The immune mechanisms of joint disease in MRL/*lpr* are not known. T cell–mediated arthritis can be induced in susceptible strains of mice and rats by immunization with type II collagen (the type found in cartilage), and the disease can be adoptively transferred to unimmunized animals with collagen-specific T cells. However, in the human disease there is no convincing evidence for collagen-specific autoimmunity. Experimental arthritis can also be produced by immunization with various bacterial antigens, including mycobacterial and streptococcal cell wall proteins. However, such diseases bear only a superficial resemblance to human rheumatoid arthritis.

terized by arthritis, endocarditis resulting in lesions of heart valves, myocarditis, and neurologic abnormalities, but no kidney abnormalities. The myocardial injury is thought to be due to an antibody against a streptococcal cell wall protein that binds to a cross-reactive antigen in cardiac muscle cells.

Despite the numerous examples of circulating autoantibodies associated with immunologic diseases, it is important to reiterate that it is often not clear whether a particular antibody is the cause of the disease or is produced as a result of cell or tissue injury. Furthermore, autoantibodies may be present but may not be responsible for pathologic abnormalities. For instance, patients with **rheumatoid arthritis** (Box 20–1) frequently have a circulating IgM antibody that is specific for their own IgG molecules, usually the Fc portions of these molecules. Such autoantibodies are called rheumatoid factors. Although their presence is a useful diagnostic test for rheumatoid arthritis, there is no evidence that rheumatoid factors are involved in the formation of injurious immune complexes or contribute to the joint lesions in this disease.

DISEASES CAUSED BY T CELLS

The potential importance of T lymphocytes as mediators of human immunologic diseases was increasingly recognized in the 1980s. This insight was largely because of two technological advances—the production of monoclonal antibodies that identify phenotypically and functionally distinct subsets of T cells, and methods for isolating and propagating T cells from lymphoid tissues and lesions. As discussed in Chapter 19, the demonstration that T lymphocytes are critical for maintaining self-tolerance to many protein antigens has led to increasing interest in their role in autoimmune disorders.

Mechanisms of T Cell–Mediated Tissue Injury

The T cells that cause tissue injury may be autoreactive, or they may be specific for foreign protein antigens that are present in, or bound to, one's own cells or tissues. T lymphocyte–mediated tissue injury may also accompany strong protective immune responses against persistent microbes, especially intracellular microbes that resist eradication by phagocytes and antibodies. The pathologic lesions vary, depending on the types of T cells that produce these lesions. T cells injure tissues by the same two mechanisms that are responsible for cell-mediated immunity against microbes (see Chapter 13):

1. T cells of the CD4$^+$ or CD8$^+$ subset secrete cytokines that activate macrophages, giving rise to **DTH reactions.** Acute tissue injury results from the products of activated macrophages, such as hydrolytic enzymes, reactive oxygen species, and pro-inflammatory cytokines. Chronic DTH reactions often produce fibro-

sis as a result of the secretion of cytokines and growth factors by the macrophages (see Chapter 13).

2. CD8$^+$ **cytolytic T lymphocytes** (CTLs) directly lyse target cells bearing class I major histocompatibility complex (MHC)–associated foreign antigens, without the participation of macrophages or any other effector mechanisms.

A role for T cells in causing a particular immunologic disease is suspected largely because of the demonstration of T cells in lesions and the isolation of T cells specific for self antigens from the tissues or blood of patients. Furthermore, cytokines secreted by activated T cells induce alterations in adjacent tissues that are used as indicators of local T cell stimulation. One such cytokine is interferon-γ (IFN-γ), which induces the expression of class II MHC molecules on cells that do not express these molecules constitutively. Abnormal expression of class II MHC molecules in a tissue suggests that T cells have been activated in the immediate environment. Aberrant expression of class II MHC molecules may also lead to excessive T cell activation because many more cells may acquire the ability to present antigen. However, the importance of aberrant MHC expression in exacerbating immunologic tissue injury is unclear because epithelial and mesenchymal cells that are induced to express class II molecules may not produce the costimulators necessary for T cell activation and, therefore, may not be efficient at stimulating T cells (see Chapter 7).

The presence of activated T cells in the blood or tissues of patients is not always associated with disorders of cell-mediated immunity. As mentioned previously, CD4$^+$ helper T cells may be abundant in lesions that are mediated by antibodies and not by the T cells themselves. Moreover, as for antibodies, the identification and even isolation of T cells are not, by themselves, proof of their pathogenic role. The most definitive proof is the ability to adoptively transfer the disease to normal recipients, and this is not possible in the clinical situation. However, in experimental models of several immunologic diseases, the lesions have been transferred to normal syngeneic animals by purified T cells or by antigen-specific cloned lines of T cells (Table 20–4). The similarities between these experimentally induced lesions and clinical diseases further support a primary pathogenic role of T cells in the latter. Finally, alterations in the ratio of circulating CD4$^+$ and CD8$^+$ cells (normal being about 2 : 1) have been used as diagnostic indices for T cell–mediated immunologic diseases. Such assays, however, are of limited usefulness because they are not specific for particular immunologic abnormalities.

Diseases Caused by Delayed Type Hypersensitivity

A variety of cutaneous diseases that result from topical exposure to foreign antigens or are sequelae of skin infections are due to T cell–mediated DTH reactions. These include skin rashes as a result of *contact*

TABLE 20-4. Identification of Antigen-Specific T Cells in Immunologic Diseases

Disease	Specificity of T Cell Clone/Line	Specific T Cells Isolated from Lesions or Blood of		Ability to Transfer Disease in Animal Models
		Patients	*Animal Models*	
Insulin-dependent (type I) diabetes mellitus	Islet cell antigens (including glutamic acid decarboxylase)	No	Yes	Yes
Experimental allergic encephalomyelitis	Myelin basic protein, proteolipid protein		Yes	Yes
Experimental allergic neuritis	P2 protein of peripheral nerve myelin		Yes	Yes
Experimental autoimmune myocarditis	Myosin		Yes	Yes
Myasthenia gravis*	Acetylcholine receptor	Yes	Yes	Yes
Some cases of Graves' disease,* autoimmune thyroiditis	Thyroid follicular epithelial cells	Yes	Yes	Yes

* In these cases, the T cells may be helper cells that stimulate local production of autoantibodies, which are responsible for inducing lesions.

sensitivity to chemicals, such as drugs, cosmetics, and environmental antigens. The rashes usually appear hours or even days after exposure to the contact sensitizing agent. The lesions may be due to T cell responses to neo-antigens created by binding of the chemicals to normal cell surface proteins on epidermal keratinocytes or Langerhans cells. Skin biopsy specimens show dermal perivascular infiltrates of lymphocytes and macrophages, and edema and fibrin deposition resulting from leakage of plasma from dermal capillaries and venules (see Chapter 13). Vascular endothelial cells in the lesions may express enhanced levels of cytokine-regulated surface molecules, such as class II MHC molecules. These DTH reactions are quite different mecha-

nistically and morphologically from two other types of immunologic skin lesions, IgE-mediated immediate hypersensitivity and immune complex–mediated Arthus reactions (Table 20–5).

Many organ-specific autoimmune diseases are caused by autoreactive T cells. In some patients with **insulin-dependent diabetes mellitus** (IDDM) (see Box 19–2, Chapter 19), there are infiltrates of lymphocytes and macrophages around islets of Langerhans in the pancreas, with destruction of insulin-producing β cells in the islets and a resultant deficiency in insulin production. Residual islet cells in these lesions express class II MHC molecules, again suggesting local cytokine production. Similar findings have been observed in

TABLE 20-5. Lesions and Mechanisms of Different Forms of Immunologic Reactions in the Skin

	Immediate Hypersensitivity	Immune Complex–Mediated Injury	Delayed Type Hypersensitivity
Induced by	Antigens that evoke IgE response (genetic predisposition?)	Antigens that induce IgM, IgG antibodies	Protein antigens; chemicals that bind to self proteins
Form of cutaneous reaction	Urticaria, wheal	Arthus reaction	Contact sensitivity, tuberculin reaction
Onset after antigen challenge	Minutes*	Usually 2–6 hours	Usually 24–48 hours
Pathologic lesion	Edema, vascular dilatation, local smooth muscle contraction	Necrotizing vasculitis	Perivascular cellular infiltrates and edema
Transferred to normal animals by	Serum	Serum	Lymphocytes
Antibody involved	IgE	IgG (usually complement-fixing subclasses), IgM	None
Effector cells	Mast cells with IgE bound to Fc receptors	Neutrophils, monocytes (recruited by complement-dependent and complement-independent mechanisms)	CD4+ T cells, macrophages (activated by cytokines)
Secreted mediators, effector molecules	Mast cell–derived mediators: vasoactive amines, lipid mediators	Products of complement activation: membrane attack complex, C3a, C5a	Cytokines, particularly IFN-γ and TNF

* Note that the late phase reaction of immediate hypersensitivity is a cytokine-mediated inflammatory reaction that develops in 6–24 hours.
Abbreviations: Ig, immunoglobulin; IFN, interferon; TNF, tumor necrosis factor.

BOX 20-2. EXPERIMENTAL ALLERGIC ENCEPHALOMYELITIS

Experimental allergic encephalomyelitis (EAE) in mice, rats, and guinea pigs is probably the best characterized experimental model of an organ-specific autoimmune disease mediated exclusively by T lymphocytes. The disease is induced by immunizing animals with guinea pig, bovine, or mouse myelin basic protein (MBP) or proteo-lipid protein (PLP) with an adjuvant containing pertussis bacteria. About 1 to 2 weeks after immunization, the animals develop encephalomyelitis, characterized by perivascular infiltrates composed of lymphocytes and macrophages associated with demyelination in the brain and spinal cord. The neurologic lesions can be mild and self-limited or chronic and relapsing. The chronic form of the experimental disease bears some, albeit superficial, resemblance to multiple sclerosis in humans. This similarity is often quoted as evidence to support the hypothesis that multiple sclerosis is an autoimmune disease. However, neither the antigen or antigens that cause multiple sclerosis nor the role or nature of pathogenic immune responses in this disease are definitively established.

In mice, EAE is caused by CD4$^+$ T cells specific for MBP or PLP. This has been established by many lines of experimental evidence. Mice immunized with either myelin antigen contain CD4$^+$ T cells that produce IL-2 and proliferate in response to that antigen in vitro. The disease can be transferred to unimmunized animals by CD4$^+$ T cells from MBP- or PLP-immunized syngeneic animals, or with MBP- or PLP-specific cloned CD4$^+$ T cell lines. Development of the disease can be prevented by injecting antibodies specific for CD4 or for class II MHC molecules into immunized mice. All disease-producing clones belong to the IL-2 and IFN-γ–producing T$_H$1 subset, and the lesions of EAE usually have the characteristics of DTH reactions. Encephalitogenic clones also express high levels of the β1 integrin VLA-4. The infiltration of T cells into the central nervous system is thought to depend on the binding of VLA-4 to its ligand, VCAM-1, on microvascular endothelium. This is one of the mechanisms responsible for the homing of activated and memory T cells to peripheral tissues (see Chapter 11). The VLA-4–VCAM-1 interaction may also provide costimulatory signals for the activation of the T cells and the production of cytokines. Why immunization with autologous or heterologous myelin antigens induces specific autoimmunity is still not clear. It has been postulated that T cells specific for autologous myelin antigens are not deleted during thymic maturation. Immunization with a myelin antigen together with an adjuvant leads to a T cell response directed against epitopes of autologous myelin proteins. As the T cells respond to these proteins adjacent to blood vessels in the central nervous system, cytokines are released that recruit and activate macrophages. This leads to destruction of the myelin.

Much interest in this disease has focused on the analysis of the fine specificity of MBP–reactive encephalitogenic T cells in different inbred mouse strains. For instance, in mice of the H-2^u strain, most encephalitogenic T cells recognize an MBP peptide consisting of the 9 amino terminal residues in association with the I-A^u molecule. The encephalitogenic T cells in these strains express a limited set of Vα, Jα, and Vβ genes. Mutational analysis of various MBP peptides, similar to the studies described in Chapter 6, has shown that some amino acid residues are critical for binding to MHC molecules and others for recognition by T cells. For instance, in MBP(1-20), an alanine substitution at position 4 enhances binding to I-A^u, whereas an alanine substitution at position 3 abolishes recognition of this peptide by MBP-specific T cells. Based on these findings, the ability of MBP(1-20) Ala 3,4 to inhibit the development of EAE was tested. If the peptide was injected in 10- to 100-fold excess together with MBP at the time of the first immunization, the incidence of EAE was significantly reduced. It is likely that the synthetic peptide binds avidly to I-A molecules and competitively inhibits the binding of the T cell–stimulating processed fragment of native MBP. This antigenic competition blocks activation of MBP-specific T cells and prevents the disease. Such findings provide an elegant in vivo demonstration of the phenomenon of antigenic competition at the level of binding to MHC molecules, which was described in Chapter 6. These results also raise the exciting possibility that if one can identify self antigens that cause autoimmune diseases, administration of mutated forms of these antigens may be a rational and specific immunotherapy for the diseases. Alternatively, if one can identify MHC molecules that bind and present self antigens, synthetic peptides that bind to these molecules but do not stimulate T cells may inhibit the binding of self antigens and, therefore, the activation of MHC-restricted autoreactive T cells. Theoretically, such an approach is feasible even without identifying the self antigen that initiates the autoimmune response. However, in outbred populations, such as humans, many MHC molecules may present many epitopes of self antigens to different T cell clones, so that competition with any one or few peptides may not be beneficial.

EAE has also been induced spontaneously, i.e., without immunization, by expressing an MBP-specific T cell receptor as a transgene in H-2^u mice. This proves that MBP-specific T cells can escape clonal deletion, mature, and enter peripheral tissues. Interestingly, in this model, only a proportion of the transgenic mice develops the disease, suggesting that factors other than expression of the self antigen–specific T cell receptor are required to initiate lesions. Such factors might include infections, which may enhance T cell activation.

Finally, because EAE is induced by well-defined antigens, it is possible to administer these antigens in ways that might induce peripheral T cell tolerance and ameliorate disease. Oral administration of MBP has already been shown to inhibit T cell responses and reduce the severity of EAE. Clinical trials of oral tolerance with MBP in patients with multiple sclerosis are now under way.

spontaneous diabetes in rats and mice, in which the lesions have been adoptively transferred to normal animals with CD4$^+$ T cells from diseased animals. CD8$^+$ CTLs may also contribute to insulitis and islet cell destruction in human and experimental diabetes mellitus. The specificity of the T cells that cause insulitis and destroy islet cells, and the nature of the initiating antigen, are largely unknown. In the NOD animal models, the initial T cell response is against an islet cell surface enzyme called glutamic acid decarboxylase. **Experimental allergic encephalomyelitis** (EAE) (Box 20-2) is a neurologic disease that can be induced in experimental animals by immunization with myelin basic protein in adjuvant. Such immunization leads to an autoimmune T cell response against myelin, culminating in activation of macrophages around nerves in the brain and spinal cord, destruction of the myelin (Fig. 20-7), abnormalities in nerve conduction, and neurologic deficits. EAE can be transferred to naive animals with myelin antigen–specific CD4$^+$ T cells, and the ex-

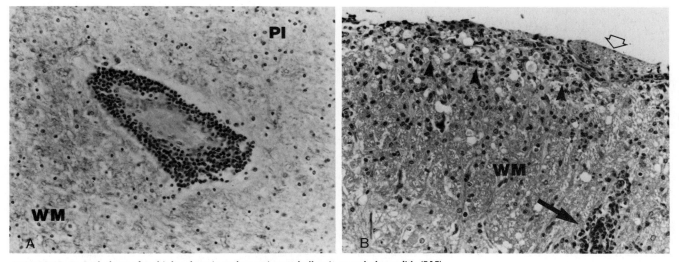

FIGURE 20–7. Pathology of multiple sclerosis and experimental allergic encephalomyelitis (EAE).
A. *Multiple sclerosis: perivascular mononuclear cell infiltrate at the edge of a demyelinated plaque (Pl) in the brain. Myelin is intact in the white matter (WM) but is lost in the plaque (pale staining).*
B. *EAE: Perivascular mononuclear cell infiltrate (black arrow) associated with demyelination (arrowheads) in a mouse immunized with a peptide of myelin proteolipid protein with adjuvant.*
(Courtesy of Dr. Raymond A. Sobel, Department of Pathology, Stanford University School of Medicine, Palo Alto, CA.)

perimental disease can be blocked by antibodies specific for class II MHC or for CD4 molecules, indicating that CD4$^+$ class II MHC–restricted T cells play an obligatory role in this disorder. A role for CTLs in this experimental disease is also suspected but remains unproved. It has been postulated that EAE is an experimental counterpart of the progressive neurologic disease multiple sclerosis.

Cell-mediated immune responses to microbes and other foreign antigens may also lead to considerable injury of the tissues at the sites of infection or antigen exposure. Intracellular bacteria such as *Mycobacterium tuberculosis* induce strong T cell and macrophage responses, resulting in the formation of granulomas, and fibrosis due to the production of cytokines that stimulate fibroblast proliferation and collagen synthesis (described in Chapter 13). Therefore, mycobacterial infections often result in extensive tissue destruction and scarring that can cause severe functional impairment, for instance in the lungs. Tuberculosis is a good example of a disease in which protective cell-mediated immunity and tissue injury due to DTH may co-exist (see Chapter 16). Sarcoidosis is a disease of unknown etiology in which granulomas develop in the lungs, lymphoid tissues, liver, and spleen. This disease is probably due to a T cell–mediated immune response to a foreign antigen that has eluded identification.

Diseases Caused by Cytolytic T Lymphocytes

The principal physiologic function of CTLs is to eliminate intracellular microbes, primarily viruses. It follows, therefore, that infected cells are lysed during CTL-mediated protective immune responses. Some viruses directly injure infected cells or are cytopathic, whereas others are not. Since CTLs cannot *a priori* distinguish between cytopathic and non-cytopathic viruses, they lyse virally infected cells whether or not the infection itself is harmful to the host. *Therefore, CTL responses to viral infections can lead to tissue injury even if the virus itself has no pathologic effects.* Examples of viral infections in which the lesions are due to the host CTL response and not the virus itself include lymphocytic choriomeningitis in mice and certain forms of viral hepatitis in humans (see Chapter 16).

There are few documented examples of autoimmune diseases mediated by CTLs. In mice infected with the coxsackievirus B, myocarditis develops, with infiltration of the heart by CD8$^+$ T cells. These animals contain virus-specific, class I MHC–restricted CTLs as well as CTLs that lyse uninfected myocardial cells. It is postulated that the heart lesions are initiated by the virus infection and virus-specific CTLs, but myocardial injury leads to the exposure or alteration of self antigens and the development of autoreactive CTLs. As mentioned above, CTLs may also contribute to tissue injury in many of the disorders that are caused primarily by CD4$^+$ T cells, such as insulitis in IDDM. It is likely, however, that extracellular tissue antigens preferentially stimulate CD4$^+$ T cells and that CD8$^+$ CTLs recognize and respond to endogenously synthesized antigens, such as viral proteins. One would, therefore, predict that these two forms of T cell–mediated responses would be involved in pathologic immune reactions against distinct types of antigens.

PRINCIPLES OF THERAPY FOR IMMUNE-MEDIATED DISEASES

Therapy for immune-mediated diseases is modeled after approaches that are used to prevent graft rejection, another form of injurious immune response (see Chapter 17). The mainstay of treatment for diseases caused by immune responses is anti-inflammatory drugs, particularly corticosteroids. Such drugs are targeted at reducing tissue injury, i.e., the effector phases of the pathologic immune responses. Antagonists against pro-inflammatory cytokines, such as IL-1 and TNF, and agents that block leukocyte emigration into tissues are also being tested for their anti-inflammatory effects. In severe cases, immunosuppressive drugs like cyclosporin A are used to block T cell activation. Plasmaphoresis has been used during exacerbations of antibody-mediated diseases to reduce circulating levels of antibodies or immune complexes.

Many experimental therapies are being attempted in cases that are resistant to conventional regimens. T cells can be depleted by injecting antibodies against CD3 or the T cell receptor. Immunoconjugates of IL-2 and toxins (e.g., ricin) may bind to activated T cells that express high-affinity IL-2 receptors and kill these cells. More specific treatment aimed at the disease-producing T cell clones or the antigen that initiates the disease requires accurate identification of the antigen. Approaches include attempts to induce tolerance, e.g., by oral administration of antigens that cause autoimmunity, or peptide competition, as in EAE (Box 20–2). Although the value of such therapies has been demonstrated in various experimental (animal) models, their application to clinical disease has not been established.

Summary

Diseases in which tissue injury and pathophysiologic abnormalities are due to immunologic mechanisms may be initiated by immune responses to foreign or self (autologous) antigens. Pathogenic mechanisms include antigen-antibody complexes formed during humoral immune responses, autoantibodies against fixed tissue or cell surface antigens, and T lymphocytes. The effector mechanisms by which antibodies and immune complexes induce tissue injury include activation of the complement system and various host inflammatory cells. Antibodies against physiologic agents such as hormones or against cell surface receptors for hormones induce functional abnormalities without the involvement of any other effector systems. T lymphocytes recruit and activate macrophages as the principal effectors of DTH and tissue injury, and CD8$^+$ cytolytic T lymphocytes themselves lyse antigen-bearing target cells. The therapy of immune-mediated diseases is aimed at reducing immune responses and the attendant inflammation.

Selected Readings

Bruijn, J. A., P. J. Hoedemaeker, and G. J. Fleuren. Pathogenesis of anti-basement membrane glomerulopathy and immune complex glomerulonephritis: dichotomy dissolved. Laboratory Investigation 61:480–488, 1989.

Castano, L., and G. S. Eisenbarth. Type diabetes: a chronic autoimmune disease of human, mouse and rat. Annual Review of Immunology 8:647–679, 1990

Charreire, J. Immune mechanisms in autoimmune thyroiditis. Advances in Immunology 46:263–334, 1989.

Harris, E. D. Rheumatoid arthritis: pathophysiology and implications for treatment. New England Journal of Medicine 322:1277–1289, 1990.

Lindstrom, J., D. Shelton, and Y. Fujii. Myasthenia gravis. Advances in Immunology 42:233–284, 1988.

Naparstek, Y., and P. H. Poltz. The role of autoantibodies in autoimmune diseases. Annual Review of Immunology 11:79–104, 1993.

Zamvil, S. S., and L. Steinman. The T lymphocyte in experimental allergic encephalomyelitis. Annual Review of Immunology 8:579–621, 1990.

CONGENITAL AND

ACQUIRED

IMMUNODEFICIENCIES

The integrity of the immune system is essential for defense against infectious organisms and their toxic products and, therefore, for the survival of all individuals. Defects in one or more components of the immune system can lead to serious and often fatal disorders, which are called immunodeficiency diseases. These diseases are broadly classified into two groups. The **primary** or **congenital immunodeficiencies** are genetic defects that result in an increased susceptibility to infections that is frequently manifested early in infancy and childhood but is sometimes clinically detected later in life. It is estimated that in the United States approximately 1 in 500 individuals is born with a defect in some component(s) of the immune system, although only a small proportion are affected severely enough to develop life-threatening complications. **Secondary** or **acquired immunodeficiencies** develop as a consequence of malnutrition, disseminated cancers, treatment with immunosuppressive drugs, or infections of immunocompetent cells, most notably with the human immunodeficiency virus (HIV), the etiologic agent of the acquired immunodeficiency syndrome (AIDS). This chapter describes the major types of congenital and acquired immunodeficiencies, with an emphasis on their pathogenesis and on the components of the immune system that are involved in each.

Before beginning our discussion, it is important to emphasize some general features of immunodeficiencies:

1. *The principal consequence of immunodeficiency is an increased susceptibility to infections.* The nature of the infection in a particular patient depends largely on the component of the immune system that is defective. For instance, deficient humoral immunity usually results in increased susceptibility to infections by pyogenic bacteria, whereas defects in cell-mediated immunity lead to infections by viruses and other intracellular microbes. Specific examples of these will be mentioned later in the chapter.

2. *Patients with immunodeficiencies are also prone to certain types of cancers, many of which are caused by oncogenic viruses.* This is generally seen in T cell immunodeficiencies because, as we discussed in Chapter 18, T cells play an important role in surveillance against tumors. In addition, somewhat paradoxically, certain immunodeficiencies are associated with an increased incidence of autoimmunity.

3. *Clinically and pathologically, immunodeficiency diseases are extremely heterogeneous.* In large part, this is because different diseases involve different components of the immune system. However, such heterogeneity is also seen in various diseases involving the same cells or molecules and even in different patients suffering from the same disorder. The reason for this variability is not well understood.

Deficient immune responses may result from abnormalities in specific or natural immunity. Defective specific immunity is due to abnormal development, activation, or function of specific T or B lymphocytes, or both. Among the examples of impaired natural immunity are defects in phagocytes and the complement system. We first describe congenital immunodeficiencies, dividing our discussion into defects in B cells, T cells, and both, and in phagocytes. In each group, the current understanding of the cellular or molecular basis of the immunodeficiency will be illustrated with selected examples. We conclude this chapter with a discussion of AIDS and other acquired immunodeficiencies.

PRIMARY DEFECTS IN B LYMPHOCYTES AND ANTIBODY PRODUCTION

Congenital abnormalities in B lymphocyte development and function result in deficient antibody production. These diseases have been recognized for many years, because assays for measuring serum antibodies have been in routine clinical use since the 1950s. A large number of congenital deficiencies that selectively affect humoral immune responses are now known (Table 21–1). Clinically, these disorders are characterized by recurrent infections with pyogenic organisms, such as pneumococcus, *Haemophilus influenzae,* and streptococcus. In addition, patients are susceptible to certain viral infections, such as polio, and to intestinal parasites such as *Giardia.* Not surprisingly, immunity to these microbes is normally mediated principally by antibodies (see Chapter 16).

In different antibody deficiencies, the primary abnormality may be at different stages of B lymphocyte maturation or in the responses of mature B cells to antigenic stimulation (Fig. 21–1). Abnormal helper T cell function may also result in deficient antibody production. One of the impressive recent achievements of molecular immunology is the identification of the genetic basis of several immunodeficiency diseases; these are mentioned below. In the following section we describe some examples of antibody immunodeficiencies, emphasizing the mechanisms of B cell defects.

X-linked Agammaglobulinemia

This disease, also called Bruton's agammaglobulinemia, is characterized by the absence of γ globulins in the blood, as the name implies. It is one of the most common congenital immunodeficiencies and the prototype of selective B cell defects. It was also the first immunodeficiency to be recognized, in 1952, and studies of these patients were useful in proving that plasma cells produced antibodies (both of which are absent in the patients). It is an X chromosome–linked disease, so that females who carry the defective gene on one X chromosome are phenotypically normal because the other X chromosome has a normal gene, but males who inherit the abnormal X chromosome manifest the disease. (In addition to X-linked agammaglobulinemia, four other human immunodeficiency diseases are

TABLE 21–1.   Examples of Congenital B Cell Immunodeficiencies

Disease	Functional Deficiencies	Presumed Mechanism of Defect
X-linked agammaglobulinemia	All Ig isotypes decreased; reduced B cells	Mutation in Bruton's tyrosine kinase Block in pre-B to B cell maturation
Selective IgA deficiency	Decreased serum IgA1 and IgA2; normal B cells	Failure of terminal differentiation of IgA⁺ B cells
Ig deficiency with increased IgM (hyper-IgM syndrome)	Increased IgM; normal or increased IgD; other Ig isotypes decreased	Mutation in gp39 T cell ligand of CD40 Defect in heavy chain isotype switching
Selective IgG subclass deficiencies	Decrease in one or more IgG subclasses	Defect in isotype switching or terminal B cell differentiation
Ig heavy chain deletions	IgG1, IgG2, or IgG4 absent; sometimes associated with absent IgA or IgE	Chromosomal deletion at 14q32 (Ig heavy chain locus)
Transient hypogammaglobulinemia of infancy	IgG and IgA decreased; detectable levels of antibacterial antibodies; normal B cells	Unknown; ? delayed maturation of helper T cells in some patients
Common variable immunodeficiency	Variable reductions in multiple Ig isotypes; normal or decreased B cells	Defect in B cell maturation, usually due to intrinsic B cell abnormality

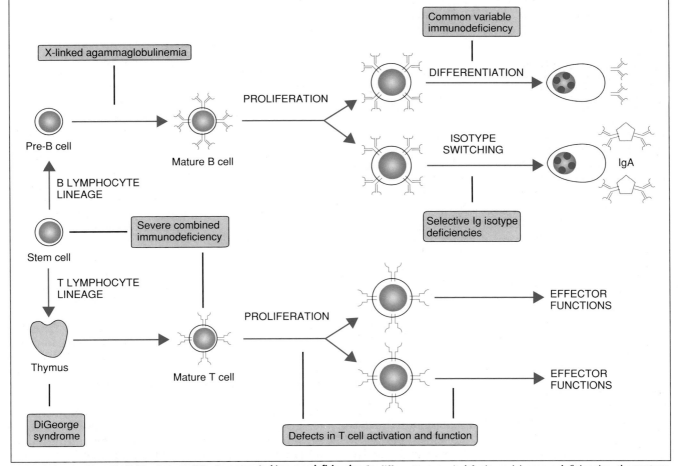

FIGURE 21–1. Sites of cellular abnormalities in congenital immunodeficiencies. *In different congenital (primary) immunodeficiencies, the maturation or activation of B or T lymphocytes may be blocked at different stages.*

linked to the X chromosome.) Thus, X-linked agammaglobulinemia is transmitted from phenotypically normal female carriers to their male offspring. All somatic cells in females randomly inactivate one or the other X chromosome ("lyonization"). B cells of female carriers of X-linked agammaglobulinemia mature only if they inactivate the X chromosome bearing the mutant allele, whereas T cells and other somatic cells show a normal random pattern of lyonization. Thus, by assessing X chromosome utilization in B cells, it is possible to identify carriers of the disease. Affected boys are susceptible to bacterial and some viral infections, whereas infections by most intracellular microbes and fungi are handled normally. These children suffer from recurrent pyogenic bacterial infections of the conjunctiva, throat, skin, middle ear, bronchi, and lungs. Newborn infants are often normal because maternally derived antibodies provide adequate protection, and the disease is usually recognized late in the first year of life. If untreated, the disease is usually fatal.

Patients with X-linked agammaglobulinemia usually have low or undetectable serum immunoglobulin (Ig), reduced or absent B cells in peripheral blood and lymphoid tissues, no germinal centers in lymph nodes, and no plasma cells in tissues. In most patients, the numbers of pre–B cells in the bone marrow are normal, and these cells synthesize normal μ heavy chains. Thus, the disease is due to a block in the maturation of pre–B cells to surface IgM-positive B cells. Some patients do have mature peripheral B cells and even have elevated levels of serum IgG and IgA. However, in these patients, B cell numbers may be 100-fold lower than normal, and antibody responses to immunization are seriously deficient, suggesting that only a very limited repertoire of B cells is present. The maturation, numbers, and functions of T cells are generally normal. Some studies have revealed reduced numbers of activated T cells in patients, which may be a consequence of reduced antigen presentation due to the lack of B cells. Almost 20 per cent of patients develop autoimmune disorders, the mechanisms of which are unknown.

The gene that is defective in X-linked agammaglobulinemia is on the long arm of the X chromosome and encodes a protein tyrosine kinase that is normally expressed in all stages of B cell differentiation and is called Bruton's tyrosine kinase (Btk). Patients with X-linked agammaglobulinemia have point mutations or deletions in this gene and therefore do not produce a functional form of this protein kinase. In pre–B cells of these patients, VDJ rearrangements and μ chain production are normal, but subsequent light chain gene rearrangements do not occur. It is therefore likely that Btk is involved in signaling events that are essential for light chain gene expression. A mutant mouse strain called **CBA/N** has an X-linked defect in B cell development that is also a result of a point mutation in the Btk gene. Another demonstration of the likely importance of protein phosphorylation events and signaling in lymphocyte maturation is provided by the mutant strain of mouse called **motheaten.** The phenotype of this mouse is inherited as a homozygous recessive trait and

is associated with severe impairment of T and B cell development. The defective gene has been identified, and it encodes a protein phosphatase.

The infectious complications of X-linked agammaglobulinemia are greatly reduced by periodic (e.g., monthly) intravenous or intramuscular injections of pooled gamma globulin preparations. Such preparations contain pre-formed antibodies against common pathogens and provide effective passive immunity.

Selective Immunoglobulin Isotype Deficiencies

Many immunodeficiencies that selectively involve one or a few Ig isotypes have been described. The most common is **selective IgA deficiency,** which affects about 1 in 700 individuals of Caucasian descent and is thus the most common primary immunodeficiency. The inheritance pattern of IgA deficiency is variable, different cases being autosomal dominant or recessive. In some patients, the disorder may not be inherited but may occur as a result of embryonic rubella infection or drug exposures. The clinical features are also extremely variable. Many patients are entirely normal, others have occasional respiratory infections and diarrhea, and, rarely, patients have severe, recurrent infections leading to permanent intestinal and airway damage, with associated autoimmune disorders.

IgA deficiency is characterized by abnormally low serum IgA, usually less than 50 μg/ml, with normal or elevated levels of IgM and IgG. The defect in these patients is a block in the differentiation of surface IgA-expressing B cells to antibody-secreting plasma cells. The α heavy chain genes and the expression of membrane-associated IgA are normal. It is not known whether the block of B cell differentiation is due to an intrinsic B cell defect or to an abnormality in T cell help, such as the production of cytokines that enhance IgA secretion (e.g., transforming growth factor–β [TGF-β] and interleukin-5 [IL-5]), or in B cell responses to these cytokines. No gross abnormalities in the numbers, phenotypes, or functional responses of T cells have been noted in these patients.

Selective IgG subclass deficiencies have been described in which total serum IgG levels are normal but concentrations of one or more subclasses are below normal. Deficiency of IgG3 is the most common subclass deficiency in adults, and IgG2 deficiency is the most common in children. These are not usually associated with significant disease. Selective IgG subclass deficiencies are usually due to abnormal B cell differentiation and, rarely, are due to homozygous deletions of various constant region (C_γ) genes. Individuals with single C_γ gene deletions are usually normal, which attests to the capacity of the immune system to compensate for selective antibody deficiencies.

IgG and IgA deficiency with increased IgM (hyper-IgM syndrome) is usually inherited as an X-linked disorder. Affected male children produce only IgM antibodies and are therefore susceptible to severe bacterial infections. Furthermore, many of the IgM antibodies are autoantibodies reactive with the patient's own red blood cells, leukocytes, and platelets. This leads to secondary deficiencies of these blood cells, further reducing resistance to infections. The C_γ and C_α genes are structurally normal, as are the switch regions located 5′ of these genes. However, heavy chain class switching to IgG and IgA does not occur, so that the patients lack B cells with surface IgG or IgA and do not produce these isotypes. The X-linked form of this disease is due to mutations in the gene encoding the CD40 ligand, gp39. The mutant forms of gp39 produced in these patients do not bind CD40 and therefore do not stimulate B cells to differentiate and undergo switch recombinations (see Chapter 9).

Common Variable Immunodeficiency

This group of antibody deficiency disorders is usually inherited in an autosomal manner. Hypogammaglobulinemia may develop in affected children at different ages, but the increased susceptibility to bacterial infections is usually manifested in late childhood or early adult life. (For this reason, the disease is also called **acquired agammaglobulinemia.**) Patients as well as relatives have a high incidence of lymphoid and gastrointestinal malignancies as well as autoimmune diseases, including pernicious anemia, hemolytic anemia, and rheumatoid arthritis.

Common variable immunodeficiency has been attributed to multiple abnormalities, including intrinsic B cell defects, deficient T cell help, and excessive "suppressor cell" activity. It is likely that in the majority of patients the primary abnormality responsible for low antibody production is a defect in the terminal differentiation of B lymphocytes to antibody-secreting cells. In lymphoid tissues, the B cell areas (i.e., lymphoid follicles) are often hyperplastic but plasma cells are absent. These findings suggest that B cells proliferate in response to antigenic stimulation but fail to differentiate normally. It is not known whether this is due to defective responses to helper T cell–derived stimuli or to more distal block(s) in the program of B cell activation. In some patients, IgM production can be induced *in vitro* by transformation with Epstein-Barr virus, which functions as a T cell–independent stimulus. However, even in these individuals, switching to other isotypes, such as IgG and IgA, usually does not occur. There are some indications that common variable immunodeficiencies and selective IgA deficiency are caused by the same genetic defects since they often occur in the same families and both are associated with mutations or rare alleles in the major histocompatibility complex.

PRIMARY DEFECTS IN T LYMPHOCYTES

Severe defects in T cell maturation, such as the DiGeorge syndrome (discussed below), have been recognized for many years. More subtle immunodeficiencies attributable to primary T cell abnormalities are now being appreciated, as our assays for T cell maturation and function are improving. In the previous section of the chapter, we mentioned that some antibody deficiencies may, in fact, be due to abnormal T cell help. We shall now describe immunodeficiencies that primarily influence T lymphocytes and, therefore, lead to impaired cell-mediated immune reactions (see Fig. 21–1; Table 21–2).

TABLE 21–2.   Examples of Congenital T Cell and Combined Immunodeficiencies

Disease	Functional Deficiencies	Presumed Mechanism of Defect
DiGeorge syndrome	Decreased T cells; normal B cells; normal or decreased serum Ig	Anomalous development of 3rd and 4th branchial pouches, leading to thymic hypoplasia
SCID X-linked	Markedly decreased T cells; normal or increased B cells; reduced serum Ig	IL-2Rγ chain gene mutation, defective T cell maturation
Autosomal recessive	Decreased T and B cells; reduced serum Ig	Defective maturation of T and B cells
ADA deficiency	Progressive decrease in T and B cells (mostly T); reduced serum Ig	ADA deficiency leading to accumulation of toxic metabolites
PNP deficiency	Decreased T cells; normal B cells and serum Ig	PNP deficiency leading to accumulation of toxic metabolites in developing T cells
Class II MHC deficiency	Normal lymphocyte numbers; normal or decreased serum Ig; deficient cell-mediated immunity	Deficiency of X-box binding factors causing defective transcription of class II MHC genes
Reticular dysgenesis	Markedly decreased T and B cells and other blood cells; reduced serum Ig	Defective maturation of hematopoietic stem cells
Wiskott-Aldrich syndrome	Progressive decrease in T cells; normal B cells; decreased IgM; deficient antibody responses to polysaccharide antigens	Defective glycosylation of membrane proteins, defective maturation of hematopoietic stem cells
Ataxia-telangiectasia	Decreased T cells; normal B cells; variable reduction in IgA, IgE, and IgG subclasses	?Defect in DNA repair

Abbreviations: SCID, severe combined immunodeficiency disease; ADA, adenosine deaminase; PNP, purine nucleoside phosphorylase; Ig, immunoglobulin; MHC, major histocompatibility complex.

Cellular immune deficiencies are manifested by increased susceptibility to infections with viruses, fungi, intracellular bacteria, and protozoa. Such microorganisms are often capable of surviving and even replicating inside cells, including phagocytes (which is why their eradication is dependent on T cell immunity, as discussed in Chapter 16). As a result, these infections are usually severe and difficult to control and may be fatal. Patients with T cell deficiencies may also be susceptible to malignancies. These aspects are discussed more fully later in this chapter when we discuss the clinical features of AIDS, the prototypical acquired T cell immunodeficiency. T cell immunodeficiencies are diagnosed by reduced numbers of peripheral blood T cells, abnormally low proliferative responses to polyclonal T cell activators, e.g., phytohemagglutinin (PHA), and deficient cutaneous delayed type hypersensitivity (DTH) reactions to ubiquitous microbial antigens, such as *Candida* antigens.

The DiGeorge Syndrome (Thymic Hypoplasia)

This selective T cell deficiency is due to a congenital malformation that results in defective development of the third and fourth pharyngeal pouches. These structures give rise to the thymus and the parathyroid glands at weeks 6 to 8 of gestation and to the aortic arch and portions of the lips and ears at 12 weeks of fetal life. Developmental anomalies induced at this stage of gestation lead to partial or complete DiGeorge syndrome, manifested by hypoplasia or agenesis of the thymus (leading to deficient cell-mediated immunity), absent parathyroid glands (causing abnormal calcium homeostasis and muscle twitching, or tetany), abnormal development of the great vessels, and facial deformities. Different patients may show varying degrees of these abnormalities. The nature of the developmental insult is usually not known. Some cases are associated with maternal alcohol consumption, and rare cases show autosomal dominant patterns of inheritance or are associated with translocations involving chromosome 22.

The hypoplasia of the thymus leads to defective maturation of all T lymphocytes, because of which peripheral blood T lymphocytes are absent or greatly reduced in number. Sometimes the total peripheral blood lymphocyte count is near normal, but most of the cells are B lymphocytes (which make up only 10 to 20 per cent of the blood lymphocytes in normal individuals). Peripheral blood lymphocytes do not respond to polyclonal T cell activators or in mixed leukocyte reactions (MLRs). Antibody levels are usually normal but may be reduced in severely affected patients. In the peripheral lymphoid tissues, the B cells appear normal. As in other severe T cell deficiencies, patients are susceptible to mycobacterial, viral, and fungal infections.

The disease can be corrected by fetal thymic transplantation or by human leukocyte antigen (HLA)-identical bone marrow transplantation. This is usually not necessary, however, because T cell function tends to improve with age and is often normal by 5 years. This is probably because of the presence of some thymic tissue or because extrathymic sites assume the function of T cell maturation. The existence of extrathymic sites of T cell development has been suspected, but no such tissue has been defined anatomically. It is also possible that as these patients grow older, typical thymus tissue develops at ectopic sites (i.e., other than the normal location). Similarly, ectopic parathyroids develop with age, with consequent improvement of tetany.

An example of T cell immunodeficiency in animals is the **nude (athymic) mouse.** These mice have an inherited defect of epithelial cells in the skin, leading to hairlessness, and in the lining of the third and fourth pharyngeal pouches, causing thymic hypoplasia. The disorder is due to a recessive gene on chromosome 11 and is therefore manifested in homozygotes (called nu/nu). Affected mice have rudimentary thymuses in which T cell maturation cannot occur normally. As a result, there are few or no mature T cells in peripheral lymphoid tissues and a failure of all cell-mediated immune reactions, including allograft rejection, DTH, and antibody responses to T cell–dependent protein antigens. As the mice age to about 1 year, some mature T cells do develop, but the site of T cell maturation is not defined. Nu/nu mice are susceptible to many infections, but somewhat surprisingly they are able to eradicate some intracellular bacteria. This is because of normal or even increased numbers of natural killer (NK) cells, which produce interferon-γ (IFN-γ), which activates macrophages and serves to eliminate the microbes. NK cells may also account for the lack of susceptibility of nu/nu mice to spontaneous tumors (see Chapter 18). A similar inherited abnormality has been observed in rats, but nu/nu rats have not been analyzed in as much detail. Several mouse strains have been developed with targeted knockout of genes required for T cell development (see Chapter 8), and these mice are useful models for T cell immunodeficiency diseases.

Defects in T Cell Activation and Function

In the late 1980s, isolated case reports of abnormalities in T cell responses to antigenic or mitogenic stimulation began to appear. These defects are associated with T cell immunodeficiencies of varying clinical severity. They may be due to multiple mechanisms, including (1) defective surface expression of the T cell receptor (TCR):CD3 complex; (2) abnormal signal transduction by the TCR:CD3 complex; (3) defective production of cytokines such as IL-2 and IFN-γ (in some cases due to defects in transcription factor expression); and (4) defective expression of receptors for IL-2. These patients may have selective T cell or mixed T and B cell immunodeficiencies despite normal or even elevated numbers of blood lymphocytes. It is likely that such abnormalities will be recognized more frequently in coming years and their molecular basis as well as clinical significance understood in much more detail.

COMBINED IMMUNODEFICIENCIES (MIXED B AND T CELL DEFECTS)

Combined immunodeficiencies affecting both the B and T cell compartments may arise as a result of primary lymphoid abnormalities or in association with other congenital diseases. In both situations, the immunodeficiencies are clinically and mechanistically heterogeneous (see Table 21–2).

Severe Combined Immunodeficiencies

The term severe combined immunodeficiency disease (SCID) is given to a heterogeneous group of disorders characterized by defective development or function of B and T lymphocytes, profound lymphopenia, and deficient humoral and cell-mediated immunity. The first example of the disease was discovered in Switzerland in the 1950s (because of which this disorder was originally called Swiss type agammaglobulinemia). The transmission of the disease may be autosomal recessive or X-linked recessive; many cases of the former are due to known enzyme deficiencies, described below.

SCID is usually due to an abnormal development of B and T lymphocytes from bone marrow stem cells. In most cases, the mechanisms of abnormal lymphocyte development are not known. The thymus as well as the peripheral lymphoid organs contain few or no lympho-

cytes. Infants show markedly reduced blood lymphocyte counts and antibody titers, and are deficient in all immune functions. Unless treated, they usually succumb to infections during the first year of life.

About 50 per cent of the autosomal recessive form of SCID (and about 20 per cent of all cases) are due to deficiency of an enzyme called **adenosine deaminase** (ADA). ADA catalyzes the irreversible deamination of adenosine and deoxyadenosine to inosine and 2′deoxyinosine, respectively (Fig. 21–2). The ADA gene is located on chromosome 2, and deficiency of the enzyme can be due to deletions or mutations in the gene. The enzyme is widely distributed but is particularly abundant and active in lymphocytes. Its deficiency leads to the accumulation of deoxyadenosine, deoxy ATP (adenosine triphosphate), and S-adenosyl homocysteine in cells, particularly in developing T and B lymphocytes. These metabolites are toxic to lymphocytes because they block DNA synthesis by inhibiting ribonucleotide reductase activity and by causing the accumulation of compounds that inhibit transmethylation reactions. Thus, ADA deficiency leads to reduced numbers of B and T cells, and a resultant immunodeficiency. Some patients may have near normal numbers of T cells but defective responses of these cells to antigenic stimulation. ADA deficiency is a prime candidate for treatment by specific gene transfer. The ADA gene has been cloned, and constitutively expressed in transfected cells. The disease is manifested in bone marrow–derived cells and may thus be treatable by transfection of a functional gene into autologous self-renewing marrow cells and transplantation of these cells back into the patient.

A rarer autosomal recessive form of SCID is due to the deficiency of another enzyme, called **purine nucleoside phosphorylase** (PNP), that is involved in purine

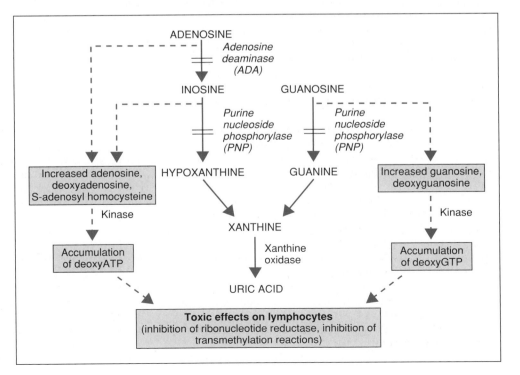

FIGURE 21–2. Congenital abnormalities in purine metabolism. *The major pathways for metabolism of purines (adenosine and guanosine) are shown in solid lines. Deficiencies of the enzymes adenosine deaminase (ADA) and purine nucleoside phosphorylase (PNP) block these metabolic pathways at different steps. This leads to shunting into secondary metabolic pathways, indicated by dashed lines, and the accumulation of toxic metabolites (in boxes).*

catabolism. PNP catalyzes the conversion of inosine to hypoxanthine and guanosine to guanine. Deficiency of PNP leads to accumulation of deoxyguanosine and deoxy GTP (guanosine triphosphate), with toxic effects more on T cells than on B cells (see Fig. 21–2). The gene for PNP is located on chromosome 9. Enzyme deficiency due to deletions or mutations in this gene usually result in deficient T cell immunity of variable severity, with normal B cell function. Patients present with variable susceptibility to infections.

Recently, an autosomal recessive form of SCID with deficiency in class II major histocompatibility complex (MHC) gene expression has been recognized, and is called the **bare lymphocyte syndrome.** These patients express little or no HLA–DP, DQ, or DR on B lymphocytes, macrophages, and dendritic cells and fail to express class II MHC molecules in response to IFN-γ. They express normal or only slightly reduced levels of class I MHC molecules and β_2-microglobulin and do synthesize the invariant (γ) chain upon stimulation with IFN-γ. In some patients the defect is due to an abnormality in a DNA-binding protein that normally stimulates transcription of class II genes by binding to the "X box" regulatory element located 5' of the class II locus (see Chapter 5). In the bare lymphocyte syndrome, either the production of this *trans*-acting DNA-binding protein is reduced, or it is structurally abnormal and, therefore, inactive. This results in reduced transcription of class II MHC genes. The consequence of deficient class II expression is a failure of antigen presentation to CD4+ T cells. As a result, affected individuals are deficient in DTH responses and in antibody responses to T-dependent protein antigens, and they are susceptible to infections, particularly viral infections. In some patients, the numbers of mature CD4+ T cells in peripheral blood and tissues are reduced. This may be because in the absence of class II MHC expression in the thymus, positive selection of CD4+ T cells cannot occur (see Chapter 8).

Several cases of X-linked SCID have recently been shown to be due to mutations in the gene encoding the γ chain of the interleukin-2 receptor (IL-2Rγ). In these patients, the mutations result in a lack of expression of the IL-2Rγ chain which is a component of high-affinity receptors for IL-2, IL-4, and IL-7 (see Chapter 12). This results in deficient T and B cell development and growth, probably because IL-7 is an important growth factor for B and T cell progenitors.

Apart from the specific disease entities mentioned above, the cellular and molecular bases of many other forms of SCID are not known. It is suspected that many of these cases may be due to defects in the rearrangement and expression of antigen receptor genes, but such defects have not been identified in humans. An instructive experimental model is the **SCID mouse,** which arose as a spontaneous mutant of an inbred strain called CB-17. In the SCID mutant strain, both B and T cells are absent because of an early block in maturation from bone marrow precursors. The defect in SCID mice is an abnormality in the DNA repair mechanisms that are required for rearrangement of TCR and

immunoglobulin (Ig) genes. In cell lines derived from immature B and T cells of SCID mice, the J_H exons of Ig genes and J_β exons of TCR genes are often deleted because of an aberrant recombination of the D segment directly to one of the constant (C) region genes. As a result, VDJ rearrangements do not occur, and antigen receptors are not expressed. Developing lymphocytes that fail to produce antigen receptors are eliminated *in vivo*. The *scid* mutation has been localized to chromosome 16, but the protein product of this gene is not identified yet. About 15 per cent of inbred *scid* mice are "leaky," in that they produce reduced but readily detectable numbers of mature B and T cells. The lymphocytes in these mice express limited repertoires of antigen receptor genes, suggesting that normal Ig or TCR rearrangements can occur in some developing clones.

Recently, two genes called RAG-1 and RAG-2 (for "recombination activating genes") have been identified that trigger VDJ recombination when transfected into cells that normally lack recombinase activity (see Chapters 4 and 8). RAG-1 or RAG-2 gene knockout mice have a phenotype similar to that of the SCID mouse.

Immunodeficiency Associated with Other Defects

Variable degrees of B and T cell immunodeficiency occur in certain congenital diseases in which there is a wide spectrum of abnormalities involving multiple organ systems. One such disorder is called the **Wiskott-Aldrich syndrome,** an X-linked disease characterized by eczema, thrombocytopenia (reduced blood platelets), and susceptibility to bacterial infections. In the initial stages of the disease, lymphocyte numbers are normal, and the principal defect is an inability to produce antibodies in response to polysaccharide antigens, which are typical thymus-independent antigens (see Chapter 9). These patients are especially susceptible to infections with encapsulated pyogenic bacteria. The lymphocytes (and platelets) are smaller than normal. With increasing age, the patients show reduced numbers of lymphocytes and more severe immunodeficiency. The gene (or genes) responsible for the Wiskott-Aldrich syndrome has been mapped to band p11.1 in the short arm of the X chromosome. The protein product of this gene is not defined. In patients with this disease, there is a defect in the glycosylation of membrane proteins, resulting in reduced expression of many cell surface glycoproteins. One such protein is a sialic acid–rich 115 kD glycoprotein called CD43 (or sialophorin), which is normally expressed on lymphocytes (both B and T), macrophages, neutrophils, and platelets. The role of CD43 deficiency in the abnormal lymphocyte function associated with this disease is not clear. It is unlikely to be the primary defect, because CD43 is encoded by a gene on chromosome 16.

Another disease associated with immunodeficiency is **ataxia-telangiectasia,** an autosomal recessive disorder characterized by abnormal gait (ataxia), vascular malformations (telangiectasias), various neurologic deficits, increased incidence of tumors, and immunodeficiency. The immunologic defects are of variable severity and may affect both B and T cells, the latter usually being more impaired. Patients experience infections, multiple autoimmune phenomena, and increasingly frequent cancers with advancing age. Multiple genetic defects may give rise to this constellation of clinical and pathologic abnormalities. The cells, including lymphocytes, of some patients contain numerous chromosomal deletions and translocations that may involve Ig or TCR loci. DNA repair mechanisms in all cells may be defective, as suggested by an increased susceptibility of patients' cells to ionizing radiation. Such defects may contribute to abnormal lymphocyte development as well as abnormal proliferative responses to antigenic stimulation.

CONGENITAL DISORDERS OF PHAGOCYTES AND OTHER CELLS OF NATURAL IMMUNITY

Natural immunity is mediated principally by phagocytes and complement, and it constitutes the first line of defense against infectious organisms. In addition, phagocytes and complement participate in the effector phases of specific immunity. Therefore, congenital disorders of phagocytes and the complement system result in recurrent infections of varying severity. Complement deficiencies have been described in Chapter 15. In this section of the chapter, we discuss some examples of congenital phagocytic disorders.

Chronic Granulomatous Disease

Chronic granulomatous disease (CGD) is rare, estimated to affect about 1 in 1 million individuals in the United States. About two thirds of the cases show an X-linked recessive pattern of inheritance, and the remainder are autosomal recessive. The disease is characterized by recurrent bacterial and fungal infections, usually from early childhood. The infections are usually not controlled by neutrophilic inflammation and may result in the formation of granulomas composed of activated macrophages. The disease is often fatal, even with aggressive antibiotic therapy.

CGD is due to a defect in the production of superoxide anion, which constitutes a major microbicidal mechanism of phagocytes. In response to an encounter with bacteria, neutrophils and macrophages rapidly consume oxygen and liberate superoxide, which is a precursor of the reactive oxygen species that serve to kill bacteria. Superoxide generation is mediated by an enzyme called nicotinamide adenine dinucleotide phosphate (NADPH)-oxidase, which upon activation catalyzes the one-electron reduction of oxygen (O_2) to superoxide (O_2^-). A neutrophil-specific protein, called neutrophil cytochrome, b245, is part of the enzyme complex that catalyzes this reaction. The neutrophils of patients with X-linked CGD are defective in this b type cytochrome and, therefore, fail to produce superoxide. It is now known that cytochrome b is a heterodimer composed of a 91 kD and a 22 kD chain. In the majority of X-linked CGD patients, the defect involves the gene encoding the 91 kD chain, which is located in band p21 of the X chromosome. The gene may be absent, truncated, or mutated so that either it is not transcribed or the RNA is unstable. Failure to produce the 91 kD protein often leads to diminished synthesis of the coordinately regulated 22 kD chain as well. The defect in most cases of the autosomal recessive form of CGD does not involve the genes encoding the cytochrome b protein. There is evidence that two other components of the NADPH-oxidase system, a 47 kD or a 67 kD cytosolic protein, are affected in some autosomal recessive forms. In both the X-linked and autosomal recessive forms, the end result is severe impairment of neutrophil superoxide generation.

It has been found that IFN-γ stimulates the production of superoxide by normal neutrophils as well as CGD neutrophils, especially in cases where the cytochrome b genes are present but their transcription is reduced. IFN-γ enhances transcription of the cytochrome b genes and also stimulates other components of the enzyme system that catalyze superoxide generation. Once neutrophil superoxide production is enhanced to within 10 to 12 per cent of normal, there is greatly improved resistance to infection. Clinical trials of IFN-γ treatment of X-linked CGD have had mixed results. The granulomatous reactions to infections seen during the natural history of the disease may reflect the body's attempt to mount a T cell response, with increased IFN-γ production and macrophage activation, to compensate for the neutrophil defect.

Leukocyte Adhesion Deficiencies

Leukocyte adhesion deficiency-1 (LAD-1) is a rare autosomal recessive disorder characterized by recurrent bacterial and fungal infections and impaired wound healing. In these patients, most adhesion-dependent functions of leukocytes are abnormal. These functions include adherence to endothelium; neutrophil aggregation and chemotaxis; phagocytosis; and cytotoxicity mediated by neutrophils, NK cells, and T lymphocytes. The molecular basis of the defect is absent or deficient expression of the β_2 integrins, or the CD11CD18 family of glycoproteins, which includes leukocyte function–associated antigen–1 (LFA-1 or CD11aCD18), Mac-1 (CD11bCD18), and p150,95 (CD11cCD18). These proteins participate in the adhesion of leukocytes to other cells (see Box 7–3, Chapter

7) and in the phagocytosis of complement-coated particles (see Chapter 15). In all patients studied so far, the defect has been mapped to the 95 kD β chain (CD18). The gene encoding this chain may be mutated, producing an aberrant transcript, or its transcription may be reduced. In fact, even in the limited number of cases analyzed, the reduced biosynthesis of the β chain has been shown to result from different molecular abnormalities.

Leukocyte adhesion deficiency–2 (LAD-2) is another disorder described in a very small number of patients that is clinically indistinguishable from LAD-1 but is not due to integrin defects. In contrast, LAD-2 results from an absence of sialyl-Lewis X, the carbohydrate ligand on neutrophils that is required for binding to E-selectin and perhaps P-selectin on cytokine-activated endothelium (see Chapter 11, Box 11–1). It is likely that LAD-2 patients have mutations in genes encoding enzymes involved in fucose metabolism.

To date, fewer than 100 patients with these disorders have been described. Like other genetic defects affecting leukocytes, leukocyte adhesion deficiencies are candidates for bone marrow transplantation and ultimately specific gene therapy.

Chédiak-Higashi Syndrome

This rare autosomal recessive disorder is characterized by recurrent infections by pyogenic bacteria, partial oculocutaneous albinism, and infiltration of various organs by non-neoplastic lymphocytes. Early studies showed that the neutrophils, monocytes, and lymphocytes of these patients contained giant cytoplasmic granules. It is now thought that this disease is due to a more generalized cellular abnormality leading to increased fusion of cytoplasmic granules. This affects the lysosomes of neutrophils and monocytes (causing reduced resistance to infections), melanocytes (causing albinism), cells of the nervous system (causing nerve defects), and platelets (leading to bleeding disorders). The molecular basis of the defect is not known. It may be due to abnormal membrane fluidity, which causes uncontrolled granule fusion and also defects in cell motility and microtubule function.

The giant lysosomes found in neutrophils form during the maturation of these cells from myeloid precursors. Some of these neutrophil precursors die prematurely, resulting in moderate leukopenia. Surviving neutrophils may contain reduced levels of lysosomal enzymes, which function in microbial killing. These cells are also defective in chemotaxis and phagocytosis, further contributing to their deficient microbicidal activity. NK cell function in these patients is impaired, probably because of an abnormality in the cytoplasmic granules that store proteins that mediate cytolysis (see Chapter 13). Interestingly, cytolytic T lymphocyte (CTL)–mediated killing is normal. A mutant mouse strain called the **beige mouse** is an animal model for the Chédiak-Higashi syndrome. This strain is characterized by deficient NK cell function and giant lysosomes in leukocytes.

THERAPEUTIC APPROACHES FOR CONGENITAL IMMUNODEFICIENCIES

In theory, the therapy of choice for congenital disorders of lymphocytes is to replace the defective gene in self-renewing precursor cells. This remains a distant goal for most human immunodeficiencies at present, despite considerable effort. Thus, current treatment for immunodeficiencies has two aims—to minimize and control infections, and to replace the defective or absent components of the immune system by adoptive transfer and/or transplantation. Among the agents that have proved useful as replacement therapy are the following:

1. Pooled gamma globulins are enormously valuable for agammaglobulinemic patients and have been life-saving for many boys with X-linked agammaglobulinemia.

2. Bone marrow transplantation is currently the treatment of choice for SCID, with careful T cell depletion from the marrow and HLA matching to prevent graft-versus-host disease (GVHD) (see Chapter 17). If a child with SCID is given a transplant of semi-syngeneic marrow cells from a parent (also called a "haploidentical" transplant because it is identical to the recipient at one of the two HLA haplotypes), the T cells that arise from the marrow must now develop in the partly foreign host. These T cells become restricted to recognizing foreign antigens in association with HLA molecules of the host, which are the HLA molecules that the donor T cells encounter during their maturation in the thymus. This, of course, is analogous to mouse bone marrow chimeras, which provided the initial evidence for the role of MHC molecules in the thymus in determining the selection of the T cell repertoire (see Chapter 8).

3. Enzyme replacement therapy for ADA and PNP deficiencies has been attempted using red blood cell transfusions as a source of the enzymes. This approach has produced temporary clinical improvements in several SCID patients. Ultimately, enzyme replacement therapies will have to be based on stable expression of a transfected gene encoding ADA or PNP in self-renewing bone marrow stem cells.

HUMAN IMMUNODEFICIENCY VIRUS AND THE ACQUIRED IMMUNODEFICIENCY SYNDROME

Acquired immunodeficiency syndrome is a disease first described in the early 1980s, characterized by profound immunosuppression with diverse clinical features, including opportunistic infections, malignancies, and central nervous system (CNS) degeneration. AIDS is one of a group of clinical syndromes caused by a retrovirus called HIV. *HIV primarily infects CD4-ex-*

pressing T cells, including helper T cells, and macrophages, as well as follicular dendritic cells in lymph nodes. The degree of morbidity and mortality caused by HIV and the global impact of HIV infection on health care resources and economics are already enormous and continue to grow. The number of people worldwide who are infected with HIV is estimated to be about 20 million, and many of these people will likely die of HIV-related disease. More than 3 million people have already developed AIDS. Currently, there is no prophylactic immunization or cure for HIV related disease. In this section of the chapter we describe the molecular and biologic properties of HIV, the nature and possible causes of HIV-induced immunosuppression, and the clinical and epidemiologic features of HIV-related diseases.

Molecular and Biologic Features of HIV

HIV is considered to be a member of the lentivirus family of animal retroviruses, on the basis of genomic sequence homologies, morphology, and life cycle. Lentiviruses, including the visna virus of sheep, and the bovine, feline, and simian immunodeficiency viruses, are capable of long-term latent infection of cells or short-term cytopathic effects, and they all produce slowly progressive, fatal diseases. Two closely related types of HIV, designated HIV-1 and HIV-2, have been intensively studied, but there may be other forms as well. Although HIV-1 and HIV-2 differ in genomic structure and antigenicity, both types cause similar clinical syndromes. HIV-1 is a far more common cause of AIDS than HIV-2 in the United States, and HIV-2 is more common in West Africa.

An infectious HIV particle consists of two identical strands of RNA, each approximately 9.2 kilobases (kb) long, packaged within a core of viral proteins, surrounded by a phospholipid bilayer envelope derived from the host cell membrane but including virally encoded membrane proteins (Fig. 21–3). The HIV genome shares the basic structure of all known retroviruses, including nucleotide sequences called *gag*, which encode core structural proteins; *env* sequences encoding envelope glycoproteins; and *pol* sequences encoding reverse transcriptase, endonuclease, and viral protease enzymes required for viral replication. In addition to these typical retrovirus genes, HIV also includes at least six other genes, including *vpr, vif, tat, rev, nef,* and *vpu* genes, whose products regulate viral reproduction in various ways, to be discussed below (Fig. 21–4).

HIV infection occurs when viral particles in blood, semen, or other body fluids from one individual bind to cells of another individual. *Two HIV envelope glycoproteins, gp120 and gp41, are critical for HIV infection.* (Conventional notation of viral and cellular proteins includes a "p" for protein, or "gp" for glycoprotein, followed by a number designating the molecular weight in kilodaltons.) The first step in HIV infection is the *high-affinity binding of gp120 to CD4 molecules* on the surface of a primate T cell or mononuclear phagocyte.

HIV does not bind to CD4 molecules in non-primate species. Free HIV particles released from one infected cell can bind to an uninfected cell. Alternatively, gp120, which is expressed on the plasma membrane of infected cells before virus is released, can bind to CD4 on another cell, initiating a membrane fusion event, and HIV genomes can be passed between the fused cells directly. The role of gp41 is discussed below.

Detailed molecular mapping studies, including x-ray crystallographic analysis, have defined which regions of the CD4 and gp120 molecules are involved in binding to one another. This information is potentially useful in the design of therapeutic agents that block virus interaction with CD4-expressing cells. Three well-conserved, noncontiguous regions in the carboxy terminus of gp120 of HIV-1 and HIV-2 are required for CD4 binding. Interestingly, these regions are separated by sequences that are extremely variable from one HIV isolate to another; this is significant to the way HIV may evade the host immune system, which we will discuss later. Such studies have already determined that various residues in the amino terminal IgV-like domain of human CD4 are critical for binding. Genetically engineered soluble CD4 molecules can block HIV infection of cells, but genetically engineered soluble CD4 has not proven to be effective in the treatment of AIDS patients.

HIV particles that bind to CD4 enter cells by direct fusion of the virus membrane with the host cell membrane, and this process is facilitated by gp41 molecules on the viral membrane. In a current model of HIV infection, gp120 binding to CD4 permits the associated viral gp41 molecule to insert its hydrophobic amino terminal head into the adjacent cell membrane, initiating fusion of the virus envelope with the cell. Other cellular factors may be critical for infection besides the CD4 molecule, as is suggested by the fact that murine cells expressing transfected human CD4 genes cannot be infected by HIV.

Once an HIV virion enters a cell, the enzymes within the nucleoprotein complex become active and begin the viral reproductive cycle (Fig. 21–5). The nucleoprotein core of the virus becomes disrupted, the RNA genome of HIV is transcribed into a double-stranded DNA form by viral reverse transcriptase, and the viral DNA enters the nucleus. The viral integrase also enters the nucleus and catalyzes the integration of the viral DNA into the host cell genome. There is evidence that the integration event is enhanced by concomitant T cell activation by antigens or super-antigens. The integrated DNA form of HIV is called the **provirus.** The provirus may remain transcriptionally inactive for months or years, with little or no production of new viral proteins or virions, and in this way HIV infection of an individual cell can be latent.

Transcription of the genes of the integrated DNA provirus is regulated by long terminal repeat (LTR) sequences, which flank either side of the viral structural genes. The LTRs contain polyadenylation signal sequences, TATA box promoter sequence, and *cis*-acting regulators of transcription of the viral genes. These *cis*-acting sequences include tandemly repeated enhancer elements that are known to bind at least two nuclear

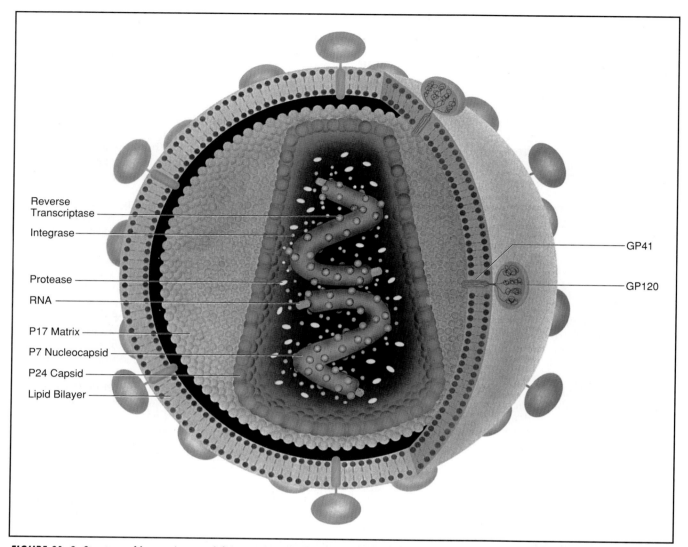

FIGURE 21–3. Structure of human immunodeficiency virus–1 (HIV-1). *HIV-1 consists of two identical strands of RNA (the viral genome) with associated reverse transcriptase and integrase, packaged in a cone-shaped core composed of p24 capsid protein with a surrounding p17 protein matrix and surrounded by phospholipid membrane envelope derived from the host cell. Virally encoded membrane proteins (gp41 and gp120) are bound to the envelope. (Redrawn with permission from Greene, W. C. AIDS and the immune system. Scientific American 269:98–105, 1993.)*

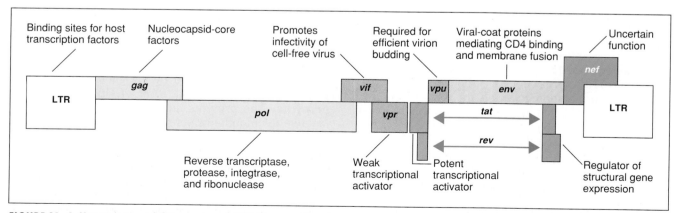

FIGURE 21–4. Human immunodeficiency virus–1 (HIV-1) genes. *The positions of the genes along the linear genome are indicated as differently shaded blocks. Some genes use some of the same sequences as other genes, as shown by overlapping blocks, but are read differently by host cell RNA polymerase. Similarly shaded blocks separated by arrows indicate genes whose coding sequences are separated in the genome and require RNA splicing to produce functional messenger RNA (mRNA). LTR, long terminal repeat. (Redrawn with permission from Greene, W. C. AIDS and the immune system. Scientific American 269:98–105, 1993.)*

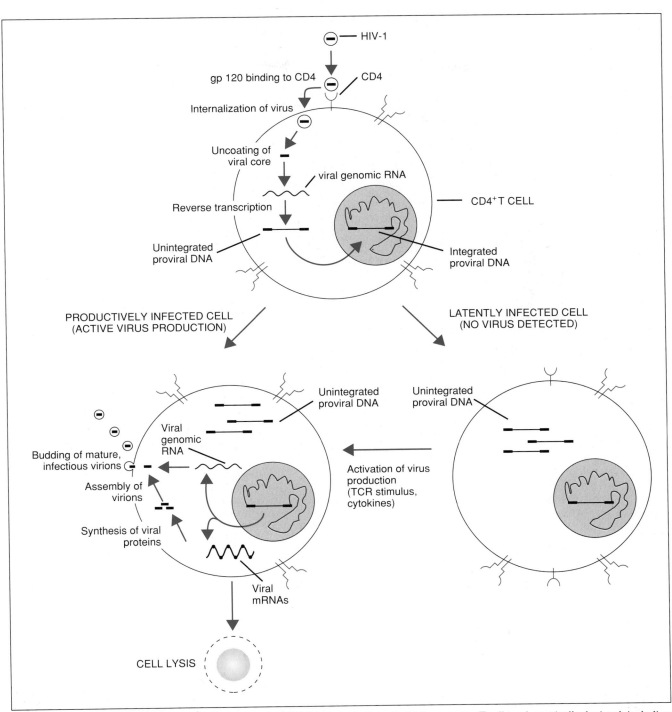

FIGURE 21–5. Life cycle of human immunodeficiency virus–1 (HIV-1). *HIV-1 infection of a CD4-expressing T cell is schematically depicted, including the relationship between latent infection and productive, lytic infection.*

regulatory factors, including NF-κB and SP1. NF-κB/rel family–like nuclear regulatory proteins, which bind to sequences in the regulatory regions of IL-2 and IL-2 receptor genes, can also bind to similar sequences in HIV LTRs and activate HIV transcription.

Initiation of HIV gene transcription in T cells is probably linked to physiologic activation of the T cell by antigen or cytokine stimulation. The LTRs of HIV are influenced by TCR and cytokine stimulation of the host cells. For example, TCR-binding lectins, tumor necrosis factor (TNF), and lymphotoxin all stimulate HIV gene expression in T cells; and interleukin-1, interleukin-3, interleukin-6, TNF, lymphotoxin, interferon-γ and granulocyte-macrophage colony-stimulating factor stimulate HIV gene expression and viral replication in monocytes and macrophages. TCR and cytokine stimulation of HIV gene transcription probably involves the induction of nuclear factors that bind to the NF-κB–binding sequences in the viral LTR. This phenomenon may be significant to the pathogenesis of AIDS in two ways. First, physiologic activation of a latently infected T cell may be the way in which latency is ended and virus production begins. Second, the multiple infections that AIDS patients acquire lead to elevated TNF production; this, in turn, may stimulate HIV production and infection of additional cells. *Thus, HIV replication is stimulated by the same mechanisms that promote growth of the host T cell.* It is interesting that when the regulatory sequences of the HIV LTR are linked to other genes and transfected into various cell types, they work efficiently. Therefore, the tissue specificity of productive HIV infection is not a function of these regulators but, rather, reflects the specificity of virus binding to and internalization by CD4$^+$ cell types.

Synthesis of mature, infectious viral particles begins after the various viral genes are expressed as proteins, and full-length genomic viral RNA transcripts are produced. The *pol* gene product is a precursor protein that is sequentially cleaved to form reverse transcriptase, protease, ribonuclease, and integrase enzymes. As mentioned above, the reverse transcriptase and integrase proteins are required for establishment of the integrated DNA proviral form of HIV. The *gag* gene encodes a 55 kD protein that is then proteolytically cleaved into p24, p17, and p15 polypeptides by the action of the viral protease encoded by the *pol* gene. These polypeptides are the mature core proteins that are required for assembly of infectious viral particles. The primary product of the *env* gene is a 160 kD glycoprotein (gp160) that is cleaved by cellular proteases within the endoplasmic reticulum into the CD4 binding protein, gp120, expressed on the external surface of the envelope, and the gp41 transmembrane glycoprotein. Gp120 does not contain a transmembrane domain, but it remains bound to the cell surface by non-covalent interactions with gp41. As mentioned above, both these molecules are crucial for viral infectivity. In addition, a soluble (virus-free) form of gp120 may be responsible for some of the immunopathology caused by HIV (see below).

In addition to the conventional retroviral genes described above, namely *gag, pol,* and *env,* at least two other HIV genes are essential for viral replication. First, the *tat* gene encodes a 14 kD protein that is reported to have transcriptional, post-transcriptional, and translational effects. This protein binds to sequences present in the LTR called the *trans*-activating response element (TAR), resulting in stimulation of expression of all HIV genes. Binding of the Tat protein to the viral LTR causes a 1000-fold increase in cellular RNA polymerase II catalyzed transcription of the provirus. *Tat* is also secreted from HIV-infected cells and may activate transcription of endogenous genes of other cells such as endothelium. Second, the *rev* gene encodes a 20 kD protein that acts post-transcriptionally to ensure proper transport and processing of viral messenger RNA (mRNA) transcripts of the *gag, pol,* and *env* genes. At the same time, the *rev* product down-regulates expression of the HIV regulatory genes, including *tat, nef,*

and *rev* itself. Thus, HIV gene expression may be divided into an early stage, during which the regulatory genes are expressed, and a late stage, during which structural genes are expressed (Fig. 21–6). The *rev* protein is apparently critical for the transition from the early to late stage. This two-stage sequence of viral gene transcription probably serves to limit the duration of the expression of viral structural proteins, thereby diminishing the chance that the host immune system will recognize these proteins and destroy the virally infected cells in which they are expressed.

The *nef* gene encodes a 27 kD myristoylated protein found predominantly in the cytoplasm of infected cells. The *nef*-encoded protein is not essential for viral replication or cytopathic effects. This protein may serve a negative regulatory function, slowing down viral replication, but its mode of action is unknown.

Three other HIV genes, which are not essential to the viral life cycle and whose functions are still poorly characterized, have been identified. The *vif* gene encodes a 23 kD protein that is involved in controlling the infectivity of HIV by an unknown mechanism. A functional *vif* gene is required for efficient infection of cells by viral particles, but it may not be involved in infection occurring by direct cell-cell contact. The *vpu* gene encodes a 16 kD protein that may be involved in assembly of new virions. The *vpr* gene encodes an approximately 110 amino acid long protein, which is apparently involved in regulation of viral replication early in the HIV life cycle, but details of how it works are not known.

In addition to their functions in the viral life cycle, the protein products of the various HIV genes are also significant because they stimulate immune responses in the host that may be either beneficial or detrimental (discussed below).

After transcription of these various viral genes, viral proteins are synthesized in the cytoplasm. Assembly of infectious viral particles then begins by packaging full-length RNA transcripts of the proviral genome within a nucleoprotein complex that includes the *gag* core proteins and the *pol*-encoded enzymes required for the next cycle of integration. This nucleoprotein complex is then enclosed within a membrane envelope and released from the cell by a process of budding from the plasma membrane. Production of mature virus is associated with lysis of the cell.

HIV-2 has basically the same molecular organization and reproductive biology as HIV-1. There are, however, several molecular differences. First, HIV-2 contains a gene called *vpx,* not present in the HIV-1 genome, which encodes a 14 kD protein of unknown function. Second, HIV-2 does not contain the *vpu* gene, which is present in the HIV-1 genome. Third, there is a large insertion in the HIV-2 *rev* gene. Fourth, distinct differences in the *env* genes between the two types of HIV result in the fact that antibodies against one type will not react with the other. This is important, since some diagnostic tests for HIV rely on antibodies that may recognize only HIV-1 and not HIV-2.

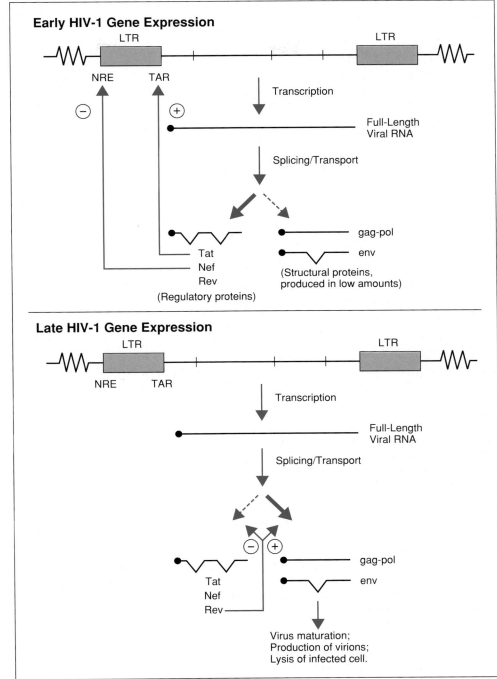

FIGURE 21-6. Early and late phases of human immunodeficiency virus-1 (HIV-1) gene expression. *During early HIV-1 gene expression, the predominant type of transcripts transported out of the nucleus are multiply spliced messenger RNA (mRNA) species encoding regulatory proteins tat, nef, and rev. Tat and nef act on genomic sequences to regulate further transcription. Rev causes a change to late phase gene expression by altering the balance of mRNA transport out of the nucleus. Specifically, rev causes a relative increase in the transport and translation of singly or unspliced mRNAs encoding viral structural and enzymatic proteins that are required for production of mature viral particles. LTR, long terminal repeat; NRE, negative regulatory element; TAR, trans-acting responsive sequences. (Modified with permission from Greene, W. C. Regulation of HIV-1 gene expression. Annual Review of Immunology 8:453–475, 1990.)*

Immunology of HIV Infection

The clinical course of HIV infection reflects a complex interplay between the effects of the virus on the function of immunocompetent cells and the host's immune response to the virus. We next describe what is known or hypothesized to be the basis for HIV-induced immunosuppression and discuss the role of the host's immune response in both aggravating and limiting the pathologic effects of the virus (Table 21–3).

NATURE AND MECHANISMS OF IMMUNOSUPPRESSION

HIV infection ultimately results in impaired function of both the specific and natural immune systems. A hallmark of the progression of HIV-induced disease is the diminishing number of $CD4^+$ T cells in the peripheral blood, from a normal amount of about 1000/mm^3 to less than 100/mm^3 in fully developed AIDS. Since $CD4^+$ helper T cells are essential for both cell-mediated and

TABLE 21-3. Mechanisms of Human Immunodeficiency Virus (HIV)-Induced Pathogenesis

Pathologic Effect	Mechanism
Immunodeficiency	
Depletion of CD4+ T cells: direct effects on infected cells	Lysis of CD4+ T cells caused by viral budding and/or *env* glyco-protein insertion or syncitium formation
	Cytopathic effect of unintegrated viral RNA and DNA
	Cytopathic effect of intracellular binding of gp120 to newly synthesized or recycled CD4
Depletion of CD4+ T cells: indirect effects	Inhibition of CD4+ T cell matura-tion
	Autoimmune destruction of unin-fected CD4+ T cells due to presence of normal T cell surface molecules that cross react with viral proteins
	gp120 cross-linking of CD4 priming cells for apoptosis
	Super-antigen effect of viral proteins on subsets of T cells
Functional impairment of im-mune system	Soluble gp120 blocks interaction of CD4+ T cells with class II MHC on APCs
	Impaired macrophage and NK cell function, unknown mechanism
	Destruction of follicular dendritic cell network and architecture of lymph nodes
Central Nervous System (CNS) Damage	Release of inflammatory cytokines from HIV-infected CNS macro-phages; soluble gp120 may interfere with neurotransmitter action on neurons

Abbreviations: MHC, major histocompatibility complex; APC, antigen-pre-senting cell; CTL, cytolytic T lymphocyte.

humoral immune responses to various microbes, the loss of these lymphocytes is a major reason why AIDS patients become susceptible to so many infections. However, the mechanisms underlying HIV-induced loss of CD4+ T cells are not fully understood. In fact, most CD4+ T cells in the blood of HIV-infected individuals do not contain provirus, and many of those that do are not actively producing viral proteins or new virus. There-fore, there are likely to be both direct and indirect mechanisms underlying the depletion of CD4+ T cells in HIV-infected individuals. Furthermore, even uninfected or viable latently infected cells not producing virus do not function effectively in AIDS patients, implying that immunodeficiency is in part a result of functional dis-turbances of the immune system independent of HIV-induced cytolysis of lymphocytes.

Several direct cytopathic effects of HIV on infected cells have been described:

1. The process of virus production with expres-sion of gp41 in the plasma membrane and budding of viral particles may lead to increased plasma membrane permeability, and influx of lethal amounts of calcium or osmotic lysis of the cell.

2. The plasma membranes of HIV-infected cells fuse with uninfected CD4+ T cells by virtue of gp120-CD4 interactions, leading to the formation of multinu-cleated giant cells or syncytia. The process of HIV-in-duced syncytial formation can be lethal to the HIV-infected T cells as well as the uninfected CD4+ T cells that fuse to the infected cells. The phenomenon has largely been observed *in vitro*, and syncytia are rarely seen in the tissues of AIDS patients.

3. Unintegrated viral DNA in the cytoplasm of in-fected cells, or large amounts of nonfunctional viral RNA, may be toxic to the infected cells.

4. Viral production may interfere with cellular pro-tein synthesis and expression, leading to cell death. Gp120 binding to newly synthesized intracellular CD4 may have toxic effects.

CD4+ T cells may also be eliminated as a result of host immune responses to HIV infection. Antibodies against HIV envelope proteins may bind to HIV-infected CD4+ T cells and mediate antibody-dependent cellular cytotoxicity directed against these cells. In addition, HIV-specific cytolytic T lymphocytes (CTLs) are pres-ent in many AIDS patients, and these cells may kill infected CD4+ T cells.

HIV may also cause the depletion of CD4+ T cells by stimulating signals that lead to apoptosis. For exam-ple, there is evidence from *in vitro* experiments that cross-linking CD4 on mature T cells primes these cells for apoptotic death upon subsequent exposure to anti-gen. Soluble gp120 released from HIV-infected cells may have the same effect on uninfected CD4+ T cells. Some data suggest that one or more HIV proteins may act as super-antigens, binding to T cell receptor β chains and inducing apoptotic signals in the T cells. HIV-induced apoptosis has also been postulated to cause the loss of developing T cells in the thymus.

There is evidence that the proportion of IL-2 and IFN-γ secreting (Th1) T cells decreases gradually in HIV-infected patients and the proportion of IL-4 and IL-10 secreting (Th2) T cells increases. This may partially explain the susceptibility of HIV-infected individuals to infections by intracellular microbes since IFN-γ acti-vates, and IL-4 and IL-10 inhibit, macrophage-mediated killing of such microbes.

In addition to depletion of CD4+ T cells, which becomes most significant late in the course of HIV in-fection, *the virus also causes functional impairment of CD4+ T cells in ways not directly related to cytotoxic effects or T cell depletion.* Uninfected T cells in HIV-infected patients have a decreased expression of IL-2 receptors and diminished secretion of IL-2 in response to soluble antigens both *in vivo* and *in vitro*. Humoral responses to soluble antigens and CTL responses to certain viruses are also impaired, probably as a conse-quence of the failure of CD4+ helper T cells to secrete adequate amounts of the appropriate cytokines re-quired for functional differentiation of B cells and CTLs.

As with the cytolytic effects, many of these func-tional abnormalities of CD4+ T cells are most likely due to the binding of HIV or free gp120 to CD4 molecules on helper T cells. Such binding could have numerous con-sequences. CD4 that has bound gp120 may not be avail-able to interact with class II MHC molecules on antigen-presenting cells (APCs), and thus T cell responses to soluble antigens would be inhibited. Alternatively, gp120 binding to CD4 may down-regulate surface expression of a variety of molecules required for T cell activation, including CD3 and CD4 itself. This down-regulation may be due to gp120-induced modulation of CD4 and, perhaps, associated CD3, as well as inhibition of transcription of CD4 and CD3 genes. In addition, the HIV Tat protein can also block antigen-induced responses of T cells, presumably by interfering with intracellular T cell activation pathways.

The immunosuppressive effects of HIV may also be partly related to effects the virus has on cells other than $CD4^+$ T cells. Abnormalities in B lymphocyte activation are frequently observed in HIV-infected individuals. Paradoxically, these patients typically have elevated serum Ig levels resulting from polyclonal activation of B cells. This may be a result of a polyclonal activating effect of HIV or gp120 itself. Polyclonal activation of B cells may also be caused by Epstein-Barr virus (EBV) infection, which can be largely uncontrolled in HIV-infected individuals as a result of poor T cell immune responses. Despite this generalized B cell hyperactivity, humoral immune responses to newly introduced antigens are greatly impaired. Diminished T cell help and refractoriness of the B cells themselves may both play a role in this deficit.

Macrophages express much lower levels of CD4 than helper T lymphocytes, but they are still susceptible to HIV infection by the gp120-CD4–dependent route described previously. Nonetheless, macrophages are relatively resistant to the cytopathic effects of HIV. This may be because high CD4 expression is required for virus-induced cytoxicity. Macrophages may also be infected by a CD4 independent route, such as phagocytosis of other infected cells or by Fc receptor–mediated endocytosis of antibody-coated HIV. Since macrophages can be infected but are generally not killed by the virus, they are probably a major reservoir for the virus. In fact, the quantity of macrophage-associated HIV far exceeds T cell–associated virus in most tissues from AIDS patients, including brain and lung. Despite macrophage resistance to HIV-induced cytolysis, macrophage functions are often impaired in HIV-infected individuals. These impairments include decreases in chemokinesis, cytokine production and reactive oxygen–dependent killing of microbes. In addition, antigen-presenting functions of macrophages are reduced in AIDS patients, possibly as a result of down-regulation of class II MHC expression.

Lymph nodes are the site of continuous HIV replication and progression of HIV-induced disease even during the long clinically silent period after acute infection. Although most of the studies of HIV-induced effects on the immune system have focused on depletion or functional impairment of peripheral blood $CD4^+$ T cells, more than 98 per cent of the body's T cells are normally found in lymphoid tissues, such as lymph nodes and spleen. Early in HIV disease, only a few $CD4^+$ T cells in the germinal centers of lymph node cells are positive for the virus. As the disease progresses, HIV is found in progressively more lymph node T cells as well as on follicular dendritic cells. HIV-positive follicular dendritic cells may facilitate infection of neighboring $CD4^+$ T cells. Thus, the lymphoid tissues are sites of continual viral production, T cell infection, and T cell destruction, even during the long clinical latent period between acute infection and overt AIDS. This accounts for the steady decline in peripheral blood $CD4^+$ T cell numbers during the latent period, since blood T cells and lymph node T cells are part of the same recirculating pool of lymphocytes. In advanced disease, lymph node architecture is markedly abnormal, the follicular dendritic network is lost, and few HIV positive cells or free virions are present.

IMMUNE RESPONSES TO HIV

Both humoral and cell-mediated immune responses specific for a wide variety of HIV gene products have been observed in HIV-infected patients. Given the extremely high fatality rate among HIV-infected individuals, it is clear that these immune responses to the virus do not confer adequate protection. This is, of course, partly due to the fact that the $CD4^+$ T cells required to initiate protective immune responses are killed or inactivated by the virus, and therefore the immune responses may be too compromised to eliminate the virus. In addition, the HIV genome displays a remarkable degree of genetic variability, largely as a result of the high error frequency intrinsic to reverse transcription. This results in antigenic variations that may serve to evade the host immune system as well as to development of drug-resistant strains of HIV. Despite the poor effectiveness of immune responses to the virus, it is important to characterize them for three reasons. First, the immune responses may be detrimental to the host, as we have alluded to previously; they result in autoimmune killing of uninfected T cells, or they may stimulate uptake of opsonized virus into uninfected cells by Fc receptor–mediated endocytosis. Second, antibodies against HIV are diagnostic markers of HIV infection widely used for screening purposes. Third, the design of effective vaccines for immunization against HIV requires knowledge of the viral epitopes that are most likely to stimulate protective immunity.

The most immunogenic molecules on HIV appear to be the envelope glycoproteins, and high titers of anti-gp120 and anti-gp41 antibodies are present in most HIV-infected individuals. A region of the gp120 molecule, called the V3-loop, is one of the most antigenically variable components of the virus. Other immunoglobulins found frequently in patients' sera include antibodies to p24, reverse transcriptase, and *gag* and *pol* products. The effect of these antibodies on the clinical course of HIV-related diseases is probably minimal. Interestingly, the anti-envelope antibodies are generally poor inhibitors of viral infectivity or cytopathic effects, supporting the hypothesis that the most immunogenic epitopes of the envelope glycoproteins are least important for the functions of these molecules. Furthermore, the antibodies are usually virus strain–specific, so that antibodies from one infected individual often do not recognize HIV isolated from other infected individuals. It is possible that the host immune response may work as a selective pressure that promotes survival of the most genetically variable viruses. Low titers of neutralizing antibodies that can inactivate HIV are present in HIV-infected patients, as are antibodies that can mediate antibody-dependent cell-mediated cytotoxicity (ADCC). These antibodies are usually specific for gp120. Whether there is a correlation between the titer of these antibodies and the clinical course remains controversial.

Experimentally produced neutralizing antibodies, made by immunizing animals with HIV or purified HIV–encoded proteins, are potentially useful for treating infected individuals. Since HIV can spread by cell-cell fusion, antibodies that block fusion as well as neutralize free virus particles would be needed. Furthermore, such antibodies would need to recognize nonvariable parts of the virus.

The role of T cell–mediated immune responses to HIV infection is also incompletely understood. MHC-restricted CTLs specific for *env*, *gag*, and *pol* gene products have been detected in HIV-infected individuals. In addition, NK cell activity against HIV-infected targets is present in these patients. These effector mechanisms are clearly important in the immunologic control of other types of viral infections, and their role in HIV infection requires more research. CD4+ T cell responses to HIV-derived peptide antigens are poorly characterized.

Clinical Features of HIV Infection

Because of the complex biology of HIV, the clinical manifestations of infection are quite variable. Although initial infection may occur without accompanying symptoms, many patients experience an **acute HIV syndrome** within 2 to 6 weeks of exposure to the virus. This syndrome is characterized by fever, headaches, sore throat with pharyngitis, generalized lymphadenopathy, and rashes. No aspect of this acute illness is specifically diagnostic for HIV infection. During this initial period after infection, the virus is replicating abundantly and is detectable in blood and cerebrospinal fluid. After the initial phase, a clinically latent phase begins, which may last up to 10 years. Although extracellular virus practically disappears from body fluids during this latent phase, and the majority of peripheral blood T cells do not harbor the virus, there is steady progression of the disease in lymphoid tissues with increasing numbers of infected CD4+ T cells, macrophages, and follicular dendritic cells. Generalized lymphadenopathy may develop during this period, but the immune system remains competent at handling most infections. A heterogeneous subset of patients develop a group of signs and symptoms which may persist for some time but do not fit the definition of clinical AIDS. These clinical features constitute **AIDS-related complex (ARC),** and include persistent fevers, night sweats, weight loss, diarrhea, inflammatory skin conditions, and generalized lymphadenopathy. ARC can persist for months or years before progression to AIDS. HIV-infected individuals who develop herpes zoster, oral candidal infection, and oral hairy leukoplakia are likely to succumb to full-blown AIDS relatively quickly.

The diagnosis of AIDS can be made based on a combination of laboratory evidence of infection (discussed below) and the presence of many possible combinations of *opportunistic infections, neoplasias, cachexia (HIV wasting syndrome), and CNS degeneration (AIDS encephalopathy).* AIDS patients acquire numerous infections that can be life-threatening, often with organisms that are not normally pathogenic for immunocompetent individuals. Pneumonia caused by the protozoan *Pneumocystis carinii* is the most commonly acquired opportunistic infection in AIDS, affecting up to 75 per cent of patients, and is perhaps the most common cause of death in AIDS. Other protozoal organisms that frequently infect AIDS patients include *Cryptosporidium* and *Toxoplasma.* Bacteria that often cause infections in AIDS patients include *Mycobacterium* species such as *M. avium* and *M. kansasi, Nocardia,* and *Salmonella.* Fungal infections with *Candida, Cryptococcus neoformans, Coccidioides immitis,* and *Histoplasma capsulatum* are common, as are viral infections with cytomegalovirus, herpes simplex, and varicella-zoster. The inflammatory responses to these various organisms are often unlike those seen in immunocompetent individuals; this probably reflects the lack of T cells that would normally secrete cytokines, which promote acute and chronic inflammation. For example, well-formed granulomas with activated macrophages are not seen in mycobacterial or fungally infected tissues in AIDS patients.

AIDS is also characterized by progressive weight loss (cachexia) and diarrhea with or without identifiable enteric infections. These symptoms are often called HIV wasting syndrome; the pathogenesis is not understood.

Various malignant neoplasms are frequently found in AIDS patients, and these represent another major cause of AIDS-related morbidity and mortality. Up to 30 per cent of AIDS patients develop Kaposi's sarcoma, a mesenchymal tumor histologically characterized by vascular spaces and malignant spindle cells. AIDS-related Kaposi's tumors, unlike sporadic forms of this neoplasm, are highly aggressive and disseminated, involving skin, mucosa, lymph nodes, and multiple visceral organs. The cause of this tumor in the setting of AIDS remains obscure, and there is some evidence that the incidence of Kaposi's sarcoma is declining. AIDS patients also develop malignant lymphomas at a much higher rate than immunocompetent individuals. Burkitt's lymphoma and other B cell tumors are most frequent, and they are often positive for EBV. The development of these tumors may result from immunologically unchecked EBV infections leading to polyclonal B cell proliferation and subsequent malignant transformation (see Box 18–1, Chapter 18). Primary lymphomas of the CNS are also common in AIDS patients.

The brain is a major site of HIV infection, and up to 66 per cent of AIDS patients suffer from a form of dementia called AIDS encephalopathy or AIDS dementia complex, characterized by memory loss and various other nonspecific neuropsychiatric disturbances. Macrophages are the cells most likely to be infected in the brain, although some evidence suggests direct infection of cerebrovascular endothelium and neurons. Neuronal damage is seen on pathologic examination of brains from AIDS autopsies, but the causes are not clear. It is possible that HIV-infected macrophages secrete cytokines that are toxic to neurons or that HIV interferes with neurotropic peptide factors or neurotransmitters.

A variety of clinical immunology laboratory techniques are used to diagnose and follow the progression of HIV infection. Antibodies to HIV proteins, including p24 and gp120, appear in the serum usually between 2 and 12 weeks after primary infection (Fig. 21–7). Standard screening protocols for HIV utilize immunofluorescence or enzyme-linked immunoassays to detect these antibodies. Positive screening tests are often followed up by Western blot or radioimmunoassay determination of the presence of serum antibodies that bind to specific viral proteins. Viral antigens (usually p24) are usually present in the serum for up to 3 months after infection, and then reappear years later when AIDS develops. These antigens can be detected using enzyme-linked immunoassays. Polymerase-chain reaction (PCR) assays are particularly sensitive in detecting the presence of viral genomes in cells or body fluids and may occasionally demonstrate HIV infection when other tests are negative. Culturing virus from infected individuals is possible but technically difficult. Diagnosis of asymptomatic infants born of HIV-infected mothers poses a special problem since maternal anti-HIV antibodies cross the placenta and will give false-positive results on screening tests. Neonatal diagnosis

therefore requires viral antigen detection, viral culture, or PCR detection of viral genomes.

The peripheral CD4$^+$ T cell count is the most commonly used laboratory test for the progression of HIV disease. After an initial transient drop in the number of CD4$^+$ T cells in the blood, there follows a steady decline over years. When the count drops below 250 cells/mm^3, the risk of full-blown AIDS with opportunistic infections becomes high.

Transmission of HIV and Epidemiology of AIDS

The modes of transmission of HIV from one individual to another are the major determinants of the epidemiologic features of AIDS. The virus is transmitted by three major routes:

1. Intimate sexual contact is the most frequent mode of transmission, either between homosexual male partners or heterosexual couples. The virus is present in semen and gains access to the previously uninfected partner either through traumatized rectal mucosa or vaginal mucosa. Transmission from infected females to males may also occur.

2. Inoculation of a recipient with infected blood or blood products is the second most frequent mode of

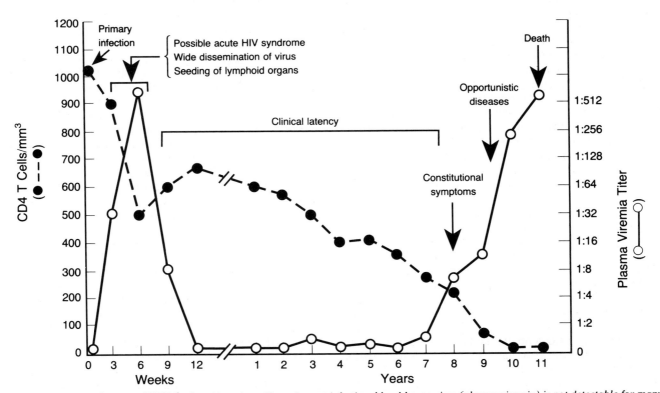

FIGURE 21–7. Typical course of HIV infection. *After about 12 weeks post-infection, blood-borne virus (plasma viremia) is not detectable for many years. Nonetheless, CD4$^+$ T cell counts steadily decline during this clinical latency period, probably because of active viral replication and T cell infection in lymph nodes. When CD4$^+$ T cell counts drop below a critical level (about 250/mm^3), there is a high risk of infection. (Reproduced with permission from Pantaleo, G., Graziosi, C., and Fauci, A. S. The immunopathogenesis of human immunodeficiency virus infection. New England Journal of Medicine 328:327–335, 1993.)*

HIV transmission. Needles shared by intravenous drug abusers account for most cases of this form of transmission. With the advent of routine laboratory screening, transfusion of blood or blood products, in a clinical setting, accounts for a very small portion of HIV infections. Patients infected in this way may then infect other individuals by sexual contact.

3. Mother to child transmission of HIV accounts for the majority of pediatric cases of AIDS. This occurs most frequently *in utero* or during childbirth, although transmission through breast milk is also possible.

Major groups at risk for developing AIDS in the United States include the following:

1. Homosexual or bisexual males
2. Intravenous drug abusers
3. Heterosexual partners of members of other risk groups
4. Babies born from infected mothers

There is a small increased risk of infection among health care workers.

In Africa, the vast majority of HIV infections occur by sexual transmission from one heterosexual partner to another, with no identifiable risk factors.

Treatment of AIDS and Vaccine Development

Treatment of HIV infection and AIDS remains largely experimental and no satisfactorily effective intervention has been developed. The only antiviral drugs approved for treatment of HIV infection in the United States are nucleotide analogs that inhibit reverse transcriptase activity. These drugs include 3'-azido-3'-deoxythymidine (AZT), 2',3'-dideoxyinosine, and 2',3'-dideoxycytidine. Unfortunately, several studies indicate that these drugs are often ineffective in halting or even slowing the progression of HIV-induced disease, largely because of the rapid evolution of mutated forms of reverse transcriptase that are resistant to the drugs. There have been active research efforts aimed at developing reagents that interfere with other parts of the viral life cycle besides reverse transcription and HIV entry into cells. Both *tat* and viral protease inhibitors have been developed and are now being used in limited clinical trials.

The individual infections experienced by AIDS patients are treated with the appropriate antibiotics and support measures. More aggressive antibiotic therapy is often required than for similar infections in less compromised hosts.

The development of an effective vaccine for immunoprophylaxis against HIV has become a major priority for biomedical research institutions worldwide. The task has been complicated by the genetic potential of the virus for great antigenic variability. Furthermore, although we know many of the viral gene products that induce naturally occurring humoral responses, these responses are ineffective in preventing disease. Perhaps vaccine development will require identification of viral epitopes that stimulate effective cell-mediated immune responses. Vaccines effective in preventing simian immunodeficiency virus (SIV) infection of macaques have already been developed. This is encouraging because SIV is molecularly closely related to HIV and causes a disease similar to AIDS in macaques.

OTHER ACQUIRED IMMUNODEFICIENCIES

Overall, acquired immunodeficiencies caused by other factors besides HIV infection are still more common than AIDS. These immunodeficiency states fall into two general etiologic categories. First, immunosuppression may occur as a biologic complication of another disease process. Second, so-called iatrogenic immunodeficiencies may develop as complications of the therapy for other diseases.

Diseases in which immunodeficiency is a common complicating element include malnutrition, neoplasias, and infections. Protein-calorie malnutrition is extremely common in developing countries and is associated with impaired cellular and humoral immunity to microorganisms. Much of the morbidity and mortality that afflicts malnourished people is due to infections. The basis for the immunodeficiency is not well defined, but it is reasonable to assume that the global metabolic disturbances in these individuals, caused by deficient intake of protein, fat, vitamins, and minerals, will adversely affect the maturation and function of the cells of the immune system.

Patients with advanced widespread cancers are often susceptible to infections because of impaired cell-mediated and humoral immune responses to a variety of organisms. Bone marrow tumors, including cancers metastatic to marrow and leukemias that arise in the marrow, may interfere with the growth and development of normal lymphocytes. Alternatively, tumors may produce substances that interfere with lymphocyte development or function, such as TGF-β. An example of malignancy-associated immunodeficiency is the impairment of T cell function commonly observed in patients with a type of malignant lymphoma called Hodgkin's disease. This defect was first characterized as an inability to mount a DTH reaction upon dermal injection of various common antigens to which the patients were previously exposed, such as *Candida* or tetanus toxoid. Other *in vitro* measures of T cell function, such as proliferative responses to polyclonal activators, are also impaired in Hodgkin's disease. Such a generalized deficiency in DTH responses is called **anergy.** The basis for these T cell abnormalities is currently unknown.

Various types of infections lead to immunosuppression. Viruses other than HIV are known to impair immune responses and lead to complicating infections by other organisms. Examples include the measles virus and human T cell lymphotropic virus–1 (HTLV-1). Both viruses can infect lymphocytes, and this may be a basis for their immunosuppressive effects. Like HIV,

HTLV-1 is a retrovirus with tropism for CD4$^+$ T cells; however, instead of killing helper T cells, it transforms them, producing an aggressive T cell malignancy called adult T cell leukemia/lymphoma (ATL). In ATL patients, typically there is severe immunosuppression with multiple opportunistic infections. Chronic infections with *Mycobacterium tuberculosis* and various fungi frequently result in anergy to many antigens. Chronic parasitic infections may also lead to immunosuppression. For example, African children with chronic malarial infections have depressed T cell function and this may be important in the pathogenesis of EBV-associated malignancies (see Box 18–1, Chapter 18).

Iatrogenic immunosuppression is most often due to drug therapies that either kill or functionally inactivate lymphocytes. Some drugs are given intentionally to immunosuppress patients, either for treatment of inflammatory diseases or to prevent rejection of tissue allografts. The most commonly used immunosuppressive drugs are corticosteroids and cyclosporin A, discussed in Chapter 17. The level of immunosuppression that is therapeutic in transplantation is usually not sufficient to cause clinically significant immunodeficiency. Various chemotherapeutic drugs are administered to cancer patients, and these drugs are usually cytotoxic to both mature and developing lymphocytes as well as to granulocyte and monocyte precursors. Thus, cancer chemotherapy is almost always accompanied by a period of immunosuppression and risk of infections. Radiation treatment of cancer carriers the same risks.

One final form of acquired immunosuppression that should be mentioned results from the absence of a spleen, caused by surgical removal of the organ after trauma or for the treatment of certain hematologic diseases or as a result of infarction in sickle cell disease. Patients without spleens are more susceptible to infections by some organisms, particularly encapsulated bacteria such as *Streptococcus pneumoniae.* The spleen is apparently required for the induction of protective humoral immune responses to the "thymus-independent" capsular polysaccharide antigens of such organisms.

SUMMARY

Immunodeficiency diseases are caused by congenital or acquired defects in lymphocytes, phagocytes, and other mediators of specific and natural immunity. These diseases are associated with an increased susceptibility to infections, the nature and severity of which depend largely on which component of the immune system is abnormal and the extent of the abnormality. In addition, patients with immunodeficiencies often show an increased incidence of cancers and autoimmune diseases.

Congenital (or primary) immunodeficiencies may be due to defects in B or T lymphocytes or both. An example of a selective B cell deficiency is X-linked agammaglobulinemia, an inherited block in the maturation of pre–B cells to B lymphocytes that results in an absence of mature B cells and antibodies and is due to mutations in a B cell progenitor tyrosine kinase gene. Congenital disorders selectively affecting the production of one or a few Ig isotypes, including IgA, IgM, and various IgG subclasses, are usually due to a failure of mature B cells to switch to particular Ig heavy chain isotypes. One example is IgG and IgA deficiency with increased IgM (hyper-IgM syndrome), and this is due to mutations in the gene encoding the gp39 ligand for B cell CD40. Common variable immunodeficiency is most often due to an intrinsic defect in the Ig secretory responses of mature B cells to antigenic stimulation.

The best-defined congenital T cell immunodeficiency is the DiGeorge syndrome, caused by a genetic abnormality in the development of the thymus. This results in a failure of T cell maturation. Diverse abnormalities in the functional responses of mature T lymphocytes to receptor-mediated stimulation have been described, but their underlying mechanisms are not known yet.

Severe combined immunodeficiencies constitute a group of disorders with defects in the development or function of both B and T lymphocytes. Some cases are due to inherited deficiencies of enzymes, such as adenosine deaminase, that are involved in purine metabolism. Other cases are attributable to poorly understood blocks in the development of antigen receptor–expressing lymphocytes from precursors in the bone marrow. Deficiencies of B and T lymphocytes are also associated with diseases that affect multiple organ systems, such as the Wiskott-Aldrich syndrome and ataxia-telangiectasia.

AIDS is a severe T cell immunodeficiency caused by infection with HIV. This virus has a tropism for CD4$^+$ T lymphocytes, causing depletion of these cells by direct lysis as well as several indirect mechanisms that lead to death, defective maturation, and abnormal function of uninfected T cells. The depletion of T cells results in greatly increased susceptibility to infection by a number of opportunistic microorganisms, including *Pneumocystis carinii,* mycobacteria, and various fungi and viruses. In addition, patients have an increased incidence of tumors, particularly Kaposi's sarcoma and Epstein-Barr virus–associated B cell lymphomas, and frequently develop an encephalopathy, the mechanism of which is not fully understood. Despite enormous effort, an effective cure or prophylactic vaccine for this disease is not available.

Acquired immunodeficiencies are also associated with malnutrition, disseminated cancers, and immunosuppressive therapy for transplant rejection or autoimmune diseases.

SELECTED READINGS

Anderson, D. C., and T. A. Springer. Leukocyte adhesion deficiency: an inherited defect in the Mac-1, LFA-1, and p150,95 glycoproteins. Annual Review of Medicine 38:175–194, 1987.

Cournoyer, D., and C. T. Caskey. Gene therapy of the immune system. Annual Reviews of Immunology 11:297–329, 1993.

Greene, W. C. Regulation of HIV-1 gene expression. Annual Review of Immunology 8:453–476, 1990.

Johnston, M. I., and D. F. Hoth. Present status and future prospects for HIV therapies. Science 260:1286–1293, 1993.

Ochs, H. D., and R. J. Wedgwood. IgG subclass deficiencies. Annual Review of Medicine 38:325–340, 1987.

Orkin, S. H. Molecular genetics of chronic granulomatous disease. Annual Review of Immunology 7:277–307, 1989.

Pantaleo, G., C. Graziosi, and A. S. Fauci. The immunopathogenesis of human immunodeficiency virus infection. New England Journal of Medicine 328:327–335, 1993.

Rosen, F. S. (chairman). Primary immunodeficiency diseases: report of a WHO scientific group. Immunodeficiency Reviews 3:195–236, 1992.

Rotrosen, D., and J. I. Gallin. Disorders of phagocyte function. Annual Review of Immunology 5:127–150, 1987.

Shultz, L. D., and C. L. Sidman. Genetically determined murine models for immunodeficiency. Annual Review of Immunology 5:367–403, 1987.

Weiss, R. A. How does HIV cause AIDS? Science 260:1273–1279, 1993.

APPENDIX: PRINCIPAL FEATURES OF KNOWN CD MOLECULES

CD Designation	Common Synonym(s)	Molecular Structure	Main Cellular Expression	Known or Proposed Function(s)
CD1a*†	T6	49 kD; β_2 microglobulin–associated	Thymocytes, dendritic cells (including Langerhans cells)	? Ligand for some $\gamma\delta$ T cells
CD1b	—	45 kD; β_2 microglobulin–associated	Same as CD1a	Same as CD1a
CD1c	—	43 kD; β_2 microglobulin–associated	Same as CD1a	Same as CD1a
CD2	T11; LFA-2; sheep red blood cell receptor	50 kD	T cells, NK cells	Adhesion molecule (binds LFA-3); T cell activation
CD3	T3; Leu-4	Composed of five chains (see Chapter 7)	T cells	Signal transduction as a result of antigen recognition by T cells
CD4	T4; Leu-3; L3T4 (mice)	55 kD	Class II MHC–restricted T cells	Adhesion molecule (binds to class II MHC); signal transduction
CD5	T1; Lyt-1	67 kD	T cells; B cell subset	? Adhesion molecule
CD6	T12	100–130 kD	Subset of T cells; some B cells	?
CD7	—	40 kD	Subset of T cells	?
CD8	T8; Leu-2; Lyt-2	Composed of two 34 kD chains; expressed as $\alpha\alpha$ or $\alpha\beta$ dimer	Class I MHC–restricted T cells	Adhesion (binds to class I MHC); signal transduction
CD9	—	24 kD	Pre-B and immature B cells; monocytes, platelets	? Role in platelet activation
CD10	CALLA	100 kD	Immature and some mature B cells; lymphoid progenitors, granulocytes	Structurally identical to neural endopeptidase (enkephalinase)
CD11a‡	LFA-1 α chain	180 kD; associates with CD18 to form LFA-1 integrin	Leukocytes	Adhesion (binds to ICAM-1)
CD11b	Mac-1; CR3 (iC3B receptor) α chain	165 kD; associates with CD18 to form Mac-1 integrin	Granulocytes, monocytes, NK cells	Adhesion; phagocytosis of iC3b-coated (opsonized) particles
CD11c	p150,95; CR4 α chain	150 kD; associates with CD18 to form p150,95 integrin	Monocytes, granulocytes, NK cells	Adhesion; ? phagocytosis of iC3b-coated (opsonized) particles
CDw12§	—	? 90–120 kD	Monocytes, granulocytes	Phosphoprotein; no known function
CD13	—	150 kD	Monocytes, granulocytes	Aminopeptidase; ? role in oxidative burst
CD14	Mo2	55 kD; PI-linked	Monocytes	LPS receptor; ? role in oxidative burst
CD15	Lewis^x	Carbohydrate epitope	Granulocytes	Sialyl form is a ligand for selectins
CD16	FcγRIII	50–70 kD; PI-linked and trans-membrane	NK cells, granulocytes, macrophages	Low-affinity Fcγ receptor: ADCC, activation of NK cells
CDw17	—	Carbohydrate epitope (lactosylceramide)	Granulocytes, macrophages, platelets	?
CD18	β chain of LFA-1 family (β_2 integrins)	95 kD; non-covalently linked to CD11a, CD11b, or CD11c	Leukocytes	See CD11a, CD11b, CD11c
CD19	B4	90 kD	Most B cells	? Role in B cell activation or regulation
CD20	B1	Heterodimer: 35 and 37 kD chains	Most or all B cells	? Role in B cell activation or regulation
CD21	CR2; C3d receptor; B2	145 kD	Mature B cells	Receptor for C3d, Epstein-Barr virus; ? role in B cell activation
CD22	—	135 kD	B cells	? Role in cell adhesion and B cell activation
CD23	FcϵRIIb	45–50 kD	Activated B cells, macrophages	Low-affinity Fcϵ receptor, induced by IL-4; function unknown
CD24	—	Heterodimer of 38 and 41 kD chains; PI-linked	B cells, granulocytes	?
CD25	IL-2 receptor α chain; TAC; p55	55 kd	Activated T and B cells; activated macrophages	Complexes with IL-2R$\beta\gamma$ high-affinity IL-2 receptor; T cell growth

CD Designation	Common Synonym(s)	Molecular Structure	Main Cellular Expression	Known or Proposed Function(s)
CD26	—	120 kD	Activated T and B cells; macrophages	Serine peptidase; ? role in HIV infection
CD27	—	Homodimer of 55 kD chains	Most T cells; ? some plasma cells	? Role in B cell growth; member of Fas, CD40 family
CD28	Tp44	Homodimer of 44 kD chains	T cells (most CD4$^+$, some CD8$^+$ cells)	T cell receptor for costimulator molecule(s) B7-1, B7-2
CD29	β chain of VLA antigens (β1 integrins)	130 kD; non-covalently associated with VLA α chains (CD49)	Broad	Adhesion to extracellular matrix proteins, cell-cell adhesion (see CD49)
CD30	Ki-1	105 kD	Activated T and B cells; Reed-Sternberg cells in Hodgkin's disease	?
CD31	PECAM-1; platelet gpIIa	140 kD	Platelets; monocytes, granulocytes, B cells, endothelial cells	Role in leukocyte-endothelial adhesion
CD32	FcγRII	~40 kD	Macrophages, granulocytes, B cells, eosinophils	Fc receptor for aggregated IgG; role in phagocytosis, ADCC; feedback inhibition of B cells
CD33	—	67 kD	Monocytes, myeloid progenitor cells	?
CD34	—	105–120 kD	Precursors of hematopoietic cells	?
CD35	CR1; C3b receptor	Polymorphic; four forms are 190–280 kD	Granulocytes, monocytes, erythrocytes, B cells	Binding and phagocytosis of C3b-coated particles and immune complexes
CD36	Platelet gpIIIb	90 kD	Monocytes, platelets	? Platelet adhesion
CD37	—	Composed of two or three 40–52 kD chains	B cells, some T cells	?
CD38	T10	45 kD	Plasma cells, thymocytes, activated T cells	?
CD39	—	70–100 kD	Mature B cells	?
CD40	—	Heterodimer of 44 and 48 kD chains	B cells	Role in B cell activation induced by T cell contact
CD41	gpIIb component of gpIIb/IIIa complex (gpIIIa is CD61)	Complex of gpIIb heterodimer (120 and 23 kD) and gpIIIa (CD61)	Platelets	Platelet aggregation and activation: receptor for fibrinogen, fibronectin (binds to R-G-D sequence)
CD42a	Platelet gpIX	23 kD; forms complex with CD42b	Platelets, megakaryocytes	Platelet adhesion, binding to von Willebrand factor
CD42b	Platelet gpIb	Dimer of 135 and 25 kD chains, forms complex with CD42a	See CD42a	See CD42a
CD43	Sialophorin	95 kD, highly sialylated	Leukocytes (except circulating B cells)	? Role in T cell activation
CD44	Pgp-1; Hermes	80–>100 kD, highly glycosylated	Leukocytes, erythrocytes	May function as homing receptor; receptor for matrix components (e.g., hyaluronate)
CD45	T200; leukocyte common antigen	Multiple isoforms, 180–220 kD	Leukocytes	Role in signal transduction (tyrosine phosphatase)
CD45R	Forms of CD45 with restricted cellular expression	CD45RO: 180 kD CD45RA: 220 kD CD45RB: 190, 205, and 220 kD isoforms	CD45RO: memory T cells CD45RA: naive T cells CD45RB: B cells, subset of T cells	See CD45
CD46	Membrane cofactor protein (MCP)	45–70 kD	Leukocytes; epithelial cells, fibroblasts	Regulation of complement activation
CD47	—	47–52 kD	Broad	?
CD48	—	41 kD; PI-linked	Leukocytes	?
CD49a	VLA α1 chain	210 kD; associates with CD29 to form VLA-1 (β1 integrin)	T cells, monocytes	Adhesion to collagen, laminin
CD49b	VLA α2 chain; platelet gpIa	170 kD; associates with CD29 to form VLA-2 (β1 integrin)	Platelets, activated T cells, monocytes, some B cells	Adhesion to extracellular matrix: receptor for collagen

CD Designation	Common Synonym(s)	Molecular Structure	Main Cellular Expression	Known or Proposed Function(s)
CD49c	VLA α3 chain	Dimer of 130 and 25 kD; associates with CD29 to form VLA-3 (β1 integrin)	T cells; some B cells, monocytes	Adhesion to fibronectin, laminin
CD49d	VLA α4 chain	150 kD; associates with CD29 to form VLA-4 (β1 integrin)	T cells, monocytes, B cells	Peyer's patch homing receptor, binds to VCAM-1; adhesion to fibronectin
CD49e	VLA α5 chain	Dimer of 135 and 25 kD; associates with CD29 to form VLA-5 (β1 integrin)	T cells; few B cells and monocytes	Adhesion to fibronectin
CD49f	VLA α6 chain	150 kD; associates with CD29 to form VLA-6 (β1 integrin)	Platelets, megakaryocytes; activated T cells	Adhesion to extracellular matrix: receptor for laminin
CD50	—	108–140 kD; ?PI-linked	Leukocytes	?
CD51	α chain of vitronectin receptor	140 kD heterodimer, associates with CD61	Platelets	Adhesion: receptor for vitronectin, fibrinogen, von Willebrand factor (binds R-G-D sequence)
CD52	—	? 21–28 kD	Leukocytes	?
CD53	—	32–40 kD	Leukocytes, plasma cells	?
CD54	ICAM-1	80–114 kD	Broad; many activated cells (cytokine-inducible)	Adhesion: ligand for LFA-1, Mac-1
CD55	Decay accelerating factor (DAF)	70 kD; PI-linked	Broad	Regulation of complement activation
CD56	Leu-19	Heterodimer of 135 and 220 kD chains	NK cells	Homotypic adhesion; isoform of neural cell adhesion molecule (N-CAM)
CD57	HNK-1, Leu-7	110 kD	NK cells, subset of T cells	?
CD58	LFA-3	55–70 kD; PI-linked or integral membrane protein	Broad	Adhesion: ligand for CD2
CD59	Membrane inhibitor of reactive lysis (MIRL)	18–20 kD; PI-linked	Broad	Regulation of complement (MAC) action
CDdw60	—	Carbohydrate epitope	Subset of T cells, platelets	?
CD61	β chain of vitronectin receptor (β3 integrin); gpIIIa	110 kD; associates with CD51 (α chain of vitronectin receptor) or CD41	Platelets, megakaryocytes	See CD51, CD41
CD62E	E-selectin, ELAM-1	115 kD	Endothelial cells	Leukocyte-endothelial adhesion
CD62L	L-selectin, LAM-1	75–80 kD	T lymphocytes, other leukocytes	Leukocyte-endothelial adhesion; homing of naive T cells to peripheral lymph nodes
CD62P	P-selectin, gmp140, PADGEM	130–150 kD	Platelets, endothelial cells	Leukocyte adhesion to endothelium, platelets
CD63	—	53 kD; present in platelet lysosomes, translocated to cell surface upon activation	Activated platelets; monocytes, macrophages	?
CD64	FcγRI	75 kD	Monocytes, macrophages	High-affinity Fcγ receptor: role in phagocytosis, ADCC, macrophage activation
CDw65	—	Carbohydrate epitope	Granulocytes	? Role in neutrophil activation
CD66	—	180–220 kD phosphorylated glycoprotein	Granulocytes	? Role in homotypic cell-cell adhesions (carcinoembryonic antigen, or CEA, is called CD66e)
CD67	—	100 kD; PI-linked	Granulocytes	?
CD68	—	110 kD, intracellular protein, weak surface expression	Monocytes, macrophages	?
CD69	—	Homodimer of 28–34 kD chains, phosphorylated glycoprotein	Activated B and T cells, macrophages, NK cells	?
CDw70	—	?	Activated T and B cells	?
CD71	T9; transferrin receptor	95 kD homodimer	Activated T and B cells, macrophages, proliferating cells	Receptor for transferrin: role in iron metabolism, cell growth

CD Designation	Common Synonym(s)	Molecular Structure	Main Cellular Expression	Known or Proposed Function(s)
CD72	Lyb-2 (mouse)	Heterodimer of 39 and 43 kD chains	B cells	Ligand for CD5; ? role in T cell–B cell interactions
CD73	—	69 kD; PI-linked	Subsets of T and B cells	Ecto-5'-nucleotidase, regulates nucleotide metabolism
CD74	Class II MHC invariant (γ) chain; I$_i$	Three protein species: 35, 41, and 53 kD	B cells, monocytes, macrophages; other class II$^+$ cells	Associates with newly synthesized class II MHC molecules
CDw75	—	53 kD	Mature B cells	?
CD76	—	Heterodimer of 67 and 85 kD chains	Mature B cells, subset of T cells	?
CD77	—	Carbohydrate epitope	Follicular center B cells	?
CDw78	Ba	?	B cells	?
CD79a	Igα, MB1	32–33 kD	Mature B cells	Component of B cell antigen receptor
CD79b	Igβ, B29	37–39 kD	Mature B cells	Component of B cell antigen receptor
CD80	B7-1, BB1	50–60 kD	Dendritic cells, activated B cells and macrophages	Costimulator for T lymphocyte activation; ligand for CD28 and CTLA-4
CD81	TAPA-1	22 kD	Broad	Associated with CD19 and CD21; ? role in B cell activation
CD82	—	50–53 kD	Broad	?
CD83	—	40–43 kD	Some B cell lines, others	?
CDw84	—	73 kD	Monocytes, lymphocytes	?
CD85	—	120 kD	B cells, monocytes	?
CD86	—	80 kD	B cells, monocytes	?
CD87	—	50–65 kD	Neutrophils, monocytes, endothelial cells	?
CD88	C5a receptor	40 kD	Neutrophils, macrophages, mast cells, eosinophils	Receptor for complement component; role in complement-induced inflammation
CD89	Fcα receptor	55–70 kD	Neutrophils, monocytes	IgA-dependent cytotoxicity
CDw90	Thy-1	25–35 kD; PI-linked	Thymocytes, peripheral T cells (mice), neurons (all species)	Marker for T cells; ? role in T cell activation
CD91	α2-macroglobulin receptor	600 kD	Macrophages and monocytes	?
CDw92	—	70 kD	Broad	?
CD93	—	118–129 kD	Neutrophils, monocytes, endothelial cells	?
CD94	—	Dimer of 43 kD units	NK cells	?
CD95	Fas antigen, APO-1	42 kD	Multiple cell types	Role in programmed cell death
CD96	—	160, 180, 240 kD forms	T cells	?
CD97	—	74, 80, 89 kD forms	Broad	?
CD98	—	Dimer of 40 and 80 kD subunits	Broad	?
CD99	—	32 kD	Broad	?
CD100	—	150 kD	T cells, B cells, granulocytes, monocytes, NK cells	?
CDw101	—	Dimer of 140 kD subunits	Granulocytes, monocytes	?
CD102	ICAM-2	55–65 kD	Endothelial cells, monocytes, other leukocytes	Ligand for LFA-1 integrin
CD103	HML-1	Dimer of 150 and 25 kD subunits (integrin)	Some T lymphocytes, other cell types	? Role in T cell homing to mucosa
CD104	β4 integrin chain	205–220 kD	Lymphocytes, others	Adhesion
CD105	Endoglin	Dimer of 95 kD subunits	Endothelial cells, activated macrophages	?

CD Designation	Common Synonym(s)	Molecular Structure	Main Cellular Expression	Known or Proposed Function(s)
CD106	VCAM-1	90–95 kD	Endothelial cells, macrophages, follicular dendritic cells, marrow stromal cells	Receptor for VLA-4 integrin; role in cell adhesion, lymphocyte activation, hematopoiesis
CD107a	LAMP-1	110 kD	Broad	Lysosomal protein of unknown function
CD107b	LAMP-2	120 kD	Broad	Lysomal protein of unknown function
CDw108	—	75–83 kD	Broad	?
CDw109	—	170/150 kD	Endothelial cells, monocytes	?

In addition to the above, several cytokine receptors have been given CD designations. In this book, we refer to cytokine receptors by the more informative descriptive names, which identify them by their specificities. The following is a current list of the cytokine receptors that have been assigned CD numbers.

CD115	M-CSF (CSF-1) receptor
CDw116	GM-CSF receptor
CD117	c-Kit, stem cell factor receptor
CDw119	IFN-γ receptor
CD120a	55 kD TNF receptor
CD120b	75 kD TNF receptor
CDw121a	Type 1 IL-1 receptor
CDw121b	Type 2 IL-1 receptor
CD122	IL-2 receptor β chain
CDw124	IL-4 receptor
CD126	IL-6 receptor
CDw127	IL-7 receptor
CDw128	IL-8 receptor
CDw130	130 kD signaling component of IL-6 receptor

This list has been compiled with the assistance of Drs. T. F. Tedder, Duke University School of Medicine, and S. Shaw, National Institutes of Health. The complete listing of CD molecules will be published in *Leukocyte Typing V,* edited by S. Schlossman, L. Boumsell, W. Gilks, J. Harlan, T. Kishimoto, C. Morimoto, J. Ritz, S. Shaw, R. Silverstein, T. Springer, T. Tedder, and R. Todd, Oxford University Press, 1994. Additional details of individual CD molecules may be found in Barclay, A. N., Birkeland, M. L., Brown, M. H., Beyers, A. D., Davis, S. J., Somoza, C., and Williams, A. F., editors, *The Leukocyte Antigen Facts Book,* Academic Press, 1993.

* CD molecules to which reference has been made in the text of this book are indicated in boldface.

† The small letters affixed to some CD numbers refer to complex CD molecules that are encoded by multiple genes or that belong to families of structurally related proteins. For instance, CD1a, CD1b, and CD1c are structurally related but distinct forms of a β_2 microglobulin–associated nonpolymorphic protein.

‡ CD11a, CD11b, and CD11c are three α chains that can non-covalently associate with the same β chain (CD18) to form three different integrins, all of which are members of the "CD11CD18" family (also called the "LFA-1 family" or the "$\beta2$ integrins").

§ Antibodies that have been submitted recently, or whose reactivity has not been fully confirmed, are said to identify putative CD molecules, indicated with a "w" (for "workshop") designation.

Abbreviations. ADCC, antibody-dependent cell-mediated cytotoxicity; GMP, granule membrane protein; GP, glycoprotein; ICAM, intercellular adhesion molecule; Ig, immunoglobulin; IL, interleukin; kD, kilodalton; LFA, lymphocyte function–associated antigen; LPS, lipopolysaccharide; MAC, membrane attack complex; MHC, major histocompatibility complex; NK, natural killer; PI, phosphatidylinositol; TAC, T cell activation antigen; VCAM, vascular cell adhesion molecule; VLA, very late activation.

INDEX

Note: Numbers in *italics* refer to illustrations. Numbers followed by "t" indicate tables; numbers followed by "b" indicate boxed material.

437